Walter and Miller's
Textbook of Radiotherapy

Dedicated to all our families

For Churchill Livingstone

Publisher: Mary Law
Project Editor: Dinah Thom
Copy Editor: Rosaline Crum
Production Controller: Mark Sanderson
Sales Promotion Executive: Hilary Brown

Walter and Miller's
Textbook of Radiotherapy
Radiation Physics, Therapy and Oncology

C. K. Bomford
BSc MPhil CPhys FInstP FIPSM

Head of Radiation Physics,
Central Sheffield University Hospitals,
Department of Medical Physics and Clinical Engineering,
Sheffield;
Honorary Lecturer, University of Sheffield;
Visiting Lecturer, Sheffield Hallam University

I. H. Kunkler
MA MB BChir MRCP(UK) DMR(T) FRCR

Consultant Radiotherapist and Oncologist,
Weston Park Hospital, Sheffield;
Honorary Clinical Lecturer, YCRC Department of Clinical
Oncology, University of Sheffield

S. B. Sherriff
DCR(T) MMedSci PhD FIPSM

Consultant Medical Physicist,
Central Sheffield University Hospitals,
Department of Medical Physics and Clinical Engineering
Sheffield;
Honorary Lecturer, University of Sheffield;
Visiting Lecturer, Sheffield Hallam University

Foreword by

H. Miller *OBE* MA PhD FInstP DSc(Hon)

Former Chief Physicist, Trent Regional Health Authority;
Emeritus Professor Associate, University of Sheffield

FIFTH EDITION

CHURCHILL LIVINGSTONE
EDINBURGH LONDON MADRID MELBOURNE NEW YORK AND TOKYO 1993

CHURCHILL LIVINGSTONE
Medical Division of Longman Group Limited

Distributed in the United States of America by Churchill
Livingstone Inc., 650 Avenue of the Americas, New York,
N. Y. 10011, and by associated companies, branches and
representatives throughout the world.

First edition 1950
Second edition 1959
Third edition 1969
Fourth edition 1979
Fifth edition 1993
　Reprinted 1994
　Reprinted 1995

ISBN 0-443-02873-7

British Library Cataloguing in Publication Data
A catalogue record for this book is available from the
British Library.

Library of Congress Cataloging in Publication Data
Bomford, C. K.
　　Walter and Miller's textbook of radiotherapy : radiation physics,
therapy, and oncology, – 5th ed. / C. K. Bomford, I. H. Kunkler,
S. B. Sherriff; foreword by H. Miller.
　　　　p.　cm.
　　Rev. ed. of: A short textbook of radiotherapy / J. Walter,
H. Miller, C. K. Bomford. 4th ed. 1979.
　　Includes bibliographical references and index.
　　ISBN 0-443-02873-7
　　1. Cancer–Radiotherapy.　2. Radiotherapy.　3. Medical physics.
I. Walter, J. (Joseph)　II. Miller, H. (Harold), 1909–　.
III. Kunkler, I. H.　IV. Sherriffs, S. B.　V. Walter, J. (Joseph).
Short textbook of radiotherapy.　VI. Title.　VII. Title: Textbook of
radiotherapy.
　　[DNLM: 1. Health Physics.　2. Neoplasms–radiotherapy.　QZ 269
B695w]
　RC271.R3B65 / 1993
　616.99′40642–dc20
　DNLM/DLC　　　　　　　　　　　　　　　　92-48182
　for Library of Congress　　　　　　　　　　　　CIP

The
publisher's
policy is to use
**paper manufactured
from sustainable forests**

Produced by Longman Singapore Publishers Pte. Ltd.
Printed in Singapore

Contents

Contributors

R. E. Coleman MB BS MRCP MD
Senior Lecturer and Honorary Consultant Medical
Oncologist, YCRC Department of Clinical Oncology,
Weston Park Hospital Trust, Sheffield

36   *Medical complications of malignant disease*

J. R. Goepel MB ChB FRCPath
Senior Lecturer in Pathology, University of Sheffield;
Honorary Consultant Pathologist, Weston Park
Hospital Trust and Central Sheffield University
Hospitals Trust

14   *Biological and pathological introduction*

A. J. Kunkler SRN BSc MPhil PhD CPsychol AFBPS
Chartered Clinical Psychologist, Rosslynlee Hospital,
Roslin, Midlothian

Co-author for:
34   *Quality of life*

I. H. Manifold MA MB BChir MD FRCP FRCR
Consultant Radiotherapist and Oncologist and Medical
Director, Weston Park Hospital Trust, Sheffield;
Honorary Clinical Lecturer, YCRC Department of
Clinical Oncology, University of Sheffield

Co-author for:
20   *Mouth, secondary nodes of neck, tonsil, nasopharynx,*
     paranasal sinuses, ear, salivary glands

21   *Larynx, lower pharynx, postcricoid, thyroid*

28   *Soft tissues and bone*

D. J. Radstone BA DipDroit, Compare-Solicitor of the Supreme
Court MB BS DMRT FRCR
Consultant in Clinical Oncology, Weston Park
Hospital Trust, Sheffield; Honorary Clinical Lecturer,
YCRC Department of Clinical Oncology, University
of Sheffield

Co-author for:
33   *Palliative and continuing care*

Foreword

It is a pleasure to be invited to write a foreword to this fifth edition of the textbook which first appeared in 1950 as a *Short Textbook of Radiotherapy for Technicians and Students*. This new book represents a tribute to the memory of the late Dr J. Walter, a co-author of the earlier editions.

Over the years the successive editions of the book have proved popular as an introductory text for radiotherapy radiographers and for both clinicians and physicists working in radiotherapy. It has been welcomed as such not only in the UK and USA but also in many distant parts of the world.

During the 14 years since the last edition appeared the developments in radiotherapy, oncology and radiation physics have been substantial and this new text is a completely revised and up-to-date account of the subject. The expansion of Part II, dealing with Radiotherapy and Oncology, is a useful revision in the new book.

It is a pleasure to see this modern version of the book still associated with the Radiotherapy Centre at Weston Park Hospital in Sheffield. The authors are to be congratulated on the excellent new presentation of the *Short Textbook of Radiotherapy*. I hope and expect it will continue to have a wide appeal in all branches of this field of clinical work.

H. M.

Preface

It is a privilege and somewhat awesome responsibility to be invited to revise a widely accepted text which has stood the test of time over four editions and 40 years. During this time this book has become affectionately known around the world simply as Walter and Miller and it is fitting therefore that the names of its creators will be perpetuated by their inclusion in its new title.

The fifth edition keeps the basic format of the fourth, namely to deal with Radiation Physics in Part 1 and with Radiotherapy and Oncology in Part 2. In recognition of the continuing expansion of the whole field of radiotherapy, the publishers have allowed us a modest increase in the overall length of the text and, for the first time, the inclusion of full colour plates, albeit grouped together and in general a little remote from the text to which they relate. We hope the cross-referencing should minimise any inconvenience.

The Physics section, Part 1, is divided into 12 chapters, many with the same titles as before, although their content has been completely revised and updated. Chapter 1 is a rather more complete summary of the basic knowledge assumed in the remaining chapters. Chapter 11 is devoted to neutron and proton therapy. The former has never lived up to expectations, except in a few particular areas, whereas the latter is an exciting field and bigger and better facilities are being developed around the world. Chapter 12 seeks to marry the existing statutory requirements on radiation protection with the more recent recommendations of the International Commission on Radiological Protection published shortly before this book went to press. We must apologise if the marriage proves a little shaky in places as the interpretation of the new recommendations becomes clearer over the coming months. As previously, some aspects of radiation protection are fitted more logically into the earlier chapters.

The section on Radiotherapy and Oncology has been virtually completely rewritten. In order to provide a practical guide to clinical radiotherapy and to satisfy the examination requirements of both radiographers and radiotherapists, the text on radiotherapy technique is more detailed than in the previous edition. The general format of chapters dealing with tumours by anatomical site has been retained. There has been an increase in the number of diagrams illustrating relevant anatomy and treatment volumes. New chapters have been included on interstitial implantation, palliative and continuing care and quality of life, reflecting their importance in clinical practice and on new developments in oncology. While the emphasis of the clinical section is still on radiotherapy, the section on medical oncology has been considerably expanded in recognition of the role played by cytotoxic therapy in a wide range of malignancies, with an additional section on the medical complications of malignant disease.

The basic aim of the book remains as it has always been, namely a basic but comprehensive text covering the uses of radiation and cytotoxic drugs in the treatment of patients with malignant disease. As such it is seen to be a study book for those seeking to qualify as therapy radiographers or as medical technical officers as well as an introductory text for the Fellowship of the Royal College of Radiologists (Radiotherapy and Oncology) and for clinical physicists.

Every effort has been made by the authors to ensure the accuracy of recommended doses of radiotherapy and chemotherapy. However, practice will vary from centre to centre, and it must be the responsibility of the practising clinician to check that the dosage is correct. Patients undergoing treatment with more complex regimes of radiotherapy and chemotherapy should be managed in a specialised cancer centre. If in doubt, expert advice should always be sought before treatment is undertaken.

Sheffield, 1993

C.K.B.
I.H.K.
S.B.S.

Acknowledgements

In writing a book of this nature, one becomes increasingly aware of how dependent one is on the advice, help and forbearance of others. We think of those who taught us all we know, and of those from whom we have learned so much in the process of teaching over many years. We must acknowledge the fact that we have built on the foundations of Dr J. Walter and Professor H. Miller who have established this title over the years. We are indebted to Harold Miller, who is still so very active in his retirement, for looking at this new script and contributing the foreword.

In preparing the script we are conscious of the help of so many who have discussed the material at various points in its development and contributed very helpfully during the drafting stages. Amongst these, we wish to acknowledge those from within and without our respective Departments, including: Professors W. Duncan and B. W. Hancock; Drs D. Addy, D. Ash, D. C. Barber, J. J. Bolger, D. Bonnett, A. E. Champion, R. E. Coleman, J. Conway, K. S. Dunn, M. Gerrard, J. Goepel, M. Greaves, M. Kesseler, I. H. Manifold, R. Nakielny, F. E. Neal, T. Powell, D. J. Radstone, L. Turnbull, A. C. Underwood, M. J. Whipp and D. Winfield; Messrs R. D. E. Battersby, S. T. S. Beggs, D. Forster, S. M. Loft, I. G. Rennie; Miss N. J. Whilde; and Mrs A. Duxbury, C. Griffiths, T. Heath and E. Steinkamp. We would also like to thank the staff of the Medical Illustration Departments of Weston Park, Royal Hallamshire and Rotherham District General Hospitals and M. Hart of Nucletron for the preparation of most of the artwork. In particular, we are indebted to Mr P. Elliott, Medical Artist, for many of the illustrations.

Our thanks are due, too, to the staff of Churchill Livingstone for their encouragement and advice throughout the preparation of this text.

The script would never have been produced without the help and expertise of our secretaries, Mrs M. Roadhouse and Mrs L. Wragg, and indeed would never have been written without the support, patience and tolerance of those at home who allowed us the freedom to work long hours in quiet solitude.

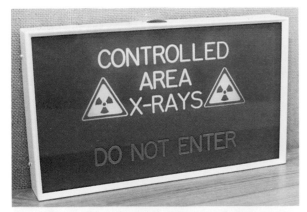

Plate 1 Controlled Area sign for use outside an X-ray therapy room (p. 54). (Courtesy of Philip Payne Ltd, Solihull.)

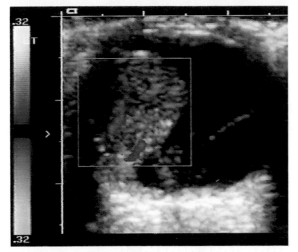

Plate 2 Colour flow Doppler image of a superficial femoral artery (flow in red) and vein (flow in blue) (p. 139).

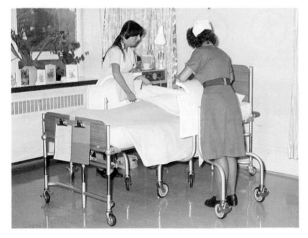

Plate 3 Colour flow Doppler image of the blood supply to an ocular tumour (p. 139).

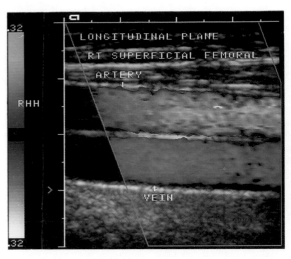

Plate 4 The radiation warning sign for the side ward (p. 157).

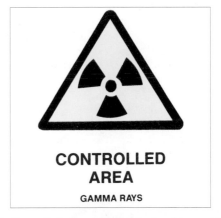

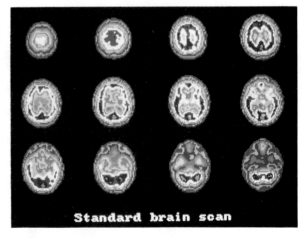

Plate 5 The use of mobile lead screens for the protection of staff attending brachytherapy patients (p. 157).

Plate 6 Tomographic scan of the regional cerebral blood flow following injection of [^{99m}]HM-PAO (p. 188).

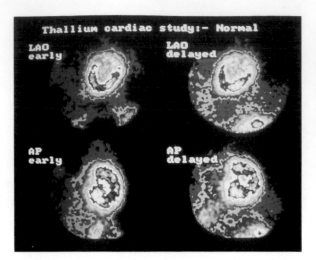

Plate 7 Normal thallium-201 distribution in the left ventricle of the heart both after exercise (early) and at rest (delayed) (p. 191).

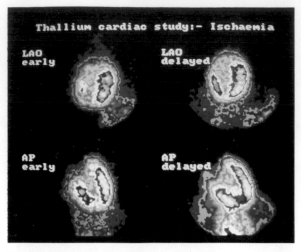

Plate 8 Thallium-201 study of the heart showing areas of reduced uptake after exercise (early) with redistribution at rest (delayed) (p. 191).

Plate 9 (left) The finger of a pioneer radiation worker (p. 210).

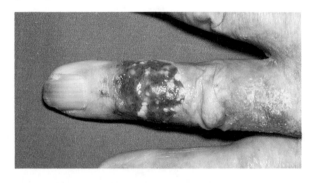

Plate 10 (below) Some safety signs (p. 223).

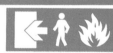

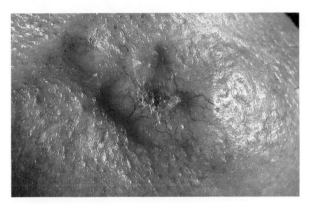

Plate 11 Basal carcinoma on the nose, showing pearly edge, telangiectasia over the surface and central ulceration (p. 293).

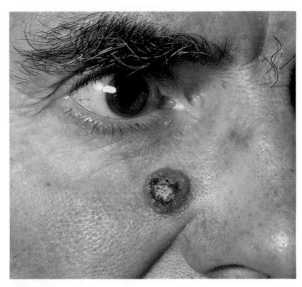

Plate 12 Squamous cell carcinoma of the skin (p. 294). (Courtesy of Dr D Gawkrodger, Sheffield.)

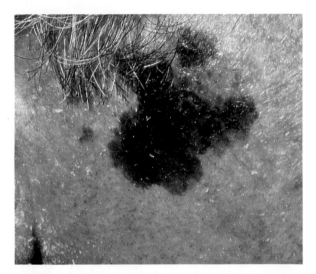

Plate 13 Skin melanoma (lentigo maligna) (p. 299) (Courtesy of Dr M Kesseler, Rotherham.)

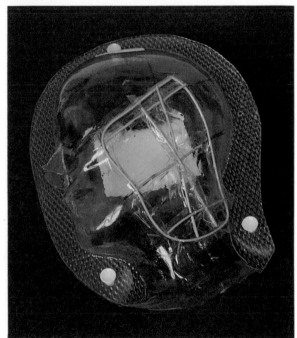

Plate 14 Mould for treating carcinoma of the parotid with anterior and posterior oblique wedged pair of fields. Catheters on the surface showing the oblique plane for CT reconstruction of 'beam's eye' view (p. 340) (Courtesy of Dr I Manifold and Dr J Conway, Sheffield.)

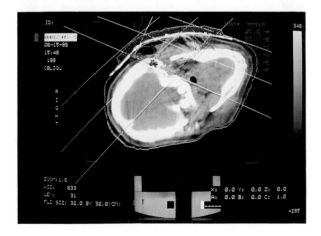

Plate 15 (left) CT reconstruction of oblique plane. The catheter on the upper surface is the central catheter seen in Plate 14, the correct obliquity of the reconstruction (p. 340). (Courtesy of Dr I Manifold and Dr J Conway, Sheffield.)

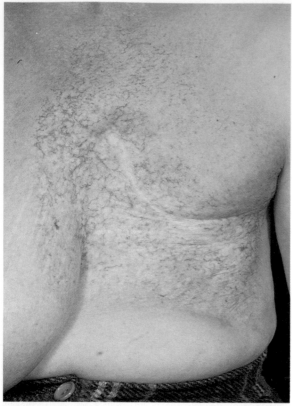

Plate 16 Telangiectasia of the chest wall, a late side-effect of postmastectomy radical radiotherapy with bolus (p. 393).

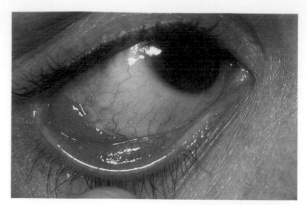

Plate 17 Pink fleshy deposits of non-Hodgkin lymphoma of the conjunctiva (p. 457). (Courtesy of Mr I Rennie, Sheffield.)

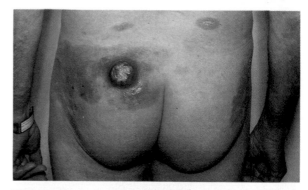

Plate 18 Typical eczematous lesions of classical early mycosis fungoides (p. 458). (Courtesy of Dr M Kesseler, Rotherham.)

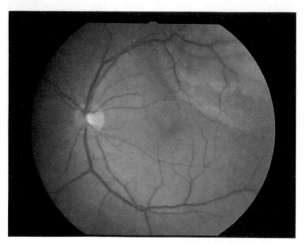

Plate 19 Choroidal melanoma (p. 496). (Courtesy of Mr I Rennie, Sheffield.)

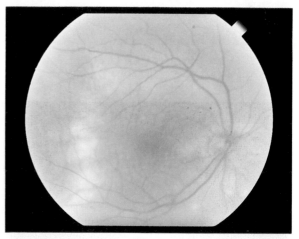

Plate 20 Choroidal metastases, showing typical honeycomb pattern of fundus (p. 499). (Courtesy of Mr I Rennie, Sheffield.)

PART 1

Radiation physics

1. Fundamentals of radiation physics

INTRODUCTION

Before proceeding into concepts of radiation physics relating to radiotherapy, it is important to grasp some fundamentals on which to build. In this first chapter, therefore, we restate some of the fundamentals with which the reader will probably be already familiar and seek to build bridges into the new areas to be studied in later chapters.

Facts about matter

The smallest identifiable quantity of an element is the atom. There are 90 naturally occurring elements and an additional 14 artificially produced elements. Combinations of elements form compounds and these may be organic or inorganic. The organic compounds found in living matter are mainly composed of carbon, nitrogen, oxygen and hydrogen together with traces of other elements. The smallest unit of a compound is known as a molecule. Organic molecules are very complex and contain very many atoms.

Solid matter is made up of atoms or molecules arranged in a regular pattern (or lattice). The forces which hold the atoms or molecules together in the lattice are very strong and give the matter its hardness and rigidity. If a solid is heated, the heat energy is transferred to the atoms or molecules, they vibrate about their equilibrium position more vigorously and the solid expands. A further increase in heat energy causes the breakdown of the forces holding the solid together and at a defined temperature the solid melts, i.e. at the melting point.

In the liquid state the interatomic forces remain strong but relative movement between the atoms or molecules is possible, the stronger the force the greater the viscosity of the liquid. Some supercooled liquids are so viscous they appear as solids, e.g. glass.

The further application of heat reduces the forces between the atoms or molecules until there is a free and random movement between them, and matter takes the form of a gas. Their constant movement inevitably means there are collisions between them and with the containing walls. This bombardment of the walls constitutes the gas pressure.

All atoms are made up of three subatomic particles: the negatively charged electron, the positively charged proton and the neutron, which carries no electrical charge. (There is an electrostatic force of attraction between unlike charges, and therefore protons and electrons will move towards each other; conversely the like charges of two electrons or of two protons tend to force them apart—the force of repulsion.) Normally an atom contains an equal number of protons and electrons and is therefore electrically neutral. If the atom is electrically charged by the addition or removal of an electron, it is called an ion. The forces holding the atoms and molecules together are electrostatic. If this sharing of ions results in free or loosely bound electrons, the matter will conduct electricity when a potential difference is applied. If the electrons are not free to move, even under the pressure of an applied potential difference, then we have an insulator. There are a few elements which exhibit both the properties of conduction and insulation. When a crystal of one of these semiconductor materials is placed in contact with a conductor, the junction allows a free flow of electrons in one direction but not in the other, i.e. the junction behaves like a diode valve or rectifier. These solid state rectifiers have largely replaced the vacuum diode valve in rectification circuits (p. 36ff) but because an X-ray tube is, to all intents and purposes, electrically the same as a vacuum diode valve, some understanding of its method of operation is important (p. 4).

Facts about electrons

The electron is a small negatively charged particle. Its charge (1.6×10^{-19} coulombs) is equal to that of a proton but opposite in sign. Its mass (9×10^{-31} kg) is

1840 times smaller than the mass of the proton (or neutron, 1.7×10^{-27} kg). Electrons may be released from gas molecules by applying a voltage between two electrodes in a partially evacuated discharge tube or from a metal by heating in a vacuum.

Dry air at normal atmospheric pressure (760 mmHg or 101.3 kPa) is a good insulator and only breaks down with a violent spark in very high electric fields. At 10 mmHg (1.3 kPa) pressure a gas will conduct electricity smoothly and is accompanied by the emission of light, the colour of which is characteristic of the gas, e.g. neon. At 0.01 mmHg (1.3 Pa) pressure, the emission is confined to streamers from the cathode to a point where the streamers strike the walls of the glass vacuum container. These streamers appear to come from the cathode but in fact trace the paths of the electrons which cause the gas to fluoresce. These electron streams are called cathode rays.

Alternatively electrons may be produced by a process known as thermionic emission. When a substance is heated the electrons vibrate and the material expands. Before the melting point is reached, the vibration of the surface electrons is sufficient to cause them to leave the surface completely. They leave the surface positively charged and are consequently pulled back by the force of electrostatic attraction. If, however, the heated surface is in a vacuum together with a second positively charged electrode (the anode), the electrons released by the heated surface may be attracted to that electrode and a stream of electrons will flow from the heated cathode to the positive anode. The student should note this electron flow is in the opposite direction to conventional electric current. Providing the anode remains cold there will be no electron flow in the reverse direction. With the gas pressure being much lower than in the discharge tube, there are insufficient gas molecules to produce the fluorescence associated with the cathode rays in a vacuum tube.

Cathode rays generated in a vacuum tube form the basis of the television set, video display and the cathode ray oscilloscope, and therefore it is worth noting their principal properties.

1. They travel in straight lines in a vacuum. Cathode rays are emitted at right angles to the surface of the cathode and may be focused using a concave cathode.
2. They carry electrical charge. Electrons carry negative charges and therefore their path may be deflected in either an electrostatic field or a magnetic field. The deflection is along the electrostatic field towards the positive electrode or at right angles to the magnetic field, following Fleming's left-hand rule.

3. They carry energy. They can cause suitable light objects to move. Their energy is proportional to the accelerating voltage and their velocity proportional to the square root of the accelerating voltage. They will penetrate thin metal foils, but if stopped in a metal target they produce heat or X-rays. When they strike glass or certain other crystals (e.g. zinc sulphide) they cause fluorescence.

Figure 1.1A shows a simple diode (vacuum tube) consisting of a heated wire filament (cathode) surrounded by a cylindrical anode contained in an evacuated glass envelope. The filament is heated by passing an electric current through it. The anode voltage V_a with respect to the cathode may be about +100 volts and the anode current I_a through the diode about 1 mA. Since the number of electrons leaving the filament depends on the filament temperature, the maximum anode current is determined by the value of the filament voltage V_f. The actual value of the anode current will depend upon whether the anode voltage is sufficient to draw all the electrons released from the filament across the gap to the anode. A graph of this variation of anode current with anode voltage is known as the characteristic curve of the diode and shown in Figure 1.1C. At

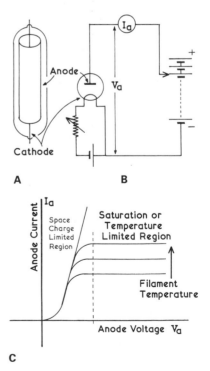

Fig. 1.1 **A** The cathode and cylindrical anode of a diode valve and **B** a simple diode in circuit to measure **C** the characteristic curves of the diode.

lower anode voltages a cloud of electrons—the space charge—forms around the filament, and being negatively charged encourages the recapture of the electrons released by the filament. As the anode voltage increases, the effect of the space charge is reduced and the anode current increases in what is known as the space charge limited region of the characteristic curve. Under saturation conditions, an increase in V_a does not increase the anode current because all the available electrons are being collected on the anode. The saturation (anode) current can only be increased by raising the temperature of the filament (by increasing V_f) to release more electrons. The number of electrons leaving a metal surface at a given temperature is very dependent on the surface conditions. Metal surfaces coated with the oxides of calcium or barium release electrons freely and are used in thermionic valves and some linear accelerators, described as having 'oxide coated cathodes'. Such cathodes are usually heated indirectly, that is, by a filament in close proximity behind the coated surface.

The arrangement of the electrodes may enable the cathode rays to bombard a fluorescent screen, thereby producing a spot of light (Fig. 1.2). If a variable electrostatic or magnetic field is applied, the spot of light can be made to move over the fluorescent screen as in a cathode ray oscilloscope (CRO). The waveform of a voltage which varies with time may be displayed by applying two signals: the voltage connected to the Y plates to cause a vertical deflection on the screen and a time signal to the X electrodes to cause a horizontal deflection. A television picture is produced on a cathode ray oscilloscope by applying time signals both vertically and horizontally so that a *raster* covers the screen; the picture, in different shades of grey from black to white, is then produced by varying the anode current as the spot moves over the screen. (A colour television uses three spots of light, each contributing one of the primary colours, which mix to make up the full spectrum of colour on the screen.)

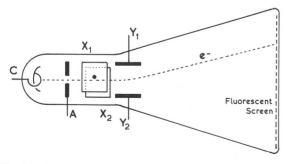

Fig. 1.2 The cathode ray tube.

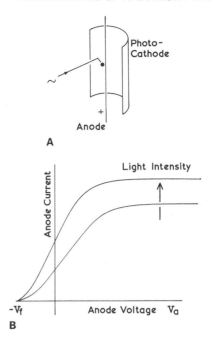

Fig. 1.3 **A** The photo electric cell and **B** its characteristic curves.

Television systems are widely used in the modern radiotherapy department—as a means of observing the patient in the treatment room through what is called closed circuit television, as an output device for the images off a simulator image intensifier, a computerised tomography (CT) or magnetic resonance (MR) scanner. The video display from the treatment planning computer or the computer controlled linear accelerator is simply a television with a special screen format.

The photoelectric cell (Fig. 1.3) is similar to the diode in its operation. Two electrodes are enclosed in an evacuated glass container and a positive potential applied to the anode. (By definition an anode is always at a positive potential with respect to the cathode.) The cathode is not heated, but made of a metal which will release its surface electrons when exposed to light of a suitable wavelength. This is the *photo electric effect*. Visible light, especially ultraviolet light, gives up its energy to the electrons on the surface of the (photo) cathode and releases them from the surface. The anode absorbs the electrons under the influences of its positive potential and causes the photocell to pass an electric current. The photoelectric cell may therefore be used as a switch operated by a beam of light—for example to terminate the exposure of a therapy machine if a radiographer inadvertently interrupts the light beam guarding the maze entrance to the treatment room (p. 54). A

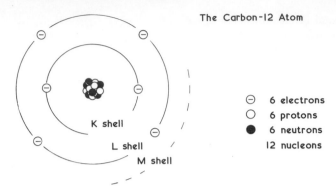

Fig. 1.4   The carbon-12 atom ($Z = 6$).

semiconductor known as a photodiode may also be used in a similar manner.

ATOMIC STRUCTURE

The atom is a miniature solar system consisting largely of empty space. At the centre of the system is the nucleus (approximately 10^{-15} m diameter) and around that centre the electrons move in orbits (approximately 10^{-11} m diameter) (Fig. 1.4). The simplest atom, hydrogen, consists of one positively charged particle (a proton) and one electron in orbit.

The number of positive charges, protons, in the nucleus is called the atomic number Z and equals the number of electrons orbiting the nucleus. Since a proton is some 1840 times heavier than an electron, practically all the mass of the atom lies in the nucleus. In all atoms, except hydrogen, the nucleus contains both protons and neutrons, in almost equal numbers. The neutron has almost the same mass as the proton but no charge. Since the number of neutrons is approximately the same as the number of protons, the number of electrons per unit mass for hydrogen is almost twice that for any other element (a fact we shall come back to in Chapter 4). The atomic weight, A, of an atom is related to the mass of the

hydrogen atom taken as 1, or one-twelfth of the mass of the carbon-12 atom.

The electrons around the nucleus are located in a few specific orbits, the nearest to the nucleus is labelled the K orbit or shell and subsequent ones are given the labels L, M, N, etc. The K orbit is the one with the least energy (but the greatest binding energy, see below). Each orbit can hold only a limited number of electrons, the maximum number in the nth orbit is $2n^2$ (e.g. the M shell is the third and can only have up to 18 electrons), but in general the electrons occupy the innermost orbits. There are exceptions to this rule, for example the outermost shell will never have more than eight electrons, before the next outer shell starts to fill (Table 1.1). (Note. We often use the words orbit or shell interchangeably. The atom is a three-dimensional solar system and each electron orbit is in a different plane—it is only for convenience that their orbits are depicted as concentric circles.)

This rather simple picture of the atom, referred to as the Rutherford–Bohr picture, helps to explain the similar chemical properties of different elements, e.g. the six inert gases (radon and xenon among them) are those elements whose outermost orbits have their full complement of eight electrons, and the four halogen gases, fluorine, chlorine, bromine and iodine, all have

Table 1.1   The atomic structure of selected atoms

Element	Symbol	Atomic no.(Z)	Nuclear charge	No. of electrons in shell			
				K	L	M	N
Hydrogen	H	1	+1	1	–	–	–
Helium	He	2	+2	2	–	–	–
Lithium	Li	3	+3	2	1	–	–
Neon	Ne	10	+10	2	8	–	–
Sodium	Na	11	+11	2	8	1	–
Calcium	Ca	20	+20	2	8	8	2

only one vacancy in their outer shell. Elements in which there are one or two loosely bound electrons in the outer shell are good electrical conductors, whereas those with a few vacancies in the outer shell are good insulators. The semiconductor elements of silicon and germanium are quadrivalent, having four electrons in their outer shell making them both poor conductors and poor insulators.

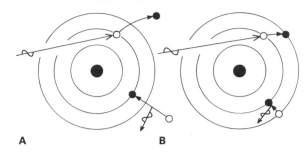

Fig. 1.5 A Ionisation and **B** excitation.

Solid state rectifiers

These are P–N junction diodes made by fusing together P-type silicon with N-type silicon. N-type silicon is pure silicon to which a small quantity of an impurity has been added, the impurity being pentavalent, i.e. having five outer electrons (e.g. phosphorus). The impurity therefore donates a spare electron which can be readily released into the conduction band and take part in electrical conduction. (This donation of a *n*egatively charged particle gives the silicon the name of N-type.) Conversely, P-type silicon carries a small trivalent impurity leaving the crystalline structure short of electrons and therefore rich in 'holes' ready to accept any free electrons from the surrounding silicon. The fusing together of P-type and N-type materials results in the surplus electrons crossing the barrier from the N-type silicon and falling into the 'holes' in the P-type silicon, thereby leaving a *depletion layer* between the two materials in which there are no surplus electrons and no surplus 'holes'. When a potential difference is applied to the junction a current will flow when the P-type is positive and the N-type is negative. If the polarity is reversed no current will flow because it increases the potential barrier across the junction and extends the depletion layer. The P–N junction therefore passes current only in one direction. This solid state rectifier is very rugged in operation, smaller in size than the thermionic diode and does not require a filament supply.

Ionisation and excitation

If an atom or a molecule has a surfeit of electrons, it is called a negative ion. A positive ion is an atom or molecule with a shortage of electrons. Ions may be produced by a variety of external agents. A solution of sodium chloride in water will conduct an electric current because the NaCl readily splits in to Na^+ and Cl^- ions. Gas at normal pressures will conduct electricity when the gas is ionised by irradiation with X-rays.

At the atomic level, the atom is said to be ionised when an electron is completely removed from the electrostatic field around the nucleus, and the process

is known as ionisation (Fig. 1.5). If the electron is only partially removed, i.e. moved from one orbit to a more distant orbit, the atom is said to be in an excited state, and the process is known as excitation. The ionised or excited atom will resume its stable state by attracting another electron into the vacant space in the orbit concerned. This movement of the electron through the shell structure is accompanied by the emission of electromagnetic radiation which may be visible, as in the fluorescence in the discharge tube, or invisible X-radiation.

Binding energy

In our solar system there are gravitational forces of attraction pulling the planets towards the sun exactly compensated by the centrifugal forces due to the rotation of the planets round the sun. The exact orbit a planet takes round the sun is determined by this balance, which may be affected to a greater or lesser degree by the other planets in the system; for this reason the orbits are not circular.

If we imagine two ions, a single positive charge and a single negative charge separated by an infinite distance, the force of attraction is zero and the total energy of the system is zero. (The force is proportional to the product of the two charges and to the inverse square of the distance between the charges—the force is zero when the distance is infinite.) As the distance between the ions is reduced, the force of attraction increases and the two ions accelerate towards each other. The kinetic energy (the energy of movement) is therefore increasing, and providing no energy has been given to or taken from the system we must assume the potential energy (the energy of position) is decreasing (from zero). The potential energy is therefore now *negative*. At some distance from the positive ion, the negative ion will find the electrostatic force of attraction is balanced by its centrifugal force due to its rotation round the positive ion (the nucleus), thereby fixing the electron in orbit round the nucleus. Now, having established its orbit, it is clear that the electron is bound to that nucleus with an energy, which we call the *binding energy*. To move the electron to an orbit further from the nucleus, we must *add* energy to the system, and if we are to remove the electron completely we must add an amount of energy equal to or in excess of its binding energy. Any energy surplus after overcoming the binding energy will be given to the electron in the form of kinetic energy. Conversely, if the electron moves to an orbit closer to the nucleus, it will have surplus energy which must be removed from the system—often in the form of an emission of electromagnetic radiation.

This simple picture is complicated by the fact that different electrons in the same shell will follow slightly different orbits giving rise to slightly different binding energies, K_A, K_B, L_I, L_{II}, L_{III}, etc., but the student is referred to more advanced texts for a detailed explanation of this phenomenon.

In the single atoms described above, the energy levels are discrete, but when the atoms are brought closer together, as in a solid material, the energy levels of each orbit are influenced by the proximity of others. This results in the broadening out of the discrete levels into *energy bands* (Fig. 1.6). The outermost band normally occupied by electrons is known as the *valence band*. The next outer band which may be occupied is the *conduction band*. In a conductor (e.g. copper) these bands overlap and electrons can move freely between them, whereas in an insulator there is a broad *forbidden zone* between them. (Remember these are energy bands, and any forbidden zone can be crossed if an electron is given sufficient energy to cross it.) Once in the conduction band an electron can move freely through the material. In semiconductors there is only a narrow forbidden zone.

Structure of the nucleus

The simplest nucleus—of hydrogen—consists of a solitary proton. All other nuclei contain a mixture of protons and neutrons in approximately equal numbers. The number of protons in the nucleus (equal to the atomic number, Z) determines the arrangement of the outer electrons and therefore the chemical properties of the element. The mass number, A, is the number of nucleons in the nucleus, that is, the number of protons and number of neutrons added together. It is possible for atoms to exist with the same atomic number (Z) and chemical properties but with different atomic weights or mass numbers, because the number of neutrons present in the nucleus can vary slightly. These are called isotopes. Some isotopes are stable, while others are unstable or radioactive. The unstable nucleus is not influenced by the chemical state of the element or by changes in temperature or pressure or by a change of state. The instability is entirely due to the number of neutrons in the nucleus. Stability will be restored by the emission of any surplus energy as electromagnetic radiation—called gamma radiation.

Both X-rays and gamma rays are electromagnetic radiations and as such may be considered either as waves or particles (photons or quanta). An X-ray photon is indistinguishable from a gamma ray photon of the same energy unless its source is known. The former results from the electron bombardment of a target, whereas the latter results from the spontaneous disintegration of an unstable nucleus.

WAVE THEORY

A wave is a progressive disturbance of a medium by which energy is transferred through the medium without any transfer of the medium.

Ripples on an otherwise still water surface are transverse waves because the oscillation of the water is at right angles to the direction of travel. Sound waves on the other hand are called longitudinal or compression waves because their oscillations are along the direction of travel. The general properties of waves are summarised in Figure 1.7. The frequency of the wave is the number of oscillations of an element of the medium in 1 second. For example, middle C on the piano is a sound wave of frequency of 256 cycles per second or 256 Hz (hertz). The wavelength is the distance, measured in the direction of travel, between two successive peaks. For example a helium–neon laser emits a beam of red light of 632.8 nm wavelength (1 nm = 10^{-9} m). The velocity, c, is the rate at which the disturbance is transmitted through the medium and related to frequency (v) and wavelength (λ) by the formula

$$c = v\lambda$$

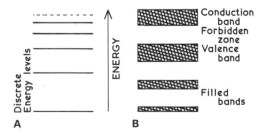

Fig. 1.6 **A** Electron energy levels in an atom and **B** electron energy bands in a solid.

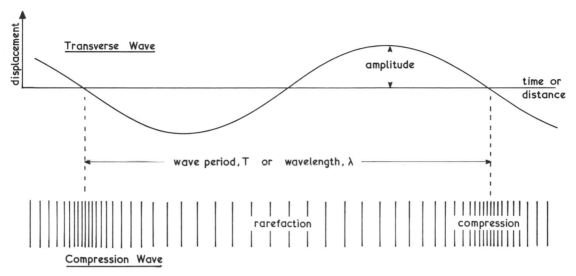

Fig. 1.7 Transverse and longitudinal waves.

The amplitude of the wave is the maximum value of the disturbance from its equilibrium value. This point of maximum disturbance is referred to as the *antinode*, whereas the point of zero disturbance is the *node*.

A single wave will have a unique wavelength and frequency, but many waves of different wavelengths may coexist in a spectrum. For example sunlight contains all the colours of the rainbow, but the individual colours only become evident when the wavelengths are separated out (or dispersed) within the raindrops. White light is a *continuous spectrum* of all the wavelengths from approximately 400 nm (violet) to 800 nm (red). Other light sources may emit only one wavelength, like the helium–neon laser, or several discrete wavelengths which then make up a *line spectrum*.

In the laboratory, a prism will demonstrate that white light is only a small part of a much bigger spectrum of wavelengths spreading to even shorter wavelengths (ultraviolet) and longer wavelengths (infrared). In fact this *electromagnetic spectrum* extends from wavelengths of many kilometres (10^3 m) to less than a picometre (10^{-12} m), these invisible waves being called radiowaves and X-rays respectively (Fig. 1.8). These electromagnetic waves travel in straight lines in free space with a velocity of 3×10^8 m s^{-1}.

Waves penetrate matter to a degree which varies in a complicated manner with the wavelength and the nature of the matter. Long radio waves penetrate non-conducting materials but are reflected by electrical conductors, such as overhead power lines. Radiations in or near the visible spectrum penetrate optically transparent materials like glass. X- and gamma rays have

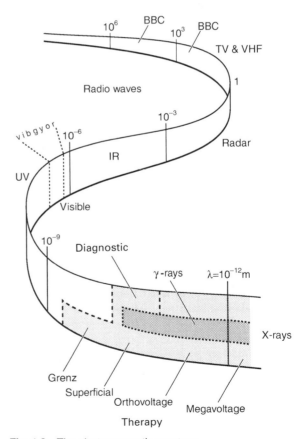

Fig. 1.8 The electromagnetic spectrum.

penetrating powers which increase with decreasing wavelength (p. 79).

Inverse square law

In general, a point source of electromagnetic radiation emanates waves isotropically, i.e. equally in all directions. If the total energy remains constant as the wave spreads out spherically, then the energy passing through a unit area of the spherical surface is inversely proportional to the square of the radius. The *intensity* of the wave is the energy carried across a unit area (in J m^{-2}) perpendicular to the direction of travel. The intensity of the radiation is therefore inversely proportional to the square of the distance from the source. This is known as the inverse square law and holds true providing the source can be regarded as a *point* source and there is no energy loss by absorption in the medium.

QUANTUM THEORY

When considering the properties of atoms it is sometimes more convenient to think of radiation as small packets of energy—called photons or quanta. The energy of each quantum (or photon) is proportional to the frequency.

$$\text{Quantum energy} = h\nu$$

where h is Planck's constant ($h = 6.626 \times 10^{-34}$ J s). The electron volt (eV) is the unit of energy of electrons in motion or the energy of quanta of radiation, and equal to the energy acquired by an electron when accelerated through a potential difference of one volt. In practice the MeV (10^6 eV) and keV (10^3 eV) are more common (1eV = 1.602×10^{-19}J).

In an atom, the electrons orbit the nucleus in precisely defined shells and any transfer of an electron from one shell to another will be accompanied by the absorption or emission of energy equal to the difference in the binding energy between the shells. Where the energy is being emitted, the energy is lost to a single photon of frequency ν where:

$$E_1 - E_2 = h\nu = hc/\lambda$$

Since the energy of each electron shell is unique to the atom, the emitted wavelengths are characteristic of the element, and therefore known as the *characteristic spectrum*.

This effect is demonstrated in the photoelectric cell, as described earlier. In the graph of anode current against anode voltage (Fig. 1.3), it will be noticed that a small anode current flows when the anode voltage is zero and the current is only reduced to zero when a negative (retarding) voltage is applied. The electrons are emitted from the cathode with a finite energy and this energy does not change when the intensity of illumination is increased. The change of intensity simply changes the number of electrons emitted.

PRODUCTION OF X-RAYS

X-rays are produced whenever fast electrons are slowed down in passing through matter. In a conventional tube, X-rays are produced when the beam of electrons is stopped in the metal target, the anode of the tube. The interactions between the impinging electrons and the target atoms occur in three main ways. Most of the electrons (Fig. 1.9A) interact with the electron clouds around the target nuclei before coming to rest, and at each deflection transfer a little of the electron's energy to a target electron in the form of heat. In many of these interactions, the orbiting electrons are removed with sufficient kinetic energy of their own to produce further ionisations and excitations of the target atoms—these tracks are known as *delta rays*. At accelerating voltages up to 500 kV, most of the energy of the impinging electrons appears as heat in the target, and cooling of the target is a major requirement of X-ray tube design (p. 33).

A second type of interaction that occurs leads to the emission of X-rays. Some of the impinging electrons interact with the inner orbital electrons of the target and cause ionisation or excitation of the target atoms. The vacant spaces so created in the electron orbits are then filled by electrons transferring from outer orbits or beyond (Fig. 1.9B). This transfer of an electron to

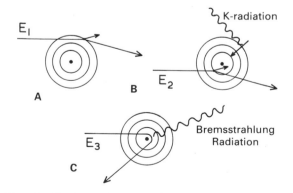

Fig. 1.9 The interactions occurring within an X-ray target. **A** The emission of a delta ray, **B** the emission of an electron and a characteristic photon and **C** the emission of bremsstrahlung radiation.

an inner orbit results in the emission of a photon of electromagnetic radiation, and within the tungsten target the photon energy is high enough to be in the X-ray region of the electromagnetic spectrum. These photons therefore contribute a line spectrum of X-rays characteristic of the target element. This second type of interaction therefore gives rise to *characteristic radiation*. For a tungsten target, characteristic X-ray photons of about 69 keV will be added to the continuous X-ray spectrum whenever the accelerating voltage exceeds 69 kV.

A third type of interaction between the impinging electron and the atoms of the target, however, is more significant in that the energy lost by the impinging electron appears directly as a photon of bremsstrahlung radiation. (The literal translation of the German word Bremsstrahlung is braking radiation, i.e. radiation produced by the sudden slowing of fast electrons.) The fast electron may lose all its energy in one 'collision' with the electric field round the target nucleus (Fig. 1.9C). It is more likely, however, that it will lose only a part of its energy in that collision and then proceed further, interacting with other target atoms before coming to rest. A beam of electrons interacting with the target in this way therefore produces X-ray photons with energies spread over a complete range, from very small values up to the maximum energy of the electrons in the beam. This gives rise to the *continuous spectrum* of X-rays and it is this process which accounts for most of the emission of X-rays from the target.

Efficiency of X-ray production

The efficiency of X-ray production, that is the proportion of the total energy of the incident electron beam energy that appears as X-rays, is normally very small, while the majority of the energy appears as heat. The efficiency of X-ray production is proportional, approximately, to both the tube voltage and the atomic number of the target. A target of high atomic number material therefore is very advantageous and tungsten ($Z = 74$) is generally used in therapy tubes. It is also a suitable material because of its high melting point, reasonable heat conductivity and good mechanical properties. For a tungsten target in an X-ray tube at 100 kV the efficiency of X-ray production is approximately 0.5%—that is 99.5% of the electron beam energy goes into heat. The X-ray production efficiency at 200 kV is approximately 1%. Accelerating voltages of 20–40 million volts are required before the X-ray production becomes very efficient, at say 60–70%.

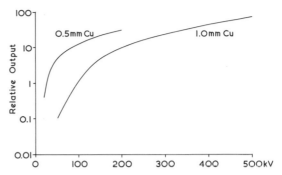

Fig. 1.10 The output dose rate increases rapidly with increasing tube voltage.

The energy of the individual electrons bombarding the tube target is determined by the voltage applied to the tube and is expressed in terms of the *electron volt*. When a potential difference V volts is applied across the tube, the electrons arrive at the target with an energy V electron volts. The efficiency of conversion of this electron energy to X-ray energy is approximately proportional to the applied tube voltage, and the energy of the electrons is also proportional to this voltage. The total X-ray emission will therefore increase approximately proportionally to the square of the applied tube voltage if the tube current is kept constant, that is, if the number of electrons striking the target per second is constant. There is thus a rapid change of X-ray output with tube voltage and much attention must be given in the design of X-ray equipment to ensure the constancy of the voltage applied to the X-ray tube (Fig. 1.10).

Distribution of X-rays round the target

When electrons strike a metal target which is just thick enough to bring them to rest, X-rays are found to be emitted from the target in all directions. The distribution of the X-radiation depends, however, very much on the tube voltage. For tube voltages of about 50 to 100 kV the maximum intensity of emission is approximately at right angles to the electron beam, but as the beam voltage increases the direction of maximum intensity moves more and more towards that of the bombarding electrons, and for beams in the megavoltage range most of the X-ray emission is confined to a narrow cone near the forward direction of the electron beam. Figure 1.11 illustrates, by polar diagrams, the distribution of X-ray energy from a target for four representative electron energies. The curves are such that the radius from the target is proportional to the intensity of the beam in that direction. It can be seen that for electrons of 100 kV

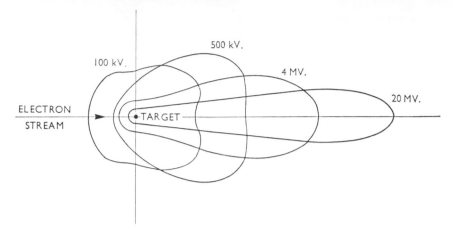

Fig. 1.11 The spatial distribution of X-rays from a thin target. (Reproduced with permission from Meredith & Massey 1977.)

energy the X-ray intensity at right angles to the electron stream is greater than in the forward direction, whereas at 20 MV the forward intensity is 10 times that at right angles.

The actual distribution of X-ray intensity round the targets of practical X-ray tubes is different from that shown in Figure 1.11 because of the attenuation of the X-ray beams in the target material, especially for beams generated at low voltages. The design of targets for X-ray tubes is, however, influenced by the distribution of X-rays illustrated in this figure. At low voltages it is advantageous to use the X-ray beam coming from the target at right angles to the electron stream and most diagnostic and therapy X-ray tubes up to 300 kV therefore use a *reflection target*, in which the useful beam is taken from the front of the target. At tube voltages of 1 million or more, however, it is advantageous to use the X-ray beam in the same direction as the incident electron stream in spite of the attenuation in the target. Such targets, which are made just thick enough to stop all the bombarding electrons, are known as *transmission targets*.

The variation of X-ray beam intensity with direction means that at low energies the target angle has to be chosen carefully if large fields are to be irradiated uniformly (p. 33), while at megavoltage energies, field flattening filters have to be introduced to compensate for the concentration of the X-ray emission in a very narrow angle round the direction of the electron beam (p. 41).

Continuous spectrum

As seen above, the X-ray beam consists mainly of photons arising from multiple interactions of many electrons with the target atoms. Photons are present, therefore, of all energies up to a maximum value corresponding to the energy of the electrons accelerated by the maximum voltage applied to the tube. This forms the continuous spectrum. The continuous spectrum has a maximum photon energy equal to the tube voltage when the energy is expressed in electron volts. Photons of maximum photon energy have the *minimum wavelength* in the spectrum. This minimum wavelength may be calculated thus:

$$\text{Minimum wavelength} = \lambda_{\min} = \frac{hc}{kV_{\max}}$$

where h is Planck's constant, v the frequency of the radiation and λ its wavelength and c the velocity of light. Incorporating the appropriate physical constants, and if appropriate energy units are used, this formula becomes

$$\text{Minimum wavelength} = \frac{1.24}{kVp} \text{ nanometres}$$

where kVp is the peak tube voltage expressed in kilovolts. (1 nanometre = 10^{-9} metre.) This relationship is sometimes referred to as *Duane–Hunt's law*.

The distribution of the relative intensity of the radiations in the continuous spectrum as a function of photon energy expressed in kilo-electron volts is shown in Figure 1.12 for three representative tube voltages in the superficial X-ray range. In this diagram the ordinate represents the energy flow per unit interval of energy, as expressed by the number of photons with that particular energy multiplied by the energy of those photons. The three curves show the continuous spectrum for tube voltages of 60 kV, 90 kV and 120 kV. Note that in these curves the characteristic radiations

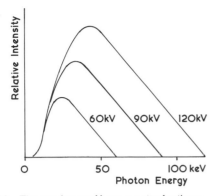

Fig. 1.12 The continuous X-ray spectra for three accelerating voltages (60, 90, 120 kV).

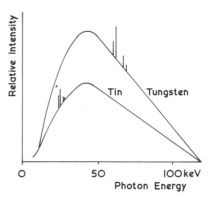

Fig. 1.13 The 120 kV X-ray spectra for tungsten and tin targets.

have not been shown, and the beam current is assumed constant for the three curves. Note the following properties of these curves:

1. The existence of a maximum photon energy (minimum wavelength) for each tube voltage.

2. The existence of a peak in the relative intensity distribution at a photon energy about one-third of the maximum value.

3. The low intensity of low energy photons, which arises because of the decrease in penetrating power of the photons as the photon energy decreases so that they escape less readily from the target.

4. An increase in tube voltage increases the intensity of emission at all photon energies and introduces higher energy photons not present at lower voltages. The total intensity of the radiation emitted from the target is easily seen to be proportional to the area under the appropriate curve and the family of curves illustrates that the total emission is approximately proportional to the square of the voltage applied to the tube.

5. With the increase in applied voltage the proportion of high energy photons increases and the peak of the curve moves to higher photon energies. Since normally higher energy photons have greater penetrating power (p. 79), the figure also illustrates the fact that increases of voltage on the tube give increased penetration power of the beam.

Characteristic radiation

The curves of Figure 1.12 are drawn for a fixed beam current with an arbitrary intensity scale. They represent the continuous spectrum from a target of any element arising from multiple interactions of the bombarding electrons with the target atoms.

For a tungsten target, orbital electrons can be

ejected from the K shell if the bombarding electrons have an energy of 69 keV or more. The resultant characteristic radiation, consisting of photons with energies in one of a small group of discrete energies of nearly the same value, appears as a line spectrum superimposed on the continuous spectrum for all tube voltages above 69 kV. If the target material were of some other element the voltage needed to dislodge the K electron would be different and the characteristic radiation would have a different wavelength. Figure 1.13 shows the two spectra including both continuous and characteristic radiation for a tungsten (W) target and a tin (Sn) target for the same tube voltage (120 kV) and the same tube current. Note the following points:

1. The continuous spectrum from tin ($Z = 50$) is less intense than from tungsten ($Z = 74$)—the total emission being approximately proportional to the atomic number of the target.

2. The characteristic radiation from tungsten appears between 57 keV and 69 keV photon energy whenever the tube voltage exceeds 69 kV, while that from the tin target appears between approximately 25 keV and 29 keV whenever the tube voltage is above 29 kV.

3. Note that although the intensity of the lines of the characteristic radiation may be high compared with that of the continuous spectrum, its contribution to the total emission of X-ray energy from the tube is relatively small.

4. The characteristic line spectrum of the target material will also include photons of lower energies appropriate to the binding energies of the L orbital electrons, but these are rarely shown as they are readily absorbed by the target and the inherent filtration of the tube and housing.

FILTRATION OF THE X-RAY BEAM

An X-ray beam is of practical use only after it has

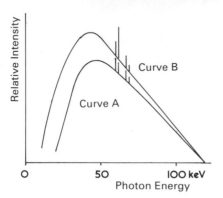

Fig. 1.14 X-ray spectra showing the effect of filtration.

emerged from the target and passed through the (glass) wall of the tube, the tube shield, and any material inevitably or deliberately placed in its path. Since the attenuation of the photons increases with decrease in photon energy, the spectral distribution of the X-ray beam changes in passing through any material between the target and the point of use. Figure 1.14 illustrates the effect, however, by plotting the spectral distribution of a beam generated at 120 kV from a tungsten target with (curve A) and without (curve B) additional filtration. It will be noted that the total intensity, as represented by the area under the curve, is reduced by the addition of the filter but at the lower energies the reduction in intensity is proportionately greater than at the higher energies. This process is known as beam hardening and is dealt with in more detail later in Chapter 5.

2. Radioactivity and production of radioactive materials

An understanding of radioactivity is possible only if we have some concept of the nature of the atom. We can explain the behaviour of atoms in simple terms by the use of simple models.

ATOMIC STRUCTURE

We have seen in Chapter 1 that the Bohr model divides the total region of the atom into two parts, nuclear and extranuclear. The extranuclear region comprising of free space and the orbital electrons and the nuclear region of the protons and neutrons. These are the primary building blocks of an atom although we will see later in this chapter that other particles exist within the nucleus. The properties of various particles are given in Table 2.1.

Extranuclear region of the atom

The extranuclear region is where chemical bonding takes place, and where the majority of interactions between matter and radiation take place. The electrons orbiting around the nucleus are grouped together in shells. Electrons in a given shell of a particular nuclide experience a specific binding energy. The electrons in the K shell have the greatest binding energy; those farthest away at the periphery of the atom are free, loosely bound, electrons. The magnitude of the binding

Table 2.2 Binding energies of the electrons in the K, L and M shells for various elements

Element	Z	Chemical symbol	Binding energy (keV)		
			K	L	M
Copper	29	Cu	9.0	1.1	0.12
Iodine	53	I	33.2	5.1	1.07
Lead	82	Pb	88.0	15.9	3.8

energy is dependent on the atomic number of the nuclide and the electron shell location. The binding energy is equivalent to the amount of energy necessary to remove that electron from its location. Examples of binding energy are given in Table 2.2.

Atomic mass, weight and size

Three scales of atomic mass are recognised.

1. The absolute scale, related to the kilogram.
2. The physical scale measured in atomic mass units (a.m.u.).
3. The chemical scale or atomic weight which takes into account the normal isotopic mix of the element.

The atomic mass unit has been defined by setting the mass of one atom of the nuclide carbon-12 equal to

Table 2.1 Properties of the elemental particles

Particle	Symbol	Rest mass (kg)	Rest energy (a.m.u.)	(MeV)	Charge*	Radius (m)
Proton	p	1.672×10^{-27}	1.0073	938.2	1	1.45×10^{-15}
Neutron	n	1.675×10^{-27}	1.0087	939.2	0	1.45×10^{-15}
Electron	e^- or β^-	9.108×10^{-31}	0.00055	0.511	−1	2.82×10^{-15}
Positron	e^+ or β^+	9.108×10^{-31}	0.00055	0.511	+1	2.82×10^{-15}
Neutrino	ν	1.000×10^{-34}	1.0×10^{-6}	1.0×10^{-3}	0	0
Photon or gamma ray	$h\nu$ or γ	—	—	—	0	0

* The unit of charge, +1, is $+1.6 \times 10^{-19}$ coulombs.

12.000. . . such units. Carbon-12 has six protons and six neutrons and since protons and neutrons have nearly the same mass each elemental particle on this scale has a mass of nearly 1. For example, hydrogen, with one proton in its nucleus and one orbiting electron, has a mass of 1.008, while bismuth, with 83 protons, 125 neutrons and 83 electrons, has a mass of 208.98.

Atomic weights as used in chemistry are usually different from the atomic masses because most naturally occurring elements have a number of stable isotopes. For example, chlorine consists of a mixture of two isotopes, chlorine-34 and chlorine-36. They occur with an abundance of 75.5% and 24.6% respectively, giving an atomic weight of 35.46.

The relationship between the absolute scale and the physical scale can be obtained with the aid of Avagadro's number (i.e. the number of atoms in a mole of a substance: 6.0225×10^{23}). Hence 12.000 g or 1 mole of carbon-12 will contain 6.0225×10^{23} atoms. (One mole is the amount of substance which contains as many elementary parts as there are in 0.012 kg of carbon-12.) Therefore:

$$1 \text{ a.m.u} \equiv \frac{1 \times 10^{-3}}{6.0225 \times 10^{23}} \text{ kg}$$
$$\equiv 1.66 \times 10^{-27} \text{ kg}$$

The mass of the electron is only 1/1840 that of a proton or neutron so a good estimate of the mass of an atom can be obtained by multiplying the number of nucleons or the atomic number by 1.66×10^{-27} kg.

Yet another physical aspect of an atom is its dimension or size. The radius of a proton or neutron is 1.45×10^{-15} m and for an electron 2.82×10^{-15} m. If we assume the nucleus is a sphere then the radii of nuclei vary from 1.45×10^{-15} m for nuclei with mass number 1, to 9×10^{-15} m for nuclei with mass number 257. The radius of the atom is much greater, varying from 0.9×10^{-10} to 1.6×10^{-10} m. This means that the nucleus, whilst containing most of the mass of the atom, occupies only one part in 3×10^{13} of its total volume. The remaining space is occupied by the electrons. These electrons must be widely spaced because electrons are about the same size as atomic nuclei. Indeed if the atom is pictured as being as large as a sports stadium then the nucleus in the centre of the stadium is about as big as a fly. This picture helps us to understand how the atomic radiations can penetrate many layers of atoms without undergoing an interaction.

Equivalence of mass and energy

In 1905 Albert Einstein put forward his famous theory of relativity. The most important concept of Einstein's theory is that mass is a form of energy, the two being related by the simple formula:

$$E = mc^2$$

where c is the velocity of light in metres per second, m is the mass in kilograms and E is the energy measured in joules.

If 1 g of matter is converted into energy the energy released will be:

$$E = (1 \times 10^{-3}) \times (3 \times 10^{8})^2$$
$$= 9 \times 10^{13} \text{ J}$$

This is an enormous amount of energy for such a small mass, being sufficient to supply the daily power requirement of 1.5 million homes.

A more convenient energy unit in nuclear reactions is the electron volt, which is equivalent to 1.6×10^{-19} J. From Chapter 1 we learnt that the rest mass of an electron is 9.1×10^{-31} kg, the equivalent energy value therefore is:

$$\frac{9.1 \times 10^{-31} \times (3 \times 10^{8})^2}{1.6 \times 10^{-19}}$$
$$= 0.511 \text{ MeV}$$

similarly, 1 a.m.u. = 931 MeV.

Energy and mass can be considered as two manifestations of the same entity and in certain circumstances are interchangeable. For example as we shall see in Chapter 4 a gamma ray whose energy is greater than 1.02 MeV may interact with the electric field around the nucleus, may disappear and simultaneously create two particles of matter, one negative electron and one positive electron or positron. This process is known as pair production. Conversely when the positron is brought to rest in matter it combines with a neighbouring negative electron, the two charges neutralise one another and the mass of the two electrons is converted back into two photons of electromagnetic radiation, each of 0.511 MeV energy.

THE NUCLEAR REGION

Atoms are classified according to the number of protons, Z, and nucleons, A, in their nuclei. Each different combination of Z and A identifies a distinct species of *nuclide*, symbolised as $^{A}_{Z}X$, where X is the element symbol. Thus hydrogen, which has only a single proton in its nucleus, is expressed as $^{1}_{1}H$ while deuterium, which has one proton and one neutron, is expressed as $^{2}_{1}H$.

All nuclides with the same atomic number (Z), and therefore the same number of electrons and chemical properties but different neutron (N) and mass (A) numbers, are known as *isotopes* ('same place'). Most elements found in nature have more than one isotope. Isotopes may be stable or unstable. For example hydrogen and deuterium, cited above, are both stable but tritium, $^3_1$H, with one proton and two neutrons, is unstable and hence radioactive.

Nuclides with the same A, but different Z and N are known as *isobars* ('equal weight'), e.g. $^{40}_{18}$Ar, $^{40}_{19}$K, $^{40}_{20}$Ca. There are several sets of triple isobars where the middle one is radioactive, and many stable pairs of isobars in which Z differs by two. This indicates that the stable nucleus favours even numbers of protons and neutrons.

Now just as a shell model can be used to describe the arrangement of electrons in the extranuclear region an analogous model can be used for the arrangement of neutrons and protons in the nucleus. In this case the shell closures occur at particle numbers 2, 8, 20, 28, 50, 82, 126.

These are known as magic numbers and apply separately to neutrons and protons. Nuclei with full shells are unusually stable, e.g. $^{208}_{82}$Pb which has 82 protons and 126 neutrons, that is it contains two magic numbers. Helium ($^4_2$He), which has two neutrons and two protons, also has a very stable nucleus and it is this feature which explains why it is ejected from the atom as a particle during alpha decay.

Nuclear energy levels

The nucleons also occupy definite energy levels in the nucleus. For each nuclide there is one set of energy levels available to the neutrons and a second set available to the protons. A nucleus is in its 'ground state' when its lowest energy levels are filled. Occasionally the nucleus may exist in an excited state, that is a proton or neutron is raised to a higher, unoccupied energy level. When such a nucleus returns to its stable state electromagnetic radiations known as gamma ray photons are emitted. The energy may be released as a single photon or as a cascade of several smaller gamma rays.

Two nuclei having the same values for Z and A but different nuclear configurations are known as *isomers*, e.g. $^{99m}_{43}$Tc, $^{99}_{43}$Tc. It is important to distinguish between nuclear and atomic excitation. Nuclear excitation is associated with the configuration and energy of the particles within the nucleus. Atomic excitation refers to the state of the electrons. Similarly while gamma rays and X-rays are both forms of electromagnetic radiation, the gamma rays originate from nuclear energy changes, whereas the characteristic X-rays arise from electron shell energy change.

Nuclear forces

As has already been stated the nucleus is very small and

consists of neutrons and protons. Protons have a positive electrical charge and, since like charges repel, there must be a large electrostatic force of repulsion resulting from the high density of like charges. We might therefore expect the nucleus to 'explode' but it does not. This can only be explained if there is an attractive force present which is greater than the electrostatic force of repulsion. This attractive force is known as the nuclear force and is some 100 times greater than the electrostatic force.

The nuclear force is greater between neutron and proton than between neutron and neutron, which is greater than that between proton and proton. This binding energy varies from element to element but the average is approximate 8 MeV per nucleon. The nuclear force is only effective over a very limited range of 0.4×10^{-13} cm to 2.4×10^{-13} cm, being at its strongest when nucleons are 1×10^{-13} cm apart. This is less than the radius of a large nucleus. In contrast the electrostatic repulsive forces work over a relatively large range. This means that in heavier atoms, in order to keep the nucleus stable, extra neutrons are required to increase the total attractive force while not altering the repulsive force. This is shown graphically in Figure 2.1 where the number of neutrons has been plotted against the number of protons for all the stable nuclides.

Nuclear binding energy

If we return to our atom of carbon-12 and try to create a new atom out of its constituent parts as follows:

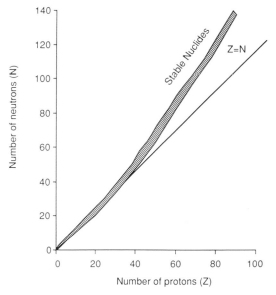

Fig. 2.1 The number of protons versus the number of neutrons with increasing atomic number.

$$n = 6 \,(1.0087 \text{ a.m.u.}) = 6.0522 \text{ a.m.u.}$$
$$p = 6 \,(1.0073 \text{ a.m.u.}) = 6.0438 \text{ a.m.u.}$$
$$e^- = 6 \,(0.00055 \text{ a.m.u.}) = 0.0033 \text{ a.m.u.}$$

we find that the sum   = 12.0993 a.m.u.

But we have already stated that the nuclide mass of carbon-12 is 12.000. . . a.m.u. which is 0.0993 less than the sum of the constituent parts. This is known as the mass defect and is not in fact lost but is converted into the nuclear binding energy. The converted energy for carbon-12 is:

$$0.0993 \text{ a.m.u.} \times 931 \text{ MeV/a.m.u.} = 92.448 \text{ MeV}$$

and the nuclear binding energy is

$$\frac{92.448}{12} = 7.7 \text{ MeV/nucleon}$$

The average binding energy per nucleon for different nuclides is shown plotted as a function of the mass number in Figure 2.2. This demonstrates: (1) A rapid increase in binding energy per nucleon for the light nuclei with a notable peak at $A = 4$ (^{4}He); (2) approximately the same binding energy (7.5 to 8.8 MeV) for all nuclei with A greater than 16; (3) the maximum binding energy per nucleon occurring at about $A = 60$ for iron, nickel and cobalt; and (4) a gradual decrease in binding energy with A greater than 60 to 7.3 MeV/nucleon at $A = 238$. This is associated with the disruptive effect of the nuclear charge.

Nuclear stability

From the previous discussions it is apparent that the requirements for a stable nucleus are that it complies with one or more of the following statements.

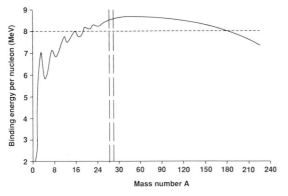

Fig. 2.2   Average binding energy per nucleon as a function of mass number.

1. There should be even numbers of neutrons and protons.
2. The shells of the nucleus should be full.
3. There should be a slight excess of neutrons.
4. The nucleus should have no more than 200 nucleons.

RADIOACTIVITY

Although many elements have several naturally occurring isotopes the number of stable arrangements of neutrons and protons is rather limited and any other configuration results in an unstable nucleus. Sooner or later such nuclei will spontaneously emit ionising radiations in the form of charged particles or photons of electromagnetic radiation in order to achieve a more stable proton neutron configuration. In so doing the atom changes its atomic number and so its chemical identity.

This phenomenon is called *radioactive decay*, and the nucleus is said to be *radioactive*. The change from one nuclide, known as the parent, to another nuclide, known as the daughter, is called a *disintegration*. The new atomic nucleus may be a stable form of the element or it may itself be unstable and radioactive.

The periodic table lists 103 elements. For most elements both stable and unstable isotopes are known. The total number of nuclides available is in excess of 1900 but of these only 266 are stable, that is, the elements exist in both non-radioactive and radioactive forms. The radioactive nuclides are those in which the number of neutrons present in the nucleus falls short of, or is in excess of, the number present in the stable nuclides. For example, the element carbon of atomic number $Z = 6$ is known to have isotopes with the following mass numbers: 10, 11, 12, 13, 14, 15. Of these the isotopes of $A = 12$ and 13 are stable and exist in nature with six and seven neutrons respectively in the nuclei. The isotope $A = 10$ and 11 are neutron deficient and those with $A = 14$ and 15 have a neutron excess. All four are radioactive. For most elements, radioactive isotopes can be produced by various techniques of nuclear bombardment, to be described later (p. 25).

Some radioactive nuclides do occur in nature, however, either because their rate of disintegration is extremely low or because they are being produced continuously by the disintegration of other very slowly disintegrating nuclides. An example of the former is the radioactive isotope of potassium ($Z = 19, A = 40$) which occurs as part of the normal naturally occurring element. An example of the latter is the radioactive element radium ($Z = 86, A = 226$) which occurs in nature as a radioactive by-product of the slow disintegration of the radioactive element uranium.

Units of activity

There are three ways of expressing disintegration rates: in disintegrations per second, in curies, or in becquerels. The curie (Ci) and the becquerel (Bq) are practical units for expressing the activity of a quantity of radioactive material.

The original definition of the curie was the amount of radiation in equilibrium with 1 g of radium. This could only be applied to radium-226 and its decay products. The curie was therefore redefined in terms of the actual phenomenon of interest, that is the number of disintegrations per second from the 1 g of radium.

$$1 \text{ Ci} = 3.7 \times 10^{10} \text{ disintegrations/second}$$

This somewhat strange unit for expressing activity has been superseded by the SI unit, the becquerel, where:

$$1 \text{ Bq} = 1 \text{ disintegration/second}$$

Thus 1 curie is equivalent to 37 gigabecquerels.

It will be appreciated that the becquerel or its sub-multiples are not a measure of the mass of the radio-active material present. In a radionuclide with a slow disintegration rate a large mass of substance will be necessary to provide 37 GBq of activity. As has already been stated, for radium-226 with a half-life of 1600 years, 37 GBq of activity will be provided by 1 g of radium. In a rapidly decaying radionuclide, however, a very much smaller mass of material will be equivalent to 37 GBq of activity. For example 37 GBq of carrier-free iodine-131 with a half-life of 8 days will have a mass of 8×10^{-6} g.

Radioactive decay

Disintegration of a radioactive nucleus is spontaneous and random. The break-up of any particular nucleus is not predictable but the proportion of nuclei in any particular radionuclide which disintegrate in unit time depends on the instability of the nucleus. The fraction of the total number of atoms of a particular radio-nuclide which disintegrate per unit time is a constant for that nuclide and is known as the decay constant or transformation constant.

It can easily be demonstrated that the disappearance of a constant fraction of the atoms per unit time can be represented mathematically by the exponential law:

$$N = N_o e^{-\lambda t}$$

where N is the number of atoms remaining at time t, N_o is the initial number present at time $t = 0$ and λ is the transformation constant.

This is the *law of exponential decay*. Since the intensity of emission from a radioactive sample is directly pro-

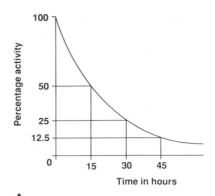

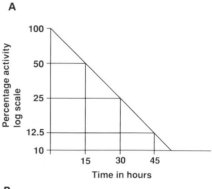

Fig. 2.3   Radioactive decay of sodium-24: **A** linear, **B** logarithmic.

portional to the number of radioactive atoms present, the exponential law of decay can be observed readily by measuring under fixed geometrical conditions the variation with time of the number of beta particles emitted per unit time or the gamma ray intensity. Figure 2.3A shows a radioactive decay curve for sodium-24.

If the exponential curve represented by the above equation is plotted logarithmically, that is, if log intensity is plotted against time, a straight line results, as shown in Figure 2.3B. This is an important aspect of the curve since if an experimentally determined logarithmic decay curve is not a straight line this is strong evidence that two or more radionuclides are present which are decaying at different rates.

Half-life

The time taken for the activity, i.e. the intensity of the emitted radiation or the number of radioactive atoms present, to be reduced to one half of the original value is a constant. Physically this means that any radionuclide has a characteristic transformation constant leading to a fixed time for the number of atoms of the nuclide to be reduced to half its original value. This time is the *half-life*. It can be shown that the half-life is related to the transformation constant by the simple relationship:

$$T_{\frac{1}{2}} = \frac{0.693}{\lambda}$$

where $T_{\frac{1}{2}}$ is the half-life.

Half-lives of radionuclides vary enormously, corresponding to a wide range of instability of the radioactive nucleus. For example, the isotope polonium-210, has a half-life of 138 days, sodium-24 15.0 hours and sodium-22 2.6 years—but extreme values of half-life are represented by potassium-40, 1.3×10^9 years, and polonium-214 (radium-C'), 1.6×10^{-4} seconds. It will be seen later (p. 179) that the half-life of a radionuclide has an important bearing on its use in clinical practice.

Mean life

It can be demonstrated mathematically that the law of radioactive decay is a statistical law and radioactive decay is subject to the laws of probability. The average number of atoms disintegrating per second is N, but the actual number disintegrating will fluctuate around this value.

The *mean life* of a radionuclide is a measure of the average life expectancy of the atoms of that nuclide. Since the decay process is statistical, any single atom could have a lifetime from zero to infinity. Based upon this, the mean life is simply the reciprocal of the decay constant.

$$\text{Mean life } \overline{T} = \frac{1}{\lambda} = \frac{1}{0.693} \cdot T_{\frac{1}{2}} = 1.44 \cdot T_{\frac{1}{2}}$$

Mean life is useful for calculating the dose due to 'infinite exposure'.

Radiations from radioactive nuclides

Radioactive nuclei may give off one of four different types of particulate radiation and may at the same time give off photons of electromagnetic radiation. The particulate radiations, alpha particles, beta particles, positrons or neutrons, are described below in more detail. Electromagnetic radiation from the nuclei of radioactive atoms is called gamma radiation. In a small number of radioactive nuclides only gamma radiation is emitted and in this case, since no charged particle leaves the nucleus, the atomic number of the disintegrating atom does not change. The resulting atom in this case is of the same chemical element as the initial one and the radioactive process has merely changed the internal energy of the nucleus.

The characteristics of the various decay processes are given in Table 2.3. Each type of disintegration can be indicated by a decay scheme, as shown in Figure 2.4. A decay scheme is a combination of a graph and an energy level diagram. The atomic number of the nuclide is represented by the horizontal scale, while the vertical scale represents the energy involved in the disintegration

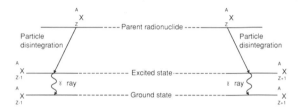

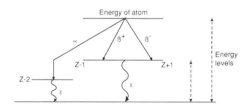

Fig. 2.4   Decay scheme diagrams.

Table 2.3   Nuclear disintegration processes

Name	Symbol	Change in nucleus		Radiation emitted
		Z	A	
Alpha decay	α	−2	−4	α
Isobaric transition				
Beta decay	β^-	+1	0	e^-, ν
Positron decay	β^+	−1	0	$e^+, \nu, (\gamma_a)$
Electron capture	EC	−1	0	$\nu, (\gamma_x, e^-_{Au})$
Isomeric transition				
Gamma ray decay	γ	0	0	γ
Internal conversion	IC	0	0	$e^-, (\gamma_x, e^-_{Au})$

ν, Neutrino; γ_a, annihilation photons; γ_x, characteristic X-rays; e^-_{Au}, Auger electrons.

process. The direction of the arrow to the right or left indicates whether the atomic number of the daughter nuclide has increased or decreased.

Alpha decay

Certain types of radionuclides, with mass number greater than 150, emit positively charged particles called alpha (α) particles. An alpha particle consists of two protons and two neutrons tightly bound together. These particles therefore have a mass of 4 on the atomic scale and a positive charge of 2 units. They are the nuclei of helium atoms. For each disintegration the energy lost by the parent atom can either be removed entirely by the alpha particle as kinetic energy or partly by the alpha particle and partly by an associated gamma ray. In each case the atomic number decreases by 2 and the mass number by 4.

$$_{Z}^{A}X \longrightarrow {_{Z-2}^{A-4}}X + \alpha + Q$$

Where Q is the energy released.

Several of the naturally occurring radionuclides, such as radium-226, are alpha emitters, as are many of the artificially prepared radionuclides of atomic numbers greater than 92, such as plutonium-239. An example of an alpha decay scheme is shown in Figure 2.5A.

Isobaric transitions

Atoms may have an imbalance in the number of protons and neutrons in the nucleus. If the excess energy is less than about 8 MeV, i.e. the binding energy of the nucleons, the nucleus may reach a stable state by changing one of its neutrons into a proton or vice versa, that is, the mass number stays the same but the atomic number either increases or decreases by one. This is called an isobaric transition. Isobaric transitions fall into three groups: beta minus (β⁻) or negatron decay, beta plus (β⁺) or positron decay and electron capture.

Negatron decay. β⁻ decay occurs when a neutron changes into a proton with the emission of an electron antineutrino pair.

$$n^{\circ} \rightarrow p^{+} + e^{-} + \nu$$

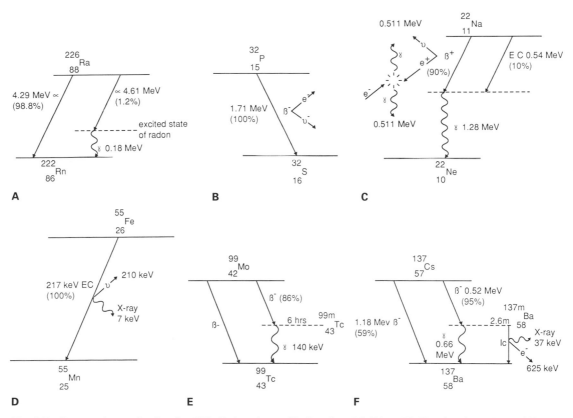

Fig. 2.5 Decay schemes for **A** radon-226, **B** phosphorus-32, **C** sodium-22, **D** iron-55, **E** technetium-99m and **F** caesium-137.

β⁻ particles are negatively charged particles with the same charge and mass as an electron. They are therefore electrons of high kinetic energy emitted from the nucleus of the atom.

Negatron decay leaves the mass number the same but the atomic number increases by one. Phosphorus-32 is a radionuclide which decays by this process, as shown in Figure 2.5B.

The beta particle ejected may have any energy from just above zero to a maximum characteristic of the parent nucleus (Fig. 2.6). A useful point to remember is that the average energy is approximately one-third the maximum energy. However the transformation within a given nuclide always results in the loss of the same amount of energy. This is achieved by the ejection of a second particle, the antineutrino, simultaneously with the β⁻ particle. Thus the total energy of the transformation may be shared differently by the two particles. The antineutrino has no electrical charge, almost no rest mass and has very little interaction with matter.

Positron decay. Positron decay is analogous to negatron decay but in this case a proton changes into a neutron, which stays in the nucleus, and a positron neutrino pair are emitted.

$$p^+ \rightarrow n^o + \beta^+ + \nu$$

The positive charge lost by the nucleus is carried off by the positron.

In this case the atomic numbers will decrease by one. Since positron emission decreases the atomic number by one the number of electrons orbiting the nucleus must also be decreased by one. Thus for positron decay to take place the difference in the energy between the parent and daughter nuclide must be at least 1.022 MeV (2×0.511 MeV).

Positrons are positive electrons, and are the same kind of particles as are produced in the pair production process when very high energy photons interact with matter (p. 66). Although the positrons have a very short life they behave in most respects exactly like negative electrons during their passage through matter, losing energy by production of ions. When the energy has been completely lost in this way the positron combines with a negative electron and the rest mass of the two particles is converted into two photons of electromagnetic radiation, each of energy 0.511 MeV. This is called annihilation radiation (p. 58). A common example of an isotope which undergoes positron decay is sodium-22 (Fig. 2.5c).

Electron capture. If the nuclear energy levels of the parent and daughter, of a proton rich nuclide, do not differ by more than 1.022 MeV, electron capture takes place. In this case the nucleus captures an electron from one of its orbits, usually the K shell, the electron and proton combine in the nucleus to form a neutron and a neutrino. The neutrino is ejected from the nucleus carrying away any excess energy.

$$p^+ + e^- \rightarrow n^o + \nu$$

If K capture occurs, the 'hole' in the K shell must be filled by another electron. This will give rise to K radiation. An example of such a decay scheme is given in Figure 2.5D.

In many cases both positron decay and electron capture will take place, as was seen in Figure 2.5C for the decay of sodium-22. The higher the Z of the nucleus and the closer the K shell is to the nucleus the greater the probability of electron capture.

Isomeric transition

Following decay by alpha or beta particle emission the daughter nucleus is often in an excited state and possesses excess energy. Isomeric transition is the change of the excited nucleus or isomer to the stable isomer. The residual energy may be emitted as a gamma ray or passed to an orbital electron.

Gamma radiation. The nuclei may be transformed from a high energy level to a low energy level by the emission of one or more quanta of electromagnetic radiation known as gamma rays (Fig. 2.5A,C). Gamma rays are indistinguishable from X-rays, being differentiated only by their origin, that is, gamma rays are emitted from an excited nucleus; X-rays are emitted either as a result of changes in the electron shells, or as bremsstrahlung when a charged particle decelerates under the influence of the nuclear field. The gamma rays emitted have discrete energies characteristic of the daughter.

In most cases gamma emission happens virtually instantaneously but occasionally the daughter nuclide

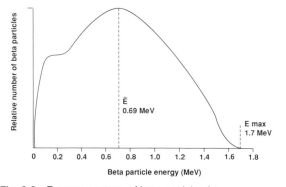

Fig. 2.6 Energy spectrum of beta particles from phosphorus-32.

can remain in the excited state for several hours. This is known as a *metastable* state. These nuclides are designated by use of the suffix or superscript 'm'. Technetium-99m (^{99m}Tc), a widely used radionuclide with a half-life of 6 hours, is an example of such a decay process (Fig. 2.5E). Metastable radionuclides are of great value in nuclear medicine as they do not emit particles only energy, in the form of gamma rays, and hence deliver a low radiation dose to the patient.

Internal conversion. In heavy atoms the electrons of the subshells, particularly the K shell, bombard the large nucleus as they orbit around it; the nucleus may then transfer its excess energy to the electron. This is known as internal conversion. The converted electron will be ejected from the atom and travel away with a discrete energy equal to the difference between the energy lost by the nucleus and the binding energy holding the electron to the atom.

The longer the half-life of the excited state the greater is the probability of internal conversion taking place. Therefore internal conversion is important in metastable decay. Barium-137m decays by a combination of gamma ray emission and internal conversion (Fig. 2.5F).

Auger electrons. Following electron conversion the atom is left with a vacancy in the K shell which will be filled by an electron from the L shell and an electron cascade will follow until the outer shell captures a free electron. These transfers will be accompanied by emission of characteristic electromagnetic radiation. Not all the X-rays produced during internal conversion are emitted from the atom; some transfer their energy to an outer electron ejecting it, as an 'Auger' electron, from the atom. The kinetic energy of the Auger electron is low, being the difference between the energy of the X-ray and the binding energy of the orbital electron.

Neutrons

The emission of neutrons during radioactive decay is quite rare. However some radionuclides, such as the artificially prepared californium-252, emit neutrons of considerable energy during their disintegration. Neutrons have no charge and are not themselves ionising radiations, being able to pass freely through the charged electron structure of the atoms of an absorbing medium. Their ionising potential arises from the collision of the fast neutron with the nuclei of the atoms of the medium, producing an efficient transfer of energy to these nuclei. Since the nuclei are charged and heavy they produce intense ionisation along their tracks.

Radioactive equilibrium

A radioactive disintegration process involving the emission of a charged particle generally results in the production of a new non-radioactive nuclide of a different element. Sometimes, however, the nuclide formed by the disintegration of a radionuclide is itself an unstable nuclide and undergoes a further radioactive transformation. This can be represented by the following decay scheme:

$$N_1 \xrightarrow{\lambda_1} N_2 \xrightarrow{\lambda_2} N_3$$

where N_1 and N_2 are the parent and daughter radionuclides respectively and N_3 is stable; λ_1 and λ_2 are the decay constants of the parent and daughter nuclides. An example of such a transformation is the decay of strontium-90 which disintegrates with the emission of a negative beta particle, forming an isotope of the element yttrium.

$$^{90}_{38}Sr \xrightarrow[T_{1/2}\ 28\ y]{\lambda_1 = 0.0000028} \ ^{90}_{39}Y \xrightarrow[T_{1/2}\ 64\ h]{\lambda_2 = 0.0108} \ ^{90}_{40}Zr$$

This isotope is itself radioactive and emits a further negative beta particle, the final product of this second disintegration process being a stable isotope of the element zirconium. Strontium-90 has a relatively long half-life of 28 years but its daughter product, yttrium-90, is much more unstable energetically and has a half-life of 64 hours. In a pure sample of strontium-90 the radionuclide yttrium-90 formed from the parent element will accumulate. The amount of yttrium-90 will grow until the number of yttrium-90 atoms breaking up per second ($\lambda_2 N_2$) equals the number being formed per second by disintegration of the parent element ($\lambda_1 N_1$). A state of radioactive equilibrium is then said to exist between the parent and daughter radionuclides. In this case the parent nuclide (strontium-90) and the daughter nuclide (yttrium-90) then decay at the same rate ($\lambda_1 N_1 = \lambda_2 N_2$), that is, the decay rate of the parent element ($T_{1/2} = 28$ years). It can be shown that the growth of the daughter product in the mixture is exponential and is governed by the decay rate of the daughter nuclide—that is, it will reach half its full equilibrium value in 64 hours and three-quarters of its equilibrium value in 128 hours, and so on.

The practical importance of this particular example arises from the fact that, though the maximum range of the beta particle from strontium-90 is only 1.2 mm in water, the beta particles from yttrium-90 are much more energetic, with a maximum range in water of 11 mm. An equilibrium mixture of the two radionuclides therefore supplies beta particles of the long range, but with an effective half-life of 28 years.

The phenomenon of radioactive equilibrium is very important in the production of short-lived radionuclides for use in medical investigations. Several of these short-lived products are available as daughter radioelements, easily separated by elution from longer-lived parent elements. These generator systems and the equations governing equilibrium will be discussed later in this chapter.

Successive disintegration

The naturally occurring radioactive elements arise from a series of decay processes producing several successive radioactive daughter products. Radioactive equilibrium is established between the primary long-lived radioactive elements—uranium, thorium, actinium and several generations of daughter products.

The most important of these is the radium series. Radium itself is one of the radionuclides in the decay chain of the parent nuclide of uranium. It is isolated chemically from uranium ores. Radium ($Z = 88$, $A = 226$) is an alpha particle emitter with a half-life of 1600 years.

Its immediate daughter product is an inert gas, radon, which is also an alpha emitting radionuclide of short life ($T_{1/2} = 3.8$ days). Radon, however, is only one step in a series of successive disintegrations leading finally to a stable nucleus at the end of the chain. This nucleus is an isotope of the element lead ($Z = 82$, $A = 206$). Figure 2.7 gives a detailed account of the successive transformations of the radium series in which some 10 different radionuclides are involved.

If the pure radium element as parent of this series is sealed in a container so that the successive radioactive products do not escape, all the radionuclides of the series accumulate until each is in equilibrium with the rest. At equilibrium each nuclide will decay at the same rate, each being produced by the decay of the radionuclide preceding it in the chain and giving rise to the nuclide following it.

At radioactive equilibrium the weight of each nuclide present is inversely proportional to the half-life of the nuclide. The importance of this radioactive family, as it is called, is that two of the radioactive nuclides in the series are emitters of penetrating gamma rays: lead-214 or radium-B, and bismuth-214 or radium-C. These two

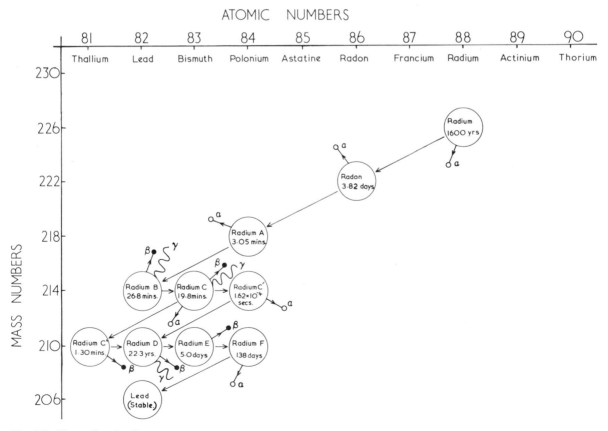

Fig. 2.7 The radium family.

nuclides have short half-lives of 26.8 and 19.7 minutes respectively but in equilibrium with the rest of the chain of radioactive products they have an effective half-life the same as the parent element radium. Radium in a sealed container in equilibrium with its products will act as a long-lived radioactive source ($T_{1/2} = 1600$ years) emitting a mixture of alpha particles, beta particles and gamma rays. A container of suitable thickness (0.5 mm of platinum), therefore, will act as a gamma emitter which is effectively constant in activity, since the half-life of radium is long enough to be considered infinite in clinical work.

It is to be noted that the first disintegration product of radium is the inert gas radon. Because it is very different chemically from the element radium it can be separated from its parent reasonably easily. If radon were itself to be sealed in a suitable container the successive radioactive products of the radium family would accumulate to equilibrium amounts, these products again including the gamma emitters lead-214 and bismuth-214. In this case the container would be an emitter of clinically useful penetrating gamma rays but with an effective half-life equal to that of radon ($T_{1/2} = 3.8$ days). Radon, sealed in thin-walled gold capsules called radon seeds, was used extensively until the late 1970s for small sealed gamma ray sources of short life. Radon seeds have now been replaced by artificially produced radionuclides of similar half-life and gamma emitting properties, particularly radioactive gold-198 ($T_{1/2} = 2.7$ days). However, the presence of radon in the sealed radium container is important since its chemical nature allows it to escape from a leaking container and this constitutes a hazard in the use of sealed radium containers which must be guarded against.

PRODUCTION OF RADIOACTIVE MATERIALS

The production of radioactive materials in forms suitable for use in medicine is an expensive and difficult matter. Amongst the naturally occurring radioactive elements radium was the only one used medically in any major way. However, approximately 0.012% of natural potassium is radioactive potassium-40. This means that approximately 7.5 Bq of potassium-40 can be found in the human body and may be monitored by means of whole body counters. The majority of radioactive isotopes used in medicine are produced artificially by bombarding a stable target nucleus with a suitable particle to produce nuclear reactions. The bombarding particles used can be positively charged, such as protons or alpha particles, or uncharged, such as neutrons. If charged particles are used they must have energies large

enough to overcome the electrostatic repulsion between themselves and the positively charged nucleus of the target atom. A charged particle accelerator, such as a cyclotron, is therefore required.

The alternative bombarding particle, the uncharged neutron, can react with the nucleus of an atom without having a high initial energy. An apparatus for the production of a suitable cloud of bombarding neutrons is the nuclear reactor.

Fission

As we discovered earlier in this chapter the very heavy elements having large nuclei tend to be unstable as the electrostatic force of repulsion between the protons overcomes the nuclear force of attraction between the nucleons. Nuclei of elements with mass number greater than 230 are unstable in a manner different from other nuclei. Under neutron bombardment, capture of a neutron takes place and the nucleus breaks up into two approximately equal parts. This *fission* is accompanied by the emission of two or three further neutrons from the broken nucleus. Other nuclei of the same type in the vicinity can be stimulated to undergo further fission by capturing these secondary neutrons. If each nucleus that undergoes fission produces two neutrons and these two are capable of causing fission in two more nuclei, the speed of the fission reaction will increase: 2:4:8:16:32:64:128; a chain reaction is thus produced. A very large amount of energy is released at each disintegration, corresponding to the conversion of a small part of the mass of the fissionable nucleus into energy. Fission and the chain reaction are the fundamental processes underlying the release of energy in the atom bomb and in the nuclear reactor.

The nuclear reactor

The nuclear reactor is an important device for releasing energy, mainly in the form of heat, from atomic nuclei. There are many different types of reactor but most are based on the nuclear fission of uranium-235 by neutron bombardment:

$$^{235}_{92}U + ^{1}_{0}n \rightarrow ^{236}_{92}U \rightarrow \begin{cases} \rightarrow \text{fission fragment A} \\ + Q + ^{1}_{0}n + ^{1}_{0}n + ^{1}_{0}n \\ \rightarrow \text{fission fragment B} \end{cases}$$

The fission fragments, A and B, are unstable nuclei of mass number between 70 and 170. They are over-rich in neutrons for their atomic number and will therefore be radioactive. Q is an energy release. The energy release can be qualitatively predicted from Figure 2.2. The binding energy or mass defect per nucleon is about 7.3 MeV for mass number 240 and 8.4 MeV for mass number 120. Division of the 240 nucleus into two 120 nuclei could result in the release of 264 MeV (240 × (8.4–7.3)).

On average 2.4 neutrons are produced for each fission. For a controlled release of energy only one of the neutrons released per fission is needed to cause further fission. The chain reaction is kept to an equilibrium controllable level by neutron absorbing control rods which prevent excessive numbers of neutrons being produced in the uranium bulk.

Natural uranium consists mainly of uranium-238; only 0.7% of the uranium nuclei are uranium-235. Unfortunately uranium-238 is not a suitable nuclide for controlled fission because it is able to capture the 'fast' neutrons (energy >0.5 MeV) produced during the fission of uranium-235 and form plutonium-239. However, the fission of uranium-235 is most efficient when bombarded by 'thermal' neutrons, that is, neutrons which have been slowed down to energies of about 0.025 eV, and these slow neutrons do not interact with uranium-238 to the same extent. The slowing down process is achieved by use of a material of low atomic mass such as graphite, which acts as a moderator.

The basic components of a typical reactor are shown in Figure 2.8. The core consists of a block of graphite which acts as the moderator into which are inserted the fuel rods. Most thermal reactors use, as fuel, enriched uranium in which the amount of uranium-235 has been artificially raised to 2–3%. Clusters of fuel elements are joined together end to end in a stringer, and placed in vertical holes in the graphite. Interleaved with the fuel rods are the control rods for absorbing the excess neutrons. The control rods are usually made of boron or cadmium and are inserted further into or withdrawn from the core depending on whether the rate of the fission reaction needs to decrease or increase. As we have already shown, each fission event releases a great deal of energy, mainly in the form of heat. Carbon dioxide gas acts as a coolant by extracting heat as it passes over the fuel in the core. It transfers its heat to water in a steam generator outside the core and the steam can be used to drive turbines coupled to an electric generator.

Around the reactor is a massive concrete shield. This protective screen is necessary to give protection not only from the large neutron emission in the reactor core but also from the beta particles and gamma rays arising from the radioactive materials produced in the core. For the production of artificial radioactive isotopes holes are made through the concrete shield into the core to allow for the insertion of the target materials to be irradiated by the neutrons.

Radionuclides produced by nuclear reactors

The fission events in the uranium result in a high neutron flux in the volume surrounding the fuel rods. Radionuclides can be produced in two ways, either by neutron bombardment of a specific target material placed within the region of high neutron flux, or by separation of the products produced by the fission of uranium.

Neutron bombardment. A 'target' is bombarded by neutrons. The neutron enters the nucleus of the target atom, thus raising the energy level of the nucleus to above ground state. The nucleus rearranges and the excess energy is given off either as a gamma photon, or by the ejection of a proton or alpha particle. The shorthand notation for these reactions is:

$$X(n,b)Y$$

where X is the target nucleus, Y is the final nucleus, n is the bombarding particle (i.e. the neutron), and b is the ejected particle (p or α) or the gamma ray (γ).

1. (n,γ) reaction. This is the most common nuclear reaction with low energy neutrons. The resultant radionuclide will be an isotope of the target material with the mass number increasing by one and the atomic number staying the same. For example the bombardment of stable phosphorus-31 with neutrons results in the production of radioactive phosphorus-32:

$$^{31}_{15}P \; (n,\gamma) \; ^{32}_{15}P$$

It is very difficult and too costly to separate the product from the target to produce a 'carrier-free' radionuclide and hence the specific activity of the radionuclide (i.e. the activity per unit mass of the element) will be low.

(n,γ) reactions generate radioactive products which

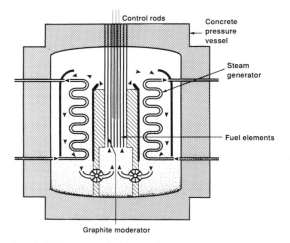

Control rods
Concrete pressure vessel
Steam generator
Fuel elements
Graphite moderator

Fig. 2.8   A gas cooled thermal reactor.

decay by beta particle emission or by electron capture, thus creating a daughter which is not an isotope of the target element. This daughter product may itself be radioactive and can be recovered 'carrier free'. Two important examples are the production of iodine-131 from tellurium-130:

$$^{130}_{52}\text{Te} \quad (n,\gamma) \quad ^{131}_{52}\text{Te} \quad \xrightarrow[T_{\frac{1}{2}}\ 25\ \text{min}]{\beta^-} \quad ^{131}_{53}\text{I}$$

and the production of technetium-99m from molybdenum-98:

$$^{98}_{42}\text{Mo}\ (n,\gamma)\ ^{99}_{42}\text{Mo} \xrightarrow[T_{\frac{1}{2}}\ 66.6\ \text{h}]{\beta^-} {}^{99m}_{43}\text{Tc} \xrightarrow[T_{\frac{1}{2}}\ 6\ \text{h}]{\gamma} {}^{99}_{43}\text{Tc}$$

The relatively long half-life of molybdenum-99 makes it ideal for use in a generator system to produce the gamma emitting radionuclide technetium-99m.

2. *(n,p) and (n,α) reactions.* These are less common reactions and require fast high energy neutrons. In (n, p) reactions the atomic number decreases by one while the mass number remains the same. An important reaction of this type is the production of carbon-14 from nitrogen-14:

$$^{14}_{7}\text{N} \quad (n,p) \quad ^{14}_{6}\text{C}$$

In (n,α) reactions the atomic number decreases by two and the mass number by three. The only example of relevance in medicine is the production of tritium from lithium:

$$^{6}_{3}\text{Li} \quad (n,\alpha) \quad ^{3}_{1}\text{H}$$

The product in these cases is easily separated from the target and hence is carrier free and has a high specific activity.

Target choice and activity. The choice of target material is obviously dependent on considerations of the final radionuclide, but several other factors also need to be considered. It should be chemically pure and contain a high proportion of the target isotope. It must be able to withstand the high temperatures generated within the nuclear reactor without giving off noxious products. It should be cheap and in a form that can be easily processed chemically to separate it from the product radionuclide.

When a target is bombarded by neutrons the atoms in the target are steadily changed into radioactive atoms. However at the same time as production is taking place some of the newly formed radioactive nuclei will disintegrate and the product material will decay. The activity of the product will therefore depend on the relative rates of these two processes. When the rate of production equals the rate of decay saturation has been achieved and equilibrium exists. The activity at time t is given by:

$$A_t = NF \cdot \lambda \cdot S$$

where N is the number of atoms of the target isotope per m^3, F is the incident neutron flux per m^2, and S is the saturation factor. S is dependent on the decay factor λ of the product material and will equal 1 at equilibrium but will equal $(1 - e^{-\lambda t})$ at any time prior to equilibrium. This is shown in Figure 2.9.

Fission products

As has been discussed already, fission is the process by which a heavy isotope such as uranium-235 splits into isotopes of two lighter elements. For example:

$$\text{n} + {}^{235}_{92}\text{U} \rightarrow {}^{236}_{92}\text{U} \rightarrow {}^{131}_{50}\text{Sn} + {}^{103}_{42}\text{Mo} + 2\text{n}$$

Fission of uranium-235 does not always produce tin and molybdenum. A whole range of fission products are formed. Figure 2.10 shows the relative amounts of materials of different mass numbers produced. One product comes from each peak. Most of the fission

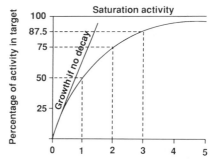

A   Time of irradiation in half lives of product

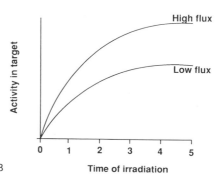

B   Time of irradiation

Fig. 2.9 A Activity in the target as a function of time. **B** Activity in target at two different levels of neutron flux.

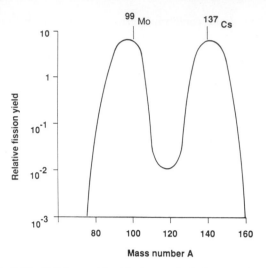

Fig. 2.10 Relative yields of fission products from uranium.

fragments can be chemically separated to provide carrier-free radionuclides. Like all heavy elements, uranium has considerably more neutrons than protons in its nucleus. The medium mass fission products will therefore have a neutron excess and will decay by beta particle emission.

Fission products such as the long-lived caesium-137 are extracted from spent fuel rods. However the short-lived radionuclides such as molybdenum-99 and xenon-133 are normally obtained by neutron bombardment of a uranium target.

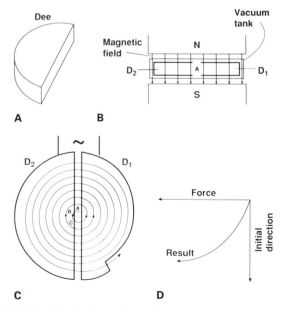

Fig. 2.11 The cyclotron (see text).

The cyclotron

The cyclotron consists of two hollow semicircular electrodes called Dees (Fig. 2.11A). The Dees, in an evacuated container, are placed between the pole pieces of an electromagnet such that the magnetic field runs perpendicular to the plane of the electrodes (Fig. 2.11B). An alternating electric field is applied between the two electrodes. Positive particles of the kind to be accelerated (e.g. protons) are produced at point A in the centre of the gap between the electrodes (Fig. 2.11C). With the electric field between the electrodes D_1 and D_2 in the right direction (i.e. D_2 negative and D_1 positive) the particles are accelerated towards point B. The charged particles are then under the influence of the magnetic field and any charged particle moving in a magnetic field will have a force exerted on it in a direction perpendicular to the magnetic field and to the direction of motion (Fig. 2.11D). Hence, the particles move in a circular path and arrive at the gap between the electrodes at C. Correct adjustment of the frequency of the electric field between D_1 and D_2 will ensure that the charge on the Dees reverses as the particles reach point C (i.e. D_2 becomes positive and D_1 negative). The particles will then be accelerated across the gap into the opposite electrode. They then move again in a circular orbit, arriving at the gap again in time to receive a further acceleration. This is possible because the time taken to travel round the semi-circular paths under the influence of the magnetic field remains constant, with increasing velocity of the charged particles only the radius of the path increases. The particles therefore travel on a spiral path of gradually increasing radius and are accelerated by the peak potential difference between the electrodes each time they cross the gap. In a typical cyclotron the peak potential difference between the electrodes might be 20 000 volts but particles are accelerated across the gap 800 times in electrodes of 30 inch (75 cm) radius, thus producing an energy equivalent to an acceleration by 16 million volts. At the edge of the electrodes the beam is no longer under the influence of the magnetic field and emerges tangentially. The high energy positive ion beams produced in the cyclotron can be used to bombard directly a suitable target in which nuclear reactions then result in the production of radionuclides.

Radionuclides produced by cyclotrons

Beams of protons (p or $^1_1$H), deuterons (d or $^2_1$H) or alpha (α or $^4_2$H) particles are used in the cyclotron. The nomenclature we employed to describe the reactions from neutron bombardment is also used to specify charged particle nuclear reactions. These include the following:

(p,n)	(d,n)	(α,n)
(p,pn)	(d,p)	(α,pn)
(p,d)	(d,α)	(α,2n)

(d,α) reaction. The bombarding particle is a deuteron and an alpha particle is released.

$$^{24}_{12}Mg + ^{2}_{1}H \rightarrow ^{22}_{11}Na + ^{4}_{2}\alpha$$

$$^{24}Mg \quad (d,\alpha) \quad ^{22}Na$$

(p,pn) reaction. Here a proton is used as the bombarding particle and two particles are released, a proton and a neutron.

$$^{58}_{28}Ni + ^{1}_{1}H \xrightarrow{EC} ^{57}_{27}Co + ^{1}_{1}p + ^{1}_{0}n$$

$$^{58}Ni \quad (p,pn) \quad ^{57}Co$$

(α, 2n) reaction. In this case an alpha particle is used as the bombarding particle and two neutrons are released.

$$^{121}_{51}Sb + ^{4}_{2}He \rightarrow ^{123}_{53}I + ^{1}_{0}n + ^{1}_{0}n$$

$$^{121}Sb \quad (\alpha,2n) \quad ^{123}I$$

The two main features of cyclotron produced radionuclides are (1) the product is a different element to the target and can therefore be separated chemically to produce a high specific activity carrier free radionuclide and (2) since the bombarding particle always includes at least one proton, most of the radionuclides produced will be proton rich and will therefore decay by positron emission or electron capture.

Radionuclide generators

A generator is a system which contains a long-lived parent radionuclide which decays to a short-lived daughter radionuclide. The parent and daughter radionuclides are different elements so chemical separation of the two can take place. A number of generator systems have been developed and some of these are listed in Table 2.4.

Table 2.4 Radionuclide generator systems

Parent	$T_{1/2}$	Daughter	$T_{1/2}$	$E_\gamma{}^*$	Decay product
^{99}Mo	67 h	^{99m}Tc	6 h	140 keV	^{99}Tc
^{81}Rb	4.7 h	^{81m}Kr	13 s	190 keV	^{81}Kr
^{132}Te	78 h	^{132}I	2.3 h	Several	^{132}Xe
^{68}Ge	280 days	^{68}Ga	68 min	511 keV	^{68}Zn

* E_γ = Energy of gamma radiation.

The activity of the daughter radionuclide, A_2, at any given time depends on several factors:

1. The activity of the parent, A_1, at time zero;
2. The rate of decay of the parent, i.e. the rate of formation of the daughter proportional to the decay constant, λ_1;
3. The rate of decay of the daughter, proportional to the decay constant, λ_2;
4. The time since the last elution, t;
5. The percentage conversion of the parent to the daughter.

If initially there is no daughter product present the daughter activity can be calculated from:

$$A_2 = \frac{\lambda_2}{\lambda_2 - \lambda_1} A_1 (e^{-\lambda_1 t} - e^{-\lambda_2 t})$$

This equation can be used for any parent daughter relationship. However in special cases the equation can be simplified.

Secular equilibrium

When the parent half-life is very much greater than the

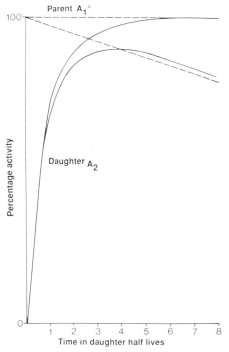

Fig. 2.12 Radioactive equilibrium: 1) secular equilibrium, uppermost curve; 2) transient equilibrium, lower curve. The dashed line represents the activity of the parent radionuclide and the solid line the activity of the daughter radionuclide.

daughter half-life ($\lambda_1 \ll \lambda_2$) the radionuclides are said to be in 'secular equilibrium'. An example of such a generator system is germanium-68 half-life 275 days gallium-68 half-life 68 minutes. The decay of the parent can be ignored relative to the decay of the daughter so the above equation can be simplified to:

$$A_2 = A_1 (1 - e^{-\lambda_2 t})$$

This is shown graphically in Figure 2.12. As can be seen, if the time t is short compared to the $T_{1/2}$ of the parent but long, 5 to 6 half-lives, compared to the half-life of the daughter, then $A_2 = A_1$ and thereafter activity decays with the half-life of the parent.

Transient equilibrium

When the parent half-life is just greater than the daughter half-life, as in the case of molybdenum-99 and technetium-99m, then the radionuclides are said to be in *transient equilibrium*. In this case the time to reach equilibrium is not short compared to the parent half-life so that at equilibrium:

$$A_2 = \frac{\lambda_1}{\lambda_2 - \lambda_1} A_1$$

and hence from this time on the activity is greater than the parent activity, but once again it decreases with the half-life of the parent (Fig. 2.12).

Technetium generator. The growth and decay of the molybdenum-99–technetium-99m transient equilibrium generator system is shown in Figure 2.13. The maximum activity is present in approximately 24 hours (4 daughter half-lives). However the total activity is not greater than the activity of the parent as we expected, and as is indicated by the dotted line, but is in fact slightly less than the activity of the parent. This is due to the fact that molybdenum-99 is converted to the metastable technetium-99m for approximately 90% of the disintegrations; the other 10% convert straight to technetium-99.

Separation of daughter radionuclides. The most common method of separating daughter nuclides from their parents is by chromatography. The parent is adsorbed on to some binder substance such as ion exchange resin, alumina or other organic exchanger. The daughter is in a different chemical form to the parent and has less affinity for the binder so it can be separated from the parent by washing the column with a suitable eluting solution. In the case of the molybdenum-99–technetium-99m generator the molybdenum, as ammonium molybdate, is adsorbed on to alumina. As the molybdenum-99 decays, technetium-99m is formed as pertechnetate. When saline is passed through the column, ion exchange takes place between the chloride and pertechnetate ions and the technetium-99m is washed off, or eluted from the column as sodium pertechnetate.

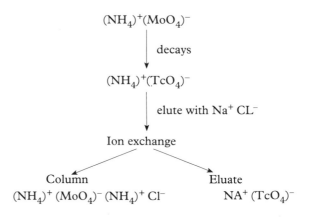

The use of technetium-99m and its pharmaceuticals will be discussed later in this book (Ch. 10).

Fig. 2.13 Activity time curves for a molybdenum-99–technetium-99 m generator.

3. The production of X- and gamma ray beams

INTRODUCTION

We have seen that X-rays are produced whenever an electron stream travelling at high speed is brought to rest in a solid target. To produce an X-ray beam it is necessary to have an evacuated tube in which the electron stream can be produced and accelerated on to a suitable target by a voltage generator. Thus the basic components of an X-ray set are:

— An evacuated tube
— An electron stream
— A target
— A voltage generator.

Gamma rays are in nature identical to X-rays except that they are spontaneously emitted from certain radioactive isotopes. A gamma ray beam may be produced by suitably housing such an isotope in a substantial shield and permitting the intense gamma radiation to emerge through an appropriate aperture in the shield. Gamma ray beam units will be described later in this chapter.

X-RAY TUBE INSERT

The X-ray tube insert is a highly evacuated envelope containing two electrodes and, as such, its electrical behaviour is the same as a diode valve (p. 4). In construction, however, there are important differences. The accelerating voltage used to generate X-rays is very large and, therefore, great care has to be taken to insulate the anode from the cathode. For this purpose the electrodes are shaped to avoid sharp corners—the electrostatic field strength is very intense at sharp corners and would give rise to sparking—and the surfaces are as smooth as possible. The two electrodes are usually sealed into a re-entrant glass or ceramic envelope so that the insulating path is as long as possible.

The electron stream is produced by thermionic emission from a heated tungsten filament (the cathode). The filament is either a flat spiral or a helix of tungsten wire at the centre of a conical or semicylindrical *focusing cup* (Fig. 3.1). This cup is maintained at the same potential as the filament and so focuses the electrons on to the X-ray target (anode). As in the case of the thermionic diode under saturation conditions, the number of electrons emitted is controlled by the temperature of the filament and increases rapidly with that temperature. The filament of an X-ray tube is heated using a highly stabilised circuit and the tube current is controlled by varying the current through the filament (Fig. 3.2).

So far the word *target* and the word *anode* have been used interchangeably, but it is important now to differentiate between the two. The *anode* is the positive

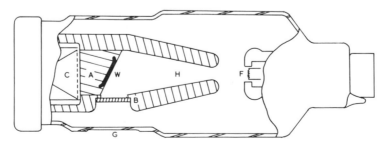

Fig. 3.1 A 250 kV X-ray tube showing the copper anode A, the tungsten target W, the cooling oil spray C, together with the copper anode hood H and the beryllium window B. The filament F and the thin window in the glass G are also shown. (Adapted from a diagram supplied by Philips Medical Systems Ltd.)

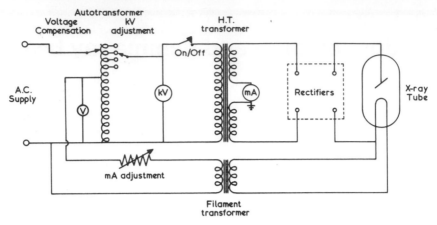

Fig. 3.2   A simple X-ray generator circuit.

electrode in the X-ray tube and the *target* is the piece of tungsten bonded to the surface of the anode (Fig. 3.1). The electrons bombard the tungsten to produce the X-rays. Tungsten is chosen as a target material for its high atomic number ($Z = 74$), which leads to a relatively efficient conversion of electron energy to X-ray energy, and for its high melting point (3387°C), which reduces the chance of the target melting under the bombardment of the electrons. Furthermore, the target material must not evaporate readily when heated in a vacuum since, if it did, it would become deposited on the tube walls, causing absorption of X-rays and a breakdown in the electrical insulation of the tube. In the hooded anode, this deposition is on the hood and so rendered harmless.

Target angle and heel effect

It has been seen in Chapter 1 (p. 12) that for con-

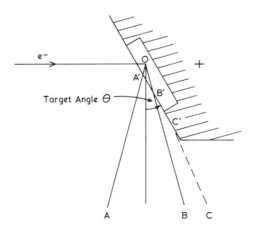

Fig. 3.3   The definition of target angle and the heel effect.

ventional energies X-rays are produced in a *reflection target* and the useful beam is considered to be at right angles to the electron beam. No mention has been made about the target angle. The *target angle* is the angle between the axis of the X-ray beam and the face of the target (Fig. 3.3). The effect of this angle is threefold.

The thin target theory suggests that although the (low energy) X-rays are produced predominantly in the direction at right angles to the electron beam (Fig. 1.11), the X-ray intensity is greater at angles of less than 90° than at angles of more than 90° to the direction of the electrons. In order, therefore, to achieve some degree of symmetry to the X-ray beam it is necessary to attenuate the radiation on the anode side of the X-ray beam axis to a greater extent than that on the cathode side. Figure 3.3 shows the effective source of X-rays at a point O below the surface of the target and the two X-rays OA and OB. From this simple construction, it can be seen that OA is attenuated by a thickness of target material OA′ and OB by a thickness of OB′. In particular, OB′ is greater than OA′. Since the relative length of OA′ and OB′ is dependent on the target angle, the angle can be chosen to produce a symmetrical beam of radiation by attenuating the more intense beam OB by a suitably greater thickness OB′.

Attenuation is, however, dependent on photon energy as well as atomic number. It follows, therefore, that a particular target angle will only produce a symmetrical beam of radiation for one photon energy, and to operate the X-ray tube at energies below the design energy will result in an asymmetric beam—with the anode edge of the beam being relatively less intense (Fig. 3.4). Over small changes in accelerating voltage this may not be clinically important for deep X-ray therapy, while the effect is less pronounced at super-

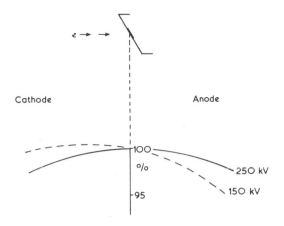

Fig. 3.4 The effect on beam symmetry of using a kilovoltage lower than that for which the target angle was designed.

ficial X-ray energies. At voltages between 200 and 300 kV, the target angle is usually about 30°.

The second important criterion which is dependent on target angle is the overall field size or maximum beam divergence. It can be seen from Figure 3.3 that as the beam divergence increases, the thickness OC′ increases rapidly and the intensity at C falls, producing a beam edge. It follows that the half angle of beam divergence cannot exceed the target angle and, in practice, the useful beam is limited to a few degrees less than the target angle.

Thirdly, the geometry of the target is such that the area of the tungsten bombarded by the electrons is larger than either the cross-sectional area of the electron beam or the area from which the X-rays are seen to emanate (Fig. 3.5). The latter is known as the *effective focal spot size* and decreases with target angle. In diagnostic X-ray tubes, where the effective focal spot size is of paramount importance, very small target angles are used—15° is common and some are as low as 7°. In therapy, however, large symmetrical beams are of greater importance than the size of the focal

spot. In either discipline, the larger the area of target bombarded by electrons the larger the area for the dissipation of heat—an important subject which will now be discussed.

Cooling the X-ray target

The generation of heat in the target by the bombardment of electrons leads to real problems of cooling in X-ray tubes. In the conventional X-ray tube only about 1% of the energy dissipated in the target is converted into X-rays and 99% is converted into heat. The method of cooling depends on the design of the target and the voltage at which it operates (Fig. 3.6). Those X-ray tubes which have a target at earth potential can be cooled directly by a flow of cold water through the anode behind the target (Fig. 3.6B). Where the X-ray tube is immersed in oil to provide additional electrical insulation around the envelope, the oil itself will be used to cool the target, either by natural or forced convection. The oil is then passed through a heat exchanger, thus transferring the heat either to water or to atmosphere and so to waste. The heat exchanger may be incorporated in the X-ray head assembly (Fig. 3.7), or in a separate unit connected to the X-ray head using flexible oil pipes. At megavoltage energies where the generation of X-rays is a more efficient process (about 50%), less heat is produced and cooling is not a major problem. The target is at earth potential and a simple flow of water through the target assembly is all that is required.

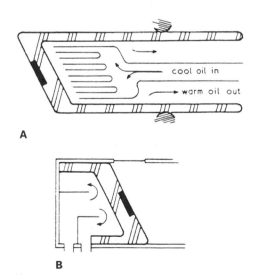

A

B

Fig. 3.6 The cooling of X-ray targets using forced convection: **A** hollow anode cooled with oil and **B** earthed anode cooled with water.

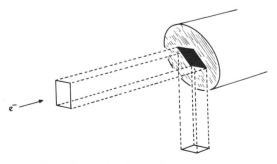

Fig. 3.5 The effective focal spot size.

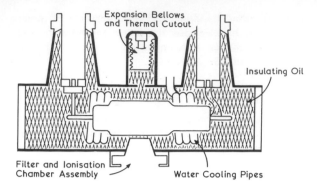

Fig. 3.7 A simple X-ray tube housing.

Warming the X-ray target

The need to cool the target is readily understood when the heat dissipation is several kilowatts per square centimetre but there is another adverse effect to be taken into account. This quantity of heat dissipated in a cold anode can cause mechanical damage, particularly where the tungsten target is inlaid into the surface of the copper anode. Dissimilar metals have different coefficients of expansion. If the tungsten expands more than the copper recess in which it fits, then it will buckle and crack. A severe example of this is shown in Figure 3.8 where the target is seen partially detached from the anode. (This radiograph was taken using an 8 MV linear accelerator and clearly shows the cooling spray behind the anode and the structure of the anode hood.)

To overcome this problem of differential heating, it is important to *slowly* increase the heating of a cold tube insert. This warming up process should be carried out first thing in the morning and repeated during the day if the workload is insufficient to keep the tube warm. The manufacturer's guidance should

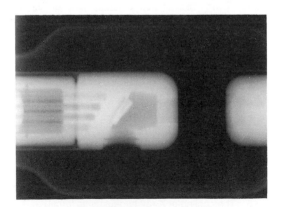

Fig. 3.8 An 8 MV radiograph of a 250 kV tube insert showing the damaged target.

Table 3.1 Permitted leakage radiation from X-ray therapy tube housings

Maximum operating potential	At 1 m from the target	At 5 cm from the housing surface
150 kV to 500 kV	10 mGy h⁻¹	300 mGy h⁻¹
50 kV to 150 kV	1 mGy h⁻¹	—
Less than 50 kV	—	1 mGy h⁻¹

be followed, but in general the warm-up period will be between 20 and 30 minutes.

X-RAY TUBE HOUSING

The X-ray tube itself is often referred to as *the insert* and is the main component contained in the X-ray head. The X-ray head is a metal tank in which the insert is rigidly mounted and connected to the high tension (HT) supply. The head contains the insulating transformer oil and some temperature sensitive device which will prevent the use of the tube when its temperature rises above a predetermined safe level. In a sealed system, this may be a diaphragm which operates a microswitch as it takes up the expansion of the heated oil (Fig. 3.7).

Other essential features of the X-ray head include:

1. The X-ray window and primary collimator through which the useful X-ray beam emerges.
2. Lead protection around the head to reduce the leakage radiation to a safe level (Table 3.1).
3. An assembly on the primary collimator to house and electrically interlock the added filtration (p. 80).
4. An ionisation chamber (p. 37) or diode to monitor the output beam dose rate.
5. An assembly to mount the secondary collimation in the form of an adjustable diaphragm or interchangeable applicators (p. 46).
6. A mounting for beam direction devices (p. 111).

The X-ray head will be mounted on a gantry or tube stand to enable the beam to be positioned and directed in a way appropriate to the treatment in hand. The gantry may be ceiling mounted to suspend the tube housing from an adjustable column; it may be wall or floor mounted with the tube housing on the end of a horizontal arm, the latter being raised or lowered on a fixed vertical column; or it may be mounted on a more complex isocentric gantry like the linear accelerator (p. 111). Whatever the type of gantry, the tube housing will need to be adjustable in three orthogonal directions and through two or three rotations, each with a reliable braking system.

X-RAY GENERATOR CIRCUITS

A simple X-ray generator circuit is shown in Figure 3.2. The input voltage is fed to the *autotransformer* via a voltage compensation circuit, which may be manually controlled at the control desk or automatically controlled. Compensation is essential because the supply voltages can vary by typically ± 6% and the local demand can also influence the supply to the X-ray unit. In the manual system illustrated in Figure 3.2, the voltage appearing across a fixed number of turns on the primary is monitored on a voltmeter V. If the indicated value is low, the supply is connected across a smaller number of turns. A larger supply voltage is applied across more turns so that the incoming volts per turn is constant, as indicated by the reference mark on the meter.

The autotransformer is a transformer with only one winding, acting as both primary and secondary, and its function is to provide an output voltage only slightly above or below the primary. Having ensured the volts per turn is correct on the primary, it is now possible to obtain the required output voltage by selecting the correct number of turns on the 'secondary' winding— and because the HT transformer has a fixed turns ratio, the selector can be calibrated in kilovolts although only a few hundred volts exist at that point in the circuit.

The safety interlocks built into the X-ray control are in the secondary circuit of the autotransformer. These will include the door interlocks, filter interlocks, the treatment timer, overtemperature interlocks, etc., along with the prereading kV meter (if fitted). The X-ray beam on/off switches will operate a heavy duty contactor in the primary circuit of the HT transformer because switching an inductive circuit at high power causes considerable sparking. In higher energy machines the contactor will be immersed in insulating oil and will often only switch on at a low kV setting, the kV being increased to the required value during the first few seconds of the exposure. In this case, the kV meter must be connected to the HT primary to ensure the correct value is reached after switch-on.

The high tension (HT) transformer is a heavy fixed turns ratio transformer increasing the normal supply voltage to tens or hundreds of kilovolts. The primary circuit carries a high current at the supply voltage through relatively few turns to be transformed into a very high voltage, low current supply for the X-ray tube. If the supply is at the normal frequency (50 Hz in the UK) then a massive soft iron core is required to maximise the flux linkage with the primary and secondary windings. Some units are now available with high frequency generators, that is to say, the frequency is increased to typically 25 kHz, thereby reducing the need for a massive core. The high frequency generators are therefore comparatively smaller and lighter in weight than the conventional ones.

The filament transformer is situated in the same housing as the HT transformer but for very different reasons. It is a step-down transformer reducing the supply voltage to a few volts to heat the tube filament (typically 60 watts). So what makes it so special? The tube filament is invariably at half or the full kilovoltage *below* earth potential, so although neither the primary nor the secondary voltage is difficult to manage, the potential difference between the primary and the secondary is considerable, requiring complete electrical isolation one from the other. Secondly, because the X-ray tube operates under saturation conditions the tube current is determined by the temperature of the filament, and the thermionic emission varies rapidly with small changes in temperature and filament voltage. The filament transformer, therefore, must guarantee a very stable voltage supply to the filament once its primary voltage has been set by the 'mA adjust' control. The filament transformer is therefore more accurately described as a *stabilised isolation* transformer.

HT cables

The HT generator and the X-ray head may both be contained in the same assembly, but more frequently they are separate assemblies connected by shockproof HT cables. The cathode cable requires two inner conductors to carry the heating supply and the negative HT connection to the filament. Although the anode cable only requires one inner conductor to carry the positive HT connection, it is common practice to use a cable with two inner conductors connected in parallel. The two HT cables may, therefore, be identical— reducing the cost of manufacture and the cost of periodic replacement. (Where an earthed anode tube is used, the anode HT cable is not required.) The inner conductors are individually insulated and then surrounded by flexible solid rubber insulation covered by a strong earthed metal sheath (of less than 1 ohm m^{-1} resistance) connected to the X-ray head at one end and to the transformer tank at the other. Electrical or mechanical failure of the rubber insulation can result in an electrical breakdown between the inner HT conductors and the earthed sheath. It will be accompanied by the smell of burning and the sound of sparking. Because of the high voltages involved all the principal components of an X-ray unit will be bonded to a common electrical *earth reference terminal* by a thick continuous copper wire or tape to minimise the risk of electric shock to staff or patient. (The sheath of

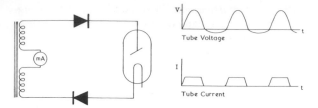

Fig. 3.9   The half-wave rectified circuit.

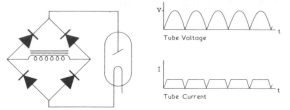

Fig. 3.10   The full-wave rectified circuit.

the HT cables must not be relied upon for this purpose.) These earth connections must not be tampered with under any circumstances.

Half-wave rectified circuit

Although the X-ray tube itself behaves as a rectifier, a circuit without additional rectifiers is of little practical value for two reasons: (1) the X-ray tube must be made to withstand the full reverse voltage; and (2) the heated anode can become a source of electrons—by thermionic emission—which will bombard and damage the filament when the potential is reversed during the negative half cycle of the applied voltage. The circuit will usually incorporate a rectifier network of diode valves or (more likely) solid state rectifiers; one or two rectifiers producing half-wave rectification, a bridge network of four rectifiers producing full-wave rectification, or a more complex circuit of rectifiers and capacitors (e.g. the Greinacher circuit). These will now be briefly dealt with in turn.

The half-wave rectified circuit is shown in Figure 3.9. During the half cycle of the applied voltage that makes the anode positive, current flows through the rectifiers and the X-ray tube. (Remember the electron flow is in the opposite direction to the conventional current. The symbol used for the rectifier indicates the direction of conventional current flow.) The voltage drop across the rectifiers is small so the voltage applied across the X-ray tube rises and falls in the same way as the transformer voltage. During the reverse half cycle, the voltage is divided between the high resistance of the rectifiers and the X-ray tube. The voltage developed across the tube is, therefore, considerably less than that produced by the transformer. The graphs in Figure 3.9 show that electrons are bombarding the target during practically the whole of the half cycle in which the anode is positive. The majority of these electrons will, however, be accelerated by voltages considerably less than the peak voltage. The radiation from a tube energised by such a circuit will, therefore, contain a larger proportion of low energy photons than if the tube was excited by a steady potential.

Full-wave rectified circuit

The use of four rectifiers connected as a bridge network (Fig. 3.10) enables current to flow through the tube during both half cycles of the applied alternating potential and gives full-wave rectification. During each half cycle, one pair of rectifiers (on parallel sides of the square) allows current to pass through the X-ray tube. The potential applied to the X-ray tube is thus unidirectional but pulsating at twice the frequency of the half-wave rectified circuit. If a capacitor is added in parallel to the X-ray tube, then the capacitor is charged to the full peak voltage during each half-cycle. As the transformer voltage falls, the capacitor begins to discharge through the tube. Providing the capacitor is large and the tube current small, the discharge will also be small. The potential of the anode will therefore not fall to zero between each pulse but it will be maintained at a value close to the peak. This slight drop in voltage every half cycle is called *ripple*. If the operating conditions of the X-ray tube are carefully chosen, the reduced anode voltage due to the ripple will not take the tube out of saturation and, therefore, the current through the tube will be steady. The output exposure rate from this *constant potential* tube will be considerably greater than that from a tube energised by the half-wave rectified circuit for the same nominal kilovoltage and, in addition, the number of low energy photons will be reduced.

In each circuit described so far, the peak voltage applied to the anode has been equal to, or a little less than, the voltage developed in the secondary winding of the transformer. In the circuit to be described now the anode voltage is twice that of the transformer and again almost constant. It is sometimes known as a voltage doubling circuit.

Greinacher circuit

The circuit is illustrated in Figure 3.11. Two rectifiers R_1 and R_2 are connected in series with the X-ray tube. Two series connected capacitors C_1 and C_2 are in parallel with the tube. The transformer secondary is connected to the midpoints of the two capacitors and

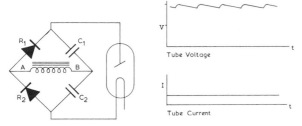

Fig. 3.11   The Greinacher circuit.

of the two rectifiers. During the half cycle, in which end A of the transformer winding is positive, the capacitor C_1 is charged through the rectifier R_1 to the full peak voltage of the transformer, while rectifier R_2 is not conducting. During the next half cycle C_2 is charged to the same potential through R_2. Now C_1 and C_2 are series connected and their potentials are additive; thus, a voltage equal to twice that of the transformer is seen across the X-ray tube. As before, the capacitors discharge through the tube, but providing their capacitance is large and the tube current small, the fall in the voltage applied to the tube will be small. So once again there will be a ripple on the tube voltage (of say 5%) but the tube current will be steady.

Control desk

The basic design (Fig. 3.2) of an X-ray installation usually necessitates a control panel remote from the HT generator and the X-ray head. (Only for generators with a maximum operating potential of less than 50 kV can the operator be in the same room as the X-ray tube.) The control may be with the traditional meters, switches and indicators or with a microprocessor and keyboard, in either case it will feature the following:

Mains voltage compensator

Some units will have an automatically controlled mains voltage compensator, while others will be controlled manually to a datum line on a meter.

Kilovoltage control and the kV meter

This may be a stepped control or a continuous smooth control. There may not be a control if the kV is automatically selected when the filter is fitted to the tube housing, but the kV and filter must be indicated at the control desk.

Tube current control and the mA meter

Again the mA may be automatically selected, but its

value must be indicated on the desk. Fluctuations in the value of mA are the first signs of an HT failure such as the tube insert or HT cable.

X-ray switch

While there may be many means by which the beam can be switched off (e.g. by opening the treatment room door), there must be only one beam-on control and that must be located on the control desk.

Treatment timers

Switching on the X-ray beam starts two independent exposure timers, the purpose of which is to switch off the X-rays automatically after a preset exposure time, measured in minutes and decimal minutes. Recent legislation suggests that the timers should count up from zero to the time prescribed—continuing beyond that preset time if, for any reason, the beam is not switched off. The second, back-up timer is independent and designed to terminate the exposure at a preset interval above the set time. It should only terminate the exposure in the event of a failure of the primary timer, but its ability to do so is to be checked in the timer reset procedure. Where the exposure is controlled by the use of timers alone, the output dose rate should be checked daily using an appropriate instrument.

Dose meter

Where possible, an ionisation chamber or solid state detector is fitted in the beam close to the target (but on the patient side of any additional filtration) to monitor the intensity of the emerging X-ray beam. The chamber should feed into a calibrated integrating dose meter (p. 75) or a dose rate meter circuit, the latter being used in conjunction with a timer to determine the dose delivered to the patient. The output dose rate is predetermined by the voltage waveform, target material and inherent filtration and controlled by the choice of added filtration, kilovoltage and tube current. Since the output is proportional to $(mA) \times (kV)^2$, the two parameters need to be continuously monitored. An uncalibrated meter is a valuable means of continuously monitoring the output dose rate, especially when the exposure is only otherwise controlled by a timer.

Indicator lamps and interlocks

There are several safety devices which can protect an X-ray unit against overheating, overvoltage, overcurrent, etc., all of which may be indicated on the control desk. The essential indicator lamps are those to indicate and interlock the added filtration or wedge filter and to indicate the excitation of the tube. It is common practice to interlock the filter, kilovoltage and the tube current so as to prevent a wrong combination from being used—this is particularly important at the grenz ray and superficial X-ray energies where units are frequently used under more than one set of operating conditions. 'Beam on' warning lights should be duplicated outside the treatment room door and also inside the treatment room. They should be energised on completion of all the interlocks but *before* the beam-on switch is operated for they are intended to indicate the unit is in a state of readiness to emit radiation as well as staying lit for the duration of the exposure.

Safety fuses or circuit breakers safeguard the equipment from electrical failure. Any failure of this sort must be identified and corrected by a competent engineer.

The generators and control circuits described above have been used over the full range of X-ray energies from 10 kV to 500 kV. They therefore cover the ranges of energies commonly known as

Grenz rays	10–50 kV
Superficial X-rays	50–150 kV
Orthovoltage X-rays	200–500 kV

The need for X-ray energies greater than this has been recognised for many years, but the problems of the insulation, the weight of the transformer and of the thickness and flexibility of HT cables prevented the widespread use of the circuits described above. Other techniques have to be used to generate *megavoltage*

X-rays. X-ray energies between 500 and 1000 kV are of no value in radiotherapy for reasons to be explained in Chapter 5.

LINEAR ACCELERATOR

Megavoltage X-rays in the range 4 MV to 25 MV for radiotherapy are generally produced by a linear accelerator (Fig. 3.12). As the name implies, the electrons are accelerated in a straight line and this is achieved using *radio frequency* (rf) waves of approximately 10 cm wavelength. These radio waves are generated in a specially designed vacuum diode valve called a *magnetron* which operates in an intense magnetic field, or in an rf oscillator called a *klystron*. In either case, the radio waves pass down a smooth rectangular waveguide containing air or gas under pressure and through an *rf window* to the evacuated corrugated waveguide.

When a radiofrequency wave passes along a smooth tube of conducting material with a diameter comparable to the wavelength, an electric field is established, as in Figure 3.13. Electrons on the axis of the tube at point A for instance will be accelerated to the right by the electric field but they will only continue in that direction if the electric field moves with them. (At B, they would not move whereas at C they would move to the left.) As the electron accelerates, so the electric field will need to move more quickly. Now, radiofrequency waves in free space travel at the velocity of light—and cannot be accelerated. They can, however, be made to move more slowly by the introduction of *iris diaphragms*

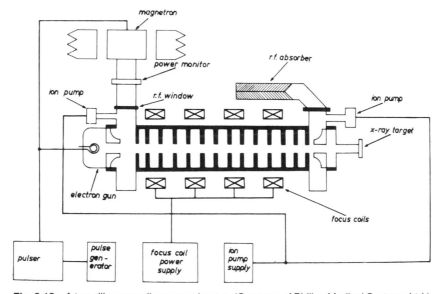

Fig. 3.12 A travelling wave linear accelerator. (Courtesy of Philips Medical Systems Ltd.)

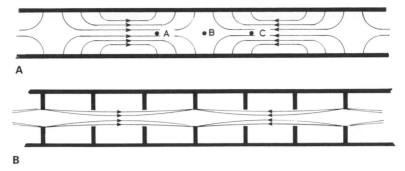

Fig. 3.13   The electric field pattern created by an rf wave passing down **A** a smooth tube and **B** a corrugated waveguide.

into the waveguide, which is then referred to as a *corrugated waveguide*. The hole diameter and the spacing of the iris diaphragms control the wave velocity (Fig. 3.13B) and in particular can slow the wave initially and then allow it to accelerate. The source of electrons may be a directly heated filament or an indirectly heated oxide–coated cathode in an *electron gun* and mounted in line at the input end of the corrugated waveguide.

Travelling wave accelerator

In the travelling wave accelerator, the (negative) voltage pulse applied to the magnetron is also applied to the gun so that the electrons enter the guide with the rf wave. The wave velocity is reduced in the *bunching section* where the iris diaphragms are close together to about 0.4*c*, but as the wave travels down the guide, the wider spacing of the diaphragms allows it to accelerate, carrying the electrons with it. (This phenomenon is familiar to those who enjoy surf-boarding!) At the end of the guide the rf wave will be diverted and absorbed (i.e. the wave energy is converted into heat in an *rf load* which in turn is water cooled), while the electrons enter a field free region prior to striking the target.

In Figure 3.14, the electrons to the left of A will experience a stronger field and therefore a greater acceleration while electrons to the right experience a lesser acceleration, thereby adding to the bunching

effect. But the mean acceleration will depend on where the bunch is centred on the wave, or to put it more technically, the acceleration of the electrons depends on the phase relationship between the wave and the electron pulse. The final energy achieved by the electrons will also be determined by the length of the corrugated waveguide and the frequency of the rf wave.

Standing wave accelerator

If the corrugated waveguide is closed at each end then the rf wave will be reflected at both ends and, at the resonant frequency, a standing wave will be established. In such a system the radiofrequency power may be applied at any point along the guide. In the standing wave accelerator, the wave pattern established is as shown in Figure 3.15. In alternate cavities at the nodes of the standing wave, the electric field is always zero while in the intermediate antinode cavities, the direction of the field changes direction with time. Now if the induced field changes direction each time the electron traverses a 'node' cavity, then the electron will be accelerated through successive 'antinode' cavities, thereby gaining energy. Again the 'length' of each cavity is designed to conform to the acceleration of the electrons. (In the so-called side-coupled waveguide, the 'node' cavities are taken out of line and attached to the side of the guide, thereby shortening the overall

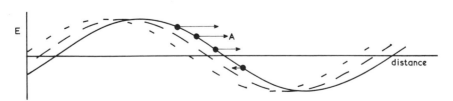

Fig. 3.14   The travelling wave accelerator .

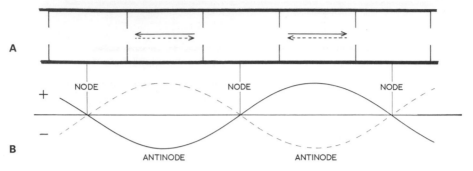

Fig. 3.15 The standing wave accelerator: **A** the waveguide and **B** the wave.

length of the guide, but the wave theory of this is beyond the scope of this book.)

The two ends of the guide have to be closed to reflect the radiofrequency wave, but in practice a small hole is left, through which the electrons are injected from the electron gun and ultimately leave the waveguide.

For low energy accelerators, the side-coupled guide is short enough to enable a transmission target to be attached to the end of the corrugated waveguide, thereby producing the X-ray beam in the *same* direction as the electron acceleration. In operation, the beam energy is more stable than with the travelling wave accelerator because the corrugated waveguide is less tolerant of small changes in the radiofrequency.

The energy of the standing wave accelerator can, however, be varied by using separate guides in tandem and varying the phase difference between the two. In fact it is possible to accelerate to a middle energy in the first guide and then, by changing the phase, either accelerate further in the second to a higher energy or decelerate to a lower energy, thereby providing very different energies.

The dimensions of the waveguide for both travelling wave and standing wave accelerators are critical, not only requiring very accurate machining during manufacture, but also temperature stabilisation during operation. In fact, the whole of the radiofrequency circuit, the magnetron or klystron, corrugated waveguide and load or feedback circuit, together with the target is temperature controlled to better than ± 1°C. This is manually achieved by pumping distilled water through cooling pipes and a heat exchanger where the surplus heat is transferred to the atmosphere or to cold water running to waste. A linear accelerator dissipates several kilowatts of heat when the beam is energised.

Within the guide there is a radial component to the electric field which would cause the electrons to disperse unless its effect was opposed by the magnetic field produced by externally mounted *focusing coils*. The final focal spot on the X-ray target should be only a few millimetres in diameter.

X-ray head

Most travelling wave and the higher energy standing wave accelerators require waveguides too long to be mounted in line with the ultimate X-ray beam. They are therefore mounted almost parallel to the axis of the isocentric gantry. The electron beam emerges from the accelerating guide into a field free 'flight tube' and then through one or several magnetic fields to steer the electrons through an angle of approximately 90° or 270° before reaching the X-ray target (Fig. 3.16). The current required by these electromagnets to steer the electrons through the required angle may be used to monitor the energy of the electrons—the higher their energy the larger the required current. Most accelerators are designed to operate at one or at most two photon energies. A variety of materials have been used for the X-ray targets in linear accelerators, including gold and platinum as well as tungsten.

Although the X-radiation from a linear accelerator is pulsed at between 100 and 500 pulses per second, the average dose rate of the flattened beam may be several grays/minute at 1 metre from the target. Each pulse lasts about 2 microseconds. The final output dose rate is determined by the gun filament temperature and the pulse rate and tuning to the optimum radio frequency.

It has been seen (p. 12) that in the megavoltage range of energies the X-rays are predominantly produced in the same direction as the electrons bombarding the target. Although this theory is based on a thin target,

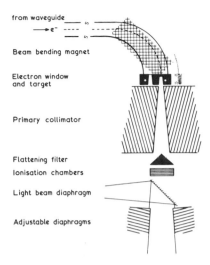

from waveguide

→ e⁻

Beam bending magnet

Electron window
and target

Primary collimator

Flattening filter
Ionisation chambers

Light beam diaphragm

Adjustable diaphragms

Fig. 3.16   The X-ray head assembly of a linear accelerator.

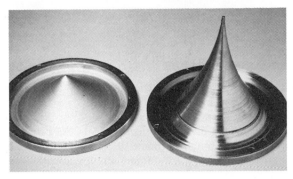

Fig. 3.17   Typical flattening filters. (Courtesy of Varian-TEM Ltd.)

the transmission target must be sufficiently thick to stop completely all the electrons bombarding it. There is, therefore, some modification of the spatial distribution. The theory, however, has two consequences particularly relevant to photon energies above 4 MV. Firstly, the photon energy sets a maximum practicable field size, in that the higher the energy the smaller the divergence of the X-rays produced. Secondly, the intensity along the central axis of the beam is greater than at the edges, that is, the dose distribution across the beam is not uniform. Beam uniformity is achieved by the use of a beam *flattening filter* close to the target (Fig. 3.17). This is a metal filter, preferably of low atomic number and conical in section, being thick at the centre to reduce the intensity of the central axis beam and tapering to zero at the edges so as not to reduce the intensity of the peripheral beam. A different flattening filter is required for each photon beam energy. The intensity distribution across the flattened beam should be such that within the central 80% of the width of the beam, it does not vary by more than ± 3% at d_{max} (Fig. 3.18). The flatness, being dependent on the distribution of the scattered radiation, varies

with depth and any definition of flatness must specify a depth. At depths less than that specified, the beam will be *over*-flattened, i.e. the central axis dose will be less than the off-axis dose, whereas at greater depths the reverse is true.

Immediately beyond the flattening filter, i.e. nearer the patient, there will be an ionisation chamber whose primary function is to provide a measure of the integrated dose at the isocentre. In practice the chamber is quite complex. It will be sealed so that its response does not vary with the ambient conditions (p. 74) and, for dual modality accelerators, the electrodes will be sufficiently thin to minimise the energy loss and attenuation of the electron beam. There will be two independent chambers feeding signals to two independent integrating dosemeters—each capable of terminating the exposure at the selected preset level, or of continuing to count up should the exposure termination circuit fail. They are independent in the sense that any failure of either circuit must not affect the operation of the other. In addition, the chamber will give a measure of dose rate. Other segmented sections of the chamber will provide signals to monitor parameters such as beam symmetry and via a servo system to correct the operating conditions.

Nearer the patient again will be the light beam diaphragm system (p. 49), the adjustable collimators (p. 48) and provision for the insertion of wedge

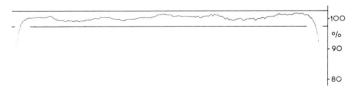

100

%

90

80

Fig. 3.18   A typical traverse across a flattened linear accelerator beam.

filters (p. 101), tissue compensators (p. 100) and local shielding blocks (p. 50).

Leakage radiation

The permitted radiation leakage through the housing of the linear accelerator is quoted as a percentage of the useful beam dose rate at 1 metre from the target, and is divided into several components. At a distance of 1 metre from *any* point along the flight of the electrons—from gun to target—the leakage dose rate shall not exceed 0.5%. Over a 2 metre radius, measured from the normal treating distance and at right angles to the beam axis, the leakage dose rate shall not exceed 0.2% except within the central area defined by the primary beam collimator. Again at the normal treating distance and at right angles to the beam axis, the area within the primary beam collimator but outside the useful beam, the transmission of the primary beam through the secondary (adjustable) collimators shall not exceed the values in Table 3.2.

Table 3.2 Leakage radiation through beam limiting diaphragms

Maximum field size (cm)	20 × 20	30 × 30	40 × 40	50 × 50
Permitted transmission (%)	2.0	1.1	0.6	0.4

At energies above 10 MV, where neutron activation may occur, the permissible leakage of neutron radiation at 1 metre from the electron beam and over the 2 metre radius beyond the limits of the primary collimator is limited to 0.05%. Maintenance staff working on these machines are advised to have a monitor available to check the radiation levels which may result from neutron activation and therefore exist after the X-ray exposure has been terminated.

Conversion to the electron beam modality

The linear accelerator is often designed for both photon and electron therapy. The conversion from the photon mode to the electron mode requires changes in the operation of the accelerator. The X-ray target is replaced by a thin window. A *scattering foil*, to disperse the finely focused electron beam, replaces the flattening filter. The electron gun temperature is reduced to lower the beam current and this in turn may require adjustments to the steering and focusing magnetic fields along the waveguide. Most of these adjustments will be made automatically when the modality switch is changed. The adjustable X-ray diaphragms will need to be wide open unless they are required at particular settings for use in conjunction with the electron beam collimators. Any material, particularly metals, in the electron beam will generate X-rays. The *X-ray contamination* of an electron beam should not contribute more than 1% of the total electron dose delivered per 5 MeV of beam energy (p. 114).

Control panel

The control panel of the linear accelerator may be of the traditional type, with a range of indicators, switches and meters, or a video display and keyboard backed by a microprocessor. Whichever type is used the control panel must clearly show the beam modality, photons or electrons, and their energy. There must be a means of presetting the dose to be delivered and the expected treatment time. In conjunction with these there will be two independent displays of the dose given and the elapsed treatment time—any one of the three displays being capable of terminating the exposure on reaching its preset value, or on developing a fault in its circuitry. Any changeable (wedge) filters or scattering foils will be interlocked and identified on the control panel. Beam on/off controls will be clearly identified. In addition to these basic requirements the control panel may display any number of parameters relating to the running conditions of the accelerator, the beam direction and couch position relating to the patient on treatment and may identify the patient as well.

Select and confirm systems

The display of patient related data is necessary if some microprocessor control is used to confirm the treatment set-up. Such a system will compare or display any serious discrepancies, for example the orientation of a rectangular field, to draw the radiographer's attention to the fact. In some cases the system will prevent treatment being given until the discrepancy is put right or reduced to an acceptable level. Sophisticated select and confirm systems of this type require some form of patient identification, often a punched card, bar code or magnetic strip, and produce a print-out of the treatment delivered.

GAMMA RAY BEAM UNITS
Choice of isotope

Gamma emitting radioactive nuclides may be used to produce a useful gamma ray beam for radiotherapy

Table 3.3 Isotopes used in gamma ray beam units

Property	Cobalt-60	Caesium-137	Radium-226 (in equilibrium)
Gamma ray energy (MeV)	1.17, 1.33	0.662	0.19–2.43
Half-life (years)	5.26	30	1620
Rate of decay (approx.)	1% per month	1% per 6 months	1% per 25 years
Air kerma rate per TBq at 1 m (Gy h^{-1})	0.307	0.078	0.195
Typical source diameter (mm)	17	20–40	40–70
Typical SSD (cm)	60–100	5–40	10

providing the photon energy is appropriately high and the specific activity is high enough to provide an adequate dose rate at the chosen treating distance. Isotopes used in this way are summarised in Table 3.3. It must be remembered that owing to the decay of activity the source will need replacing from time to time. Any one source is normally used for a period a little longer than one half of the half-life of the isotope, that is when the activity has decayed to about two-thirds of the initial activity and the treatment times have increased by about one-half. Owing to the discrete energies of gamma rays, the gamma beam is equivalent in many respects to X-ray beams generated at twice the photon energy (e.g. cobalt-60 at 100 cm source–skin distance (SSD) produces a beam equivalent to an X-ray beam of approximately 3 MV).

Early units using radium had the advantage of a long half-life and an effectively constant output dose rate. There were however three disadvantages: the potential leakage of radon gas, the low specific activity and the very high photon energy made the protection of the source housing difficult. These radium sources have been replaced with either caesium-137 or cobalt-60.

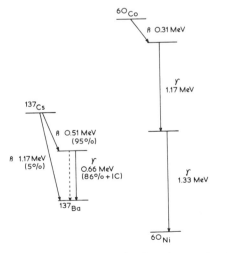

Fig. 3.19 The decay schemes of radioactive caesium-137 and radioactive cobalt-60.

Caesium-137

Caesium-137 has a long half-life (30 years) and is an attractive alternative to radium. Unfortunately, it has only a low specific activity (like radium) as well as a low gamma ray constant, which together result in relatively low output dose rates even from large sources. Caesium units, therefore, operate at SSDs of less than 40 cm and the useful beam has a wide penumbra (p. 49). The decay scheme (Fig. 3.19) shows a gamma emission of 0.66 MeV photons which is high enough to overcome the differential absorption in body tissues and low enough to make source housing a manageable size. The disadvantages of caesium, however, outweigh its advantages and it is now rarely found in teletherapy units. It is widely used as a radium substitute in brachytherapy (Ch. 8).

Cobalt-60

The effective photon energy of cobalt-60 is only slightly lower than that of radium and its half-life is relatively short, but despite this, cobalt-60 is the most widely used isotope in gamma ray beam units. It can be made to a high specific activity which combined with an air kerma rate of 0.3 Gy h^{-1} TBq^{-1} at 1 m produces a source with a high useful beam dose rate (1 TBq = 10^{12} Bq; T = tera). The half-life is such that treatment times have to be increased by approximately 1% per month and the useful life of the source is approximately 3.5 years.

Cobalt-60 is produced by neutron bombardment of cobalt-59 and decays to nickel-60 by emitting a beta particle and two gamma rays of 1.17 and 1.33 MeV.

Source design

To guard against the leakage of radioactive particles and to simplify the handling of the source, the radioactive cobalt (or caesium) is doubly encapsulated in stainless steel (Fig. 3.20). The cobalt metal is in the form of discs approximately 2 mm thick and 17 mm in diameter. These discs, probably 10 to 12 of them,

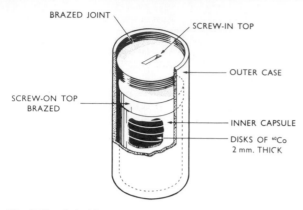

Fig. 3.20 A double encapsulated teletherapy cobalt-60 source. (Reproduced with permission from Meredith & Massey 1977.)

depending on the required activity, are inserted into the inner capsule and any remaining space is taken up by similarly sized inactive discs. The inner capsule is then closed with a screw cap which is sealed by brazing. The sealed inner capsule is then mounted in an outer case which is again closed with a screw cap and brazed.

It should be noted that although a unit may be designed to accept sources of a certain activity, say 200 TBq, the source is often specified in terms of the air kerma rate at a metre. This is directly related to the activity of a point source. In practice a long, small diameter source may have the same activity (in TBq) as a short, large diameter source but will have a lower output dose rate owing to the inherent attenuation of the photons emitted from the nuclei at the back of the source. This *self-absorption* within the source is taken into account in the specification of the air kerma rate at a metre, in that it is a measure of the output rather than the content of the source.

Source change procedure

The manufacturer of the cobalt unit provides the supplying isotope laboratory with a *source pencil* or holder which will accept the doubly encapsulated source. The laboratory will load the source into the pencil and the pencil into the manufacturer's transit container. To facilitate the changing of a source on site, two such containers are brought to the hospital. The empty container is linked to the unit, and the pencil with the spent source is transferred from the treatment head to the transit container. The container with the new source pencil is then linked to the unit and the procedure reversed. The whole procedure may take a whole day, although the actual source transfer will only take a second or two. Since this procedure is only

carried out every 3–3.5 years for cobalt, the student should watch it—preferably by closed circuit television—if the opportunity arises.

The alternative procedure is to dismantle the source housing from the unit and send it to the isotope laboratory to have the new source fitted. This results in a considerably longer 'down time' unless the isotope laboratory is only a short distance from the hospital. The spent source may be of value in another unit of shorter SSD.

Despite all the precautions, it is good practice to take a *wipe test* soon after a new source is fitted and periodically (e.g. annually) after that. To do this, all readily accessible surfaces—especially the collimating system—are wiped with a damp swab. A simple wipe is unlikely to pick up all the active dust particles and the activity measured on the swab will be only a fraction of that which has escaped from the source capsule. Providing the activity *on* the swab is less than 200 Bq the source is considered leak free. A full quality assurance check, including two independent output dose rate measurements, must be made before the new source is used to treat patients. The supplier's test report on the source will relate to specified laboratory conditions and not to the clinical application, although a comparison with test reports on previous sources should confirm the result of the output dose rate measurement.

Beam control

One fundamental difference between an X-ray unit and a gamma ray beam unit (Fig. 3.21) is that the gamma radiation cannot be switched off. If the mains supply fails or is interrupted by a switch the X-ray beam is automatically safe. The gamma ray beam is not—unless it is designed to be so—but again mechanisms may fail.

The *moving source unit* has a mechanism whereby the source can be moved from the centre of the protective shield to the apex of the collimating system—that is the point from which the useful beam emanates. The mechanism moves the source between the 'Beam Off' position and the 'Beam On' position. In the *fixed source unit*, however, the source is fixed at the apex of the collimating system and a shutter absorbs the useful beam or allows it to pass out of the head—the open shutter may form part of the collimating system. Whichever mechanism is employed, it is mandatory to provide a spring return mechanism and a manual return system to make the unit safe in the event of a failure. The failure of the electrical supply or of the spring must not leave the source stranded in the 'Beam On' position. The manual return system needs to be understood by everyone who may be required to

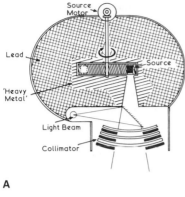

A

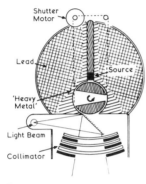

B

Fig. 3.21 Typical cobalt-60 teletherapy units of **A** the moving source type and **B** the fixed source type.

operate the unit and a written protocol must be kept readily available and rehearsed by selected members of staff. Mechanical indicators are incorporated in the design of the unit to show that the shutter (or source) is in the safe 'Beam Off' position. Supplementary electrical and mechanical indicators may also be fitted. It must be possible to mechanically lock the mechanism in the 'Beam Off' position whenever the unit is left unattended.

Since the radiation is emitted spontaneously and decays with the half-life of the isotope, the only controls required are those to operate the beam on/off mechanism. The control desk is, therefore, very simple. A double treatment timer is used to terminate the exposure after a preset time. The primary timer should measure the length of the exposure to the patient while the secondary back-up timer should measure the time the source/shutter is out of the 'Beam Off' position—the difference between the two timers on completion of the exposure is therefore the overall transit time. Any change in this overall transit time may give advanced indication of a mechanism malfunction and should be reported. To correct for the decay of the source, treatment times will need to be increased

by approximately 1% each month for cobalt-60 units (1% every 6 months for caesium-137)—but the output dose rate should be confirmed by regular measurement. Lamps are used to indicate the position of the source or shutter showing 'Source Safe', 'In Transit' or 'Beam On'. Interlock circuits will be used to confirm the use of wedges and flattening filters. A continuously energised independent gamma alarm in the treatment room should indicate when the shutter is open.

Leakage radiation

Reference has already been made to the lead protection incorporated in the tube shield of an X-ray unit and to the lead surrounding the source in a gamma ray beam unit. The function of this lead protection is primarily twofold. First to reduce the level of radiation reaching parts of the patient other than the treated area and, second, to reduce the level of radiation reaching the walls of the treatment room, thereby reducing the wall thickness required. In the case of a gamma ray beam unit there is the additional need to make the unit safe in the 'Beam Off' condition to enable the radiographers to attend to the patient and other staff (cleaners, for example) to carry out their duties in the treatment room in safety. The gamma ray source, therefore, needs to be housed in a protective shield such that the gamma ray air kerma rates at the surface and at 1 metre from the source are below the accepted safety limits (Table 3.4). The major part of the source housing will be either heavy alloy, depleted uranium or lead. The head of a 200 TBq cobalt unit may weigh 1000 kg. This protective material will surround the source in all directions except one—the direction of the useful beam.

In any new installation or following any modifications which may affect the protection surrounding the head, a complete check is required to ensure the intensity of the leakage radiation is below the accepted limits and to ensure there are no weaknesses, such as cracks or pinholes, in the material used. The former is

Table 3.4 Leakage air kerma rates permitted from gamma ray beam units

	At 1 m from source		At 5 cm from surface
	Maximum	Average	
Beam off	0.1 mGy h^{-1}	0.02 mGy h^{-1}	2.0 mGy h^{-1}
Beam on	0.1%*	—	—
Beam on (small units)	10 mGy h^{-1}	—	—

* Of the useful beam kerma rate at 1 m.

measured using a large volume (e.g. 500 ml) ionisation chamber and the latter by wrapping X-ray film around the surface of the housing. (In the context of gamma ray beam units, students should not confuse the leakage of active material from the source detected by the wipe test (p. 44) and the leakage of radiation through the limited attenuation afforded by the source housing.)

BEAM COLLIMATION

Beam collimation and collimating systems have been referred to above but will now be dealt with in greater detail. In general terms *beam collimation* means the limiting of the spread of the radiation to a predetermined direction and over a given solid angle. In practical radiotherapy it is necessary to be able to vary the size of the beam to suit the needs of each patient. This is referred to as field size or beam size. The collimation system can be divided into primary collimation and secondary collimation.

Primary collimation

Primary collimation is achieved by a conical hole in a suitably thick metal block close to the source of radiation. The axis of the hole defines the beam axis and should pass through the centre of the source of radiation. It also defines the maximum divergence of the beam and, therefore, the maximum field size at a specified distance from the source. If this primary collimator is circular then the larger square fields will have 'rounded corners'. On an X-ray unit the primary collimator will be part of the X-ray tube housing or X-ray head (Fig. 3.7); on an accelerator it will be a heavy metal block close to or incorporating the X-ray target (Fig. 3.16) and on a gamma ray unit (Fig. 3.21) it may be part of the shutter mechanism. The maximum divergence is predetermined either by the target angle in the lower energy X-ray units or by the photon energy of the linear accelerator (p. 12). When an isotope source is used the maximum field size is only limited by

Table 3.5 Effect of the inverse square law on the percentage dose at the corners of large fields

Typical unit	SSD (cm)	Field size (cm)	Dose at corner* low by (%)
Linear accelerator	100	40 × 40	4
Cobalt unit	80	40 × 40	6
Orthovoltage X-rays	50	25 × 25	6
Superficial X-rays	25	30 cm diameter	14

* This will be very dependent on the shape of the flattening filter.

the engineering problems associated with the secondary collimating system.

It needs to be remembered, however, that unless some compensation (e.g. a flattening filter) is introduced into the beam, the dose rate at the corner of a large field will be lower than that at the centre, owing to the effect of the inverse square law. Table 3.5 shows some typical values. In some centres, low atomic number flattening filters have been introduced into the superficial X-ray units for just this reason. At orthovoltage energies where scattered radiation plays an important role, the reduction of scatter further reduces the dose at the edges and in the corners.

Secondary collimation

Having defined the overall maximum field size and the beam direction, the secondary collimation provides a means of adjusting the field size to suit the particular requirements and the means of rotating square and rectangular fields about the beam axis. Secondary collimation may be achieved by either interchangeable applicators or adjustable diaphragms.

Interchangeable applicators are preferred where the SSD is short as the applicator provides an accurate means of setting up the SSD and, therefore, reducing errors due to the inverse square law. The closed ended applicators also simplify the use of bolus by presenting a surface normal to the beam axis against which the bolus can be packed (p. 100). On obese patients, the applicator can also be used as a means of applying compression, so reducing the distance between the skin surface and the treatment site. *Adjustable diaphragms* are essential where rotation techniques are to be used (as the SSD varies with the rotation) and for high energy radiation beams. In practice, applicators are used for low photon energies (below, say 500 kV) and where SSDs are short (below, say 20 cm); diaphragms are used on megavoltage units and for orthovoltage rotation techniques. (Interchangeable applicators are preferred for electron therapy but adjustable diaphragm systems are again required for rotation techniques.)

Interchangeable applicators

To provide an adequate choice of size and shape of field, up to 20 applicators may be required for each machine. Temporary shapes can be made using lead or lead rubber of adequate thickness over the end of a slightly over-large applicator. Table 3.6 shows the lead equivalence required to attenuate the incident beam to less than 2%. The actual thickness of lead rubber is several times greater than its lead equivalence, i.e. the

Table 3.6 Lead equivalence required to reduce the transmitted primary beam to less than 2%

Therapy beam	Approx. lead equivalence (mm)
50 kV 1 mm Al HVL	0.25
100 kV 2 mm Al HVL	0.5
150 kV 4 mm Al HVL	1.0
250 kV 2 mm Cu HVL	2.0
Caesium-137	31
Cobalt-60	60

thickness of lead which will produce the same degree of attenuation. Where lead is used the bare surfaces should be covered with wax or plastic film to minimise the lead contamination of both the patient and the staff. The surface dose rate will be reduced due to the change in back scatter (p. 86) and may be further reduced by the increased SSD, and appropriate corrections will be required to the treatment time (p. 115). An alternative to the moulding of lead sheet, is the use of low melting point alloy sprayed on to a plastic impression of the area to be treated (p. 52). The alloy can be built up to any desired thickness, conform to any surface contour and, of course, be recycled at the end of treatment.

Two types of X-ray applicator are shown in Figure 3.22. In both cases the applicator has a base which serves as a means of attaching the applicator to the X-ray head and incorporates a diaphragm which limits the beam to a size slightly larger than that required. The diaphragm is required to reduce the intensity outside the useful beam to less than 2% of that of the useful beam. The distal end of the applicator wall may be transparent to enable the coverage of the beam to be checked when the applicator is in contact with the patient. The final collimation is achieved at a point within approximately 5 cm of the skin surface. The face in contact with the skin indicates the actual area irradiated by the beam. In the design shown in Figure 3.22A the walls are not irradiated and can be

made of steel; however, the straight sides make large applicators particularly bulky and difficult to handle. The 'Fulfield' applicator (Fig. 3.22B), on the other hand, has lead lined walls parallel to the rays at the edge of the field and the Perspex end (typically 3 mm thick) is taken across the face of the applicator to absorb secondary electrons from the lead. The Perspex face is inscribed with the principal axes which, of course, intersect on the beam axis, simplifying the setting-up of a patient and the use of 'bolus'.

Open ended applicators are invariably used in electron therapy. Their design may be similar to that in Figure 3.22A, namely a remote diaphragm limits the electron beam to a size only marginally larger than the aperture in contact with the patient. The size of the margin is critical to the uniformity of the beam profile. Electrons striking the inner surface of the applicator will be scattered back into the beam and ideally boost the dose delivered to the edge of the field to the level on the beam axis; too many or too few contributing to a non-uniformity at the edge. Alternatively, the electron beam will be collimated through a series of apertures mounted on an otherwise open frame, the final beam being shaped by a cut-out cast into low melting point alloy.

From time to time applicators should be checked for accurate alignment. The check is twofold. First, set up an independent pointer to mark the beam axis on the surface of the applicator, then, on rotating the applicator in its mounting, the pointer should remain at the same point on the applicator surface or describe a circle less than 2 mm diameter (Fig. 3.23A). Second, a film should be exposed, with minimal back-scattering material, (to a density of about 1.5) with markers indicating the corners of the applicator—the processed film should show coincidence of the markers with the corners of the blackened area. The blackened area should be checked carefully for a 'pin-cushion' effect as 'Fulfield' applicators tend to be handled in such a way that the lead lining is deformed inwards and becomes separated from the applicator wall material. This effect is shown exaggerated in Figure 3.23B; the marker *t* simply aids the correlation of the processed film with the experimental set-up.

If these checks suggest the alignment on rotation is satisfactory, but the coincidence of the blackened area and markers is poor, then the focal spot may not be correctly aligned to the axis of rotation of the applicators. To check this requires a special device called a 'pin-hole camera' (Fig. 3.23C). This device is mounted in place of the applicator and checked for rotational accuracy. A film is then exposed and the focal spot is imaged on the film together with the shadow of the

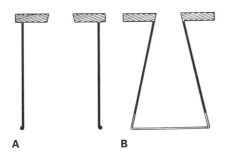

Fig. 3.22 Beam defining applicators. **A** Parallel-sided and **B** Fulfield.

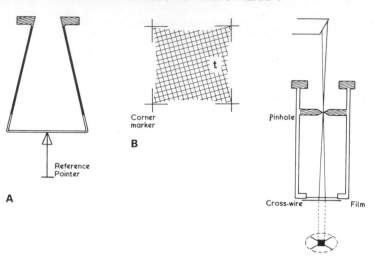

Fig. 3.23 Alignment checks on beam defining applicators. **A** The reference pointer, **B** the mechanical/photon alignment and **C** the pinhole camera.

cross-wires, the intersection of which should be close to, or in the centre of, the image of the focal spot. (A regular focal spot film can give useful information on the condition of the focal spot.)

Adjustable diaphragms

Adjustable diaphragms are used for megavoltage units as the penetrating radiation requires a large thickness of a heavy metal to reduce the transmitted intensity to less than the permitted maximum (Table 3.2). In addition, the high energy radiation produces in the diaphragms secondary electrons which have a considerable range in air and so, if the diaphragms were close to the skin, these electrons would contribute to the skin dose, negating one principal advantage of megavoltage radiation—the skin sparing or build-up effect (p. 87). The optimum diaphragm–skin distance is based on the consideration of skin dose and penumbra width and is typically not less than 20 cm, but the precise value depends on the beam energy and the design of the unit. In practice, the diaphragms are

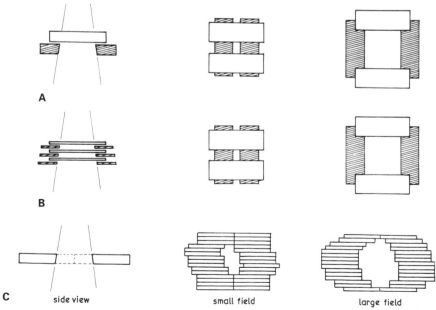

Fig. 3.24 Adjustable diaphragm systems modified: **A** double plane, **B** interleaved and **C** multileaved.

approximately halfway between the source of radiation and the patient and have a transparent electron filter over the aperture.

As with applicators, there are two designs of adjustable diaphragms in common use, they may be conveniently referred to as double plane and interleaved (Fig. 3.24A and B). These limit the choice of field shape to squares and rectangles within the overall circle defined by the primary collimator. Two design features of adjustable diaphragms are based on the requirement to minimise the size of the *penumbra*. The collimating faces of the thick diaphragm blades are made to move in such a way that they always lie along the direction of propagation of the radiation, i.e. along a radius from the source. Secondly, the collimated length—the distance from the source to the most distant part of the diaphragm blade—is made as large as possible. A compromise has to be reached between the collimated length and the range of the secondary electrons from the diaphragm blades.

The double plane system has the clear disadvantage in that the collimated length of the two pairs of blades—which may be 10 to 12 cm thick—is different, giving rise to different penumbra widths on the two principal axes of the beam. The interleaved system poses considerable engineering problems, particularly for the higher energy beams where the overall thickness of the blades is large.

There is increasing interest in multileaf diaphragms in an effort to overcome the limitation of beam shape. If, for example, blades are mounted to move in a plane parallel to the beam axis, then the displacement of each blade can be adjusted to configure any shape of field (Fig. 3.24C). The computer control of this complex diaphragm system is essential for conformation therapy techniques. Such a system may replace the secondary collimation or may be an accessory used in conjunction with the secondary collimation.

Since the diaphragm system is some distance from the patient, a light beam is incorporated in the unit to indicate the area covered by the radiation. The light beam (Fig. 3.25) is provided by a small filament lamp positioned in such a way that its virtual image is coincident with the source of X- or gamma rays. In this way, the visible light is seen to emanate from the same source as the radiation beam and therefore illuminates the area irradiated and defined by the diaphragm system. The thin surface-silvered mirror does not appreciably affect the photon beam. A specially constructed mirror is required if it is to be used in conjunction with an electron beam. A suitable cross-hair 'object' is incorporated to produce an 'image' on the patient, identifying the principal axes of the beam and their intersection on the beam axis. A simple optical SSD pointer may project one or more spots of light to coincide with the beam axis at a predetermined SSD or an illuminated scale on which the SSD may be read at the point indicated on the beam axis.

Periodic checks are carried out to confirm the accuracy of the light beam and the adjustable diaphragm system. First, a reference mark—a cross on a piece of paper—is attached to the couch at the isocentre. The cross is aligned to the beam axis as delineated by the light beam. Rotating the diaphragm should not cause a deviation of greater than 2 mm. Second, check with a ruler that the light beam delineated correlates correctly with the set field size at the normal SSD. Then, using film or radiation sensitive paper and radio-opaque corner markers, check the optical/photon alignment by making an appropriate exposure as described above. The setting-up is simplified if the corner markers are incorporated into the surface of say 12 mm Perspex. The markers are then in close contact with the film and the Perspex provides the necessary build-up. This test should be repeated over a range of field sizes. Close examination of the films should confirm the coincidence of all four corner markers, the orthogonality of adjacent diaphragms and the parallelism of opposing diaphragms—both to better than 1°.

The light beam gives a sharp image of the beam edge, which is misleading as the photon beam will have a penumbra edge of finite size.

Penumbra

If the source of radiation in the therapy unit was a point source, the precise direction of the radiation would be known and the size of the beam would be

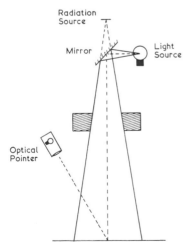

Fig. 3.25 The principle of the light beam diaphragm and optical front pointer.

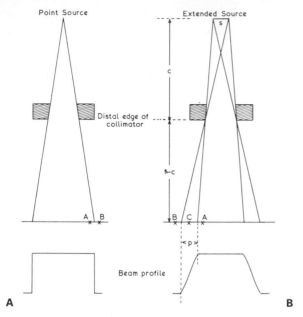

Fig. 3.26 The effects of geometric penumbra **A** from a point source and **B** from a finite source.

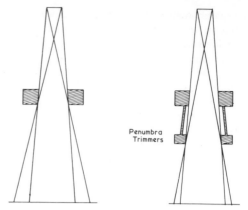

Fig. 3.27 The reduction of geometric penumbra by the use of penumbra trimmers.

uniquely defined. In practice it is not a point source. The X-rays may emanate from a small area on the target. Gamma rays, on the other hand, emanate from all points within a finite cylindrical source. This presents a problem. In Figure 3.26A the point marked A is in the beam of radiation and point B is outside the beam. In Figure 3.26B this is also true, but point C is neither inside nor outside the beam; it is said to lie in the *geometric penumbra*. It is in a region where it can receive radiation from some parts of the source but not from the whole source. In the case of a point source, the dose gradient between points A and B is sheer, while in the case of a finite source, the dose gradient is gradual and depends principally on the size of the source. Applying the principle of similar triangles to Figure 3.26B, the geometric penumbra p is defined by:

$$p = s\frac{(f - c)}{c}$$

where s is the diameter of the source, f the SSD and c the collimated length. The geometric penumbra is independent of field size. It is easy to see from the equation above that to reduce the size of the geometric penumbra the source diameter must be reduced ($s = 0$ for a point source) or the collimated length must be increased and made more nearly equal to the SSD. The collimated length is measured to the distal edge of the diaphragm blade from the source. It should be noted that although the diagrams show the geometric penumbra as defined at the skin surface, it increases

as the beam passes through the patient. If the penumbra is to be calculated at any other depth, then f should be taken as the distance from the source to the depth of interest.

In practice, the diaphragm blade may be very thick and unless its face is parallel to the rays from the source of radiation, the rays 'just outside the beam' will not traverse the full thickness of the collimator blade and will give rise to a further blurring of the edge of the beam, which can be referred to as a *transmission penumbra*. By changing the angle of the collimator face as the field size is changed, the face can be maintained parallel to the rays from a point source, thereby presenting the full thickness of the blade to the rays to be absorbed. However, there will be some transmission penumbra effect when the source is of finite size as each blade can only rotate about a single point. The combined geometric and transmission penumbra width can be estimated by replacing c in the above formula by $(c - t)$ where t is the thickness of the diaphragm.

Penumbra trimmers

Where the geometric penumbra is large and where the treatment technique permits, it is possible to increase the effective collimated length by the use of *penumbra trimmers*. These are heavy metal bars mounted between the diaphragm system and the patient (Fig. 3.27) and positioned in such a way that the inner surfaces lie in the same plane as the faces of the diaphragm blades themselves. Penumbra trimmers are often offered as an accessory, particularly for cobalt or caesium teletherapy units.

Beam shaping and local shielding blocks

Adjustable diaphragms, in general, limit the choice of

field sizes to squares and rectangles. Unless a multileaf diaphragm system is used, any modification to the shape of the field must be achieved by the addition of heavy metal blocks (lead, tungsten, heavy metal or one of the special alloys). Areas in the centre of the field may be protected in a similar manner. The thickness of the blocks will be determined by the degree of protection required having taken into account the fact that the dose in the shadow will be increased by the scatter from the adjacent irradiated tissues. For megavoltage radiations the thickness will be at least 6 cm lead equivalent (Table 3.6).

In practice these blocks may be suspended from the front of the unit or mounted on a 'shadow tray' similarly suspended. Alternatively, they can be supported on a table over the patient. The shadow tray or table may be a sheet of Perspex or a perforated aluminium plate. The actual means adopted must be decided from a consideration of the penumbra width, the electron contamination and the weight of the blocks. The sharply defined shadow produced by the light beam can be deceptive in that it gives no indication of the penumbra width. Accurate shielding requires, therefore, the blocks to be close to the patient. On the other hand, electron contamination and weight considerations require the blocks to be distant from the patient.

The electron contamination can be reduced by fitting each block with a material which will absorb these secondary electrons and which will not itself produce additional contaminating electrons. Brass is often used both as a filter and a means of protecting lead blocks from damage—lead is soft and easily distorted. Brass has the further advantage that it can be tapped to accept fixing screws through a perforated shadow tray so that the blocks can be fixed in position when the beam axis is not vertical.

Lead shielding blocks intended for general use are often rectangular in section, i.e. the (collimating) faces are parallel to the beam axis and not to the radiation they are intended to absorb. These give rise to the maximum transmission penumbra and, therefore, a poor X-ray shadow. Wherever possible the blocks should be tapered to minimise the transmission penumbra effect (Fig. 3.28).

Low melting point lead/bismuth alloys are readily available and enable shielding blocks to be tailor-made to the patients' individual requirements and later melted down and recycled. The density and atomic number of the alloy are less than those of lead, about 9.7 g cm^{-3} and 75 respectively, and therefore the blocks need to be proportionally thicker. The simplicity of manufacture and the accurate shaping (in all three dimensions) far outweigh the problem of thickness. One method which

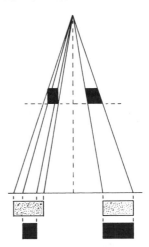

Fig. 3.28 The reduction of transmission penumbra by the use of tapered (tailor-made) shielding blocks.

may be used is as follows. A radiograph is taken using the simulator so that the SSD and field size match those to be used during treatment. The area to be shielded and the beam axis are marked carefully on the film (Figs 3.29A and 3.30). The pattern on the film is then used in conjunction with the hot wire to cut a hole in the expanded polystyrene (Fig. 3.29B) using the focus–film distance (FFD) from the simulator and the source-shielding tray distance from the treatment unit. The polystyrene is then used directly as a cast for the low melting point alloy. The cooling rate of the alloy needs to be carefully controlled to minimise the risk of cavitation—the formation of cavities in the apparently

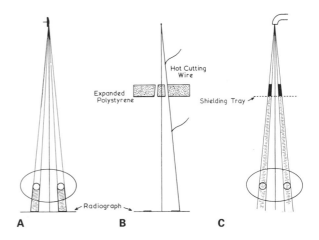

Fig. 3.29 The making of tailor-made shielding blocks. **A** Patient radiographed on simulator under treatment geometry. **B** The cast cut to shape using hot wire and marked-up radiograph. **C** Patient treated using the cast shielding blocks.

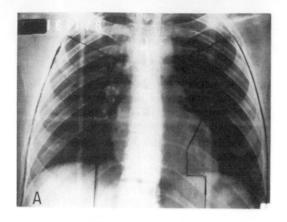

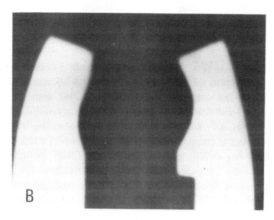

Fig. 3.30 Planning film **A** from the simulator used in the preparation of tailored shielding blocks and the check film and **B** on the linear accelerator confirms their accuracy.

solid material. The blocks then produce the precise shadows to protect the areas originally marked on the film (Figs 3.29C and 3.30). As an alternative to the alloy, lead shot may be poured into the polystyrene cast and used directly or the lead shot may be glued together using wax and then removed from the cast. Great care is needed in handling lead shot to guard against its being spilt on the floor and producing a skating rink surface!

In superficial radiotherapy, it is often necessary to shape sheet lead to the patient contour—by beating the lead on to a plaster cast—before cutting an aperture to the shape of the target area. Beating makes the lead thinner. Once beaten out the lead cannot be used again unless it is melted down and recast. A technique which is gaining popularity is to spray molten alloy on to the cast—or better still on to a plastic shell (p. 108) —to the required thickness. Providing the spraying is done carefully in an appropriate spray booth, the

alloy loss is minimal. The same technique can be used for electron therapy where irregular areas are to be treated.

Low melting point alloy can be recycled many times without any noticeable deterioration, making it ideal for all tailor-made appliances. Eventually its melting point rises as the balance of metals in the alloy is disturbed. The alloy can, however, be replenished by adding the lost component to the molten alloy. Providing the alloy is never overheated and is handled according to the manufacturer's instructions, it is not considered a health hazard.

DESIGN OF BEAM THERAPY ROOMS

Adequate protection in a beam therapy room begins with the generator itself; and the protective requirements of the equipment have been detailed earlier in this chapter.

Primary and secondary barriers

The walls of a megavoltage therapy room are frequently identified as primary barriers or secondary (or scatter) barriers. The primary barrier is the wall (and ceiling and floor) which may be irradiated by the primary beam, while those unlikely to be so irradiated are termed secondary or scatter barriers. The latter only receive the secondary (leakage) radiation from the source/tube housing (which is limited to approximately 0.1% of the primary beam dose rate) and the scattered radiation from the patient and other material in the beam. The secondary radiation will be of low intensity but high in energy. The scattered radiation will be lower in energy, depending on the angle of scatter, and of an intensity dependent on the angle, the area irradiated and to a lesser extent on the scattering material. For megavoltage radiations, the 90° scatter has an energy of about 0.5 MeV and therefore the broad beam absorption data for 1 MV radiation may be used. Table 3.7. shows the energy of the scattered radiation for a range of primary photon energies and scattering angles calculated using the formula for Compton shift (p. 63). The primary barriers are typically about six tenth value layers (TVLs) thick, and the secondary barriers about half that thickness, to bring the time averaged dose rate outside the room down to a level consistent with the dose limit applicable to those not occupationally exposed.

For example, consider a 4 MV linear accelerator producing a primary beam dose rate of 1.6 Gy min^{-1} at 1 m SSD (Fig. 3.31). If a point 5 m from the focus is to be protected to reduce the dose rate to 1 mSv y^{-1}

Table 3.7 The energy of scattered radiation: $h\nu/[1 + \alpha\,(1 - \cos ø)]$

Primary photon energy (MeV) = $\alpha = h\nu/0.511$ =		0.26 0.5	0.51 1.0	1.02 2.0	2.56 5.0	5.11 10.0	10.22 20.0	25.55 50.0
Angle ø	$1 - \cos ø$			Energy of scattered photon (MeV)				
30	0.13	0.24	0.45	0.81	1.55	2.22	2.84	3.41
60	0.50	0.20	0.34	0.51	0.73	0.85	0.93	0.98
90	1.00	0.17	0.26	0.34	0.43	0.46	0.49	0.50
120	1.50	0.15	0.20	0.26	0.30	0.32	0.33	0.34
150	1.87	0.13	0.18	0.22	0.25	0.26	0.27	0.27
180	2.00	0.13	0.17	0.20	0.23	0.24	0.25	0.25

(1 mGy y^{-1}) when the beam-on time is expected to be no more than 2 hours per day, 5 days per week, then the barrier thickness may be calculated as follows:

Primary beam dose rate at 1 m
$$= 1.6 \times 2 \times 60 \times 5 \times 52 \text{ Gy y}^{-1}$$

Primary beam dose rate at 5 m
$$= \frac{1.6 \times 2 \times 60 \times 5 \times 52}{25} \text{ Gy y}^{-1}$$

Primary beam dose rate at 5 m
$$= 2000 \text{ Gy y}^{-1}$$

Wall attenuation required
$$= 1 \text{ mGy}/2000 \text{ Gy} = 0.5 \times 10^{-6}$$
$$\text{or} = 6 \text{ TVL} + 1 \text{ HVL}$$

The data from Table 12.4 gives 1 TVL = 275 mm and 1 HVL (half value layer) = 85 mm concrete, making this primary barrier 1.75 m thick. Under these conditions, the instantaneous dose rate at the point will be $1.6 \times 0.5 \times 10^{-6}/25$ Gy min^{-1} or 35 nGy min^{-1}.

Some isocentrically mounted equipment is fitted with a primary beam-stop to absorb the exit beam emerging from the patient. Such a device radically modifies the protection requirements of the room in which it is installed. Since the primary beam is heavily attenuated before it strikes the wall, the primary barrier may not need to be any thicker than the secondary barrier.

For cobalt-60 gamma ray units and X-ray units of lower energy, the versatility of the gantry or tube stand enables the primary beam to be aimed in any direction and the distinction between primary and secondary barriers is inappropriate—and economically not justified. It is not good practice to make assumptions about what fraction of the total beam-on time is appropriate for each barrier. It is good practice, however, not to direct the primary beam at the entrance or at the observation window. Doors, as with windows, should afford the same degree of protection as the walls in which they are situated, and that protection must be continuous through the door frame by suitably lapping the lead shielding over the joints (Fig. 3.32).

Entrance doors

At megavoltage energies, doors become too heavy and are best replaced by maze entrances, through which the scattered radiation is attenuated by multiple scattering and distance (Fig. 3.33). At the outer end of the maze—which should be in full view of the operator at

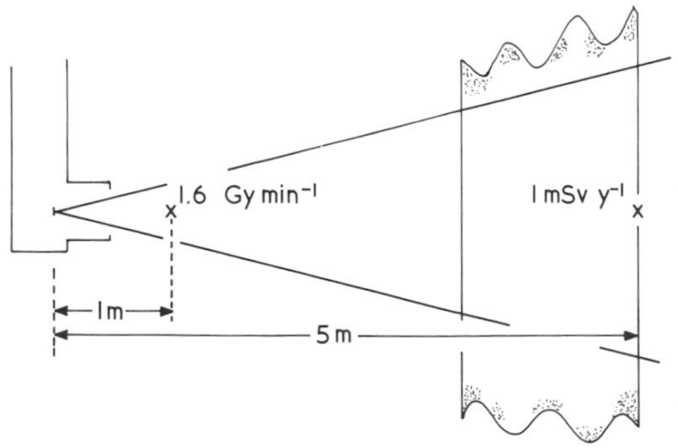

Fig. 3.31 The calculation of primary barrier thickness.

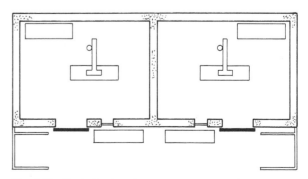

Fig. 3.32 Typical orthovoltage treatment room layout showing the transformer cabinet in the room, the protected sliding door and lead glass window.

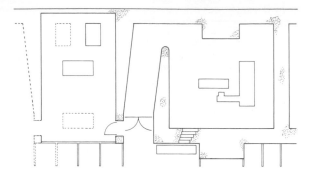

Fig. 3.33 Typical megavoltage treatment room layout showing the primary barriers, maze entrance and lead glass window. Note the adjacent accommodation for the modulator and chiller.

the control desk—there must be a full door, a gate or a light beam sensor to terminate any exposure in progress when the barrier is broken. This door interlock should be a fail-safe device which can only be reset by the positive action of the operator at the control desk—when all but the patient have left the room. A similar door interlock is required on all therapy rooms where the operator is outside the room, and on each and every door if there is more than one. Treatment simulator rooms often have more than one entrance, and although door interlocks are not mandatory on diagnostic rooms, it is good practice to have them on the treatment simulator.

All X-ray therapy rooms will be controlled areas whenever the generator is energised and warning signs, preferably electrically operated, must be displayed to that effect at each entrance. From the moment the generator is in a state of readiness to emit radiation until the termination of the exposure, an additional warning sign should display DO NOT ENTER or otherwise advise of the hazard (Plate 1). Gamma ray beam units will require the treatment room to be a controlled area at all times because of the total activity of the source, and therefore, a permanently fixed controlled area notice is appropriate, supplemented by the same DO NOT ENTER or similar warning, electrically operated. Visible and audible warnings are required inside all treatment rooms to indicate that radiation is imminent or present. In a gamma ray beam room or remote afterloading suite, these are supplemented by independently powered gamma alarms.

Observation of the patient

Both diagnostic X-ray (including the treatment simulator) and therapy rooms are controlled areas when

the beam is emitted and therefore everyone except the patient must either move out of the room or behind a protective shield. However, in the interests of safety, the patient must be kept under observation. At diagnostic energies and up to orthovoltage therapy energies, lead glass windows are commonly used. With lead as an added ingredient, glass can be made with an increased density ($\rho \sim 4000\ kg\ m^{-3}$) and effective atomic number for use in protective barriers. Glass of up to 2 mm lead equivalence is readily available and widely used. The window and its frame have to afford the same degree of protection as the surrounding wall or partition and be large enough to provide a clear view of the room and the patient for more than one operator.

For megavoltage therapy rooms, lead glass has been used but, more recently, closed circuit television (CCTV)—in black and white or in colour—has proved more convenient and somewhat cheaper. Several lead glass slabs some 200 mm thick are required to attenuate the scattered radiation to an acceptable level. To ensure there is no leakage at the edges, each slab is bigger than the one before—the smallest being on the outside. High density lead glass is very soft and easily damaged either in the handling during installation— each slab weighs some 50 kg or more—or by cleaning during normal use—the surfaces are easily scratched.

Closed circuit television, with a pan and tilt camera fitted with a zoom lens, is ideal in that the patient can be viewed either in close-up or from a distance. Two systems enable the operator to have two angles on the patient and provide some insurance against the failure of one system. The vantage points commonly used are (1) close to the sagittal laser, looking along the gantry axis, and (2) at about $45°$ to the first, to give a more lateral view without obstruction by the rotation of the gantry head. Providing the vantage points are carefully chosen, they can both pan to observe the patients having total body irradiation over against the wall. If the video signal is interrupted by the door interlock circuit, then the monitor screens can be blanked out while the radiographer is in the room attending the patient, thereby increasing their privacy. The CCTV system does not offer the patient a view of the operator and this is often cited in favour of the window.

The operator is only allowed to stay in the treatment room when the equipment cannot exceed 50 kV. Unless the equipment is specially designed to be hand-held, the operator must still stand behind the lead glass screen.

Communication with the patient

A hands-off intercom should be available so the patient

can speak to the operator during the treatment without having to move. Again, if this is linked through the door interlock circuit, it can be muted while the operator is in the room.

ACCEPTANCE TESTS

New radiotherapy equipment should only be ordered after close scrutiny of the manufacturer's technical specification and discussion about the customer's particular requirements. Compliance with local, national or international requirements should not be assumed. The equipment will then be delivered and installed by the manufacturers or their agents, but before it is accepted the customer's Medical Physicist should ensure the installation complies with the agreed specification. The acceptance tests may take from a few hours to several weeks depending on the complexity of the equipment in question.

The acceptance tests will therefore be designed to demonstrate that the details of the agreed specification have been satisfied—in five main areas:

1. The radiotherapy beams—each beam energy and beam modality—are of the specified quality, intensity and range of sizes and can be controlled and monitored in the specified manner. Wedges, filters, applicators, etc. must be interlocked.

2. All the movements of the gantry, collimators and couch cover the specified range and the brakes operate effectively throughout the range. Where motorised movements are involved the speed and control must be checked. The accuracy of the isocentre must be checked as appropriate.

3. All the electrical aspects of the equipment must be checked for safety—the connections to earth, the operation of limit switches, interlocks, built-in safety circuits, particularly where the equipment could malfunction and where maintenance staff may be put at risk. The consequences of a mains supply failure must be included.

4. The radiation safety requirements must be met—leakage radiation levels from the tube/source housing, collimator transmission, beam dosimetry and control, etc. The installer will have had the adequacy of the structural shielding checked at an early stage, but checks should be made on other aspects such as door interlocks and warning signs (unless the manufacturers have supplied and fitted these, they will not accept sole responsibility for them).

5. The inventory of the accessories, spare parts, instruction and maintenance manuals, circuit diagrams and safety manuals, etc.

A careful record of all these checks and operating parameters must be kept for future reference.

Equipment peripheral to the radiotherapy equipment, e.g. the CCTV viewing system, intercom, lasers, etc., may or may not be the responsibility of the supplier of the therapy equipment. The structural work on the treatment and control rooms may be the subject of a separate contract.

Commissioning new equipment

Once new equipment has been accepted then the customer will repeat most of the checks listed above with a view to making detailed measurements to ensure the equipment can be used safely to treat patients. This commissioning of the equipment will be the responsibility of a competent Medical Physicist and will include:

1. Full radiation protection survey of the treatment room and adjacent areas—not forgetting above and below—to ensure the requirements of the safety legislation are satisfied within the accepted use of the equipment. Any failure in structural protection may be difficult to correct at this stage and may impose limitations on the use of the equipment or the occupancy of the adjacent areas. This survey will include interlocks and warning signs and the systems for audiovisual contact with the patient during treatment.

2. Full radiation protection survey of the equipment itself—leakage radiation levels when the beam is on. Further assessments will be necessary with gamma ray beam units in the beam-off mode and with electron accelerators generating X-rays at greater than 10 MV where there may be residual radiation from the short-lived isotopes produced by neutron activation.

3. Confirmation of the accuracy of all the beam direction devices, the collimators and the coincidence of the photon/electron beams with the mechanical/optical delineators, including the isocentre and sagittal projection lasers, if fitted.

4. The measurement of depth dose, beam profiles and isodose chart data for all beam modalities in sufficient detail for the treatment planning of patients. The measurement of output factors, wedge and shadow tray correction factors, etc., to enable the correct correlation between monitor units and the delivered absorbed dose in grays.

5. The output dose calibration over the full range of the dose monitor to check linearity, over the range of available dose rates to check saturation. To check all the facets of the double dosimetry system.

In addition, the radiographers and the mould room

staff will need to familiarise themselves with the accessories supplied with the equipment, e.g. couch head rests, to assist with the setting-up of patients.

It is important that all the staff involved with the equipment are given time to become familiar with it before it is handed over for the treatment of patients. Radiographers need time to practise the controls both inside and outside the room. Maintenance staff need time to study drawings and circuits and to locate principal components within the equipment—the simplest repair can take many hours if the technician does not know where to find the faulty component.

Quality assurance

Throughout the life of the equipment, it is essential to ensure that the data collected during commissioning continues to be relevant by monitoring the performance of the equipment through a programme of regular checks. These checks will take a variety of forms and be repeated at different intervals.

A separate log book must be maintained by the radiographer (and others) of all the faults which develop on each equipment—however trivial they may appear. This is important for two reasons. Where radiographers work in shifts on one piece of equipment or when their duties rotate through several pieces of equipment, no one person will be able to remember all the quirks of that equipment. The written log will reveal the frequency at which faults occur and the dates on which major repairs have been undertaken and, over a period of time, trends will be detectable which may assist in the maintenance programme. The log book records the random and intermittent events that inevitably occur. The quality control technician and the maintenance technician should examine the log book regularly.

A planned quality assurance programme does not wait for faults to happen, but looks for consistency in general and thereby finds discrepancies before they manifest themselves as faults. The programme will usually consist of daily, weekly, monthly checks and maybe 6-monthly or 12-monthly checks. The actual frequency of a particular check will be determined for each particular item of equipment. For example, the calibration of the output dose rate of an accelerator should be repeated at least weekly for photons and at

least twice weekly for electrons. For orthovoltage and lower energy X-ray generators, the output should be calibrated at least once every 4 weeks if an output dose rate monitor is fitted, but checked daily if there is no monitor fitted. If a prescribed attenuator is then placed in the primary beam, a second measurement can confirm the quality or penetration of the beam—this type of measurement may not be a precise measurement of HVL or quality index, but over a period of months the consistency of the result builds confidence in the equipment. Other beam parameters which should be included in the quality assurance programme will include beam flatness and symmetry, wedge correction factors, photon/optical beam alignment and beam size indication—particularly where there is no mechanical indication.

All the devices used for setting-up a patient's treatment should be included in the programme. These will include the alignment of the lasers, optical and mechanical pointers, scales, rotations about the isocentre, the security and alignment of head-rests, shadow trays, etc., the security of shielding blocks, wedges and other accessories.

It should not be necessary to check indicator lamps, because any failures should have been reported previously in the log book. The operation of interlocks and limit switches should be included, particularly if they are rarely used in clinical practice. Quality assurance is a shared responsibility between radiographers and medical physics staff and close cooperation is essential.

The preventative maintenance inspection is a vital part of the overall quality assurance programme carried out by the maintenance technician. The details need not concern the radiographer but will include checking water flows and air filters and the tightness of electrical connections, as well as the more intimate operation of the equipment itself.

The quality assurance programme is vital to any radiotherapy equipment and takes time to implement. How long depends on the complexity of the equipment. Fifteen to twenty per cent of the machine time is typical for megavoltage therapy equipment, but half that may be sufficient for other equipment. This investment in time does not preclude the possibility of breakdown but can minimise the unexpected interruptions to the treatment schedule.

4. The interaction of radiation with matter

All radiations have energy, either kinetic energy as in the case of moving charged particles, or inherent energy as in the case of electromagnetic radiation. When radiation passes through matter it may interact with the material, transferring some or all of its energy to the atoms of that material. A knowledge of the fundamentals of the interaction of radiations with matter is important because it forms the basis of radiobiology, radiation protection, radiation detection and the effective use of safe and appropriate methodologies in both radiodiagnosis and radiotherapy.

The presence of a beam of radiation is only apparent if some of the energy of the beam interacts with, and is transferred to, an absorbing material. If the radiation passes straight through a detector without interacting then it will not be detected. Similarly if it passes through tissue without interacting with the tissue then it will not have transferred any of its energy and hence will not have delivered a radiation dose to the tissue. The absorbing material with which the radiation interacts, whether it is a detector or tissue, consists of atoms.

At atomic level the radiation can interact with the nuclear region, the nuclear field or the extranuclear region or, because of the wide open spaces within the atom, it may pass straight through without interacting. How radiation reacts with matter depends upon many factors including: its mass, energy and electrical charge; and the atomic number, mass number and density of the medium.

INTERACTIONS OF CHARGED PARTICLES WITH MATTER

The charged particles of radiation include the electron, positron and alpha particle. The electron and positron may be ejected from a radioactive material during radioactive decay as positive or negative beta particles, Auger electrons or internal conversion electrons or, perhaps more importantly, they may be secondary forms of radiation resulting from photon interactions. It is these secondary charged particles which are responsible for the tissue damage attributed to X- and gamma rays.

The forces operating between the charged particles and the absorbing material are the electrostatic forces of attraction and repulsion which exist between charged bodies. The negatively charged electron will experience a repulsive force in encounters with the orbiting electrons of the atom, but an attractive force when in the vicinity of the positively charged nucleus. An alpha particle will experience the opposite interactive forces. The charged particle may 'excite' the atom to a higher energy level, it may dislodge an electron from the atom to form a positive and negative ion, or it may produce electromagnetic radiations. Each of these processes deplete the charged particle of some of its energy. We will now consider these interactions in more detail.

Excitation

The high speed particle may *excite* the atom by moving one of its outer electrons into a higher energy optical suborbit (Fig. 4.1A). The energy required to do this is only a few electron volts and hence the energy lost by the colliding incident particle is small. When the excited atom returns to the ground state it will give off the excess energy acquired in the interaction as heat, UV, or visible light. This is the mechanism involved in scintillation counters (Ch. 9).

Ionisation

If the incident particle completely removes an orbital electron from the atom then *ionisation* has occurred (Fig. 4.1B). The average energy required to form an ion pair in air is about 34 eV. Actually only about 15–20% of this energy is needed for the ionisation, the remainder is dissipated as excitation energy. If the ejected electron leaves the atom with a kinetic energy of about 100 eV then it is known as a delta ray and may in turn cause further ionisation and excitation (Fig. 4.4B).

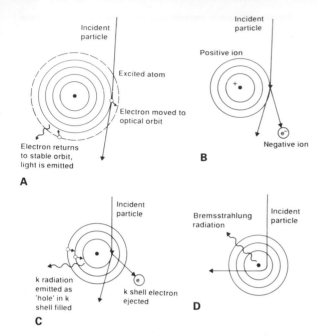

Fig. 4.1   Possible types of interaction between charged particles and the atoms of an absorbing medium. **A** Excitation, **B** ionisation, **C** characteristic radiation and **D** bremsstrahlung radiation.

Electromagnetic radiation

Characteristic radiation

If the charged particle collides with and ejects an electron from the inner K or L shells of the atom then a 'hole' will be left in the shell. When an electron falls into the 'hole' characteristic K or L radiation will be emitted (Fig. 4.1C).

Bremsstrahlung radiation

Occasionally the charged particle will pass very close to the nucleus of the atom and undergo a dramatic de-acceleration and energy loss. The energy lost is transformed into X-radiation (Fig. 4.1D). This radiation is known as *bremsstrahlung* from the German word meaning braking radiation. This process is unlikely at low particle energies but becomes increasingly more probable at higher energies.

For particles of a given energy the de-acceleration varies directly with the square of the atomic number Z of the absorber and z, the number of unit charges on the particle, and inversely with the mass of the particle M. Thus the intensity of bremsstrahlung varies between charged particles and materials as:

$$\frac{Z^2 z^2}{M^2}$$

It follows that particles of small mass such as electrons and positrons are much better producers of bremsstrahlung than the heavier alpha particles. Similarly materials of high atomic number such as lead and tungsten are more efficient producers of bremsstrahlung than low atomic number materials such as plastic and soft tissue.

The bremsstrahlung radiation appears as a continuous spectrum. Different amounts of energy are lost by the particles at each bremsstrahlung event. The maximum energy of the bremsstrahlung will equal the maximum energy of the particle and corresponds to the particle losing all its energy in one interaction. Bremsstrahlung radiations are the primary element of diagnostic X-rays. They are also a factor in radiation protection as they constitute a kind of extraneous radiation. The dependence of bremsstrahlung on Z means that a plastic shield is a more suitable material for protection against pure high energy beta particle emitters such as phosphorus-32 than the more usual high atomic number lead shields.

Annihilation radiation

A third form of electromagnetic radiation is associated with positron particles. Fast positrons interact with the orbiting electrons of the atoms without crashing into them, but as they lose energy and slow down they are pulled into contact with an electron. The opposite charges of the two particles cancel each other out and the masses of the two particles disappear or are *annihilated* (Fig. 4.2). The annihilation of the two particles results in the production of two annihilation photons; each has an energy of 0.511 MeV (Fig. 4.2). We discussed in Chapter 2 that the energy equivalence ($E = mc^2$) of a positron or an electron is 0.511 MeV. The two photons are indistinguishable from gamma rays except in one

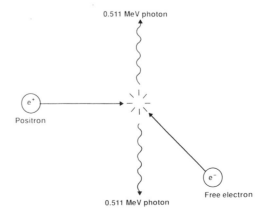

Fig. 4.2   The annihilation of a positron and an electron.

respect; they leave the site of collision in diametrically opposite directions. This feature is utilised in positron detectors.

Linear energy transfer

The energy that a particle dissipates to the absorbing medium per unit length of its path is termed the *linear energy transfer* (LET). It is usually expressed as kilo electron volts per micron (keV μm^{-1}). As a charged particle loses energy in one of the processes described above it will eventually lose all its kinetic energy until it is moving so slowly that it cannot cause further damage. At this point the electron will join a large group of free electrons, the alpha particle will pick up free electrons and become a neutral helium atom, and the positron will join with an electron and be annihilated. An inverse relationship exists between a particle's velocity and the resulting LET. The higher the velocity or kinetic energy (MeV), the lower the LET value. The LET value for a 1 MeV electron in water is 0.25 keV μm^{-1} while for a 0.1 MeV it is 0.4 keV μm^{-1}. The LET value is also dependent upon particle type; the heavy alpha particles move straight through material, dislodging atomic electrons and losing energy very rapidly. The LET of a 1 MeV alpha particle in water is 260 keV μm^{-1}.

Specific ionisation

The number of ion pairs produced per millimetre of path length travelled by the charged particle is called the specific ionisation (SI). It is directly related to the length of path along which the particle moves before being stopped and the electrical charge on the particle, and is inversely proportional to the velocity of the charged particle. Alpha particles relative to other particulate radiations are quite massive. They are not easily deflected by interactions with electrons and travel in straight lines (Fig. 4.4A). They possess a double positive electrical charge and so are highly ionising. The atomic electrons are pulled out of their orbits by the attractive force of the heavy alpha particle as it passes close by. An 8 MeV alpha particle has a range in air of 8 cm and has a specific ionisation value of about 2000 ion pairs per millimetre at the beginning of its path and about 7000 ion pairs per millimetre at the end of its track. As it slows down it literally spends more time electrically influencing the atoms along its path. This is illustrated in Figure 4.3b.

Positrons and electrons carry a single electrical charge and are relatively light, having the same mass as the atomic electrons. They are easily deflected and their path through matter is tortuous (Fig. 4.4B). For these

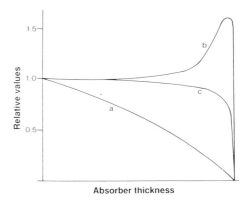

Fig. 4.3 Composite diagram of alpha particle interaction with matter. (a) Particle velocity, (b) specific ionisation and (c) range.

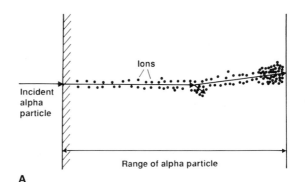

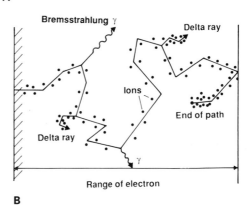

Fig. 4.4 The course through matter of **A** an alpha particle and **B** a beta particle.

reasons their specific ionisation is much less than for an alpha particle.

Particle range

The furthest distance penetrated by a charged particle from its point of origin to the position at which it no

Table 4.1 The range of some alpha and beta particles in water and in tissue

Energy (MeV)	Particle	Range in air (mm)	Range in water (mm)
8	α	7.3 x 10^1	1.0 x 10^{-1}
	β	3.4 x 10^4	4.1 x 10^1
1	α	5.0 x 10^0	7.0 x 10^{-3}
	β	3.5 x 10^3	4.2 x 10^0

longer interacts with the material is known as the range. The range of some alpha and beta particles in air and in water are given in Table 4.1. The maximum range of alpha particles in tissue is always less than 0.1 mm. They do not therefore constitute an external radiation hazard. However if alpha emitting nuclides are ingested and deposited in tissues the alpha particles which have high specific ionisation and LET values will cause significant radiation damage to the tissue.

The range of an electron or positron is much greater than the range of an alpha particle of equivalent energy. The specific ionisation is less and hence the local radiation damage to tissue is also less than for an alpha particle. However because of the very convoluted and tortuous path taken by the beta particle the straight line distance between the beginning and end of the beta particle track, i.e. the range, may be only half its path length.

INTERACTIONS OF X- AND GAMMA RAYS WITH MATTER

Photons (X- and gamma rays) react with matter in a very different way to the charged particles. They do not experience long range coulomb forces and interact only in direct collision processes. Hence the behaviour of a beam of photons differs from the behaviour of a beam of particles. Charged particles have a definite range in matter but photons are much more penetrating, have no definite range and demonstrate exponential absorption.

Intensity

The intensity of a beam of electromagnetic radiation is the amount of energy per unit of time crossing a unit area perpendicular to the beam. For example if one joule of energy passes through an area of one square metre every second then the intensity, I, equals one watt per square metre:

$$I = W\,m^{-2}$$

(watts = joules/second)

Inverse square law

When a photon beam diverges from its point of production its intensity is reduced as the distance from the source increases, in a manner determined by the inverse square law. This law indicates that for radiation spreading from a point source, in a non-absorbing medium, the intensity varies inversely with the square of the distance from the source to the point of measurement.

From an uncollimated point source the electromagnetic radiation radiates in all directions and each photon has an equal opportunity to pass through any chosen square centimetre of a sphere of radius, r, surrounding the point source, where the point source is at the centre of the sphere (Fig. 4.5). Provided there is no absorption or scattering of the beam all the photons leaving the source will pass through the surface of the sphere. The area of the surface of any sphere is given by $4\pi r^2$ cm^2. Therefore the intensity at any given distance r from the source S is given by:

$$I = \frac{S}{4\pi r^2}$$

and since S and 4π are constants the intensity is varying by $1/r^2$. If the power of the point source is 2012 W and we measure the intensity at distances of 2, 4 and 8 metres from the source then we find intensity values of 40, 10 and 2.5 W m^{-2} respectively.

The inverse square law holds for all radiations from a point source, provided there is no attenuation by

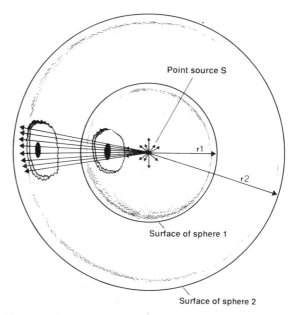

Fig. 4.5 The inverse square law.

absorption or scattering, whether it is collimated in a narrow beam or radiated in all directions.

Attenuation

When describing the attenuation of electromagnetic radiations with matter we must consider the radiations as waves, when describing their reflection and refraction, and as 'corpuscular' when considering their origin and interactions. They carry discrete quanta or packets of kinetic energy, travel at the speed of light (in vacuo), can exert forces on impact with certain objects and carry momentum. However they have no mass and therefore can only interact with the electrical fields around electrons and positrons and the electromagnetic field of the atomic nucleus. On passing through matter photons may pass straight through without interacting with the atoms of the medium, they may be totally absorbed by the medium (*photoelectric absorption*), they may be scattered from their original path without being absorbed (*classical scattering*), or they may be scattered and partially absorbed (*Compton scattering*), or scattered and partially or completely absorbed (*pair production*). Removal of radiation from the beam either by scattering or absorption is called attenuation. Before discussing the individual processes in more detail we will define the absorption coefficient and consider exponential absorption.

For homogeneous radiation, i.e. monochromatic radiation or radiation of one wavelength, the attenuation takes place according to the following law of attenuation. Equal thicknesses of the same attenuating material remove equal fractions of the radiation intensity incident on them and the fractional reduction of intensity per unit thickness of attenuator is constant.

This law of attenuation gives rise to an exponential attenuation curve (Fig. 4.6). It can be expressed by the mathematical equation:

$$I_t = I_o e^{-\mu t}$$

where I_t is the intensity transmitted through attenuator thickness t, I_o is the intensity with no attenuator present, t is the attenuator thickness, e is the mathematical constant ($=2.718$) and μ is a constant for a given material and a given photon energy of the radiation. μ is called the *total linear attenuation coefficient* and is defined as the fractional reduction of intensity per unit thickness of attenuator (for small thicknesses of attenuator). The product μt is the probability that a photon will be absorbed or scattered by a very thin absorber t.

The probability of a photon of electromagnetic radiation interacting with a single atom is very low. However in a solid substance there is a high concentration of

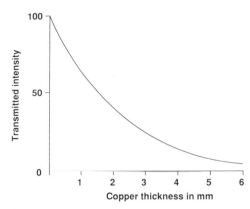

Fig. 4.6 Attenuation curve for homogeneous 100 keV X-rays being attenuated in copper.

atoms in a small volume. In any given area a proportion of this area is occupied by atoms which may block the transmission of the photons. Each atom offers a *cross-section* area, a, to the photon. The larger the value of a the greater is the chance of an interaction occurring. Figure 4.7 shows a very thin section of attenuating material having an area A, a thickness dt, and containing N atoms each of cross-sectional area a cm^2.

The total area blocking the transmission of the photons is $aNAdt$ cm^2. The product of the cross-section of each interaction centre and the number of interaction centres (aN) for a unit volume (Adt) of the target material is denoted by the symbol μ. The *cross section per unit volume* μ varies with photon energy and atomic number, as will be seen later in this chapter. You will have noticed that cross section per unit volume and total linear attenuation coefficient refer to the same physical quantity, and are measured in mm^{-1}. These two terms will be used interchangeably throughout the following text.

The mathematical form of the attenuation curve for homogeneous beams is the same as the mathematical form of the exponential decay curve of a single radioactive material (Ch. 2). The exponential attenuation curve similarly has two characteristic properties. First, if plotted logarithmically, that is, if log I_t/I_o is plotted against t, a straight line is obtained whose slope is $-\mu$, where μ is the attenuation coefficient. Second, there is a

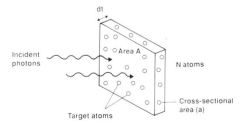

Fig. 4.7 The concept of 'cross section' of target atoms.

constant value of thickness of attenuator which reduces the incident intensity to half its initial value. This is called the *half value thickness* (HVT). It will be seen that the attenuation curve of Figure 4.6 corresponds to an HVT of 1.5 mm of copper. These two properties hold for homogeneous radiation.

The quantity μ, the attenuation coefficient, is a constant for a particular photon energy of the beam and for a particular attenuating material. It increases with the density, and the atomic number of the attenuator and decreases with increasing photon energy of the beam.

It can easily be shown that there is a simple relationship between the HVT of a homogeneous beam and the attenuation coefficient μ. This is as follows:

$$\text{HVT} = \frac{0.693}{\mu}$$

where HVT is expressed in mm and μ is expressed in mm^{-1}.

In shielding and radiation dosimetry we may refer to the *tenth value thickness* (TVT). That is the thickness of absorbing material which will reduce the radiation to one-tenth of its unattenuated value. This is given by:

$$\text{TVT} = \frac{2.3}{\mu}$$

Mass attenuation coefficient

In Figure 4.7 the absorber of thickness dt reduces the intensity of the radiation via interactions between the photons and the electrons and atoms in the absorber. The attenuation produced by a layer (dt) will depend upon the number of atoms in the layer. If the layer could be compressed to half its thickness it would still contain the same number of atoms and hence still attenuate the same number of photons. However the linear attenuation coefficient (attenuation per mm) would be doubled. Linear attenuation is therefore dependent on the density of the material. If the constant μ is divided by the density ρ of the attenuating material a quantity (μ/ρ) is obtained which is independent of the density of the attenuator. This is known as the *total mass attenuation coefficient* and gives the fractional reduction of intensity if the beam passes through an attenuating layer of thickness 1 g mm^{-2} or 1 kg m^{-2}. The significance of the word 'total' in these definitions of attenuation coefficients will be shown on page 67.

The total mass attenuation coefficient changes rapidly with the photon energy (i.e. the wavelength) of the beam and the atomic number Z of the attenuator but the relation is a complicated one. This is because attenuation, that is the loss of energy from the beam, arises from a number of processes of interaction between the beam photons and the electrons in the attenuating material. A rough guide, however, is as follows. For the low photon energy, long wavelength, region of the X-ray spectrum (i.e. for diagnostic X-rays for example) μ/ρ is roughly proportional to Z^3 and to λ^3 or $1/(h\nu)^3$. In the high photon energy, short wavelength, region of the spectrum (i.e. for high energy radiotherapy beams) μ/ρ is roughly proportional to λ or $1/h\nu$ and is largely independent of Z.

Classical scattering

For long wavelength radiations, that is soft diagnostic X-rays and in materials of high atomic numbers such as metals when the energy of the photon will be much less than the binding energy of the electrons in the absorbing medium, then the photon may be scattered or re-radiated with no loss of energy. This radiation is of the same wavelength as the incident radiation. This scattering phenomenon is similar to the scattering of light from dust particles. Since it can be explained by well-established theories which treat X-rays as a wave propagation, it is often referred to as *classical scattering*, or alternatively as *elastic*, *unmodified* or *coherent scattering*. It does not contribute any real absorption of energy to an attenuator since no fast electrons are liberated from the attenuator atoms. This type of scattering is relatively unimportant in medical uses of X-rays since low photon energy beams and high atomic number attenuators are not the normal conditions in such use.

The Compton effect

In practice it is found that when shorter wavelength, more energetic radiation beams are used to irradiate materials of low atomic number, such as tissue, the electromagnetic radiation interacts with a 'free' electron in the attenuating medium. A collision-like process occurs in which the incident photon gives up some of its energy to the electron, known as a 'recoil or Compton electron', and the remainder of the energy appears as a scattered photon of lower energy. The energy of the incident photon, therefore, is shared between the scattered photon of longer wavelength and the recoil electron. In addition the greater the angle through which the photon is scattered the longer is the wavelength of the scattered radiation. This scattered radiation is called *modified scatter* and the process is referred to as *inelastic scattering* or *Compton scattering*.

This type of interaction is represented diagrammatically in Figure 4.8. The incident photon of energy $h\nu_1$ (i.e. the product of Planck's constant and the frequency)

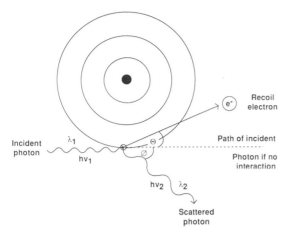

Fig. 4.8 The Compton scattering effect.

and wavelength λ_1 collides with the electron and produces a recoil electron with kinetic energy E_e at an angle θ and a scattered photon of reduced energy $h\nu_2$ and longer wavelength λ_2 at an angle ϕ.

Since total energy is always conserved $h\nu_1 = h\nu_2 + E_e$, the energy of the electron and the energy of the scattered photon depend upon the original energy of the incident photon and the angle of scattering of the Compton photon as follows:

$$h\nu_2 = \frac{h\nu_1}{1 + \dfrac{h\nu_1}{mc^2}(1 - \cos\phi)} = \frac{h\nu_1}{1 + \dfrac{h\nu_1}{0.511}(1 - \cos\phi)} \quad (4.1)$$

where mc^2 is the rest energy of the electron. As we saw in Chapter 2 this can be expressed in MeV and is 0.511 MeV. A range of energies from a maximum to a minimum are possible for the scattered photon and the recoil electron, however their values are inversely related as the total energy must remain the same as the energy of the initial incident photon. Minimum photon energy occurs when the incident photon makes a direct hit, ejecting the electron straight forward and scattering the Compton photon back through 180° (the cosine of 180° is –1 and hence $1 - \cos\phi = +2$, equation 4.1). Conversely

maximum photon energy occurs when the incident photon makes only a glancing collision with the electron ejecting it with an angle θ of 90° and scattering the Compton photon with an angle ϕ of ~0° (the cosine of 0° is +1 and hence $1 - \cos\phi = 0$). Any number of intermediate collisions is possible and Table 4.2 gives values of the energies of the scattered photon and the recoil electron for a selection of incident photon energies and scattering angles.

It can be seen from the table that low energy photons do not lose much energy upon scattering. The 50 keV photon loses at maximum only 8 keV. On the other hand the high energy 1 MeV photon loses 796 keV of energy upon 180° scattering. The proportion of photons scattered in different directions varies with the energy of the incident photon; low energy photons are scattered in all directions with almost equal probability, whilst high energy photons, greater than about 1 MeV, are scattered principally in the forward direction.

The recoil electron behaves the same as any electron, it is so named to indicate its origin. Since the recoil electron has been given kinetic energy it can now undergo the various types of electronic particle interactions described earlier in this chapter. It is indeed the recoil electron resulting from the Compton collision which causes the radiation damage to the tissue, not the initial photon interaction which has created only one ion directly.

We have stated that the photons interact with 'free' electrons. The term 'free' electron refers to those electrons in which the binding energy is small compared to that of the incident photon. The binding energy of the outer electrons in light elements, such as the primary building blocks of soft tissue, is only a few electron volts (eV). This is quite small compared to the energy of a photon of even the soft X-rays used in medical work—which is generally more than 50 keV .

Mass attenuation absorption and scatter coefficient

The Compton effect occurs with free electrons so the cross-section σ can be expressed in terms of target area

Table 4.2 Energies of Compton scattered photons and recoil electrons

Incident photon energy (MeV)	Angle ϕ of scattered photon							
	30°		90°		120°		180°	
	$h\nu_2$	E_e	$h\nu_2$	E_e	$h\nu_2$	E_e	$h\nu_2$	E_e
0.05	0.049	0.001	0.046	0.004	0.044	0.006	0.042	0.008
0.10	0.097	0.003	0.084	0.016	0.077	0.023	0.072	0.028
0.50	0.442	0.058	0.253	0.247	0.202	0.298	0.169	0.331
1.00	0.792	0.208	0.338	0.662	0.254	0.746	0.204	0.796

per electron. Therefore, with the exception of hydrogen, the Compton effect is independent of atomic number. This is because (1) all electrons have the same cross-section for interaction with photons of a given energy, and (2) the ratio of neutrons to protons is similar for all elements and hence all elements contain approximately the same number of electrons per gram (3×10^{23}). Hydrogen is an exception as it contains no neutrons and hence the number of electrons per gram is twice that of other elements (6×10^{23}). The significance of this is discussed in Chapter 5. It follows that the attenuation per gram by the Compton process, and hence the mass attenuation coefficient σ/ρ for any given photon energy, is the same for all materials except hydrogen. The mass attenuation coefficient for Compton scattering is given by:

$$\sigma/\rho = \frac{1}{h\nu} \qquad (4.2)$$

It can be seen from the above equation that σ/ρ is inversely proportional to energy and so decreases as $h\nu$ increases.

The mass absorption coefficient for Compton scattering is given by σ_a/ρ. This represents the energy transferred to the recoil electron, and hence deposited in the absorbing medium. As we saw in the previous section the higher the photon energy the greater is the proportion of that energy which is given up to the electron. The mass scattering coefficient σ_s/ρ represents the proportion of the energy removed by the scattered photon. This will decrease with increasing incident energy.

The mass attenuation, absorption and scattering coefficients for different incident photon energies are depicted graphically in Figure 4.9. The mass absorption coefficient increases with increasing energy up to about 1 MeV and then decreases again, whilst the mass scattering coefficient decreases with increasing energy. These two curves cross at about 1.5 MeV; this is the point at which the scattered photon and the recoil electron carry away equal amounts of energy. At energies below 1.5 MeV the greater fraction σ_s/σ_a is removed by the scattered photon. Above 1.5 MeV the greater fraction σ_a/σ_s is removed by the recoil electron. This latter fraction is used to determine the radiation dose to patients and the energy transfer due to Compton collision.

The mass attenuation coefficient, which is a measure of the total energy removed from the primary beam by the Compton process, is given by:

$$\sigma/\rho = \sigma_a/\rho + \sigma_s/\rho$$

It is seen to decrease with increasing energy, as predicted by equation 4.2.

Summary of the Compton process. To summarise, the important properties of the Compton process are as follows:

1. The wavelength of the scattered radiation increases as the angle of scattering relative to the incident beam increases.

2. The energy of the incident beam is shared between recoil electrons in the attenuator and scattered photons of longer wavelength. If the photon energy of the incident beam is low, the proportion of the energy appearing as scattered electromagnetic radiation is high, but for incident beams of high photon energy the majority of the energy lost from the beam appears as energy of recoil electrons.

3. As the incident photon energy increases, the scattered electromagnetic radiation is concentrated more and more in the forward direction.

4. The recoil electrons are emitted mainly in the forward direction and are increasingly concentrated in the direction of the incident beam as the energy of the incident photons increases.

5. The total attenuation of a beam produced by the Compton process is independent of the atomic number of the attenuator (except for hydrogen) but increases with the wavelength of the radiation, that is it decreases as the photon energy of the radiation increases.

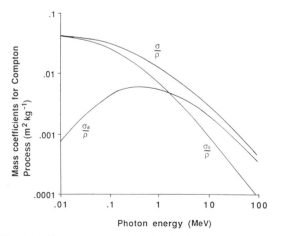

Fig. 4.9 The mass attenuation (σ/ρ), absorption (σ_a/ρ) and scattering (σ_s/ρ) coefficients for Compton scattering.

The photoelectric process

The photoelectric process involves an interaction between an incident photon and a 'bound' electron. We saw earlier that if the incident photon had low energy compared to the binding energy then classical scattering

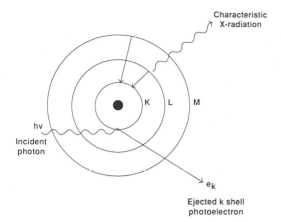

Fig. 4.10 Photoelectric absorption with the subsequent emission of characteristic X-rays.

occurs. If, however, the incident photon has an energy just greater than the binding energy of the electron a complete transfer of the photon energy to the electron occurs. This is shown schematically in Figure 4.10.

A photon of energy hv ejects a K shell electron of binding energy BE_k. The electron escapes from the atom with an energy E_k equal to that of the incident photon minus the energy required to release it from its orbit.

$$E_k = hv - BE_k$$

There is no scattered photon; all the energy has been transferred to the electron, now known as a *photoelectron*. Interactions of this kind can take place with electrons in the K, L, M and N shells.

The probability of a photoelectric process occurring depends upon the photon energy. The energy of the photon has an adverse effect on the photoelectric cross section τ. Figure 4.11 shows the mass attenuation coefficient for the photoelectric process, τ/ρ, plotted

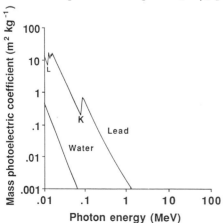

Fig. 4.11 Photoelectric mass attenuation coefficients for water and lead.

against incident photon energy for two materials, lead and (tissue equivalent) water. For water, where the graph is a rapidly falling straight line, the mass attenuation coefficient is approximately inversely proportional to the cube of the photon energy.

$$\tau/\rho \propto \frac{1}{(hv)^3}$$

For lead the picture is a little more complicated. The graph shows a series of vertical 'breaks' or 'edges' with straight portions between them. The probability of a photoelectric interaction occurring is greatest when the photon energy is equal to or just greater than the binding energy of the electron and decreases rapidly thereafter. If the photon has sufficient energy to liberate a K shell electron it will transfer its energy to that electron rather than to one further from the nucleus.

The K edge for lead occurs at 88 keV, which is the binding energy of the K shell in lead. At this point the attenuation coefficient increases by a factor of about 5. Thus there is about a 5:1 preference for the K shell electrons over the other shells. If the energy of the incident photon is less than the binding energy of the K shell the photon will transfer its energy to a less tightly bound electron, always preferring the inner to the outer shells. In the straight portions between the edges the mass attenuation coefficient is again reduced by approximately $1/(hv)^3$ as the energy of the incident photon increases. However as we have seen at the edges this law does not apply and a high energy photon may have a higher mass attenuation coefficient than a lower energy one.

Figure 4.11 also demonstrates that the attenuation coefficient in lead is approximately 1000 times greater than in water. The mass attenuation coefficient is approximately proportional to the cube of the atomic number. Hence:

$$\tau/\rho \propto \frac{Z^3}{(hv)^3}$$

This is an important factor in producing high contrast between bone and soft tissue in diagnostic radiography and in the use of lead in radiation protection.

Since the photoelectric process results in the emission of an electron from a position in one of the shells of the atom of the attenuator, a vacant space is left in that shell. A readjustment is made by electrons falling into vacancies producing characteristic X-rays and Auger electrons. This shell filling process is the same as that following internal conversion described in Chapter 2; it should also be compared but not confused with the emission of characteristic radiation from an X-ray target (Ch. 1).

The photoelectric interaction prevails over Compton scattering for low energy photons and high atomic number absorbing materials. The atom completely absorbs the photon in a photoelectric event and the energy of the photon is converted into electron energy. Once again it is the electron which transfers the energy to the absorbing material and produces the radiation damage in tissue.

Summary of the photoelectric process. To summarise, the important properties of the photoelectric effect are:

1. All of the energy of the incident beam is given up to the photoelectron.
2. Characteristic X-rays and Auger electrons may be produced.
3. The probability of occurrence increases with the cube of the atomic number of the absorbing medium.
4. The probability of occurrence decreases with the cube of the photon energy except when the energy is just greater than the binding energy of the electrons, at which point absorption edges occur.

Pair production

One further interaction process occurs for photons whose energy is greater than 1.022 MeV. Photons of energy greater than this may interact with the electric field around the nucleus. This interaction results in the complete absorption of the photon and the simultaneous creation of two electrons, one positive and one negative (sometimes referred to as a positron and a negatron respectively), as shown in Figure 4.12. The production of these two electrons represents the creation of matter from energy. The equivalence of matter and energy was set out by Einstein in quantitative form by the equation $E = mc^2$. This has been discussed in Chapter 2 where we saw that the energy equivalent to the mass of one electron is 0.511 MeV. In order to create two electrons,

therefore, a minimum energy of 1.022 MeV is necessary. Since the electrons are opposite in charge no creation of charge is involved in pair production. If the energy of the initiating photon hv is greater than 1.022 MeV then the excess energy will appear as kinetic energy, E, shared between the electrons:

$$hv = mc^2 + mc^2 + E^+ + E^-$$

Thus for an 8 MeV photon the sum of the kinetic energies for the two particles will be 8 – 1.022 = 6.978 MeV. The most probable distribution is for this energy to be shared equally between the positron and the electron. However all the energy may be given to one or other particle and a spectrum of possible particle energies exists. Just as in the case of Compton scattering and the photoelectric process the kinetic energy of each particle is then dissipated in the absorbing medium.

As we have seen previously the positive electron does not have an isolated existence when at rest and when it comes to rest it combines with a neighbouring electron. The two charges neutralise each other and the mass of the two electrons is converted back into two photons of electromagnetic radiation, each of 0.511 MeV energy, travelling in opposite directions to each other. This is annihilation radiation and is shown in Figure 4.2.

The mass absorption coefficient for pair production is usually represented by π/ρ. The pair production process occurs only for radiations of photon energy greater than 1.022 MeV. Above this energy, however, the probability of the process occurring increases rapidly with increase of photon energy. This is the only attenuation process therefore in which attenuation *increases* with increasing photon energy. The cross-section for the pair production process also increases with increasing atomic number of the attenuator. This is because pair production occurs in the nuclear field and the electric field around the nucleus increases with increasing Z. Thus

$$\pi/\rho \propto (hv - 1.02) \cdot Z$$

In practice this process is of little importance in the low atomic number elements of soft tissue except above about 20 MeV radiation. In industrial radiography, however, when high energy beams are used to penetrate metals it can become the major attenuation process.

Summary of the pair production process. To summarise, the important properties of the pair production process are:

1. An electron and a positron are produced.
2. The photon energy must be at least 1.022 MeV.
3. The probability of occurrence increases with increasing energy (hv–1.022) and with increasing atomic number.

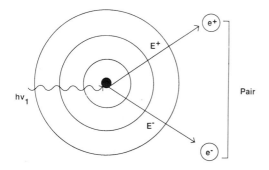

Fig. 4.12   The absorption of photons by pair production.

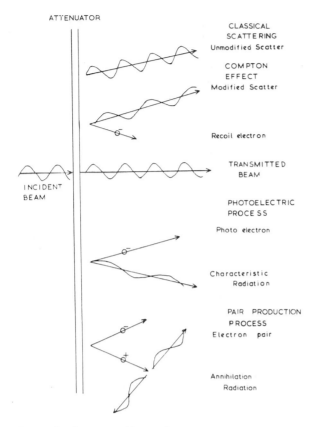

Fig. 4.13   Summary of interaction processes

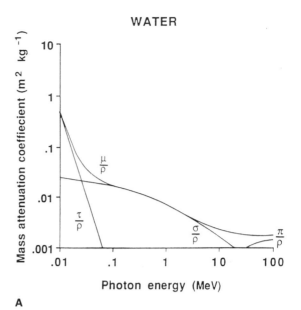

A

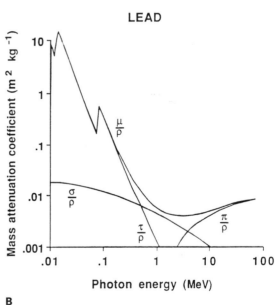

B

Fig. 4.14   Mass attenuation coefficient for **A** water and **B** lead.

Summary of interaction processes

Figure 4.13 summarises the four processes which are involved in the loss of energy from a beam of photons passing through an attenuating material.

Some of these processes give rise to deposition of energy in the attenuator, via charged particle interactions. They are: (1) the photoelectric process, (2) that part of the Compton process that gives rise to recoil electrons and (3) the pair production process. The rest of the energy lost to the main beam either escapes from the attenuator as scattered radiation or gives rise to further interactions remote from the first. This includes (a) classical scattering of long waves, (b) the characteristic radiation following the photoelectric process, (c) the scatter component of the Compton effect and (d) the annihilation radiation arising from the pair production process.

Total mass attenuation coefficient

When a *single* photon interacts with matter any one of the processes described above may occur. When a beam of photons interacts with matter all of them may occur. The total mass attenuation coefficient discussed at the beginning of this section is composed of the contributions from each of the processes. Thus:

$$\mu/\rho \;=\; \sigma/\rho \;+\; \tau/\rho \;+\; \pi/\rho$$
Total   Compton   Photoelectric   Pair Production

The total mass attenuation coefficient, being the sum

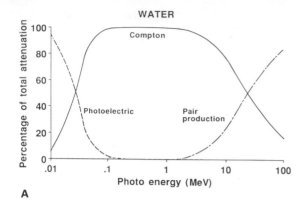

A

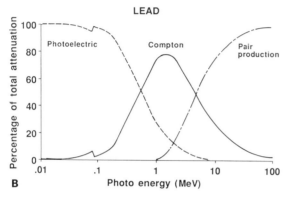

B

Fig. 4.15 The percentage contribution to the total attenuation from each of the three processes **A** in water and **B** in lead.

of the three partial attenuation coefficients, varies in a complicated way with both photon energy $h\nu$ and atomic number Z. The total mass attenuation coefficients and the relative contribution of the individual coefficients for water and for lead are shown in Figure 4.14.

Initially the rapid variation of the photoelectric effect with $h\nu$ and Z is the predominating influence and the total attenuation curves fall rapidly with increasing energy. The absorption edges are pronounced in the high atomic number materials. The curves decrease more slowly in the region where the Compton effect, σ/ρ, is the important influence. The Compton effect is independent of atomic number and is therefore similar for both tissue and lead. Finally the curve rises slightly at high energies due to pair production. For soft tissue the rise in total coefficient at high energies is negligible as the decrease in Compton effect is matched by the increase in pair production. However in lead the rise in the curve at high energies is quite marked. Hence for high atomic number materials increasing the energy of the photon results in a *less* penetrating beam. Figure 4.15 shows the

percentage contribution to the total attenuation of each of the three processes. It can be seen that for water (soft tissue) the Compton process dominates over a wide range of energies (0.03 to 20 MeV), but for lead the photoelectric effect and pair production are important. These curves have important implications for the differential absorption of photons in bone and soft tissue and for the choice of absorbing materials in radiation protection.

If photoelectric absorption predominates the bone will absorb approximately six times as much energy as soft tissue. For diagnostic X-rays operating between 60 and 140 kV this will give good contrast. When Compton absorption is the dominant process bone and soft tissue absorb approximately the same amount of energy per gram. This is advantageous in radiotherapy, particularly when treating tumours through, or overlying, bony structures. Pair production is only of importance with very high photon energies when bone will absorb approximately twice as much energy as soft tissue.

Real energy absorption

When a beam of electromagnetic radiation is attenuated in a medium all the interaction processes involved give rise to some form of electromagnetic radiation as a secondary product. This radiation does not cause the direct deposition of energy to the attenuating medium, though as scattered radiation it has important effects both in diagnostic radiology and in radiotherapy and is very important from the point of view of radiation hazard control. Energy is only transferred to the attenuating medium through the production of fast electrons which produce ionisation in the medium. Real energy absorption arises therefore from photoelectrons, the recoil electrons of the Compton process and the pair of electrons in the pair production process.

In terms of partial attenuation coefficients, therefore, real energy absorption over the main range of photon energies used in radiotherapy can be represented by the coefficients: $\tau/\rho + \sigma_a/\rho$ where τ/ρ is the mass photoelectric attenuation coefficient and σ_a/ρ is the mass attenuation coefficient representing the conversion of the incident photon energy to energy of recoil electrons in the Compton process. We have seen that σ_a is an increasingly high proportion of the coefficient σ for the whole Compton attenuation process as the photon energy increases. For very high photon energy beams where the pair production process becomes important an additional contribution to real energy absorption in the medium will arise from the kinetic energy of the two electrons produced in the interaction. Calculations on the real energy absorbed using these partial attenuation

Table 4.3 Some examples of the electron ranges involved in the attenuation processes.

Photon energy of incident radiation	Energy of electrons		Range in tissue
50 keV	Photoelectron	50 keV	42 μm
	Recoil electron	4–8 keV	0.5–1.7 μm
250 keV	Recoil electron	50 keV	42 μm
1 MeV	Recoil electron	500 keV	2 mm
8 MeV	Recoil electron	5 MeV	28 mm

coefficients are relevant to the problem of dose measurement discussed in Chapter 5.

Electron ranges in tissue

The ranges of the electrons responsible for the ionisation in the attenuating medium and therefore for the deposition of energy, vary with the incident photon energy (Table 4.3). For X-rays in the diagnostic range the ranges in tissue are very small but at high photon energies used in megavoltage therapy the electron ranges become larger and of the order of several millimetres. They thus become comparable with the size of the coarse structure of the tissues being treated. The range then has profound effects on the distribution of absorbed energy in tissues. This will be dealt with in Chapter 5.

Measurements of radiation

Later chapters of this book will describe in detail the methods by which reliable quantitative measurements of X- and gamma rays can be obtained and used in radiotherapy. It can be seen from the description of the processes of interaction between photon beams and matter given in this chapter that two concepts of measurement are possible. It is possible, for example, to seek a quantitative estimate of the total flow of photons at a point in space or in tissue being irradiated by an X- or gamma ray beam. In practice this flow of photons is measured by ionisation produced in air or in an appropriate air cavity within an irradiated medium. The quantity so measured is referred to as *exposure*. On the other hand, energy is only transferred to a medium subject to this irradiation when secondary electrons are produced which deposit energy. This energy is the absorbed energy and a quantitative estimate of this is referred to as the *absorbed dose*. Both of these two concepts of measurement are in use and it is important to distinguish them and the measurement units involved. An illustration might help to clarify the difference. When one moves round the garden in sunlight one is bombarded from all sides by photons of light of a variety of wavelengths. Some of these are the primary photons from the sun and some are scattered photons from the environment. This photon flux is equivalent to exposure, as referred to above. However some of these photons enter the eye and by producing chemical changes on the retina impart visual information. Similarly some enter the skin and produce chemical changes leading to pigmentation. This is equivalent to absorbed dose. Exposure and absorbed dose are clearly related to each other. The second is proportional to the first but the constant of proportionality will depend on a variety of conditions. In tissues being irradiated the constant of proportionality will depend on the relative magnitudes of the different processes of attenuation and therefore on the photon energy distribution in the irradiating field and on the atomic number of the medium. Figure 4.14 has illustrated that the relationship between exposure and absorbed dose can be expected to be complex.

5. The measurement of X- and gamma ray beams

INTRODUCTION

The primary interaction processes discussed in the last chapter showed that the effect of radiation on matter is to produce ionisation. It is this ionisation which precipitates biological damage in living tissues. The same processes, however, give rise to the absorption of energy from the radiation beam by the tissues. To measure the absorbed energy is therefore to measure the intensity of the radiation *and* the ability of the tissues to absorb the radiation. Both these concepts will be explored in this chapter.

The dependence of the absorption coefficients on photon energy and atomic number is seen in this chapter in two forms of differential absorption: (1) photons of the same energy will be differentially absorbed in the different tissues; and (2) photons of different energy will be differentially absorbed in the same filter.

The concept of exposure

Exposure is a measure of the photon flux (or flow of photons) to which the point of interest (the air) is subjected in a given time. It is a measure of the amount of ionisation (the number of ions) produced in a unit mass of air under standard conditions. The formal definition of exposure as adopted by the International Commission on Radiological Units (ICRU) in 1962 is as follows:

$$X = \Delta Q / \Delta m$$

where ΔQ is the sum of the electrical charge on all the ions of one sign produced in air when all the electrons liberated by photons in a volume element of air whose mass is Δm are completely stopped in air.

There is no special unit for exposure in the SI system and the units are simply coulombs per kilogram (C/kg) of dry air. Previously the special unit was the roentgen (R) and equal to 1 esu of charge per 0.001293 g of dry air or 2.58×10^{-4} C/kg. The definition quoted above is a strict and formal one. The old definition of the roentgen was less precise but helps to explain the conditions under which measurements of exposure are made. The roentgen was 'that amount of X- or gamma radiation such that the associated corpuscular emission per 0.001293 g of dry air produces, in air, ions carrying one electrostatic unit of charge of either sign.' The density of dry air at standard temperature and pressure is 0.001293 g cm^{-3}. The description of the standard free air ionisation chamber below illustrates how the measurement of exposure can be made in practice. It should be noted that the concept of exposure is confined to photon beams in air. Its advantage in radiotherapy lies in the fact that both the measurement of exposure (in air) and its conversion to absorbed dose in tissue are relatively easy.

The concept of kerma

A high energy electron can travel a considerable distance in air and produces ionisation throughout the length of its track. Since the definition of exposure demands that all such electrons liberated by photons are completely stopped in air, the collection of charge could be very remote from the mass of air where the electron originated. This meant the roentgen was never defined above about 3 MeV. However, the number of ionisations produced by a high speed electron is determined by its initial kinetic energy, since the energy required to produce one ionisation in air is constant and the energy lost in bremsstrahlung production is negligible. It follows therefore that the exposure (X) is closely related to the total kinetic energy of all the electrons liberated by the photons in the same volume element of air, namely

$$K_a = X(W/e)$$

where W is the mean energy required to produce one

ionisation in air ($W = 5.39 \times 10^{-19}$ J) and e is the charge on the electron (1.6×10^{-18} C). Therefore

$$K_a = 33.9X \text{ Jkg}^{-1}$$

This concept of the kinetic energy of the electrons liberated is given the name KERMA—an acronym for the *Kinetic Energy Released* per unit *Mass*—and defined by ICRU as follows:

$$K = \Delta E_{tr}/\Delta m$$

where ΔE_{tr} is the sum of the initial kinetic energies of all the charged particles liberated by uncharged ionising particles in a material of mass Δm. Since kerma is an energy per unit mass, its units are joules per kilogram. The reader will note that kerma is not confined to photons in air, as was the case with exposure, but *air kerma*, K_a, can be defined and is related to exposure, X, by the equation given above.

The concept of absorbed dose

While kerma is a measure of the energy released by photons in a small mass of absorber, that energy may not be totally deposited in the same small mass but carried by the energetic electrons to be deposited in neighbouring masses of the absorber. Our major interest in radiotherapy is the energy actually deposited in a small mass and this we call the absorbed dose. ICRU defines absorbed dose as

$$D = \Delta E_d/\Delta m$$

where ΔE_d is the energy imparted by ionising radiation to the matter in a volume element of mass Δm. This definition encompasses all absorbing materials and all types of ionising radiation. The special unit of absorbed dose is the gray

$$1 \text{ Gy} = 1 \text{ J/kg}^{-1}$$

The old unit of absorbed dose, the rad (= 0.01 J/kg^{-1}) has been replaced by the gray, although the centigray (1 cGy = 1 rad) has come into common usage for obvious reasons.

Absorbed dose in many cases is difficult to measure and is usually calculated from the measurement of exposure and knowledge of the real mass absorption coefficients of air and tissue.

STANDARD FREE AIR IONISATION CHAMBER

The standard free air ionisation chamber is a purely laboratory instrument and is of no practical value in the radiotherapy department. It is, however, a fundamental instrument in that it is a practical interpretation

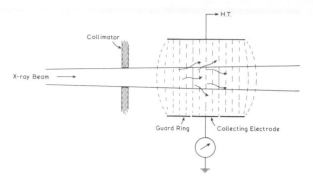

Fig. 5.1 The standard free ionisation chamber.

of the definition of exposure, enabling measurements to be made of the charge liberated from a known mass of air. Ionisation chambers of this type can be found at national standardising laboratories and form the basis for the standardisation of the day-to-day ionisation chambers used routinely in radiotherapy departments and elsewhere.

The measurements are made under strictly standardised conditions. A beam of radiation is passed between two parallel plates (electrodes) under conditions such that the volume where the primary ionisation is taking place is known accurately. The ions produced are collected and measured. The apparatus is illustrated in Figure 5.1.

A narrow and accurately defined beam of radiation passes between two parallel electrodes. Between the two electrodes a potential difference is maintained so that ions of one sign are collected on one electrode while those of the opposite sign travel to the other. The potential difference between these electrodes must be sufficient to collect all the ions liberated—and to prevent any recombination of the (negative) electrons and positive ions—that is, the ion chamber must operate under *saturation conditions*. This is a very important precaution that must be observed when ionisation chambers of any form are employed. It should also be noted that if the rate at which the air is ionised is increased then to maintain the saturation condition, the potential difference will need to be increased. This is particularly important where the radiation is pulsed, for the dose rate during each pulse can be very high compared with the mean. One electrode consists of two sections, an inner collecting electrode and, insulated from it, an annular electrode known as a *guard ring*. The collecting electrode and the guard ring are maintained at the same potential by an external connection. When an electric field is maintained between parallel plate electrodes, its strength is uniform over the central area but weaker at the edges. Alternatively, it can be said that the lines of electrostatic force over the central area are straight and perpendicular to the electrodes while at the edges they are not. Isolating the collecting electrode from the guard ring by a narrow insulated region guarantees the uniformity of the electric field and, in particular, the lines of force will be straight and perpendicular over the whole area of the collecting electrode. By this means a volume of air is defined. The cross-sectional area of the beam is predetermined by the accurate collimation and the length of the beam within the measuring system is determined by the length of the collecting electrode. The mass of air in the volume so defined can be calculated from the known ambient conditions (of atmospheric temperature and pressure) and the electric charge liberated is measured directly on the collecting electrode. This charge is small and very sensitive instruments are required.

In using the free air chamber, care must be taken to ensure that the distance between the plates is so large that the high speed electrons produced in the central region of the chamber lose all their kinetic energy in the production of ions before they hit the electrodes. For X-rays generated at 200 kV, the plates will be of the order of 20 cm apart, the separation increasing with photon energy. The overall chamber size is, therefore, large and it is this size which places the rather arbitrary 3 MeV limit on the measurement of exposure.

In addition the collimating system and the exit port of the chamber must be far enough from the prescribed air volume so that electrons released from them lose all their kinetic energy before reaching the air volume. This isolation of the volume from the surrounding components, by a wall of air of a thickness which is greater than the range of the most energetic electrons, is the reason for describing the chamber as 'free air' and an appreciation of this requirement will assist the reader to understand the need for an *air equivalent wall* in more practical chambers.

It will be appreciated that photo- and Compton electrons will be released at all points within the beam and not only in the collection volume and that these electrons will follow tortuous paths of considerable length before losing all their kinetic energy by producing further ionisations—each will produce several hundred further ionisations. It is inevitable that some electrons originating outside the collection volume will enter that volume and contribute to the collection of charge, but fortunately the converse is also true, i.e. electrons originating inside the volume will stray outside and the ions these produce will be collected by the guard ring and lost; what is gained is balanced by what is lost. A state of *electronic equilibrium* is said to exist. It

can, therefore, be assumed that the ions collected by the collecting electrode, and therefore measured, all originate from the collection volume.

PRACTICAL IONISATION CHAMBERS

Three aspects of the free air chamber must be applied to practical chambers, these are:

— The chamber must operate under saturation conditions.
— There must be an air (equivalent) wall.
— The air mass must be determined from the fixed volume and corrected for the ambient temperature and pressure.

Thimble chamber

For clinical purposes the exposure at a point can be measured using a *thimble ionisation chamber*. This term describes an ionisation chamber in which a small volume of air is enclosed in a thimble-like conducting cap with an insulated axial collecting electrode (Fig. 5.2A). The cap is often made of a unit density material such as graphite or nylon made conducting by a layer of colloidal graphite on the inner surface or Shonka plastic. The central electrode may be aluminium. The insulator may be amber but Perspex and polythene are often used. If a potential difference (usually a few hundred volts) is maintained between the cap and the collecting electrode, then radiation falling on the chamber will ionise the air and an ionisation current will flow between the two electrodes. The polarising voltage must not be so large that it causes ionisation of the air enclosed in the chamber. Such a chamber will give an accurate measure of the exposure providing (1) the walls are made of a material with the same atomic number as

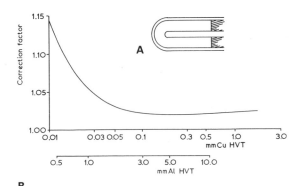

Fig. 5.2　A A thimble ionisation chamber and **B** a typical correction curve for its energy response.

air, and (2) that the wall has a thickness greater than the range of the electrons produced in the material. A chamber wall of unit density material 1 mm thick would be equivalent to approximately 75 cm of air (the density of dry air being 0.001293 g cm⁻³). The actual wall thickness required is determined by the energy of the radiation to be measured. For low energy radiations a very thin-walled chamber is required (e.g. 2 mg cm⁻²) as the electron range in the material is small and the radiation would be attenuated by a thicker wall before reaching the enclosed air. As the energy increases, the thickness of the wall must be increased; for example, for cobalt-60 radiation some 4 mm would be required.

Errors are introduced into the measurement of exposure if the wall material has an atomic number which differs from that of air, especially in measurements at depth in tissue where low energy scattered radiation is present due to the pronounced photoelectric effect. At higher energies discrepancies in atomic number are less serious.

The volume of the chamber required depends on the sensitivity of the measuring system and on the intensity (or exposure rate) of the radiation to be measured. The exposure rate in the useful beam of the therapy unit may be conveniently measured using a chamber volume of approximately 0.5 ml (Fig. 5.21), while the leakage radiation through the treatment room walls will require a chamber of about 200 ml (Fig. 12.2).

Since the measurement is dependent on the air mass enclosed by the chamber, it is important that the chamber contains either a fixed mass of air or a fixed volume of air at the ambient atmospheric pressure. In either case the electrodes must be rigid. If the chamber is sealed so as to enclose a fixed mass of air, then fluctuations in the ambient temperature and pressure will not affect the air mass enclosed and the reading obtained will not require the air mass correction factor to be applied. If the chamber is unsealed, fluctuations in the ambient conditions will affect the magnitude of the reading obtained and two correction factors will be required, namely the temperature correction and the pressure correction—together they are referred to as the *air mass correction factor*. The density of air at 0°C and 760 mmHg mercury (101.3 kPa) is 0.001293 g cm⁻³ but if the temperature rises the density falls, while if the pressure rises the density also rises. The density of air and, therefore, the reading obtained in the measurement of exposure, has to be corrected by multiplying by

$$A = \frac{760}{P} \times \frac{(T + 273)}{273}$$

when the temperature is $T°$C (or $T + 273°$K) and

the atmospheric pressure is P mmHg providing the standard pressure is also quoted in mmHg. The alternative units are kPa or mbar. Some standardising laboratories use 20°C as a reference temperature, in which case the temperature factor is

$$\frac{(T + 273)}{(273 + 20)}$$

Despite the need to apply correction factors most thimble chambers are designed to be unsealed (but see p. 76).

Methods of using thimble chambers

The use of a thimble chamber under the conditions described makes possible a measurement of the exposure at a particular point—usually the centre of the chamber. A *calibration* of the chamber is, however, required. This calibration enables the readings from the thimble chamber to be used to calculate the exposure that would be recorded at the same point using the free air chamber. Such a calibration is required because no practical chamber will have a wall which is air equivalent for more than one photon energy. The standardising laboratory will, on the other hand, compare the thimble chamber with the free air chamber over a wide range of photon energies and issue a calibration curve of the calibration factors, N, (Fig. 5.2B) for different photon energies or radiation qualities.

The thimble chamber may be used to measure *total exposure*, X, or to measure *exposure rate*, $\dot{X}$. From the definitions of exposure and exposure rate

$$X = \frac{\Delta Q}{\Delta m} \text{ and } \dot{X} = \frac{\Delta Q/t}{\Delta m}$$

it can be seen that to measure exposure, the total charge released, ΔQ, must be determined, while to measure exposure rate the ionisation current, $\Delta Q/t$ is required. Thus, to measure exposure, the potential difference developed across a *capacitor* is measured and, for exposure rate, the potential difference developed across a *resistor* is measured. It is possible to determine the exposure rate by measuring the exposure and dividing by the duration of the exposure, but this assumes the exposure rate is constant—an assumption that is not always valid.

Measurement of exposure

The two electrodes separated by a very good insulator which make an ionisation chamber may be treated as an electrical capacitor and used as a means of storing electrical charge. When the chamber is irradiated, the ionisation will cause some of the stored charge to leak away and, providing the chamber remains *saturated*, the charge leaked will be directly proportional to the total exposure given to the chamber and this may be measured by determining the *change* in the potential difference across the *capacitor-chamber*. This may be interpreted mathematically as follows. If the electrical capacitance of the ionisation chamber is C, then the storage of a charge Q will produce a potential difference across the capacitor of V where $V = Q/C$. If now an exposure X is given to the chamber resulting in an ionisation of ΔQ then the potential difference will fall by ΔV where $\Delta V = \Delta Q/C$. Thus, the exposure, X, will be given by $C\,\Delta V/\Delta m$, where Δm is the mass of air enclosed in the chamber.

This type of capacitor-chamber has the particular advantage that it is possible to use many chambers with only one charging/measuring instrument. The chambers will not be connected to the instrument during exposure. This system can, therefore, be used to measure the exposure at various points in the beam during a single irradiation.

On the other hand, the direct connection to the measuring device via a *screened lead* enables the exposure to be integrated during the irradiation, which can then be terminated at a predetermined exposure. Such a simple direct reading exposure meter is illustrated in Figure 5.3. The circuit shows a simplified version of that used in the popular Farmer exposure meter. The chamber is connected via a screened flexible cable to the exposure meter. The polarising voltage causes the ions to flow through the collecting electrode on to the capacitor C, thereby increasing the potential difference across the capacitor. This rise in the grid voltage applied to the (triode) electrometer

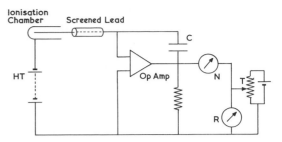

Fig. 5.4 A simplified schematic circuit for an integrating exposure meter using an operational amplifier (see text).

valve V, causes the null meter N, to deflect. This deflection is corrected by adjusting the potentiometer T (sometimes referred to as a Townsend balance) to lower the grid voltage to its initial value. The voltmeter R then measures the change in the potential difference across the capacitor C and can be calibrated in air kerma or grays, depending on whether the chamber is used in air or water, respectively. The function of the electrometer valve V is to amplify the small change in grid voltage, thereby increasing the sensitivity of the instrument. As mentioned before, the ionisation in the chamber is very small. A similar circuit using an operational amplifier in place of the electrometer valve is shown in Figure 5.4.

Measurement of exposure rate

If the integrating capacitor C in the circuit shown in Figure 5.3 is replaced by a very high resistor (say 10^{10} ohms), and the Townsend balance is omitted, then the ionisation current will flow through the resistor. The potential difference developed across the resistor is proportional to the current flowing through it (Ohm's law) and, therefore, proportional to the exposure rate. The deflection of the meter N is then a measure of the exposure rate.

Parallel plate ionisation chamber

So far only a small thimble chamber has been discussed. In fact, provided two insulated electrodes enclose a volume of air, an ionisation chamber can be almost any desired shape. In practice the radiation beam monitor incorporated into the X-ray head of a therapy beam unit is invariably a parallel plate ionisation chamber.

Two or three thin electrodes of aluminium or graphite coated Perspex are used to enclose a volume of air close to the X-ray target but on the patient side of any added filters. The electrodes of the ionisation chamber may constitute part of the added filtration. The electrodes are large enough to extend over the

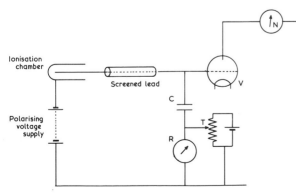

Fig. 5.3 A simplified schematic circuit for an integrating exposure meter using an electrometer valve.

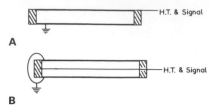

Fig. 5.5 Typical beam monitor chambers used to monitor the output from therapy units.

whole of the useful beam defined by the primary collimator. If only two electrodes are used then one will be at HT (the polarising voltage) and the other at earth potential and either one used as the collecting electrode (Fig. 5.5). Where three electrodes are used, then the centre electrode will be at HT and used as the collecting electrode, enabling the whole of the outer surface of the chamber to be connected to earth potential.

Parallel plate chambers may be used to monitor exposure or exposure rate as before, but if they are to be used to provide a measure of the dose given to the patient, during treatment on a linear accelerator for example, then the chambers must be *sealed* to obviate the need to correct for temperature and pressure changes—the temperature of the air in the chamber may be higher than that of the ambient room temperature owing to its position in relation to the target.

ALTERNATIVE METHODS OF DOSE MEASUREMENT

The primary effect of the radiations in which we are interested is the production of ionisation and this may be revealed as electrical conductivity in air, or it may be revealed in a number of other ways such as physical or chemical effects in solids or liquids. Any of these physical or chemical effects which can be estimated quantitatively can be used as a dose measuring system, and in the past most of them have been tried. A satisfactory dose measuring system requires, however, that the effect observed does not show too great a variation of sensitivity with wavelength. This is because of the continuous nature of the X-ray spectrum and the presence of scattered radiation in the beam under certain conditions. For high energy gamma rays the beam consists initially of radiation of a single wavelength or of a few discrete wavelengths but scattering again changes the spectral distribution and in measurement a reasonable wavelength independence is desirable. Some of the methods used in the past have now only a historical interest but others are quite important. A brief account of these will now be given.

Biological method

A biological method of measuring dose was attempted in the early days of radiotherapy using the property of the radiations to produce a reddening of the skin—erythema. This biological reaction is described in detail in Chapter 16. In using this reaction as a dose measuring system, a unit of dose was defined as the amount of radiation which just produced an appreciable reddening of the skin. The method was extremely inaccurate because of the difficulty of determining the threshold erythema and its variability from one person or one site to another. The method, however, could not be continued as a dose measuring system since it was soon established that different amounts of X-ray energy are necessary to produce the erythema when beams of different effective wavelength are used.

Chemical method

Chemical methods of measuring dose were in use for some time in the so-called 'Pastille dose'. A layer of crystalline barium platinocyanide changes colour from yellow to brown under exposure to an X-ray beam. A unit of dose was defined as the amount of radiation necessary to produce a given change of tint in a specimen of the material held half-way between the skin and the target. As a method of dosimetry for radiotherapy, this method has long since been abandoned because the material contained elements of high atomic number and therefore did not respond equally to radiations of different wavelengths.

The production of chemical effects by X- and gamma ray beams requires in general very large doses and chemical methods of measurement are, therefore, relatively insensitive. There has been a great revival of interest in chemical dosimeters recently, however, since they can be used under two conditions in which ionisation methods are somewhat unsatisfactory, both arise out of the development of nuclear energy. They are the measurement of doses of thousands of grays, such as might be experienced in the neighbourhood of massive radioactive sources, and the measurement of extremely high dose rates, such as might be experienced in the neighbourhood of a nuclear explosion. They can be used to advantage in radiotherapy as a means of measuring the average absorbed dose over a large or irregularly shaped volume. Chemical dosimeters can be made relatively simply to work under these conditions.

The ability of ionising radiations to promote the oxidation of ferrous compounds has been known for a long time as one of the many chemical effects of radiation. The *Fricke dosimeter* uses a solution of ferrous sulphate in sulphuric acid which is irradiated and the amount of ferric sulphate produced is estimated by making a quantitative estimate of the colour change. This is generally done by measuring the optical density before and after the irradiation in a beam of light of suitable wavelength (304 nm) using a spectrophotometer. With care, it can be accurate to approximately 2% over a range from 10 to 500 Gy.

A more complicated chemical dosimeter is a mixture of chloroform and an aqueous solution of a suitable indicator dye sealed in a glass container together with a small amount of a stabilising agent, resorcinol. Radiation produces acids in the chloroform. Shaking the mixture separates the acids into the aqueous layer and a visible colour change is produced in the dye. This type of dosimeter is much more sensitive than the ferrous sulphate one and can be used to measure doses in the range 0.50 to 100 Gy. These dosimeters are useful for measuring bursts of radiation of several gray at high intensity.

Calorimetry

A direct method of measuring the real energy absorbed from an X-ray beam in a medium would be to measure the total amount of heat developed. There are great difficulties in making a direct measurement of absorbed energy in this way, the major one being the small temperature changes involved. A beam of X-rays giving a soft tissue dose of 5 Gy, for example, causes a temperature rise of only 10^{-3} °C. In spite of the small temperature rise, however, methods of heat measurement are now sensitive enough for a new interest to be taken in this method of measuring dose. This interest arises because calorimetry provides a measurement of radiation energy in terms of fundamental energy units, that is, in units to which the gray is directly related.

$$\text{Dose (Gy)} = 4.2 \times C \times T$$

where C is the specific heat of the irradiated material in cal kg^{-1} °C^{-1} and T is the change in temperature in degrees centigrade. 4.2 is the conversion from calories to joules.

The calorimeter has been used, for example, to measure the energy in the beam of gamma rays from a cobalt-60 therapy unit. The absorber was a block of lead suspended in a vacuum inside a well-insulated box. The heat-detecting element was a thermistor—a semiconducting material whose resistance changes very rapidly with temperature—its resistance changes were detected electrically by using it as one arm of a Wheatstone bridge. Temperature changes of about 10^{-4} °C per minute were measured.

More recently there has been a considerable increase in the use of the calorimeter as an absolute dosimeter. While the technique is too difficult to contemplate for everyday use in the hospital, in the standardising laboratory it is proving to be very valuable in the megavoltage photon range—beyond the practical range of the free air chamber—and for high linear energy transfer (LET) radiations (Chapter 11). For photons, water calorimeters may be used and have the advantage of being tissue equivalent, but in practice, carbon calorimeters are easier to use, together with knowledge of the absorption coefficients to convert dose in carbon to dose in water.

Geiger–Müller tubes

The Geiger or Geiger–Müller tube is one of the most widely known radiation detectors and is extensively used in radiation protection, being very sensitive. It is, however, less effective as an accurate means of radiation measurement. It relies on the ionisation of gas at low pressure and the acceleration of the negative ions by the high polarising voltage to produce further ionisations to produce a measurable electrical signal. This process and the practical applications are described more fully in Chapter 9.

Scintillation detectors

Scintillation detectors are also discussed more fully in Chapter 9. The sensitive part of the scintillation detector is a crystal in which the photoelectric absorption of a single photon produces a photon of visible light—of a wavelength characteristic of the crystal. Because the characteristic photon is of an energy where the absorption is minimal (p. 65), it passes readily through the crystal to be captured by the photocathode of a photomultiplier tube mounted in close contact with the crystal. This detection of individual ionisations makes the scintillation crystal one of the most sensitive radiation detectors available.

Photographic methods

The effect of X- and gamma rays in producing blackening on a photographic film may also be used to estimate dose, especially if the amount of blackening is measured with a densitometer. A densitometer causes a pencil beam of light to pass through an area of the film on to a photocell which measures the intensity of the light transmitted by the film in the form of an electric current, the current being proportional to the intensity. The degree of blackening is expressed as an *optical density,* which is the logarithm (to base 10) of the light intensity transmitted by an unexposed area of the film divided by that transmitted by the exposed part of the film. Thus, an optical density of 1 means that only one-tenth of the light is transmitted, while a density of 2 transmits only one-hundredth. Over a limited range density is proportional to dose. The properties of photographic film exposed to ionising radiation are dealt with more fully in Chapter 7.

The photographic method suffers from several disadvantages. It is difficult to obtain reproducible and accurate results even though great care is taken to process films under standard and controlled conditions. For instance, variations of developer strength and temperature and of processing techniques make great differences to the density. Films also show great differences in sensitivity to radiation over the wavelength range in which measurements are needed.

The photographic method is nevertheless a very sensitive one and is very useful when small quantities of radiation are to be measured, particularly if the time involved in the exposure is long and if a high degree of accuracy is not required. These are the conditions involved in the measurement of radiation exposure for protection purposes and the use of photographic film for this purpose is described in Chapter 12.

Thermoluminescence

The transition of an electron from an outer orbit to an inner orbit and the consequent emission of a characteristic X-ray photon has already been discussed (Ch. 1). Similar transitions take place between the outer orbits with the corresponding emission of characteristic radiation. In a crystal, these outer orbits are shared by the atoms and again transitions can occur between them. If the emission is in the visible part of the spectrum the phenomenon is known as *luminescence.* For example, sodium iodide is one example of a crystal which produces scintillations under irradiation. In Chapter 7 it will be seen that intensifying screens enhance the photographic action of X-rays by emitting visible light of a wavelength to which X-ray film is particularly sensitive and fluoroscopy (or 'screening') is a means of making an X-ray image visible to the human eye. In each of these instances, the visible light emission is an immediate and instantaneous response to the absorption of an X-ray photon. This is *fluorescence.* Another form of luminescence of particular interest in this section is that of *thermoluminescence.*

Certain crystalline materials such as *lithium fluoride* can absorb X-ray energy and store that energy at room temperature for a very considerable time, many months in fact. At the atomic level this process can be explained briefly as follows. When X-ray energy is absorbed, secondary electrons are lifted from the outer electron orbits into another orbit which is normally empty in a non-conducting material. (In a conducting material, this orbit will contain a certain number of *free* electrons which carry the flow of charge we refer to as an electric current.) Since these electron orbits are not uniquely defined in a solid they are referred to as *bands,* the normally filled *valence band* and the normally empty *conduction band,* respectively, with a *forbidden zone* between them, as between any two shells (Fig. 1.6). In a pure crystal the electrons will fall back from the conduction band into the *holes* they left in the filled band. If an impurity is deliberately added to the crystal—manganese, for example—some of these electrons will fall into the *impurity traps* which now lie in the forbidden zone. Here the electron is held and the energy is stored. This energy is only released when sufficient heat is applied to lift these trapped electrons into the conduction band a second time, from where they may return to the filled band, emitting their excess energy in the form of photons of visible light. This is thermoluminescence. The intensity of the light output is small but it is proportional to the X-ray energy previously absorbed, hence the value of the technique as a means of measuring radiation dose.

The dosimeters may be in the form of *powder,* impregnated plastic *discs,* extruded *chips* or *rods,* each containing some 50 to 100 mg of phosphor material. After irradiation, the phosphor is placed in a planchet in the 'TLD Reader' where it is heated to 300°C in an oxygen-free (nitrogen) atmosphere (Fig. 5.6). The light output is measured using a photomultiplier and amplifier feeding a digital display. The system is essentially a comparator and any measurement of dose relies on the read-out of identical dosimeters exposed

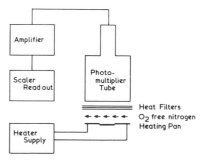

Fig. 5.6 A thermoluminescent dosimeter read-out system.

to known doses of the same quality radiation. Lithium fluoride has an atomic number close to that of soft tissue and therefore its response is almost independent of the photon energies encountered in the radiotherapy department. A wide range of doses may be measured, enabling the system to be used for measuring patient doses, doses to sensitive organs outside the treatment beam and for personnel monitoring (Ch. 12). Crystals of lithium borate and of calcium fluoride may be used as alternatives to lithium fluoride.

Solid state detectors

Silicon diode detectors are widely used for the measurement of electron beams and megavoltage photon beams. Their relatively high atomic number ($Z = 14$) makes them unsuitable for lower photon energies. The silicon diode may be thought of as a solid ionisation chamber of very small size. The radiation causes ionisations within the detector and the ions are collected in the same way as in an ionisation chamber. The principal differences are that the ionisations occur in a material of a much higher density than air—volume for volume, the silicon diode is some 20 000 times more sensitive than the air ionisation chamber—and there is no need for a large polarising voltage because the contact potentials within the diode are sufficient to prevent ion recombination. Their disadvantages are principally their (photon) energy dependence and their ultimate destruction through radiation induced damage—this is a gradual process which shows in changes in sensitivity to both dose and temperature. Careful use and frequent calibration is required.

The sensitive part of the silicon diode is the junction between the p-type and the n-type silicon. The p-type silicon is silicon with a boron ($Z = 5$) or an aluminium ($Z = 13$) impurity which absorbs electrons from the silicon leaving positive (p) 'holes' in the material. On the other side of the junction the phosphorus impurity ($Z = 16$) donates negative (n) electrons to the silicon. This imbalance results in a contact potential being set up at the junction between the dissimilar materials and a mopping up of the 'free' ions, creating a depletion layer only a few microns thick. If the atoms in this depletion layer are ionised by radiation, then the negative ions (electrons) will be attracted to the positively charged phosphorus (impurity in the n-type silicon) and the positive 'holes' will diffuse towards the boron impurity in the p-type silicon. This flow of ions constitutes an ionisation current proportional to the dose rate incident on the detector and can be measured on a sensitive ammeter (an electrometer) without the need for an external polarising voltage.

Although all these detectors use both n-type and p-type material, some are described as p-type while others are n-type. The label identifies which material forms the larger part of the junction. The junction is very small—a few millimetres square by half a millimetre thick—and has to be encapsulated in a suitable protective sheath. The sheath is usually of a material and thickness to provide full electron build-up in the photon beam. These cannot therefore be used to measure 'skin' or 'lens' dose during radiotherapy. Detectors designed for use in a water phantom will usually enable the build-up curve to be measured at least to within a millimetre of the surface.

It should be noted that where silicon diodes—with build-up material in the encapsulation—are used to monitor the patient dose during radiotherapy, there is a significant spatial error between the detector and the point at d_{max} where the dose is prescribed. These measurements therefore need careful interpretation in the light of the geometrical set-up and the energy of the radiation.

QUALITY OF AN X-RAY BEAM

To be able to measure the exposure in air at a point outside the patient is one thing, but to be able to predict the dose at a point inside the patient is another and one of equal importance. The dose at such a point depends on many factors:

— The ability of the primary radiation to penetrate the tissues.
— The contribution made by the radiation scattered by the surrounding tissues.
— The dose delivered to the surface (or just below the surface) of the patient.

The penetrating ability of the primary radiation is often referred to as the *quality* of the beam as it emerges from the X-ray head. It has been seen in previous chapters that the X-ray spectrum contains photons of many wavelengths and the extent to which any of these interact with matter depends on the wavelength and on the atomic number of the attenuating medium. If the photons are not absorbed they will be transmitted to subsequent layers of matter. Therefore, to know fully the penetrating ability of an X-ray beam requires a knowledge of the number of photons of each wavelength and the method by which each wavelength is absorbed and attenuated. Fortunately, for radiotherapeutic purposes such a detailed knowledge is not required and some approximation is adequate.

The beam quality of an X-ray beam generated at less than one million volts is stated in terms of the

HVT and either the generating voltage (kVp) or the homogeneity coefficient. Above one million volts the statement of the X-ray beam energy in MV is adequate, but there is an increasing interest in a specification in terms of a *quality index* defined in a 10×10 cm^2 field at 100 cm source–chamber distance where

$$\text{Quality index} \quad = \quad \frac{\substack{\text{Ionisation measured at a} \\ \text{depth of 20 cm (J20)}}}{\substack{\text{Ionisation measured at a} \\ \text{depth of 10 cm (J10)}}}$$
at the same source–chamber distance

Typical values of quality index are given in Table 5.4. In the case of gamma ray beams the isotope and its mass number are normally adequate, although the quality index may be specified.

The HVT is the thickness of a stated material required to reduce the intensity of the beam to half its value. The *homogeneity coefficient* is the ratio of the HVT divided by the thickness of the same material required to further reduce the intensity of the beam from 50 to 25%. This is sometimes referred to as the second HVT. For a homogeneous (monochromatic) beam (e.g. caesium-137) the first and second HVT will be the same and the homogeneity coefficient will be equal to one. For X-ray therapy beams it is generally between about 0.5 and 0.7.

The X-ray beam quality depends on various factors:

— The accelerating voltage
— The voltage waveform
— The target material
— The inherent filtration
— The added filtration.

Taking these very briefly in turn, the accelerating voltage (kVp) determines the minimum wavelength in the spectrum and all the longer wavelengths will be present. If the generator is at constant potential then this minimum wavelength will be present throughout the exposure, whereas if a half-wave rectified circuit is used, it is only present for one instant in every 1/50 s (for a 50 Hz supply), giving the spectrum proportionately more lower energy photons. The target material will superimpose on the 'white' spectral distribution its own characteristic line spectrum (Chapter 1). Filters can be used to remove the low energy photons and their effect will now be discussed in detail, with particular reference to the HVT.

Filtration

The mass attenuation graph of Figure 5.7 shows that in the photoelectric region an absorber will attenuate low energy photons more readily than the higher

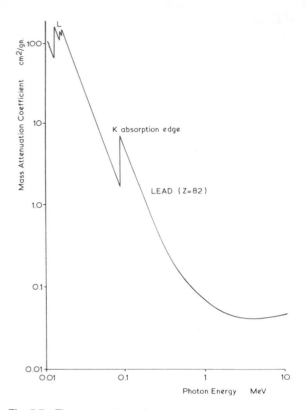

Fig. 5.7 The mass attenuation curve for lead.

energy photons. This property is exploited in the use of *beam hardening filters* applied to radiation beams accelerated at voltages of less than 1 MV. In the range from about 1 to 10 MV, the absorption graph is almost flat and there is little preferential absorption. Filters, therefore, have no beneficial effect in removing the lower energy photons. Above 10 MV in the pair production dominated region, the higher energy photons are absorbed in preference to those of lower energies. Again there is no beneficial effect. Beam hardening filters are, therefore, not used at megavoltages and must not be confused with beam flattening filters (p. 41) and beam modifying filters (p. 100f).

In Figure 5.8 the horizontal axes of the two graphs cover the same photon energy range. The upper graphs show the linear attenuation coefficients for aluminium, copper and tin. The lower graph shows a 250 kVp X-ray spectrum under different degrees of filtration. The unfiltered spectrum shows that the majority of the photons are of such low energy that they will not penetrate to a deep seated tumour but will be absorbed in the skin. In order to preserve as many high energy photons while removing the unwanted low energy photons, a filter which is highly attenuating below

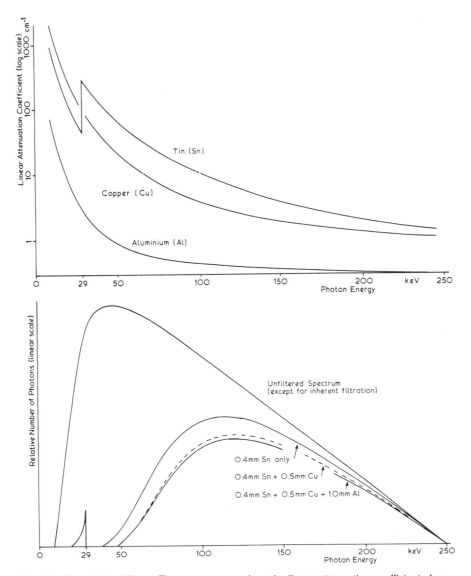

Fig. 5.8   The effect of filters. The upper curves show the linear attenuation coefficients for the filters used on the unfiltered X-ray spectrum shown below. The copper filter reduces the 29 keV peak.

40 keV and offering little attenuation to the photons in the 200 keV region is required. Aluminium ($Z = 13$) is of little value in this situation, but may be used as a filter for X-rays generated at energies up to approximately 150 kVp. Copper ($Z = 29$) may be used up to 250 kVp, but tin ($Z = 50$) is better for energies above 200 kVp. Copper and tin are never used in isolation. In the lower graphs of Figure 5.8 the upper curve represents the spectrum of a 250 kVp beam emanating from the tube housing, that is, filtered only by the inherent filtration. If a filter of 0.4 mm tin is added to the beam it hardens the beam very adequately, the spectral peak moving from 45 keV to about 115 keV, but there is still a lesser peak at 29 keV owing to the K absorption edge of tin. For this reason a copper filter, which is highly attenuating at 29 keV, is added. Copper, however, has a K-absorption edge at 9 keV which has to be filtered out using aluminium—the K edge of aluminium is less than 2 keV and is negligible. It needs to be remembered that tin and copper

not only have a low attenuation coefficient at 20 keV and 9 keV respectively, but that they can become sources of their own characteristic radiations with photon energies 1 or 2 keV below these edges. These are not shown in the diagram, but constitute an addition to the spectrum. It is important, therefore, that when using a *compound filter* the metal filters are fitted in the correct order—highest Z close to the target, lowest Z to the patient.

The tin–copper–aluminium filter is often referred to as a *Thoraeus filter* after the Swedish physicist who found the most efficient filter for his 200 kVp X-ray beam was 0.4 mm Sn + 0.25 mm Cu + 1.0 mm Al. By 'efficiency' in this connection we mean getting the desired hardening effect with the minimum loss of beam intensity. Thoraeus found that this combination gave the maximum output dose rate.

Beam hardening filters can, therefore, improve the relative penetration of the beam and raise the value of the homogeneity coefficient. The actual measurement of these parameters will now be considered.

Measurement of HVT

The method of measuring HVT is the same over the whole range of energies found in the radiotherapy department providing the characteristics of the radiation are observed, namely that the ionisation chamber wall is air equivalent over the range of photon energies being measured—the same chamber could not be used for both 10 kV and 10 MV. It should also be remembered that the penetrating ability of the beams will vary considerably and the choice of absorbing material is important—those normally used are shown in Table 5.1.

The apparatus required is shown schematically in Figure 5.9. The HVT is determined by measuring the intensity of the beam transmitted through various thicknesses of material and interpolating to find the thickness that would transmit 50% of the intensity

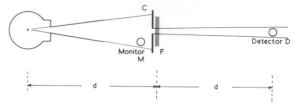

Fig. 5.9 The layout for the measurement of half value thickness.

measured with zero thickness of material added. Therefore, the following form the basic requirements: a means of collimating the beam, C, to a small size but large enough to cover the ionisation chamber, D, which will be referred to as the detector. The error resulting from the use of a large beam size will be explained later. If the exposure cannot be given very accurately a second monitor chamber, M, will be required on the tube side of the small beam collimator to detect the variation in the exposure incident on the filters, F, as they are added during the experiment. The focus-to-filter distance should be approximately equal to the filter-to-detector distance and greater than the range of the electrons emitted from the filter material. With the apparatus carefully and rigidly aligned and a table in which to record the results (Table 5.2), the measurements can begin. (If the monitor, M, is not used then it is assumed that the readings that would have been obtained would all be equal, namely $M_0 = M_1 = M_2$ etc. in Table 5.2 and columns 4 and 5 would not be required.) The maximum thickness of the filters to be added will depend on the radiation and material being used and the exact purpose of the experiment but the transmission should be reduced to between 25 and 10%. The calculation of percentage transmission for the final column of the table is:

$$\frac{D_n \times M_0 \times 100}{D_0 \times M_n}$$

where D_n and M_n are the readings taken on inserting

Table 5.1 Typical values of added filtration and beam quality

	kVp	Added filter	HVT	Effective photon energy	Equivalent wavelength (nm)
Grenz rays	10	Nil	0.02 mm Al	6 keV	0.207
Superficial	80	1 mm Al	2.5 mm Al	30 keV	0.041
Orthovoltage	250	1 mm Cu + 1 mm Al	2.1 mm Cu	108 keV	0.011
Orthovoltage	300	0.8 mm Sn + 0.25 mm Cu + 1.0 mm Al	3.8 mm Cu	155 keV	0.008
Cobalt-60	—	Nil	10.4 mm Pb	1.25 MeV	0.001

Table 5.2 Measurement of half value thickness

Added filter	Total filtration	Detector reading	Monitor reading	Ratio D/M	Percentage transmission
Nil	Nil	D_0	M_0	D_0/M_0	100.0
t_1	t_1	D_1	M_1	D_1/M_1	$\dfrac{D_1/M_1}{D_0/M_0} \times 100$
t_2 etc.	$t_1 + t_2$	D_2	M_2	D_2/M_2	etc.

a thickness t_n making the total filtration equal to t. On completion of the readings and calculations, a graph of the percentage transmission through the chosen filter material is plotted as in Figure 5.10A. If possible, the logarithm of the percentage transmission should be plotted as in Figure 5.10B. From these graphs it can be seen that 1.0 mm is required to reduce the intensity to 50%, and 2.6 mm to reduce it to 25%. The HVT is, therefore, 1 mm and the homogeneity coefficient is (1.0/1.6) or 0.63. This completes the measurement of HVT, but this graph reveals a good deal more. First, it has been said that the homogeneous radiation from a gamma ray source would obey the law of exponential absorption and would have a homogeneity coefficient of unity. The law of exponential absorption states, using the same nomenclature:

$$D_n = D_0 e^{-\mu t} \text{ or } \ln(D_n/D_0) = -\mu t$$

The straight line graph (curve B) in Figure 5.10B may be the graph of this equation and its gradient is $-\mu$. The gradient of our curve A is also $-\mu$, but the magnitude of μ varies from one point to the next; in fact μ

decreases with increasing filtration. Now consideration of the photoelectric region shows that the linear attenuation coefficient μ (or rather μ/ρ, but ρ is constant) decreases with increasing photon energy (Fig. 5.8). This, therefore, is another way of explaining that the peak of the spectrum is moved to a higher photon energy by the preferential absorption of the low energy photons by the addition of filters.

Effective photon energy and equivalent wavelength

Secondly, if $T_{1/2}$ is the HVT, then D_n/D_0 in the above equation is 0.5 by definition and the equation simplifies to:

$$T_{1/2} = 0.693/\mu \text{ or } \mu = 0.693/T_{1/2}$$

since $-\ln(0.5) = 0.693$. From the attenuation data appropriate to the filter material μ can be used to derive the energy of a homogeneous beam of photons having the same HVT as the X-ray beam under examination. This energy (in keV) is known as the *effective photon*

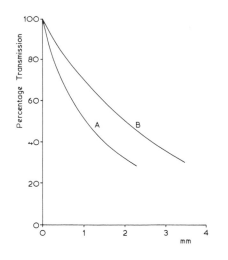

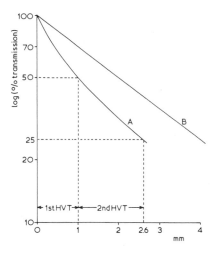

A   **B**

Fig. 5.10 The attenuation of a radiation beam by the addition of filters plotted **A** on a linear scale and **B** on a logarithmic scale. Curve A is for an inhomogeneous X-ray beam and curve B for a homogeneous gamma ray beam.

energy of the X-ray beam. This is particularly useful when attempting to compare X- and gamma ray beams.

A third alternative specification of the quality of the beam can be derived using the Duane–Hunt law (p. 12) to calculate the *equivalent wavelength*, λ, where

$$\lambda = 1.24/E \text{ nm}$$

providing E is the effective photon energy in keV. Some typical values of effective photon energy and equivalent wavelength were given in Table 5.1.

Broad beam attenuation

Thirdly, it was stated earlier that a narrow beam should be used for the measurement of HVT. This is necessary to minimise the radiation scattered by the added filters by an excessively large beam of radiation. Such scattered radiation would increase the reading D_n which, when plotted on the transmission graph, would give an overestimate of the HVT. Such *broad beam* data has its usefulness in radiation protection (Chapter 12) but for radiotherapy treatment, narrow beam attenuation is required.

DISTRIBUTION OF X-RAY DOSE IN A UNIFORM PHANTOM

In the earlier part of this chapter the quality of the beam was discussed in terms of its ability to penetrate through attenuating materials, which have been conveniently referred to as filters. Applying our understanding of the absorption processes, the photoelectric absorption process has been exploited in the use of beam hardening filters to improve the penetrating power of the beam. It is now necessary to investigate the penetration of the beam into the tissues of the body. Owing to the complex structure of the body and the problems of measuring the radiation within the body itself, most measurements are made using a *phantom* which is carefully chosen to be *tissue equivalent*.

Tissue equivalent materials

Tissue equivalent phantom materials are those materials which behave in much the same way as the body tissues when irradiated. From the analysis of the absorption processes it is clear that a phantom material must have (1) an effective atomic number very close to that of the tissue it simulates because of the dependence of photoelectric absorption and pair production processes on Z, (2) an electron density close to that of the tissue simulated because of the dependence of the Compton scattering process on the number of electrons per gram,

Table 5.3   Properties of tissue equivalent and other materials

	Effective atomic no.	Electron density	Specific Gravity
Soft muscle tissue	7.35	3.36×10^{23}	0.98–1.00
Water	7.4	3.34	1.00
Mix D	7.5	3.39	0.99
Temex rubber	7.1	3.27	1.01
'Bolus'	7.3	3.32	1.0
Perspex	6.47	3.27	1.19
Bone	13.8	3.0	1.85
Fat	5.9	3.5	0.91

and (3) because spatial measurements are to be made in the phantom material the density or specific gravity should be as close as possible to that of the tissue simulated.

Table 5.3 lists these parameters for the principal body tissues and some of the traditional phantom materials. Soft muscle tissue phantom materials are the most commonly used and water is the most common of these. In many ways, water is the ideal material in that it is homogeneous and yet permits ionisation chambers (or other radiation detectors) to be moved freely within it. Mix D is a mixture of paraffin wax, polyethylene and other materials and is often used in the form of 1 cm thick slabs. Temex rubber is a polymerised rubber and can be obtained in homogeneous slabs or moulded on to phantom bone as an actual body phantom. Temex has the advantage that it is flexible whereas Mix D is brittle. Lincolnshire Bolus is a mixture of sugar and magnesium carbonate made up into small spheres. While the density of the material is greater than that of tissue, the packing density of the spheres produces good tissue equivalence. It is important, therefore, to check from time to time the condition of the bolus and to separate fragmented or powdered spheres from it. More recently a variety of materials have become available which can be made and shaped in the laboratory to make homogeneous or heterogeneous phantoms to almost any specification by varying the relative ingredients. Phantom materials for other body tissues are not in common use, but cork and chalk have been used to simulate lung and bone respectively, where more precise equivalent materials are not available.

The calculation of dose within a patient is invariably based on the dose distribution in a uniform soft tissue equivalent phantom and the rest of this section will be devoted to this. For the purpose of measurement the phantom will be a *semi-infinite rectangular water tank* and the beam axis will be at right angles to the entry surface of the phantom. A phantom is said to be semi-infinite if the measurements being undertaken are not affected by any further increase in the size of the phantom.

Percentage depth dose

The term *percentage depth dose* (%DD) expresses the dose at any point within the phantom as a percentage of the maximum dose on the central axis of the beam, i.e.

$$\%DD = \frac{\text{Dose at a point within the phantom}}{\text{Maximum dose on the central axis}} \times 100$$
$$\text{of the beam within the phantom}$$

Apart from a few exceptions (p. 101), the percentage depth dose at all points will be less than 100%. The *central axis depth doses (d)* are often plotted against depth as a means of comparing one radiation beam with another (Fig. 5.11 and Table 5.4) or plotting the percentage depth dose at 10 cm deep against beam quality (Fig. 5.12), while a map of the dose distribution within the irradiated volume will be shown as an *isodose chart* where each line represents points of equal dose; in many respects they are analogous to height contours on a geographer's map. Typical isodose charts

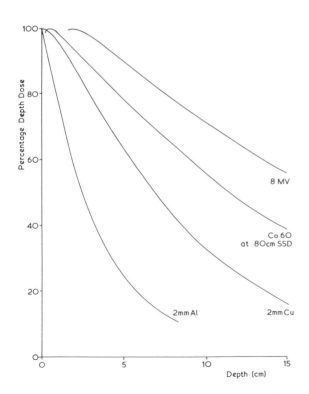

Fig. 5.11 Typical central axis depth dose curves for X-and gamma ray therapy beams.

Table 5.4 Some isodose data for 10×10 cm^2 fields

Energy	SSD (cm)	HVL/QI	d_{max} (cm)	$d_{80\%}$ (cm)	$d_{50\%}$ (cm)	$\%_{10cm}$
100 kV*	20	2 mm Al	0	0.7	2.2	5.2
250 kV	50	2 mm Cu	0	3.0	6.9	32.3
Cobalt-60	80	0.57	0.5	4.7	11.6	56.4
4 MV	100	0.58	1.0	5.9	13.7	62.7
6 MV	100	0.65	1.5	6.8	15.7	67.7
8 MV	100	0.68	2.0	7.4	17.1	71.0
10 MV	100	0.75	2.5	8.5	19.1	74.5

* 5 cm circle.

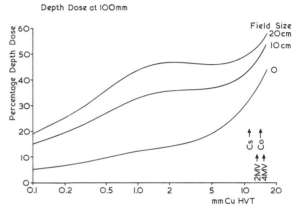

A

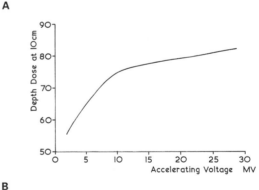

B

Fig. 5.12 Variation of depth dose at 10 cm **A** at 50 cm SSD with HVT and **B** at 100 cm SSD with accelerating voltage.

are shown in Figure 5.13, where the charts represent the distribution of dose in one of the principal planes of the beam, i.e. a plane parallel to the edge of the beam but containing the central axis. (In Figure 5.13 only half of each chart is shown.)

Central axis depth dose

There are many factors which affect the distribution of dose along the central axis of the beam. The dose

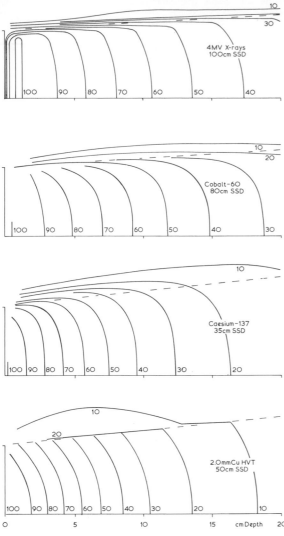

Fig. 5.13 Typical isodose charts for megavoltage, teleisotope and orthovoltage beams. The broken lines show the geometric edge.

will fall with increasing depth owing to the absorption in the successive layers of tissue and the increasing distance from the target. (The inverse square law has to be obeyed.) Superimposed on this *primary* radiation (from the target) will be the *scattered* radiation which results from the Compton scattering processes taking place within the tissues.

The magnitude of these effects will depend on the quality and the size and shape of the radiation beam and the nature of the tissue itself. Figure 5.14 shows the central axis depth dose curves for a 250 kV and a cobalt-60 beam with the contribution from scatter

plotted separately. The important role played by scattered radiation in orthovoltage therapy is clearly visible and emphasised when compared with the relatively minor role it plays in megavoltage therapy. Two other factors are also clearly shown: first, at orthovoltage energies the exposure to the surface (zero depth) is significantly affected by scattered radiation or *back scatter*; and second, at megavoltage energies the surface dose is less and builds up to a maximum at some distance below the surface. *Build-up* is a physical phenomenon which explains the *skin sparing effect* of megavoltage radiations and is one of the principal advantages of these higher energy beams in radiotherapy.

Back scatter

The exposure at the surface of the phantom is substantially greater than the exposure at the same point if no phantom were present. The phantom material is scattering back to the surface a considerable amount of radiation and this contribution is known as back scatter (Fig. 5.15). The contribution due to back scatter at the point where the beam axis enters the phantom is expressed as a percentage of the contribution due to primary radiation and called *percentage back scatter*. The percentage back scatter increases with the area of the field irradiated and with the thickness of the underlying tissues. This is to be expected, although with very large fields and very thick tissues the extremities of the irradiated tissue are a long way from the centre of the incident field and contribute very little. The back scatter, therefore, approaches a maximum. For the same reason, the back scatter from a square or circular field will be greater than that for an elongated field of the same area.

The amount of back scatter at the surface of an irradiated phantom varies in a complicated way with radiation quality. It is largest for a beam quality of 0.8 mm Cu HVT—the deep therapy region—and falls as the quality increases, that is as the Compton scatter becomes increasingly in the forward direction as well as decreasing in magnitude. It also falls with softer quality beams where Compton interactions are swamped by photoelectric interactions by which most of the radiation is absorbed. At its maximum the percentage back scatter can reach 50% and is, therefore, very important.

Equivalent square

It has been seen above that back scatter cannot be directly related to the area of the field. Elongated fields produce less back scatter as measured on the central axis than square fields of the same area.

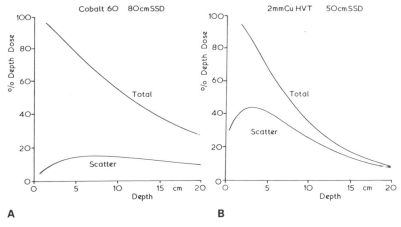

Fig. 5.14 Percentage depth dose curves for **A** cobalt-60 and **B** 250 kV beams showing the relative magnitude of the dose contributed by the scattered radiation.

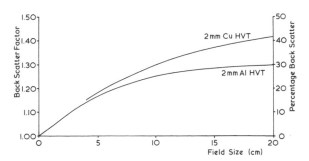

Fig. 5.15 The back scatter factor increases with the equivalent square of the field size.

Table 5.5 Abridged table of equivalent squares of rectangular fields

Long axis (cm)	Short axis (cm)							
	2	4	6	8	10	15	20	30
2	2.0							
4	2.7	4.0						
6	3.1	4.8	6.0					
8	3.4	5.4	6.9	8.0				
10	3.6	5.8	7.5	8.9	10.0			
15	3.9	6.4	8.5	10.3	11.9	15.0		
20	4.0	6.7	9.0	11.1	13.0	17.0	20.0	
30	4.1	6.9	9.4	11.7	13.9	18.9	23.3	30.0

Nevertheless, the rectangular field will give rise to back scatter of the same magnitude as a square field of *smaller* area (Fig. 5.16). It is therefore possible to define for each rectangular field an *equivalent square* field which produces the same percentage back scatter. This concept is of particular value when treating non-standard field sizes. It is not only the back scatter that is the same, but the forward scatter is also the same and this gives rise to the same central axis depth dose. The primary contribution is the same for all fields (of the same quality and SSD). The scatter contribution is the only variable.

Tables are available which give the size of the equivalent square for all rectangular fields commonly encountered; an abridged table is given in Table 5.5.

Build-up

At megavoltage energies, the scattered radiation is more in the forward direction and gives rise to less scattered radiation outside the edges of the beam. This is clear as soon as you compare the isodose charts for orthovoltage and megavoltage beams (Fig. 5.13). Analysis of the Compton scattering process also shows that the recoil electron is ejected in the more forward direction and with increasing kinetic energy. The recoil electron range at 200 kV is extremely small but at megavoltages it is considerable (Table 4.3) and electron dose build-up manifests itself below the surface of the irradiated tissue.

This may be explained in simple terms as follows. Each successive thin layer of tissue produces its quota of fast electrons which in turn deposit their energy in

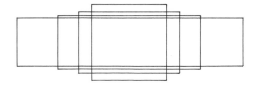

Fig. 5.16 Rectangular fields of different size and elongation having the same equivalent square.

several layers of tissue beyond their point of origin. Although the kinetic energy released in each layer (the kerma) is constant, the energy deposited in each layer (the absorbed dose) will be determined by the number of electrons passing through the layer, and that number increases as each layer adds electrons to the electron flux from the preceding layers. This increase continues until the electrons released only replace those which have come to the end of their range. The dose build-up thus reaches a maximum at a depth determined by the range of the electrons and therefore by the energy of the photon beam. In practice the kerma is not quite constant but falls as the primary radiation undergoes absorption and attenuation, with the result that the depth of the dose maximum is slightly less than the maximum range of the secondary electrons (Fig. 5.17). The depth of the peak in centimetres is approximately a quarter of the X-ray energy in megavolts (2 cm at 8 MV, etc.). Cobalt-60, being approximately equivalent to 2 MV X-rays, has a peak at approximately 5 mm (Fig. 5.17).

The shape of the dose build-up curve is primarily determined by the recoil electrons from within the tissues being set into motion in the forward direction, and therefore it will not be affected by the curvature of the skin or the obliquity of the incident beam. In general, the depth of d_{max} should be measured in the direction of the ray from the X-ray focus or gamma ray source. This has only to be modified when the angle of incidence approaches 90° (i.e. when the beam is almost tangential to the surface). Although the recoil electrons are predominantly in the forward direction, they do not travel in straight lines, but deviate and distribute their energy over a small area. This is only demonstrated at large angles of incidence. There

is still some build-up of dose below the tangential surface, but the skin dose is higher than that at normal incidence and builds up to a maximum over a depth considerably less than the normal value suggests.

This analysis of build-up suggests that the dose at the surface is zero. The surface dose in practice is variable and is mainly due to electrons scattered from other material in the beam—diaphragms, penumbra trimmers, beam shaping blocks, etc.—together with the intervening air itself. The value of the surface/skin dose and the shape of the build-up curve will therefore vary from one machine to another of the same photon energy, and with field size (Fig. 5.17). In practice the surface dose will be in the range of 20 to 50% for most megavoltage units, and lower values can be expected as the photon energy increases. This problem of electron contamination can be so pronounced that if, for example, cobalt-60 is used at very short distances (5–20 cm SSD, see p. 114), the skin sparing build-up is completely lost and may even be reversed, i.e. the contaminating electrons may raise the surface dose to a value higher than the dose at 5 mm depth, even after the effects of absorption and inverse square law are taken into account. In this situation *electron* filters may be used to advantage. Brass or copper filters are ideal, but Perspex or lead glass is used where the filter has to be transparent.

Definition of field size

Another characteristic of isodose charts is the width of the penumbra, and here we are referring to the penumbra as measured in the water phantom and, therefore, include the geometric penumbra, the transmission penumbra and the effects of scattered radiation. It will be noticed that megavoltage X-ray beams have a narrower penumbra than cobalt-60 or caesium-137 beams owing, principally, to the differences in the source diameter. The question then arises, 'how do we define field size?' The design of the diaphragm system and the light beam is such that the edge of the light beam roughly corresponds to the width of the beam defined by the 50% isodose line at the depth of the peak dose, and this is the definition used when data are published for general use. Other definitions, however, are in use in clinical radiotherapy—for example 'the 80% width at the depth of the maximum ionisation on the central axis' is common. Where detailed plans are produced the numerical size of the field is perhaps unimportant, but where one field butts up to the edge of another, knowledge of the actual percentile value defined by the light beam diaphragm is vital. In multicentre trials and where the results

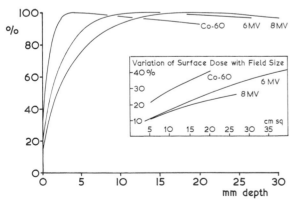

Fig. 5.17 The build-up curves for cobalt-60, 6 MV and 8 MV. The inset shows the variation in skin dose with field size for the same two beams.

of treatment are published the definition of the field size must be given alongside any statement of field size.

Asymmetric beams

In the above discussion, each radiation beam has been considered to be symmetrical about the axis of rotation of the diaphragm system. This is not always the case. Asymmetric control is widely available on one or both pairs of diaphragm blades (Fig. 3.24); and of course with multileaf collimators, size and shape are variable with respect to the axis of rotation of the diaphragm system.

The initial demand for asymmetric diaphragm systems—and probably one of their main uses—is in the treatment of the breast (Ch. 23), where the junction between the edges of the two tangential fields to the breast needs to be aligned with the edge of the anterior supraclavicular field. The alignment was technically not possible because each of the three beams was a divergent beam. By moving one collimator blade to coincide with the axis of rotation of the diaphragm system, it is possible to generate a beam of radiation which is asymmetric and, in particular, where one geometric edge follows the axis of the diaphragm system—while the other edge diverges in the normal way. (A similar beam shape can be produced by aligning a local shielding block (p. 50) with the axis—a technique sometimes known as *beam blocking*.) Now, in the case of the breast treatment above, if three such asymmetric beams are used, then the superior borders of the two tangential fields can be made to coincide with each other and with the inferior border of the supraclavicular field, all three beams being set up to a common isocentre. This opens up the possiblity of abutting the fields to deliver a more uniform dose.

The edges of the asymmetric or *beam blocked* beam will still exhibit a penumbra effect (p. 49). This must be taken into account when interpreting the area delineated by the light beam diaphragm unless that area and the field size are both defined at the 50% width.

This is but one example of the use of asymmetric collimation. With two pairs of asymmetric diaphragm blades, any large or small field can be defined anywhere within the confines of the primary collimator and may or may not contain the axis of rotation. (The asymmetric blades may cross over this axis so that both edges diverge from the axis in the same direction). Experience in the use of such systems is currently limited and there is no universally accepted definition on which to base the dosimetry—the previous reference point at d_{max} on the axis (of rotation) is no longer meaningful. To refer the relative dose to a point at d_{max} in the centre of the beam may be a logical approach. For absolute dosimetry, or dosimetry relative to the normal reference point (at d_{max} on the axis of rotation), an off-axis correction factor will need to be defined. All these data will need to be measured locally and carefully evaluated. The addition of wedges to the asymmetric beam will further complicate the dosimetry.

Multileaf collimation

Multileaf collimators enable the shape of the beam to be varied from the normal rectangular format, although all the many corners will remain right angles (Fig. 3.24c). The 'serrated' edge of the field will give rise to an effectively broader penumbra, while the isodose distribution and the absolute dosimetry will have to be defined in terms similar to those outlined above. New protocols are urgently awaited.

Effect of changes in source–skin distance

It has already been stated that the central axis depth dose is dependent on the inverse square law and, therefore, on the SSD. If primary radiation from the source alone was involved then the simple application of the inverse square law would be all that is necessary to derive depth dose data for different SSDs. However, the field width measured at depth varies with the SSD, owing to the beam divergence (Fig. 5.18). Therefore, assuming the same field size at the surface, the scatter component at depth will decrease with increasing SSD. Furthermore, at megavoltage energies the 100% reference point is at a depth d_{max} below the

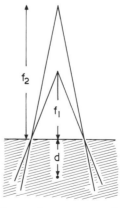

Fig. 5.18   The effect on the percentage dose at depth *d* of changing the SSD from f_1 to f_2.

surface and this must also be taken into account. To quantify the basic assumption that the *depth dose at depth d increases with source–skin distance f*, we define a factor:

$$F = \frac{(f_1 + d)}{(f_1 + d_{max})} \cdot \frac{(f_2 + d_{max})}{(f_2 + d)}$$

in which d_{max} is equated to zero when the 100% is at the surface. The modified depth dose D is then given by:

$$D(f_2,S) = D(f_1,S/F) \cdot \frac{B(S/F)}{B(S)} \cdot F^2$$

where $B(S)$ is the back scatter factor for the equivalent square field of side S. This simple formula is only approximate, giving results accurate to about 2%. Since F is a function of d, its application is usually limited to evaluating a few points in any clinical situation, e.g. the midpoint and peak dose for a parallel opposed pair.

Measurement of isodose charts

Owing to the complexities of the isodose distribution within the radiation beam, many approximation methods have been devised to minimise the number of measurements required before the isodose chart can be uniquely specified. Mathematical models have been devised which, with the help of a computer, can calculate the shape of isodose lines with the minimum of input data—and some of these models are entirely empirical. These techniques are beyond the scope of this book. The outline given below is based on a simple rectilinear system for measuring the distribution directly, which will be available in some form or another in almost every department.

The basic requirement is a water tank, probably $50 \times 50 \times 50$ cm^3 but preferably larger, in which a small detector can be moved in two directions by remote control (Fig. 5.19). The plane of movement will contain the central axis of the beam. If the output of the radiation beam is likely to fluctuate (as in any X-ray unit), a monitor will be rigidly mounted in the beam but out of the plane of movement of the detector—to avoid collisions. The movement of the detector will be followed exactly by a pen—through a mechanical or electrical linkage—which will trace the position of the detector in the phantom tank, whereas the object of the exercise is to record the magnitude of the ionisation at that position. It is at this point where the systems differ. The laborious, but very practical, method is for the operator to write alongside the pen the dose measured at each point in

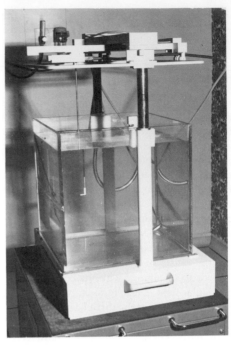

Fig. 5.19 The water phantom for use with an automatic isodose plotter. The horizontal beam to be measured enters the side of the tank on the left where the 'window' thickness has been reduced. The solid state detector may be moved in all three orthogonal directions.

the beam. Alternatively an automatic device may cause the pen (and the detector) to move along lines of equal dose, thus drawing the isodose curve directly on the paper, switching from one isodose level to another (Fig. 6.23C). Most isodose plotting systems are now based on a computer which automatically records the relative signal and the coordinates of the detector at many thousands of points, either for immediate display on the isodose plotting computer or in a compatible form for later analysis on a treatment planning computer. Whatever 'electronic black box' is used, isodose lines are charted based on the measurement of the ionisation produced at different points in the uniform semi-infinite tissue equivalent phantom.

Where a water tank is not available, useful information regarding the dose distribution in a megavoltage beam can be determined using film. If a slow radiographic film is sandwiched firmly between sheets of tissue equivalent material of adequate size and exposed in such a way that the film contains the beam axis, then isodensity lines may be plotted using a densitometer. The dose calibration of these isodensity lines must be based on ionisation measurements along the central axis. The technique may be improved by

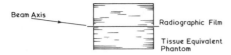

Fig. 5.20 The use of film for the measurement of megavoltage isodose charts.

darkening the room so that unwrapped film may be used to ensure good contact with the phantom and by inclining the beam axis at a few degrees to the plane of the film (Fig. 5.20) to ensure the primary radiation traverses the phantom and not only the film. This technique is equally applicable to photon and electron beams. At conventional X-ray energies, the energy response of the film and the changing X-ray spectrum with depth in the phantom make the interpretation of the film too difficult to be of any practical value.

Some isodose curve characteristics

Before leaving the subject of isodose charts it is worth summarising some of the characteristics of the different radiations met in the radiotherapy department.

Any isodose chart (Fig. 5.13) may be identified by examination of the following three aspects:

1. Central axis depth dose distribution, particularly the depth of the maximum dose and, say, the 50% depth.
2. Beam profile or the dose distribution across the beam.
3. Penumbra region.

The orthovoltage X-ray beam has a central axis dose which falls fairly rapidly from 100% at the surface to 50% at between 4 and 6 cm; the profile is curved and the penumbra is very sharp and clearly diverges from the source, while outside the penumbra there is the distinct contribution due to side scatter. The caesium-137 chart has a very rounded appearance with broad penumbra, the peak dose on the central axis is 2 mm below the surface and the beam 'edge' appears to be undefinable. Cobalt-60 is readily identified by the 5 mm depth of peak, a well-defined beam edge but fairly wide penumbra, the profile is less rounded except close to the beam edge, the 50% depth lies between 7 and 12 cm, depending on field size and SSD. Megavoltage X-ray beams are characterised by their narrow penumbra, flat profile and a depth of peak dose greater than 5 mm, the 50% depth will be between 10 and 20 cm, depending on energy and SSD but largely independent of field size.

The student should compare these isodose curves with those shown in Figure 6.23.

MEASUREMENT OF OUTPUT DOSE RATE

There have been different recommendations laid down on how to measure the output dose rate for a therapy unit. The techniques described below are those currently laid down in the U.K. The technique used is based on the use made of the therapy unit in question, namely at energies above 150 kVp the unit is generally required to treat tissues at depth and the output is measured at depth in a standard phantom. At energies below 150 kVp the unit is generally required to treat the skin surface and the output is measured in air (Fig. 5.21). In both cases an ionisation chamber is used for which a known quality correction factor, N, has already been determined by comparison with a secondary standard exposure meter (which in turn has been compared with the standard free air chamber, p. 72). The measurement is then suitably corrected to give the actual dose rate at the point of maximum ionisation on the central axis of the beam entering the patient.

In each case the output dose rate is measured under the operating conditions used clinically and using an average field size (10×8 cm² or 10×10 cm² are recommended) and standard SSD. If more than one combination of kV, mA and filter are used, then the

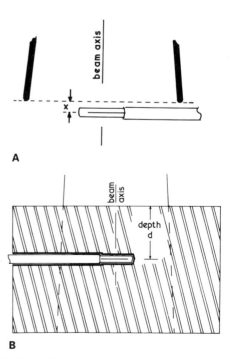

Fig. 5.21 The calibration of output dose rate **A** in air for superficial X-rays and **B** in phantom for megavoltage X-rays.

output must be measured for each combination. Regular calibrations are recommended, the frequency being at least once every 4 weeks.

Conversion from exposure to absorbed dose

From the definition of mass absorption coefficient (p. 61), we have

$$(\mu_a/\rho) = \frac{\text{Energy absorbed per unit mass}}{\text{Energy in the beam}}$$

This equation is true for any absorbing medium and therefore for tissue and air in particular. Therefore, it follows that

$$\frac{(\mu_a/\rho)_{\text{tissue}}}{(\mu_a/\rho)_{\text{air}}} = \frac{\text{Energy absorbed per unit mass of tissue}}{\text{Energy absorbed per unit mass of air}}$$

Now, if the charge on one electron is 1.6×10^{-19} C and the average energy absorption required to produce one ionisation (one electron) in air is 5.44×10^{-18} J, then one coulomb of charge will require the absorption of $5.44 \times 10^{-18}/1.6 \times 10^{-19}$ or 33.97 J. Therefore

Dose in air (grays) = 33.97 × Exposure in air (C kg)

and by substitution in the equation above

Dose in tissue (grays) = F × Exposure in air (C kg)

or

$$D_{\text{tissue}} = F \cdot X$$

where

$$F = \frac{33.97 \ (\mu_a/\rho)_{\text{tissue}}}{(\mu_a/\rho)_{\text{air}}}$$

Although for most purposes, the F-factor will be that for soft tissue (Table 5.6), it is instructive to realise that this will be different from that for other body tissues—bone and fat for instance—owing to the differences in their atomic numbers. Bone, for example, has an atomic number nearly twice that of soft tissue and a lower hydrogen content. Gram for gram, therefore, the

Table 5.6 Typical values of the F-factor for soft tissue

Beam quality	F-factor (J C⁻¹)	F-factor (cGy R⁻¹)
1 mm Al HVT	34.0	0.88
4 mm Al HVT	34.0	0.87
2 mm Cu HVT	36.5	0.94
Cobalt-60	37.0	0.95
4 MV	36.5	0.94
6 MV	36.5	0.94
10 MV	36.0	0.93

dose to bone is several times greater than that to soft tissue at low photon energies, while at higher energies it is less (Fig. 5.22). Armed with this information, therefore, a measurement of the exposure, X, at a point can be converted into absorbed dose by multiplying by an appropriate F-factor. This is true for the range of photon energies for which exposure can be measured at the standardising laboratory—up to cobalt-60 or 2 MV. At energies over 2 MV, F is replaced by C_λ to emphasise the conversion from exposure at 2 MV to dose at the operating potential.

Conversion from kerma to absorbed dose

Under conditions of electronic equilibrium all the kinetic energy released in unit mass of air (air kerma) will be absorbed in the air providing none is lost in bremsstrahlung (X-ray) production:

i.e.

$$dE_{\text{tr}} = dE_{\text{d}}$$

or

Dose in air = $K_{\text{air}} = X \ W_{\text{air}}/e = 33.97X$

But if the energy liberated, dE_{tr}, is not all absorbed then

$$\text{Dose in air} = \frac{K_{\text{air}} \ (\mu_a/\rho)_{\text{air}}}{(\mu_{\text{tr}}/\rho)_{\text{air}}}$$

where (μ_a/ρ) is the mass energy absorption coefficient and (μ_{tr}/ρ) is the mass energy transfer coefficient and the ratio accounts for the energy lost in bremsstrahlung production. (The ratio increases with energy, being approximately 1.003 for cobalt-60 photons.) It follows that:

$$\text{Dose in tissue} = \frac{K_{\text{air}} \ (\mu_a/\rho)_{\text{tissue}}}{(\mu_{\text{tr}}/\rho)_{\text{air}}}$$

Now $(\mu_a/\rho)_{\text{tissue}}/(\mu_{\text{tr}}/\rho)_{\text{air}}$ is approximately 1.10 for soft tissue over a wide range of photon energies and therefore

Dose in soft tissue (grays) = $1.10 \ K_{\text{air}}$ (grays)

$$= 1.10 \times 33.97 \times X \ (\text{Ckg}^{-1})$$

Cross-calibration of instruments

There is a hierarchy of instruments for measuring dose to ensure not only accuracy of the dose measured but also to ensure a consistency of that accuracy between radiotherapy centres. This is particularly important where patients are entered in multicentre trials or where the results of treatment are published in journals. To achieve this, there are international inter-comparisons of national standardising laboratories and their primary standards, but we do not get involved in these. The national standard for lower energy radiations is usually a free air ionisation chamber (p. 72), but for high energies calorimeters are being increasingly used. In addition to the national standards, there is a limited number of secondary standard instruments, held by competent physicists in regional centres. In the UK, some 25 secondary standard instruments are calibrated against the primary standard every 3 years over a wide range of photon energies—from 10 kV to 20 MV—and at the same time the linearity of their scale and range is checked. The calibration factor will be either in terms of air kerma in grays, N_k, or exposure in roentgens, N_x, or dose to water in grays, N.

The secondary standard instruments are then used to calibrate the dosemeters in everyday use, and in the actual radiation beams in which they are used, wherever possible. These intercomparisons are carried out annually in accordance with agreed protocols and provide each field instrument with a calibration factor, N_f, in terms of absorbed dose to water. These calibration factors will incorporate the appropriate factor for the secondary standard, N_k or N_x, and a factor to convert from air to water for megavoltage energies:

$$N_f = 1.138\, N_k C_\lambda\, R/R_f \text{ or } 0.01\, N_x C_\lambda\, R/R_f$$

and at orthovoltage energies:

$$N_f = 1.141\, N_k F\, R/R_f \text{ or } 0.01\, N_x F\, R/R_f$$

where R and R_f are the readings obtained on the secondary standard and field instruments respectively (corrected for any difference in the ambient conditions between the two chambers); F and C_λ with the numerical constants convert from the air kerma or exposure to absorbed dose in water. N_f then has the units grays per div. The values of N_k and N_x are those appropriate to the energy (HVT) of the photon beam used or 2 MV, whichever is the lower.

Where calorimetry is used as the primary standard for megavoltage energies above 2 MV (cobalt-60) the calibration factor for the secondary standard instrument is quoted in absorbed dose in water and the calibration of the field instrument is simply:

$$N_f = NR/R_f$$

Calibration of output dose rate (below 150 kV)

The ionisation chamber is aligned close to the surface of the applicator and centred on the beam axis (Fig. 5.21A). The size of the applicator should be the locally agreed standard, typically 5 cm diameter at 15 cm SSD or 10 cm diameter at 30 cm SSD. The distance, x, from the centre of the chamber to the surface must be measured accurately. The chamber is then exposed for a period of time, t, equivalent to a typical treatment of, say, 2 to 3 Gy and the ionisation charge integrated on the exposure meter as a reading, R. The ambient temperature in the treatment room and the atmospheric pressure are noted. The reading R is corrected by multiplying by the air mass correction factor, Λ, (p. 74) and then by the calibration factor, N_f (gray div^{-1}), derived from the intercomparisons with the secondary standard for the beam being measured, to give the total absorbed dose in water at the centre of the chamber.

The inverse square law correction factor $[(s + x)^2/s^2]$, where s is the SSD, corrects for the stand-off, x, of the chamber, and the back scatter factor, B, takes care of the lack of tissue behind the chamber.

Thus the dose rate, $\dot{D}$, at the surface of a patient in contact with this applicator is given by:

$$\dot{D} = R \cdot A \cdot N_f\, [(s + x)^2/s^2]\, B/t \text{ gray min}^{-1}$$

It should be noted that N_f and B are both energy dependent and the values appropriate to the HVT of the beam must be used.

It is good practice to use an average field size as standard, to take two or three readings and take an average value for R, and to ensure there is nothing significant in the beam to generate back scatter to the chamber.

Timer error

Where the treatment duration is controlled by a timer, preferably with an independent back-up timer (p. 37), the quotation of a dose rate must assume that dose rate is constant so that the product of dose rate and time is an accurate estimate of total dose. Variations in kV and mA must be minimal. However, on many units—conventional X-ray generators and teleisotope units—the dose rate is not constant because it is not immediately established on switch-on and may not fall immediately to zero at the end for technical or mechanical reasons. The error introduced in this way is constant and can be measured as follows. If the timer error is Δt and a reading R_1 is obtained during an exposure of time t using a set-up as described above, then the reading is related to the time by the equation:

$$R_1 = k(t + \Delta t)$$

where k is an unknown constant. If the exposure is

now repeated except for the fact it is deliberately interrupted once part way through, then a reading R_2 will be obtained where

$$R_2 = k(t + 2 \Delta t)$$

t is the same total exposure time as before but the interruption has increased the switch-on/switch-off procedure from once to twice and therefore the error is $2 \Delta t$. Eliminating the unknown by dividing these equations and solving for Δt, we get

$$\Delta t = \frac{R_2 - R_1}{2R_1 - R_2} \cdot t$$

Δt is usually negative and the prescribed treatment time must be increased by adding Δt to the set time and each time the beam is energised after an interruption.

Calibration of output dose rate (above 150 kV)

At the higher photon energies the 'in-air' measurement is inappropriate and the output dose rate is measured at depth. The depths used vary with the photon energy, but for most purposes a depth of 5 cm is used. The recommended depths for higher energies are given in Table 5.7 and there are proposals in hand for calibrating lower energy beams at depth in a phantom for which shallower depths will have to be defined, but until then the in-air technique described above will be used.

A phantom of adequate size, at least $20 \times 20 \times 10$ cm^3 is used such that the ionisation chamber is positioned with its centre at the appropriate depth below one of the larger faces and with at least 5 cm to the exit surface. The top face of the phantom is positioned at the normal treating distance with the ionisation chamber on the central axis (Fig. 5.21B) in a 10×10 cm^2 field. The chamber is in a close fitting Perspex sheath. The chamber is then exposed for a typical treatment time or for a known number of monitor units on the integrating dosimetry system, say 2 to 3 Gy. As before, several readings are taken and the average reading R corrected using the air mass correction factor based

Table 5.7 Recommended calibration depths

Radiation energy	Depth (cm)
150 kVp – 10 MV X-rays	5
Cobalt-60, caesium-137	5
11–24 MV	7
25–50 MV	10
Electrons	d_{max}

on the atmospheric pressure and the temperature of the phantom—if that is likely to be different from the ambient temperature of the room. The percentage depth dose factor corrects the measured value to dose rate at d_{max} without the need for inverse square or back scatter factors. The dose rate is therefore:

$$\dot{D} = \frac{R \cdot A \cdot N_f}{\%DD \cdot t}$$

where a preset dose has been used, then the calculated peak dose:

$$D = R \cdot A \cdot N_f / \%DD$$

should be within ± 1% of the monitor units set.

Output factors

The routine output dose rate measurements are made using an average field size (usually 10×10 cm^2). At the initial calibration of the unit, the output dose rate will be measured for all field sizes which will be encountered in the clinical use of the unit. The variation in output dose rate is principally due to the increase in scattered radiation with field size. It is customary to tabulate the output dose rate for each applicator size available on an orthovoltage unit or to tabulate output factors for (equivalent) square fields on megavoltage units. The output factor is unity for the reference field size. For other field sizes the output factor is defined as:

$$OF_s = \frac{\text{Output dose rate for field size, } S}{\text{Output dose rate for the reference field size}}$$

EFFECTS OF INHOMOGENEITIES ON DEPTH DOSE

The fundamental measurements on the relative distribution of dose and the absolute magnitude of the dose in a beam of radiation have all assumed that the patient is accurately represented by a rectangular water tank. This is far from true! Yet in most of our treatment planning little cognisance is given to this fact, largely because of the complexities which arise as soon as any inhomogeneity is introduced (Fig. 5.22).

Where treatment planning is carried out using manual techniques, the sheer complexity of the problem makes any adjustment of the dose distribution for the presence of inhomogeneities prohibitive. Where computer techniques are available, the ability to adjust the distribution is there but often the patient data are not. Several attempts have been made using atlases of body sections to provide data on the size and position of the

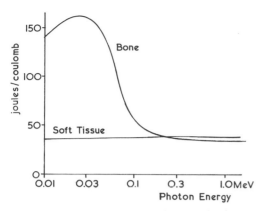

Fig. 5.22 The relative absorption in bone and soft tissue.

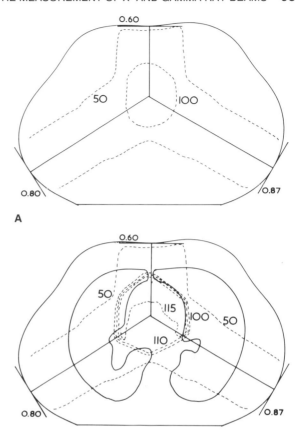

Fig. 5.23 The effect of lung correction factors. In **A** the contour is assumed to be homogeneous, whereas in **B** allowance is made for the lower density in the lungs — no other beam parameter is changed.

principal inhomogeneities. CT scanners are invaluable here. Using multiple slices through the target site, the principal inhomogeneities can be localised within the external contour automatically (Ch. 7) and the necessary information made available to the treatment planning computer. The effect of an inhomogeneity can be described in qualitative terms.

A beam of radiation passing through healthy lung will be less attenuated than it would be through soft tissue, with the result that soft tissues beyond healthy lung and within its geometric shadow will receive a greater dose than that predicted from the standard isodose charts. The effect of correcting for the lung inhomogeneities is illustrated in Figure 5.23. In (A) the contour is assumed to be homogeneous soft tissue, whereas using the same beam parameters together with lung correction an increase of more than 15% in the tissue dose is shown in (B).

Similarly, bone will absorb more radiation than soft tissue, with the result that the soft tissue beyond the bone will receive less dose. Remember that although bone and tissue may absorb equal doses of megavoltage radiation gram for gram, bone is nearly twice as dense as soft tissue. Remember too that while healthy lung tissue has a density of about 0.3 g cm^{-3}, malignant lung tissue density is closer to 1 g cm^{-3}. This relatively simple situation is further complicated by the fact that the radiation scattered by bone and lung is different and so is the electron flux. At orthovoltage energies, the dose to soft tissue beyond lung is higher due to increased transmission through the lung and lower due to the reduced scatter produced by healthy lung, while beyond a bone inhomogeneity the dose is reduced by the high

absorption in bone and increased by the increased scatter. Similarly, at megavoltage energies, the secondary electron flux is greater in bone than in soft tissue and since the electrons have a range of several millimetres, the electrons generated in the bone close to the bone–tissue interface will increase the dose to the tissue until electronic equilibrium is restored. Conversely lung. Soft tissue close to bone and, therefore, the soft tissue elements actually living within bone always receive a higher dose than they would if the bone was replaced by soft tissue. So, although there may be clearly defined interfaces between the soft muscle tissues and the inhomogeneities, their effect on the dose distribution is far from clear. The student is referred to more advanced texts for further discussion on this subject.

6. Principles of radiation treatment planning

INTRODUCTION

The phrase *radiation treatment planning* as applied to external beam therapy is used to describe the work involved in displaying graphically a dose distribution which results when one or more radiation beams converge on the target volume. It does not include any assessment of the dose fractionation or of dose rate effects (Ch. 17).

For most purposes the dose distribution is a two-dimensional distribution in the midplane of treatment which also contains the principal axes of all the treatment fields. The two-dimensional distribution has limitations, but the majority of treatment sites are cylindrical in section and the distribution in planes parallel to the midplane is not markedly different. Three-dimensional treatment planning is now available on the larger computer systems, removing the need for coplanar beam axes and introducing the possibility of viewing the distributions from any angle. The visual appreciation of the distribution becomes the principal obstacle because the three-dimensional plan has to be displayed or printed in two dimensions.

Criteria by which a dose distribution are judged vary from one centre to another, although the following give a guide as to what is required. For the sake of clarity the words *target volume* are used to refer to that volume defined by the clinician as being the tumour or lesion surrounded by any margin he or she chooses to include in the treatment; the words *treatment volume* are used to refer to that actually covered by the radiation beams and raised to a dose greater than the minimum dose in the target volume.

1. The dose throughout the target volume should be uniform to within ± 5%.
2. The treatment volume should as near as possible be the same as the target volume in position, size and shape.
3. The dose to the treatment volume should exceed that to any other area by at least, say, 20%.
4. The dose to neighbouring radiosensitive sites (e.g. eyes, spinal cord, etc.) should, where practicable, be kept below their tolerance dose.
5. The integral dose should be kept to a minimum.

These criteria also provide guidelines on how the treatment planning of any site should be approached. Criterion (3) suggests that unless the treatment volume includes the skin surface, then two or more fields should be used to converge on the treatment volume. Criteria (2) and (5) suggest that the radiation beam size should be kept to a minimum and the beams should enter the patient as close to the treatment volume as possible providing criterion (4) is not broken. To enable an assessment of the effectiveness of the plan, a calculation of the irradiated volume has been suggested, the *irradiated volume* being defined for this purpose as the volume receiving more than half the target dose. The first and foremost criterion is dose uniformity and examples will be given to show how this can be achieved.

Where treatment planning is done by hand, it is normal practice to add the percentage values displayed on the isodose chart (Fig. 6.1). The net result is that the summated isodose lines are normalised to the applied (given) dose to each field, as in Figure 6.2. Where the planning computer is used the distribution is normalised to the target dose, as in Figures 6.8 and 6.11, for example, and the applied (given) dose to each field is a percentage of the target dose.

Later, in Part 2, examples are given for different treatment sites, whilst here we concentrate on the effects of different field combinations. It should be borne in mind that the relative distribution is not altered appreciably by changes in the size of the patient section or the size of the radiation beams used, e.g. four oblique fields to the head treating the pituitary produce the same basic distribution as four oblique fields to the abdomen treating the bladder.

TREATMENT PLANNING BY HAND

This procedure is simplified if a planning table is available, i.e. a light box set into a desk top and inclined at an angle of, say, 10° to the horizontal. Each isodose chart should be available on a separate acetate sheet, so it can be adjusted to the desired position and angle under a sheet of tracing paper on which the patient contour is drawn. The resulting distribution is then drawn on the tracing paper. (If a simple beam isodose chart needs modifying, e.g. to allow for oblique incidence (p. 99) or for weighting factors (p. 103), this should be completed before attempting the following procedure.) If a three field plan is to be drawn, the third field is added to the summation of the two; a four field plan is the addition of the summation of fields one and two to the summation of fields three and four.

In Figure 6.1, two isodose charts are shown, each normalised to 100% at d_{max} with the isodose lines at 10% intervals. In practice it is easier to add the distributions of two intersecting beams, as shown, than to add parallel opposed beams, and to draw every isodose line in the resulting distribution, again at 10% intervals. Thus, to draw the 120% isodose line the planner will look for and mark the intersections of the individual isodose lines which add up to 120%, as shown, i.e. 100 + 20, 90 + 30, 80 + 40, 70 + 50, 60 + 60, 50 + 70, 40 + 80, 30 + 90, 20 + 100. Having marked

all the points, notice the marks are at the diagonally opposed corners of each quadrilateral if they are consecutive points in the above list. Now join up all the points in order as smoothly as possible *without* crossing any isodose line except at the intersection of two. Occasionally two adjacent points are the addition of the same two isodose lines and may appear inseparable—the resultant isodose line lies between the two! Occasionally, too, there are too few points of intersection to know for certain where the resultant isodose line should be drawn. To solve this the planner must interpolate the individual isodose charts to find points of the required value, e.g. 75 + 45, 63 + 57, etc. Remember isodose lines in the resultant distribution will *never* intersect and will always be continuous within the patient contour—isodose curves of low value may be discontinuous at the patient contour.

SIMPLE DISTRIBUTIONS

Parallel pair

Two directly opposing fields are known as a parallel opposed pair and the distribution is typified in Figure 6.2A. In general, the distribution is symmetrical about the beam axes. In particular, the midpoint receives the minimum dose *along* the central axes (except within the build-up region) and the maximum dose *at right angles* to the central axes. The actual variation of dose along these axes of symmetry depends on the type of radiation and on the separation of the fields (Fig. 6.3). The variation in dose is reduced by reducing the separation and by increasing the energy of the radiation. Within these limits, the tissue irradiated receives a uniform dose.

It should be remembered (Fig. 5.13) that the dose to the edges of the beam, while being lower than the central axis dose where the beams are incident normally on the skin, may be increased where there is excessive curvature of the entry surfaces, e.g. frontal and occipital fields to the head.

This technique is valuable where large volumes of tissue are to be irradiated or where the treatment is palliative. The use of very large fields will be discussed later in the chapter.

Box technique

If a parallel pair gives uniform irradiation to the enclosed tissues, then two intersecting parallel pairs will produce an even distribution over the volume enclosed by all four fields. This is true regardless of the angle between the axes of the two pairs, i.e. the box is not necessarily rectangular. For example, two pairs at right angles produce a 'square' distribution (Fig. 6.2C), while two

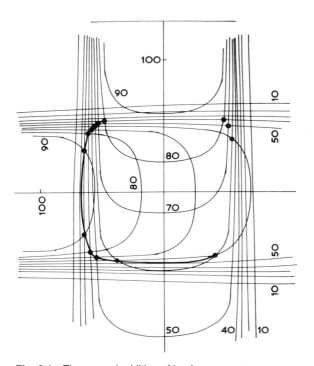

Fig. 6.1   The manual addition of isodose curves.

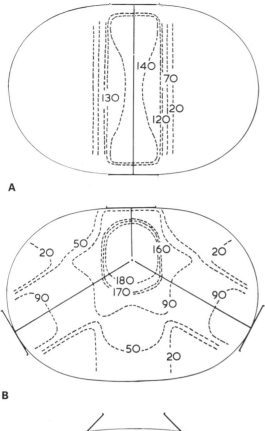

A

B

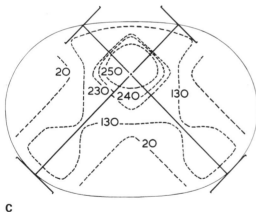

C

Fig. 6.2 **A** The parallel opposed pair distribution; **B** the three field distribution; **C** the four field box distribution.

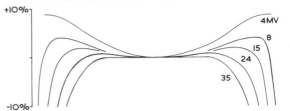

The dose distribution normalized to the mid-point along the common axis of a parallel opposed pair of 200mm separation

Fig. 6.3 The variation of dose uniformity along the common axes of a parallel opposed pair with photon energy.

Three field technique

By arranging fields so that they overlap *only* in the target volume, it may be possible to bring most of the tissue outside the target volume to less than half the dose or at least to keep the irradiated volume small and close to the target. In Figure 6.2B it will be seen that except for regions close to the target the dose in general is less than half of that to the target volume. It will be also noticed that the dose gradient at the edge of the target volume is less steep than that in the box technique. The three and four field techniques are widely used in radical treatments using quite small fields—providing the beam direction can be guaranteed and the target is close to the centre of the patient section.

Atlases of dose distribution

Where the planning work has to be minimised through lack of facilities it may be helpful to refer to an atlas of these three basic treatment techniques. Each chart in the atlas provides the dose distribution resulting from fields of a stated size, relative angle, separation and beam quality. In practice, the chart giving the 'best fit' is used and may be modified slightly as required. Atlases are not to be recommended for the routine planning of radical courses of treatment because of the limitations inherent in such distributions but may often assist in the planning of difficult cases by showing the effect on the distribution of varying one or other of the many parameters involved. The radical treatment plan demands the distribution to be tailored to the individual patient. An accurate distribution may require the use of oblique incidence corrections, compensators, wedges or weighting factors. Patient shells (moulds) or other immobilisation devices may also be required.

OBLIQUE INCIDENCE AND ITS CORRECTION

Owing to the curvature of the skin, most radiation beams

pairs at, say 120°, produce a 'diamond' distribution. The disadvantage of the box technique is seen when small fields are used at large separations since the irradiated tissue outside the target volume receives half the dose to that inside. This may violate the criterion (4) above. There is no reason against using three parallel pairs, but the improvement is rarely justified.

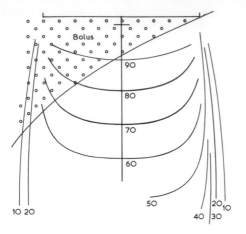

Fig. 6.4 The use of bolus to restore the normal incidence and so maintain the charted dose distribution, but note the loss of skin sparing.

Table 6.1 Isodose shift factors

Cobalt-60	0.67
5–15 MV X-rays	0.60
15–30 MV X-rays	0.50

applied to the patient will enter a curved surface at an angle of incidence which is not zero (normal incidence). Such oblique incidence may be quite deliberate or simply due to the fact that the patient's skin is not flat; in either case the dose distribution in the patient will not be that shown on the appropriate isodose chart. There are two alternative ways of dealing with this, either to correct the distribution or to correct the curvature.

At the orthovoltage energies where there is no build-up or skin sparing effect the space between the treatment applicator and the skin can be filled with 'bolus' or tissue equivalent wax, thus making up the tissue deficiency, to provide both attenuation of the primary radiation and to generate the scattered radiation so vital to the dose distribution. This may be done at megavoltage energies also where skin sparing is not required (Figs 6.4 and 6.19F). In either case normal incidence is restored and the appropriate isodose chart can be used without correction, providing the entry point is correctly positioned.

If the build-up region is to be retained to maximise the skin sparing then the isodose distribution may be corrected from that of normal incidence to that for oblique incidence. The computer will invariably use a mathematical approach to the problem and use either an exponential correction factor based on the lack of attenuation through the tissue deficiency, or an inverse square law correction factor based on the change in source skin distance. For routine manual treatment planning these approaches are too time consuming and an approximation method has to be used.

A 'rule-of-thumb' is frequently used. A rule-of-thumb is an approximation to the truth which is sufficiently accurate for the purpose in hand, providing it is used within its limitations. The rule here is to move the

charted isodose curves through a distance related to the thickness of the missing tissue. The distance moved depends on the beam energy and the depth of the isodose line (Table 6.1). The isodose lines on the chart are shifted by a fraction of the thickness of the tissue deficiency as measured along the ray from the source of radiation (Fig. 6.5). This does not apply in the build-up region where the build-up follows the expected pattern, i.e. the isodose lines remain essentially parallel to the skin surface.

Where the treating distance is measured to the skin on the central axis, it is often found that on one side there is a tissue deficiency while on the other there is excess tissue. The same correction technique may be applied— but making the reverse effect. The use of this rule-of-thumb should be restricted to small angles of incidence and small excesses or deficiencies of tissue.

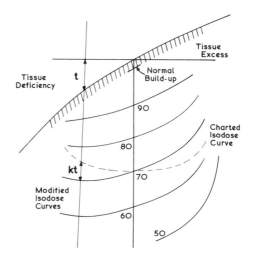

Fig. 6.5 The correction for oblique incidence using the shift technique.

Tissue compensators

The charted isodose curve may be used while maintaining the skin sparing properties of the megavoltage beam by the use of *tissue compensators*. Here the lack of attenuation in the region of tissue deficiency is made good by using an attenuator in the beam sufficiently removed from the skin that the build-up region is unaffected (Fig. 6.6). This technique is particularly

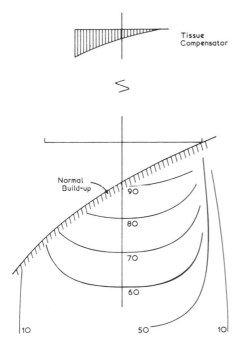

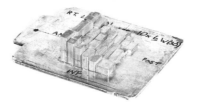

Fig. 6.7   A tissue compensator.

Fig. 6.6   Using a remote tissue compensator, the skin sparing effect and the charted dose distribution are both maintained, providing the SSD is increased by the compensated thickness.

valuable in regions where the skin curvature is complex, e.g. in the region of the neck.

Where the curvature is sufficiently great to justify a tissue compensator, the accurate alignment of the compensator and patient during the treatment demands the use of a mould or shell to immobilise the patient. The mould extends over the treated region and therefore the data required to make the compensator can be obtained from the mould—a considerably easier exercise than measuring directly from the patient. Having determined accurately the position and direction of the beam axis, the stand-off or thickness of tissue deficiency is measured at 1 cm intervals over the whole of the field area and preferably 1 cm beyond. For simplicity each measurement is rounded to the nearest centimetre. Using this information it is possible to build up the compensator with 'bricks', each equivalent to a cubic centimetre of tissue. These 'bricks' will be less than 1×1 cm^2 in area owing to the fact that the compensator will be mounted about half way between the source and the skin. Their height will be 1 g cm^{-2} in whatever material is chosen, e.g. aluminium. The bricks will be glued to a base plate, say 3 mm aluminium, which can be uniquely positioned in the beam to guarantee the correct alignment (Fig. 6.7). In most cases two or more compensators will be required, one for each treatment field. In use, the normal

SSD will be increased by the compensated distance as measured along the central axis of the beam, and an output correction factor applied based on the attenuation through the base plate.

Tissue compensators should be confined to small fields treating small body sections. Although scattered radiation plays a less significant role in megavoltage therapy, the loss of scatter generation in the tissue deficiency does result in a small reduction in dose to the first few centimetres relative to the dose to tissues at greater depth where the scatter contribution is not affected. A small correction may be required to correct for this.

WEDGES

Where the target volume is close to the surface of the patient but too thick to be adequately treated by a single field, it is often convenient to use two beams with wedges. A *wedged pair* can be used to treat regions such as the antrum, the larynx and the middle ear.

The wedge is a specially machined wedge-shaped piece of metal. It can be made of any metal, although there is some preference for those of low atomic number, especially where the wedge has to be positioned close to the patient. The wedge may be positioned in the beam immediately behind the mirror of the light beam diaphragm (Figs 3.16 and 3.25) or between the

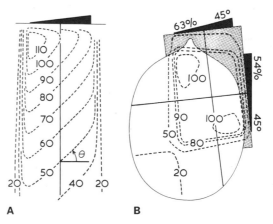

Fig. 6.8   **A** The wedged isodose chart; **B** the use of wedged beams in the treatment of the antrum.

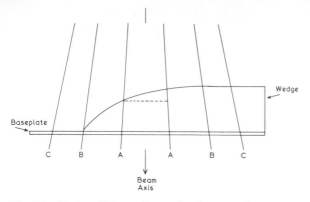

Fig. 6.9 Wedge efficiency: the wedge factor can be reduced by using a wedge no bigger than the field.

diaphragms and the shielding tray. The purpose of the wedge is to attenuate the beam on one side of the beam axis relative to the other, thereby tilting the isodose curves through an angle. This *wedge angle* is defined as the angle through which the 50% isodose line is turned (Fig. 6.8A). (Some centres define the wedge angle at a specified depth, say 10 cm, rather than the specified percentile line.) In the design of a wedge it is often expedient to straighten out the curvature of the (unwedged) beam profile as well as tilting it through the required angle. The wedge profile will take the form shown in Figure 6.9.

The wedge attenuates the beam and thereby reduces the useful beam dose rate. The treatment time or the set monitor units, therefore, has to be increased. The increase is determined by the *wedge factor* which is defined as the time required to deliver a given dose to a point on the central axis when using the wedge, divided by the time required to deliver the same dose to the same point without the wedge. Each wedge is usually designed for use up to a limited field size to maximise the wedge efficiency. A wedge which is too large requires the use of an unnecessarily large wedge factor. For example, in Figure 6.9 the field size AA requires a much thinner wedge than the field size BB to produce the same wedge angle, with the result that the wedge factor could be reduced if field AA is the maximum required. The clinical use of wedges is such that wedge angles up to 45° are required in fields up to about 20 cm wide and above 45° in fields up to about 15 cm wide. Unless the diaphragm size is electrically interlocked with the wedge, it is advisable to extend the thickest part of the wedge beyond the maximum field size BB to minimise the effects of overdosage should an over-large field be used accidentally. The wedge will usually cover the whole range of field sizes perpendicular to the wedged direction.

Where discrete wedges are used, it is usual to have a range of wedge angles available, typically 15, 30, 45 and 60°. With computer controlled linear accelerators, it is possible to produce a variety of wedge angles by other means. For example, the wedged isodose distribution for any wedge angle up to 60° can be produced by delivering a fraction of the dose with the 60° wedge in the beam and the remaining fraction without it—the larger the fraction with the wedge, the greater the effective wedge angle. Alternatively, the wedge effect can be produced by using the asymmetrical diaphragm facility—and moving one diaphragm blade relative to the other while the radiation is being delivered. Both these 'alternative wedge' systems demand very careful quality control if the dose is to be delivered accurately.

Wedged dose distribution

The ideal dose distribution is obtained when two beams of wedge angle θ are used with a hinge angle of $(180 - 2\theta)°$, where the *hinge angle* is the angle between the beam axes at their point of intersection (angle *qps* in Figure 6.10). This only applies when the beams enter a flat surface at normal incidence (Fig. 6.8B). The 'wedging effect' produced under conditions of oblique incidence invariably reduces the wedge angle and increases the optimum hinge angle.

The *wedging effect* of oblique incidence can sometimes be compensated by the use of wedges of shallow wedge angle, say 15°. For example, when treating a larynx with a parallel opposed pair it may improve the final dose distribution if wedges are used such that their thick edges are to the anterior. This is a technique of limited value but can with care be used to advantage wherever the skin curvature is predominantly in one plane. The student should note that wherever wedges are used, they are used in pairs with the 'thick edges together' irrespective of the hinge angle.

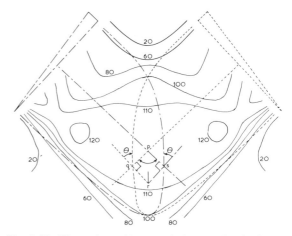

Fig. 6.10 The optimum hinge angle for a wedged pair.

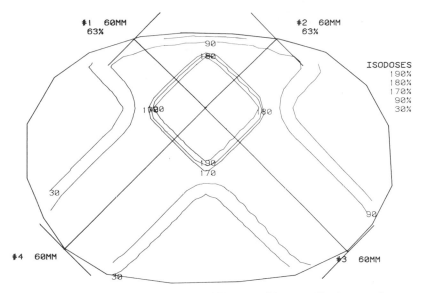

Fig. 6.11   The four field box distribution of Figure 6.2C improved by the use of weighting two fields by 63%.

WEIGHTING FACTORS

So far it has been assumed that each field in a distribution is given the same dose (100%). Some distributions may be improved by reducing the dose given to one or more fields in the multifield treatment plan. These fields are said to be weighted against the others. Weighting factors of 50% (half dose) or 75% (three-quarter dose) are simple to handle but any factor can be used. The effect is to reduce the *dose gradient* and therefore weighting factors may be used to improve the uniformity of dose. For example, if the box technique is used to treat a volume which is off-centre (as in Fig. 6.2C), then the distribution may be improved by weighting those fields closer to the treated volume so that they can contribute the same actual dose to

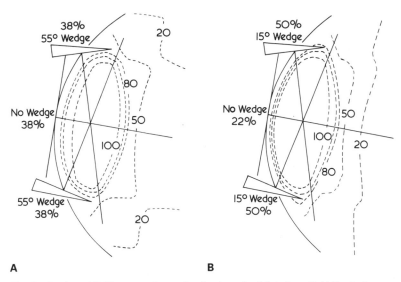

Fig. 6.12   **A** and **B** The use of a wedged pair and a third plane field illustrating how the dose to tissues outside the target volume can be modified by changing the weighting factors and wedge angle.

the centre of the volume as the more distant fields (Fig. 6.11). Alternatively, weighting factors may be used to modify the distribution of dose *outside* the target volume, as in Figure 6.12. This is particularly useful where radiosensitive tissues are close to the target volume. This introduction of a plain field between two wedged fields produces a very versatile technique for treating both superficial targets, as shown, or deep-seated targets such as the bladder and nasopharynx.

Where the dose distribution is normalised to the target dose, all the fields will carry a weighting factor; they may be equally weighted as in Figure 6.12A or differently weighted as in Figure 6.12B.

ROTATION THERAPY

A logical extension of the multiple fixed field distribution is to have an infinite number of fields all aimed at one centre. This is achieved by moving the source in an arc whilst irradiating the patient. In *arc therapy*, the source of radiation moves through a prescribed angle, while in *rotation therapy* the source moves through a full 360°. Rotation therapy was developed in the 1920s as a means of achieving an adequate dose at depth without exceeding the tolerance dose to the skin using 200 kV radiation. This was prior to the introduction of megavoltage radiation. Although skin tolerance is no longer a problem, rotation therapy is still used in some centres, particularly where cobalt-60 provides the only megavoltage radiation. The dose distribution resulting from a full rotation of the source of radiation is essentially circular or elliptical—the major axis of the ellipse

being at right angles to that of the patient contour (Fig. 6.13). There are no steep dose gradients at the edges of the target volume, the beam edges being blurred by the rotation. The actual dosimetry is complicated by two facts: (1) that the SSD will vary because the source–axis distance is constant, and, (2), that a full rotation needs to be represented by at least 18 fields (at 20° intervals)—a problem best solved using a computer. However, the maximum dose will be close to the centre of rotation, and it is often adequate to calculate the dose at that point only. This is most conveniently done using tissue–air ratios or tissue–phantom ratios.

Tissue–air ratio

The tissue–air ratio (TAR) is the ratio of the dose rate at a point in the patient to that at the same point (at the centre of a minimal mass) in air when there is no patient present. The dose rate at a point is dependent on the distance from the source (the inverse square law), the thickness of the overlying tissues and the scatter contribution which varies with field size. Since the TAR is the ratio of dose rates at the same point in space, it is independent of distance from the source—the inverse square factor cancels out. For a given field size (and, therefore, scatter contribution), it is possible to tabulate or represent graphically the TAR against the thickness of the overlying tissue (Fig. 6.14).

$$\text{TAR} = \frac{\text{Axis dose rate in tissue}}{\text{Axis dose rate in air}}$$

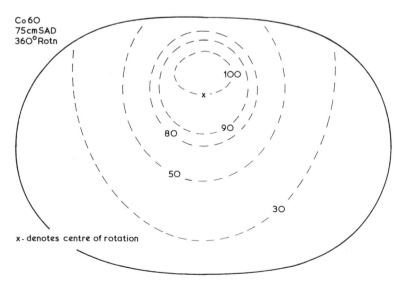

Co 60
75 cm SAD
360° Rotn

100

90

80

50

30

x - denotes centre of rotation

Fig. 6.13 A dose distribution resulting from rotation therapy.

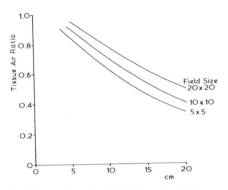

Fig. 6.14 Tissue–air ratios (TAR) for cobalt-60.

By definition the dose rate on the axis is the dose rate in air at that point multiplied by the TAR. For a given patient contour, the centre of rotation is marked and eighteen radii are drawn at 20° intervals. The length of each radius is measured from the centre to the patient's skin and the TAR noted. The mean value of the TAR is calculated and used to determine a mean dose rate on the axis of rotation.

Tissue–phantom ratio

The tissue–phantom ratio (TPR) may be used instead of the tissue–air ratio above, providing the reference dose rate is known at the reference point in the phantom. (The tissue–maximum ratio (TMR) is the special case of TPR where the reference point is at the d_{max} on the central axis.) The use of TPR is a little more straightforward in practice because the reference dose rate can be measured directly under standardised conditions and avoids the interpretation of the phrase 'minimal mass in air'.

$$TPR = \frac{\text{Axis dose rate at depth } d \text{ in phantom}}{\text{Axis dose rate at reference depth in same phantom}}$$

Using TPRs and the reference dose rate, the mean dose rate at the axis of rotation may be determined in the manner outlined for TARs above.

The calculation of dose rates at points other than the centre of rotation is complex and the student is referred to more advanced texts for a detailed explanation. Atlases of rotation dose distribution are frequently normalised so that the point at the centre of rotation is 100%, as in Figure 6.13.

If a full rotation is not possible because of the attenuation through the spine of the couch, for example, then arcing over a limited range of angles can be used. This increases the skin/tumour dose ratio and brings the maximum dose point away from the axis of rotation towards the centre of the irradiated arc.

MANTLE TREATMENTS

The treatment plans considered so far have involved radiation fields of smaller dimension than the patient so that with some modification the isodose data measured in the semi-infinite phantom can be regarded as adequate. There are situations, however, where the field size is larger than the patient—the treatment of the thorax using mantle fields, for example.

The radiation treatment planning of mantle fields is complicated because it always involves substantial lung shielding (Fig. 3.30) and the separation of the parallel opposed AP-PA pair can vary considerably over the length and breadth of the fields. Unfortunately the minimum separation is usually across the upper half of the field where the local shielding is also minimal.

The lung dose under the shielding blocks is unlikely to be much below 10%, in that the major component will be scattered radiation from the irradiated tissues. The presence of the shielding, on the other hand, reduces the scatter component to the irradiated tissues, and the equivalent square concept is not simply applied. The scatter component near the centre of the 'T' will be greater than along its three arms. At the higher photon energies, the scatter component is small and therefore variations in scatter will only have a small effect on the dose uniformity.

The effect of the variation in beam separation is also minimised by the use of higher photon energies and extended SSDs—often necessary to get the required field size. Both parameters reduce the dose gradient with depth and therefore reduce the variation of midpoint dose with field separation.

The third area of concern in this technique is the lateral aspect of the chest wall, which may be included in the field but be outside the lung shield. Here the beam separation is very small, therefore increasing the combined effect of the two, but the scatter component will be negligible—there will be no scatter generated by the photons lateral to the wall (they will shine past) and no significant scatter generated within the shielded lung. Therefore, although the primary radiation component will be increased, the lack of scatter will bring the total dose down. This qualitative account highlights the areas of uncertainty of dose and the student should refer to other texts for a more quantitative account.

TOTAL BODY IRRADIATION

The use of total body irradiation (TBI) with megavoltage (6 MV) photons has become an established preliminary to bone marrow transplants in both children and adults. This poses real practical problems as well as in radiation treatment planning. The very large field sizes and the low dose rates required usually mean the patient is treated at an SSD of several metres, assuming the treatment room is large enough! It follows that the patient is usually treated with two lateral fields with a few centres adding AP and PA fields where the necessary patient position can be maintained and reproduced with sufficient accuracy. The treatment is usually given over six or eight fractions with two fractions per day. Whatever position the patient adopts—seated or lying down—the treatment fields will be rectangular in shape and somewhat larger in both dimensions than the patient and parallel opposed.

The radiation treatment planning is usually based on the midline dose at different levels within the patient, where the effective beam separations vary from typically 10 to 40 cm. These major variations in beam separation can be accommodated using tissue compensators to the head and neck and below the hips (Fig. 6.15). Lateral beams to the thorax, however, traverse considerable thicknesses of lung, where the attenuation is less than in normal tissue, and, because the dose to the lung is critical, careful lung compensation is essential. The lung compensators are best designed using the three-dimensional data from a full CT investigation of the thorax. All the compensators are conveniently attached to a transparent (acrylic) screen close to the patient to bring the peak dose (at d_{max}) closer to the skin.

It is customary to monitor the dose given to the patient

using radiation dosimeters (TLDs or silicon diodes) attached to the patient at selected and critical points. This survey of dose may be carried out as a preliminary to the treatment using a low dose trial irradiation, or at the first fraction or at each fraction throughout the treatment. As with all patient dose measurements, the results must be interpreted carefully in the light of conditions prevailing at the time of irradiation—the presence or absence of build-up material, of secondary scatter and the direction of irradiation. Where three or four fields are used, the weighting of each field will be determined from such a dose survey.

RADIOSURGERY

In contrast to TBI, radiosurgery is the use of very small fields (less than 25 mm) to treat brain disease. For example, arteriovenous malformations are often too deep within the brain for conventional interventional surgical techniques to be used, but are readily acces-

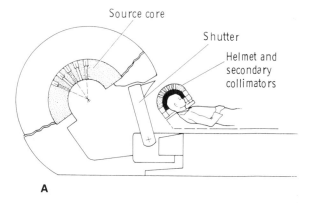

A

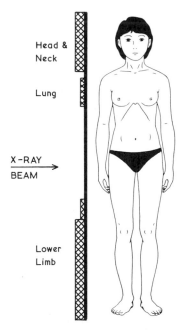

Fig. 6.15 Tissue compensation in total body irradiation.

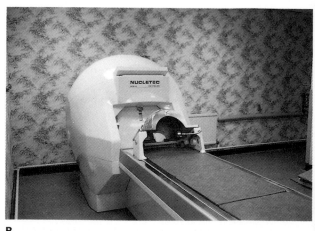

B

Fig. 6.16 **A** and **B** The Sheffield Stereotactic Radiosurgery Unit.

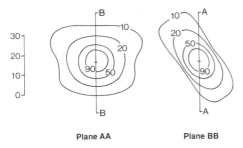

Plane AA   Plane BB

Fig. 6.17 The treatment plan for radiosurgery.

sible to accurately collimated and accurately defined radiation beams.

The technique has been established using a large number of cobalt-60 sources arrayed over a spherical sector and individually collimated to focus their radiation on to the target tissues. The unit in Sheffield (Fig. 6.16) uses 201 1 mm diameter cobalt sources to irradiate a volume of tissue at the focus as small as 4 mm diameter or as large as 18 mm. Larger targets can be accommodated using multiple foci. Figure 6.17 illustrates a typical treatment plan showing two orthogonal views of the distribution within the skull.

This level of accuracy demands the localisation, treatment planning and the treatment to be completed in a single session during which the patient 'wears' a reference frame attached rigidly to the outer table of the skull. Once attached under local anaesthetic, the frame is not removed until the final treatment is completed, usually 4–6 hours later. The patient is usually allowed to leave hospital the next day.

Radiosurgery is now being practised in some centres, using the linear accelerator as a source of radiation. To achieve the concentration of dose over such a small volume at the isocentre requires a special collimator and four or more arcs of gantry rotation, each at a different setting of couch rotation. As may be expected, the dose gradient at the edge of the irradiated volume is less steep than on the cobalt unit and the smallest irradiated volume is about 15 mm.

PATIENT CONTOURING DEVICES

The value of radiation treatment planning depends on the reproducibility of the position and shape of the patient on a day-to-day basis throughout the course of treatment. The couch where the patient contour will be taken should be identical in every respect to the couch on which that patient will be treated. The obese patient will have a contour which changes from day-to-day, while the patients with less 'padding' will find the hard top couch so uncomfortable that they will find it difficult

to lie still for the duration of the treatment. In either case immobilisation devices (e.g. patient moulds or shells) become important, especially for treatments of the head and neck. For treatments in the abdomen and thorax reliance is placed on the radiographer's ability to position the patient in the same way each day of treatment, paying particular attention to the position of the limbs and extremities. It is imperative that the patient is so positioned before the contour is taken for planning purposes. A variety of devices are available for taking patient contours. The very simple lead strip (say 10 × 3 mm² × 600 mm long) is widely used. Such a strip can be easily bent round the patient, and skin marks transferred to the lead using a piece of chalk. The lead should be varnished in preference to being covered with a plastic sheath as the latter can slide along the strip (moving the marks with respect to the contour) or stretch or crack. As with other devices, it is advisable to check the principal dimensions of the contour by an independent means, e.g. calipers or a height bridge.

Adjustable templates are valuable for taking complex contours (e.g. round the ear). These are made up of a large number of parallel rods which can be adjusted lengthwise to fit any shaped contour and then clamped in position (Fig. 6.18). The contour can then be traced on paper round the ends of the rods. Three such templates can be mounted on a frame and used to take complete contours.

A simple jig for taking the contour from the outside of a patient's shell is shown in Figure 6.19D. The shell is supported on four pins which define the plane of

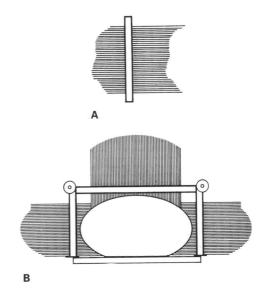

Fig. 6.18 Adjustable templates. **A** Round the ear and **B** for complete body contours.

the contour. A fifth pin is free to rotate about a vertical axis and scaled in degrees of rotation about the axis and centimetres radius from the axis. By measuring these two parameters for a variety of points round the surface of the shell, the contour can be readily plotted on polar graph paper. Providing the range finder on the simulator is sufficiently accurate it may be used in conjunction with the gantry angle in a similar manner. A simple device of similar design can reproduce the contour from the inside of the shell to represent the patient contour.

External and internal patient contours can be obtained from CT scan data, thereby enabling the anatomy to be accurately located within the external patient contour. The treatment planning computer may also be used to reconstruct the contour and the internal anatomy in a plane oblique to the normal CT scan by interpolating the data for several closely packed CT scans. Such reconstructions can be particularly useful in sites, such as the middle ear, where the complex anatomy presents particular problems. The contours produced from CT data are, however, often too detailed for planning purposes and some smoothing is required. Care has to be taken to ensure the CT couch is as flat and hard as the treatment couch and, where necessary, the patient is restrained (e.g. using a shell) in the planned treatment position.

PATIENT SHELLS

A patient shell which fits a patient and immobilises that patient enables the planning and treatment to be carried out with greater accuracy. The good shell locates on the bony protuberances of the patient and

— Enables the localisation of the lesion to be accurately determined from surface markers attached to the shell.
— Enables an accurate position of the patient to be reproduced each day.
— Provides an accurate and constant patient contour.
— Can be labelled and marked clearly and avoids the need to draw lines on the patient.
— Provides accurate beam entry and exit points.
— Provides a base on which wax build-up and local lead shielding can be built.

Space does not permit a detailed description of all the procedures involved in making a shell and the student should visit a mould room wherever possible. The principles of making a shell using a plaster bandage impression are outlined below.

1. Preparation of the patient. When the impression is taken, the patient should assume the position to be adopted in the treatment room (Fig. 6.19A) as nearly as possible. The clinician should be consulted if there is any doubt. The mould of a patient's head will be more accurate if long hair is cut short or shaved if the patient is likely to lose the hair during treatment. Hair should be covered with a tight swimming cap or stockinette and the face well coated with a separating medium. The patient should be warned that the plaster will be cold at first, but will become quite warm as it becomes hard.

2. If a full head mould is to be made, the back half should be made first. The edge of the plaster bandage should be neatly finished to define the coronal plane through the centre of the ears. The impression should be allowed to harden and then a separating medium should be put on the outside, extending about 3 cm from the edge.

3. Before commencing the front half, it must be decided how far the impression should extend—upwards and downwards—bearing in mind that the finished mould needs bony protuberances on which to locate, e.g. the nose, the eyebrows, the chin, the shoulders. Secondly, how is the patient going to breathe? He or she may breathe normally through the nose in which case the mould will be made with the mouth closed. In this case, the position of the chin will be determined by the teeth and the decision must be made at this stage whether treatment will be given with or without dentures. Furthermore, if any dental work is anticipated before the end of treatment, it should be completed before the mould is made.

Alternatively, the patient may breathe through the mouth, in which case a mouth insert with a short breathing tube should be made to fix the position of the chin and to depress the tongue.

4. The impression can now be commenced. The plaster bandage should be shaped carefully round the bony points and round the greased edge of the back half of the impression, if present (Fig. 6.19B). The two halves should fit uniquely together after they have been removed from the patient. The impression will usually require about six thicknesses of plaster bandage, suitably overlapped to give rigidity to the finished impression. Weaknesses can be strengthened after the impression has been removed from the patient—distortions cannot be corrected. Once the impression has hardened (after about 5 minutes) it should be eased off carefully. The patient will require assistance to remove the separating medium and splashes of plaster.

5. The two halves should now be fixed together by adding a further three layers of plaster bandage over the joint. If only one half has been made then the open side should be closed using plaster bandage, taking care not to distort the impression. The mouth or nose

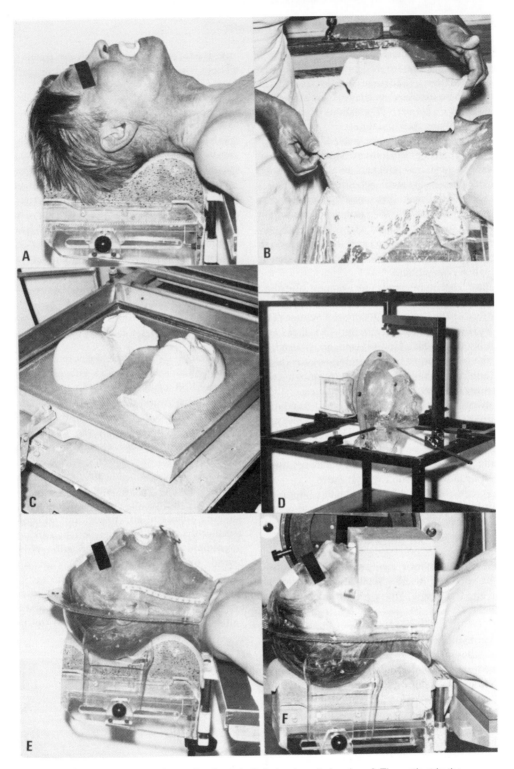

Fig. 6.19 The production and use of patient shells in treatment planning. **A** The patient in the proposed treatment position with a breathing tube; **B** the removal of the front half on completion of a whole head impression; **C** the two halves of the cast in position for vacuum forming; **D** the complete shell in the contouring jig; **E** the patient in the shell in position for the localisation films on the simulator; **F** the shell complete with tissue equivalent wax block in use on the accelerator.

aperture should also be closed. After rinsing with a separating medium, fill the impression with a fairly thin mix of plaster of Paris (adequate support round the impression must be provided so that it is not distorted under the weight of plaster). This should be allowed to set without applying additional heat.

6. The impression can now be peeled off the cast, leaving an exact replica of the patient. Small pimples on the cast resulting from air pockets in the impression can be pared away easily with a knife. The cast of a full head should be sawn into two halves along a diameter chosen to avoid the proposed treatment beams. The cut must be straight. Any deviations may cause the casts to crack, and in any case they will result in the two vacuum-formed half shells being at too great a separation when reassembled.

7. The casts are now ready for vacuum forming (Fig. 6.19C). The flat surface of each cast is placed on the platform of the vacuum forming machine. The plastic sheet is inserted, clamped around its edges and heated until it is pliable. Compressed air is used to prestretch the plastic into a bubble and the cast is raised into that bubble. The vacuum is applied, removing the air and forming the plastic tightly round the cast.

8. The plastic is trimmed off the cast, leaving a flange approximately 3 cm wide all round. Press-studs fitted into this flange will hold the two halves of the full mould together. If only a half mould is being made the excess plastic will be cut away completely. The breathing aperture can be cut away using a dental saw.

9. The patient shell is thus completed. Supports will be moulded (by hand) and attached to the shell to allow it to be fitted to a head rest or the couch of the treatment unit so that the patient is held secure (Fig. 6.19E).

10. Treatment accessories, e.g. wax, lead shielding, etc., can be attached to the shell after the tumour localisation and treatment planning has been completed (Fig. 6.19F).

If the treatment demands the skin sparing effect to be retained, the entry ports for the treatment beams will be pared away, leaving a narrow strap across the centre to uniquely define the central axis of the treatment field. The need for this should be borne in mind from the beginning as it will tend to weaken the shell, making it less effective as an immobilisation device. There is no reason why the plaster bandage impression should not be used as the mould, providing it is well made it can be similarly pared away and fixed to the head rest or couch. The plastic vacuum-formed shell is more pleasant to look at and to handle; it stands up to daily use rather better and the transparency of the plastic enables the accuracy of the fit to be checked. There is no place for a badly fitting shell. There is no place for a good shell, badly fitted.

Alternative materials

Although plaster bandage has been used exclusively as an impression material in the discussion above, other materials are available and can be used to advantage in certain cases. Invariably they are used in conjunction with plaster bandage. Certain materials (e.g. dental compression compounds) are used dry, relying on heat to soften them during the impression stage and hardening as they cool. Other water based materials (e.g. alginates) are poured on to the patient and set into a gel which reproduces the very texture of the skin. These materials are valuable if impressions are required from moist open wounds.

Immobilisation

Where a reproducible position is the only requirement, then self-hardening effervescent materials can be used. A crude frame of expanded polystyrene is formed, say round the head and shoulders. The patient is then positioned in the frame on a large empty polythene bag. The materials are mixed and introduced into the polythene bag, expand to fill the gaps between the frame and the patient, and harden, forming an accurate impression of the patient's position. Being aerated like the expanded polystyrene, the immobilisation device produces negligible attenuation of the treatment beam and, providing adequate access to setting-up marks has been left, it can be used on the treatment set without modification (Fig. 6.20). Two words of caution. The chemicals are toxic and toxic fumes may be produced, therefore the polythene bag must not be perforated. During hardening, heat is generated and, while generally acceptable, some sensitive skins may find it too much. If this technique is to

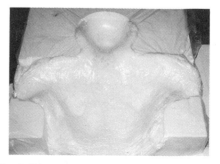

Fig. 6.20   Self-hardening foam impression.

be used regularly, then the polystyrene frame should be designed to fit uniquely to the treatment couch to further simplify the setting-up procedure.

An alternative to the foam bag is to use a sealed plastic bag loosely filled with small expanded polystyrene spheres. The same crude frame may be used and the patient positioned on top of the bag. The bag is formed round the patient whilst the air pressure in the bag is gradually reduced. At approximately half atmospheric pressure, the bag becomes rigid and 'fits' firmly round the patient, preventing any significant movement. The rigidity can be maintained throughout a course of treatment and until the vacuum is released, when the bag may be re-used for another patient. A variety of shapes and sizes of bag is available to immobilise any part of the anatomy or the whole of the patient, for TBI, for example. As with the foam, the attenuation in the polystyrene is minimal, but being opaque, consideration must be given to the beam entry ports during the initial evacuation. Radiation damage to the plastic will eventually cause the vacuum to fail and lead to the replacement of the bag.

The head may be immobilised using a *bite block*. This is a dental impression suspended from a rigid gantry attached to the couch. The patient lies supine on the couch in the treatment position with the bite block in his or her mouth. The gantry is then adjusted to fix the position of the bite block with respect to the couch. Providing its adjustment and the patient's grip on the bite block are both maintained, then the position of the patient's head will be accurately held and reproduced each day.

BEAM DIRECTION DEVICES

The radiation treatment planning and the immobilisation of the patient is of little value unless the day-to-day treatment can be set up accurately. This requires that the treatment unit and the patient are correctly aligned for each radiation field. In simple terms *beam direction devices* are those which enable the beam axis to be directed at the lesion in the planned direction at a predetermined point and distance from the source of radiation. The simplest and most widely used devices are the front and back pointers.

Front and back pointers

Front and back pointers are mounted on the unit in such a way that they lie and move along the beam axis, the front pointer being calibrated to show the distance between its tip and the source of radiation (Fig. 6.21). The accuracy of any pointer system needs to be checked periodically. In this case, this is done by rigidly mounting

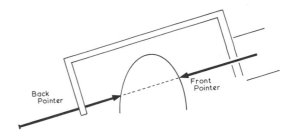

Fig. 6.21 The principle of the front and back pointer.

a reference marker such that it coincides with the tip of the pointer to be checked and rotating the beam diaphragm system about the beam axis—the tip of the pointer should not deviate from the reference marker by more than 1 mm. This check should be repeated with the pointer set at several positions along its length and at several gantry angles.

In use the front pointer is set at the SSD prescribed and the patient positioned so that the entry point (for the beam axis) on the patient coincides with the tip of the pointer. The angle of the beam is then adjusted until the back pointer coincides with the exit point, the entry and exit points being clearly marked on the patient's skin or mould. The pointers must be removed before the beam is switched on.

The front pointer may in practice be replaced by a light pointer system or by a cross-hair mark on the face of an interchangeable applicator. Similarly, back pointers have been replaced by other devices, too numerous to mention but which fulfil the same purpose, namely to define the direction of the beam in relation to the entry point on the patient.

Isocentric gantry

Reference has already been made to the isocentric gantry but its description is included here for it is essentially a beam direction facility.

The isocentric gantry has three principal axes of rotation: the beam axis or axis of rotation of the diaphragm system, the horizontal axis of rotation of the gantry and the vertical axis of rotation of the couch. These three axes of rotation intersect at a point called the *isocentre* (Fig. 6.22). The position of this point in space may also be identified by two or three light pointers or lasers mounted on the walls and ceiling of the treatment room. The third laser is better positioned high on the wall opposite the gantry so that it projects a single vertical plane of light along the axis of rotation of the gantry. This greatly assists in getting the patient straight and, if appropriate, central along that axis.

The value of the isocentric gantry lies in the fact that in setting up the patient a rotation about any of these

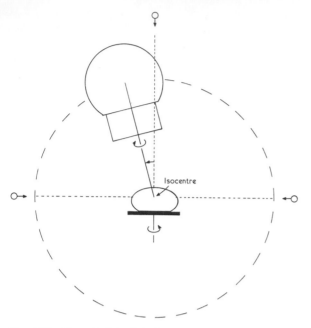

Fig. 6.22   The principle of the isocentric gantry.

three axes can be carried out knowing that the position of the isocentre is not altered. In practice, this is a considerable help whether the patient is being treated with the isocentre on the skin or inside the lesion.

To set up to a skin mark

Using the optical or mechanical front pointer the skin mark is positioned at the isocentre using the *linear* movements of the couch, i.e. couch height, lateral and longitudinal movements. This fixes the SSD. The beam direction is then set using the *rotational* movements, i.e. gantry and couch rotations to the specified angles or until the back pointer locates the beam exit mark. The diaphragm rotation completes the set-up. Do not use the linear movements after the entry mark has been set up. It is easy to remember: linear movements set the entry point, rotation movements set the exit point.

To set up to a point inside the lesion

At the planning stage the intersection of the beam axes is located as being '*d* cm vertically below' an appropriate skin mark. The front pointer is set at the source–axis distance *less* the value of *d*. With the beam axis vertical, the pointer and the skin mark are brought together using the *linear* movements as before, so positioning the planned intersection of the beam axes at the isocentre. The patient couch is now rotated to align lateral skin marks with the wall-mounted laser pointers or to define

the plane containing the planned beam axes. The gantry and diaphragm rotations can now be set for each field in turn. Once the patient has been positioned there is no need to move the patient or the couch between the treatment of different fields.

A further advantage of mounting a cobalt unit or linear accelerator on an isocentric gantry lies in the fact that the massive weight required to counterbalance the head on the gantry rotation can be put to good use in the form of a *primary beam stop*. This is a shield mounted on the gantry in such a way that it will attenuate the primary beam after it has passed through the patient, irrespective of gantry angle. In certain situations this can be more economical than providing primary barriers in the structure of the room (Ch. 3) but at the expense of some inconvenience to the radiographer setting up the patient.

Whether or not the counterbalance provides a primary beam stop, it is now common practice to have an additional laser built into the counterbalance, with a cylindrical lens to spread the laser light into a single plane containing both the axis of rotation of the gantry and the axis of rotation of the diaphragms. This is not a back pointer in the true sense, but because it defines a plane containing the beam axis, the line it casts on the patient will pass through the beam exit point only when the beam direction is correct.

The isocentre is defined as a point, whereas in practice, because of mechanical tolerances, it is usually a small sphere or ellipsoid—having a maximum diameter of less than 2 mm. Its accuracy is most readily checked by setting-up reference pointers to check each of the three rotations in turn, as follows. Fix a mechanical front pointer to the X-ray head with its tip at the isocentre, and a reference pointer horizontally and overhanging the end of the couch, again with its tip at the isocentre. With the beam axis vertical rotate the couch between its two extremes of movement, measuring the deviation from the front pointer, then repeat the procedure fixing the couch and rotating the gantry. Once that has been completed, repeat the procedure again, but this time measuring the deviation of the front pointer from the couch pointer on rotation of the diaphragms at selected gantry angles. This is a purely mechanical check because the isocentre is mechanically defined; the check on the couch rotation is more realistic if the couch is loaded with a distributed weight of 135 kg.

Finally, a word of warning. The rotational movements referred to above are those about the principal axes which define the isocentre. The unit may have other rotational facilities, the main ones being the rotation of the couch about an eccentric support and a limited 'pitch' rotation of the treatment head within its supporting arm or yoke. The latter enables the beam axis to move away from the isocentre in special circumstances—it should be returned to and locked in the isocentric position at all other times. Similarly, the eccentric rotation of the couch should be locked in its central position when it is not being used.

TREATMENT OF SUPERFICIAL LESIONS

So far in this chapter we have dealt with the treatment of deep seated lesions using two, three or four fields. If the lesion is superficial and only involves the skin or underlying tissues to a depth of a few centimetres, then a single treatment field is all that is required. Depth dose is a function of photon energy and inverse square law and it may be reduced by reducing either photon

energy or the SSD or both. Traditionally, superficial X-rays are generated at between 50 and 150 kV and used at 15 to 30 cm SSD. Owing to the dominance of photoelectric absorption in tissues at these photon energies, the irradiation of surface lesions overlying bone has led to very high doses being given to the bone. Today, higher photon energies may be used at even shorter SSDs, e.g. cobalt-60 gamma rays at 5 to 20 cm SSD. (Radium-226 at similar distances had been used for many years prior to the change to cobalt-60, see Ch. 3.) Furthermore, electron beams up to about 10 MeV and beta ray plaques are valuable in certain circumstances.

Typical isodose curves for some of these types of radiation are shown in Figure 6.23. The student should note the three characteristics mentioned earlier (p. 84f) in respect of these isodose charts. The advantages and disadvantages of each will be dealt with briefly.

Superficial X-ray beams

Superficial X-rays still treat over 90% of the superficial lesions in the radiotherapy department. The advantages are the simplicity of the X-ray unit, both in design and operation, the ease of collimation and field shaping to individual requirements with only 1 mm of lead, and a wide range of field defining applicators. The disadvantages are the high bone absorption and the minimal penetration—over the range of energies and field sizes in common use the 80% depth varies from only 6 to

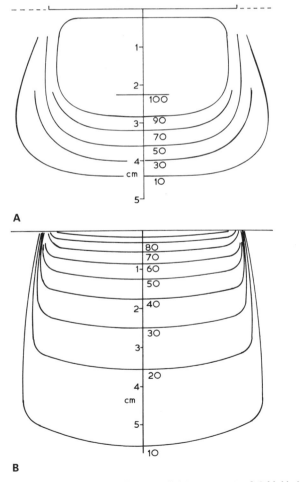

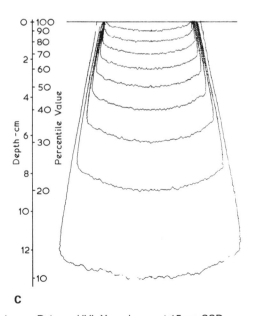

Fig. 6.23 Isodose charts for superficial treatments. **A** 9 MeV electron beam; **B** 1 mm HVL X-ray beam at 15 cm SSD; **C** cobalt-60 beam at 10 cm SSD.

16 mm (see also Fig. 5.11 and Table 5.4). Orthovoltage X-rays (say 2 mm Cu HVL) may be used at normal SSDs for the treatment of some superficial lesions.

High energy photon beams

Cobalt-60 gamma rays at 5–20 cm SSD can only be collimated adequately by using 5 cm of heavy alloy, which means there can be no individual beam shaping for each lesion to be treated. Skin sparing is not required as the lesions are superficial, although electron contamination of the gamma beam must be filtered out to prevent an excessive skin dose. The small source (say 2 TBq, 4 mm diameter) produces a narrow penumbra but the short SSD gives rise to a wide divergence of the beam. The shortness of the SSD also means that the setting up of the patient is critical. A 1 mm error in a 5 cm SSD produces a 4% error in dose rate. A patient shell is essential to maintain the SSD as well as to immobilise the patient. The use of surface applicators, i.e. the application of brachytherapy sources mounted on a tissue equivalent shell, typically 1 cm thick (Ch. 8), has largely been discontinued because of the poor depth dose and the hazards to staff.

Electron beams

High energy beams for clinical use may be produced from linear accelerators over a range of energies from about 5 MeV up to about 25 MeV. For clinical purposes the nominal energy (E) of the electron beam has been defined in terms of its half-value depth, i.e.

$$E \text{ (MeV)} = 2.5 \times HVD \text{ (cm)}$$

or

$$d_{50}\text{(mm)} = 4 \times E \text{ (MeV)}$$

where the HVD is the depth of the 50% isodose line on the central axis. A more useful parameter by which to define the electron beam is the quotation of d_{80}, i.e. the depth of the 80 percentile. The build-up curve for the electron beam is less marked, giving a skin dose of greater than 80%. The d_{80} value, beyond d_{max}, may therefore be used to define the treatable depth. The approximation that

$$d_{80} \text{ (mm)} = 3 \times E \text{ (MeV)}$$

is a useful aide mémoire, but it can vary with different methods of electron acceleration. The depth dose curve (Fig. 6.24) for electrons is characterised by its flat peak and the steep dose gradient which flattens into the X-ray tail (the X-rays being generated at the same peak energy as the electrons using the electron window, ionisation chamber, the collimators, the air and the tissue as X-ray targets). The gradient of the depth

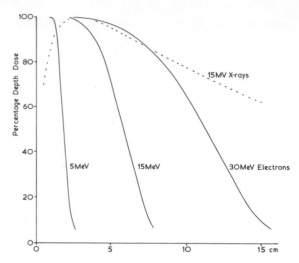

Fig. 6.24   Electron central axis depth dose curves.

dose curve is less steep for the higher energies since these electrons undergo many more interactions (ionisations and excitations) and their paths are correspondingly more tortuous.

The advantages of electron beams (up to 10 MeV) for the treatments of superficial lesions are clear. The dose is satisfactorily uniform to a depth determined by the energy of the electrons and the sharp fall-off of dose leads to the sparing of tissues at depth. Collimation is relatively simple over a wide range of field sizes; local beam shaping requires a few millimetres of lead depending on electron energy. Arc therapy with electrons offers a useful means of irradiating the post mastectomy chest wall, with minimal irradiation of the lungs.

Extensive skin disease (e.g. mycosis fungoides) can be treated using the large low energy electron beams (say 3 MeV) covering the whole surface of the patient. In this case the patient may be treated with eight very large (2×2 m^2) fields at long SSDs, or with more than four smaller overlapping fields. The minimum of four fields is required to cover the anterior, posterior and two lateral aspects of the patient. At long SSDs, the energy of the electrons incident on the patient will be less than on leaving the accelerator and the X-ray contamination of the electron beam may contribute a significant if not prohibitive whole body dose to the patient.

The higher electron energy beams (10 to 25 MeV) may be used in single or multifixed field treatments or in combination with photon beams.

CALCULATION OF DOSE

No treatment plan is complete without a specification

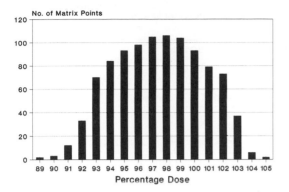

Fig. 6.25 Dose histogram.

of the dose to be given to the tumour. The dose prescription will be the responsibility of the clinician and will be quoted in terms of the target dose to a specified percentile value in a number of fractions. The number of fractions per week of treatment will be an important factor in determining the overall dose, but does not come into the calculations. The choice of dose may be the maximum, minimum, mean, average or modal dose to the target volume. While the first two are uniquely defined, the others will lie somewhere between the first two and in a good distribution they will not be significantly different. They are most easily understood by the following example.

Let us assume the dose to each of 1000 equally spaced points within the defined target volume has been rounded to the nearest 1%, and they are distributed as in the dose histogram shown in Figure 6.25.

Dose value (D)	No. of points (N)	Dose value (D)	No. of points (N)
89	2	98	106
90	3	99	104
91	12	100	93
92	33	101	79
93	70	102	73
94	84	103	37
95	93	104	6
96	98	105	2
97	105	106	0

The most frequently occurring dose is 98%, which occurs at 106 of our matrix points. This is the modal dose. The average dose is half way between the maximum and minimum and therefore equal to ½(89 + 105) or 97%. The mean dose is weighted average or Σ (DN)/N = 97464/1000 or 97.5%. The average and mean are rarely used, while the modal dose is probably most common. Where the target tissues have been treated before then the clinician may decide to prescribe to the

maximum, but if the tissue is known to be particularly radio resistant then prescribing to the minimum may be more appropriate.

As a means of standardising the choice of prescription for the purpose of multicentre comparisons of treatment, it is recommended that the target absorbed dose will be defined on the central axis or axes:

— *For single beams*: at the dose maximum (electrons) or at the centre of the target volume (photons).
— *For parallel opposed beams*: at the midpoint for equally weighted beams or at the centre of the target volume for unequally weighted beams.
— *For two or more intersecting beams*: at the point of intersection of the axes.

This statement of target dose should be supplemented by a statement of minimum and maximum dose if the dose over the target volume varies by more than ± 10%.

The prescription will be a target dose, D, to a percentile value, %TD, in F fractions.

In the simplest case of a single field treatment this means the total peak (applied) dose, P, may be obtained by rearranging the definition of percentage depth dose, viz:

$$\dot{P} = \frac{D \times 100}{\%TD}$$

and the peak (applied) dose per fraction, P/F. If the peak dose rate, say on the cobalt-60 unit, is $\dot{P}$, then the exposure time per fraction will be

$$t = \frac{P/F}{\dot{P}} + \Delta t$$

The quoted peak dose rate, $\dot{P}$, may be specified only for a standard field size, say 10 cm × 10 cm, in which case it should be modified by multiplying by the appropriate output factor before calculating the exposure time. The output factor is defined as

$$= \frac{\text{Peak dose rate for the equivalent square}}{\text{Peak dose rate, } \dot{P}, \text{ for the reference field}}$$

Similarly, on an orthovoltage or superficial X-ray unit, the dose rate quoted for the applicator should be reduced when a lead cut-out modifies the field size, by the ratio of the back scatter factors (BSF) for the cut-out and applicator respectively, i.e. $BSF_{cut-out}/BSF_{applicator}$.

If there is a small stand-off between the applicator surface and the skin, then the treatment time should be further increased by the inverse square factor $(f + x)^2/f^2$ where f is the normal SSD and x is the stand-off. (At megavoltage energies, the factor is $(f + d_{max} + x)^2/(f + d_{max})^2$.) Where the stand-off is significant, so as to

Table 6.2 Calculation of treatment time and monitor unit settings for typical treatment plans

Treatment plan shown in figure	6.2 (c)	6.12 (b)	
Prescribed target dose, D, say	50 Gy	60 Gy	
Prescribed % target dose, %TD	240%	100%	
		wedged	non-wedged
Weighting factor, W_i	100%	50%	22%
Total applied dise, P_i (Gy)	20.8	30.0	13.2
No. of fractions, F	20	25	25
Applied dose per fraction, P_i/F (Gy)	1.04	1.20	0.53
Output factors, say	0.98	0.96	1.00
Wedge factors, say		1.12	
Set monitor units, mu*	1.06	1.40	0.53
Treatment time, t (min*)	0.68	0.90	0.34

* assuming the dose rate at d_{max} for the reference field size is 1.56 Gy per minute and the integrating dose meter (mu) is calibrated in grays.

produce a change in field size, then the change in the depth dose distribution may also have to be taken into account.

In all the above examples, it has been assumed that the exposure to the patient will be controlled by time alone. Where a dual dosimetry system is being used on a linear accelerator, for example, the exposure will be determined solely by the monitor units (mu) set. (The second dose channel and the treatment timer are for back-up purposes only.) The monitor units will usually be calibrated in grays or centigrays for a reference field size (10 cm × 10 cm) at the normal treating distance (say 100 cm). As before, the peak (applied) dose per fraction, P/F, will be calculated, and for a field size other than the reference, the monitor units required will be

$$mu = (P/F)/\text{output factor}$$

The monitor units will be further increased by multiplying by the wedge factor, shadow tray correction factor, etc., as appropriate to the treatment in hand.

Providing a dose distribution involving two or more fields is based on the premise that the peak dose to each of the fields is 100%, as in Figure 6.2, then the calculations are as described above. However, if the distribution assumes the peak dose to any one of the fields is not 100%, either because weighting factors have been used or the distribution has been normalised to the target dose, then the total peak (applied) dose, P, must be calculated separately for each field using the formula

$$P_i = D \times \frac{100}{\%TD} \times W_i$$

where W_i is the weighting factor and i identifies the field. This new value, P_i, may then be used to replace P in the equations above.

In Table 6.2, the dose distributions illustrated in Figures 6.2C and 6.12B are used in conjunction with a typical dose prescription to derive the exposure time or monitor units required for each fraction of treatment.

Integral dose

Dose has been defined as the energy absorbed per unit mass of tissue in a small element of tissue, viz:

$$D = \Delta E/\Delta m$$

Integral dose is the summation of the dose to all elements of the irradiated tissue and represents the total absorbed energy, viz:

$$E = \int D \mathrm{d}m$$

The unit of integral dose is the kg-gray and equivalent to the energy absorption of 1 joule. The detailed eva-

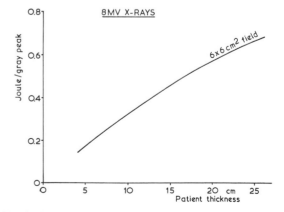

Fig. 6.26 Integral dose increases with patient thickness.

luation of the integral dose is complex in practice, but it is easily appreciated that it increases with incident dose and the volume of irradiated tissue—manually determined by field size and thickness of the patient treated (Fig. 6.26). It is less easy to appreciate that in a particular treatment situation the integral dose decreases with increasing photon energy and varies only slowly with the number of fields used.

Integral dose in this context is confined to the tissues deliberately irradiated during a course of radiotherapy. In addition, there is a component of integral dose arising from radiation scattered from the exposed tissues and the irradiation of the whole body by leakage radiation from the source/tube housing. It is in recognition of this whole body irradiation that the acceptable levels of leakage radiation are set.

7. Diagnostic radiography and the treatment simulator

INTRODUCTION

In previous chapters the word *exposure* has been given to a clearly defined scientific concept, namely the ionisation produced per unit mass of air ($X = \Delta Q / \Delta m$), while in every day usage it takes the meaning of *being exposed to*. In this chapter the word will be used in the latter sense unless it is accompanied by the symbol (X).

The most precise method of checking the accuracy of the position of a treatment field is to expose an X-ray film during treatment and so produce a picture of the tissues irradiated. This film is known as a *portal film* or *check film*. The film should show the entire treatment volume enclosed and the adjacent anatomy, thereby confirming that the treatment beam is correct in position, size and direction. In addition, it is convenient if the film can be left in position for the whole treatment fraction rather than having to disturb the patient to remove the film before completing the dose.

At orthovoltage X-ray energies, the image quality of the check film is poor but adequate, providing the exposure factors and processing combine to produce the maximum contrast. The advent of megavoltage radiotherapy brought several potential improvements in treatment, not least:

— Improved penetration (greater depth dose)
— Reduced skin dose (the build-up effect)
— More sharply defined beams (narrow penumbra)
— Reduced bone absorption.

The reduced bone absorption is advantageous to the radiotherapy but not to the check film. The only appreciable contrast on a check film taken using megavoltage beams is between the tissues and the air passages, where the density difference (in g cm^{-3}) is very great (Fig. 7.1A). One way open to continue the use of check films is to have a machine which simulates the movements of the therapy unit but uses a source of lower energy X-rays. The *treatment simulator* is, therefore, a

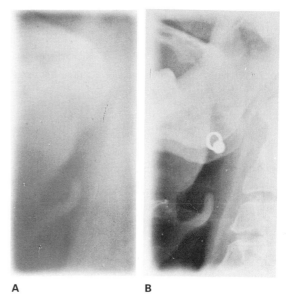

A   **B**

Fig. 7.1 Radiographs of the same patient **A** at 8 MV and **B** on the simulator.

unit incorporating a diagnostic X-ray tube in a gantry similar to the treatment unit, particularly in regard to beam collimation and direction and the patient's couch. The simulator (Fig. 7.2) is a sophisticated unit and often considered essential to the planning of any course of radical radiation treatment using megavoltage radiation. The unit is best situated close to the treatment units it simulates but, perhaps more important, it should be close to the mould and planning room facilities. It is often the focal point in the therapy department where staff in these various disciplines converge and bring their expertise to bear on the patient's treatment plan. In most departments, the simulator will be in the hands of the therapy radiographic staff.

This chapter seeks to outline some of the aspects of diagnostic radiology which are relevant to the use of the simulator. In no way is it to be taken as a comprehensive

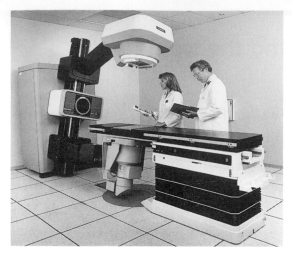

Fig. 7.2 A typical treatment simulator. (Courtesy of Varian-TEM Ltd.)

treatise on the subject. It is only an introduction to encourage the reader to begin to understand the simulator.

PHYSICAL CONSIDERATIONS
Magnification and distortion

Any X-ray image will be a magnified image. Just as an optical shadow is larger than life size, so the X-ray image is larger than the anatomy it portrays. X-rays diverge from a small focal spot and travel in straight lines through the object before reaching the image receptor, which may be the radiographic film (p. 122), the input phosphor of an image intensifier (p. 127) or an array of radiation detectors (p. 128). The simple geometry (Fig. 7.3A) shows the magnification factor(m) is defined as

$$m = \frac{XY}{xy} = \frac{f}{s} = \frac{f}{f\text{-}h}$$

providing both the object and the image are perpendicular to the central ray. If this condition is not satisfied the image will suffer *distortion*, in that the magnification at the two ends will be different (Fig. 7.3B). (It should be noted that f, h and s are measured parallel to the beam axis, not along the ray from the focal spot.)

Geometric unsharpness

If the size of the focal spot is not negligible, then the image will be unsharp due to the geometric penumbra (analogous to the geometric penumbra of the therapy beam, p. 49). Figure 7.3C shows the unsharpness at the two ends is different, due to the angle of the target.

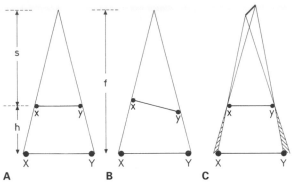

Fig. 7.3 The principles of **A** magnification, **B** distortion and **C** geometric distortion.

Geometric unsharpness may be reduced by increasing the focus–film distance (FFD) and/or by reducing the film–object distance.

These effects are simply illustrated when the object is a caesium needle or an iridium pin. On treatment simulators, the effect is most clearly shown in the image of the wire diaphragms used to define the field size (p. 130). The wires are of small diameter, a long distance from the film and cast a broad shadow on the film, particularly when a broad focus tube is used (Fig. 7.4B). Note. A double image is sometimes visible on one pair of wire diaphragms but not on the other, until the diaphragms are rotated. This is due to the nature of the focal spot. The focal 'spot' usually consists of two relatively intense line sources of X-rays separated by an area of less intense emission. When the wire of the diaphragm system is parallel to the line foci, two images of the wire are produced under conditions of large magnification. This effect is not so apparent in the tissues of the patient because the magnification is smaller and the effect reduces to one of geometric unsharpness.

The magnified image of more solid objects of a random three-dimensional shape will not only exhibit distortion but also suffer from unsharpness due to an effect analogous to the transmission penumbra considered earlier (p. 50). Cylindrical and more complex shapes present different thicknesses to the primary radiation and the transmitted intensity will vary with that thickness.

Consider the situation in Figure 7.5 where an inhomogeneity is introduced into an otherwise homogeneous medium. In mathematical terms and considering exponential attenuation only, the intensity transmitted by the homogeneous medium, I_1, is given by the equation

$$I_1 = I_0\, e^{-\mu_1 x_1}$$

while in the shadow of the inhomogeneity, the transmitted intensity, I_2, is given by

$$I_2 = I_0\, e^{-\mu_1(x_1 - x_2)}\, e^{-\mu_2 x_2}$$

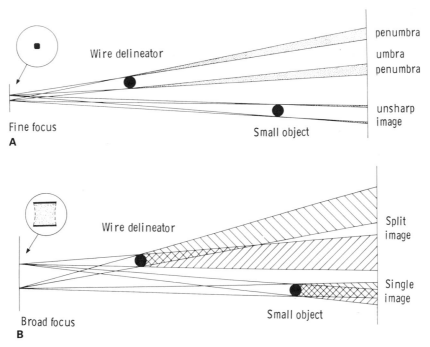

Fig. 7.4 Geometric distortion under **A** fine and **B** broad focus conditions.

where I_0 is the unattenuated intensity and μ_1 and μ_2 the attenuation coefficients in the media of thickness x_1 and x_2 respectively. Rearranging the terms in the second equation gives

$$I_2 = I_0 \, e^{-\mu_1 x_1} \, e^{(\mu_1 - \mu_2)x_2}$$

and substituting the first equation gives

$$I_2 = I_1 \, e^{(\mu_1 - \mu_2)x_2}$$

Thus the ratio of the transmitted intensities is dependent on the thickness of the inhomogeneity and on the difference in the linear attenuation coefficients. The presence of a small inhomogeneity or the thin edge of a larger inhomogeneity will only be detected when I_2 and I_1 are visualised as being different on the radiograph, i.e. when $(\mu_1 - \mu_2)x_2$ is significant. It follows that if vessels are not normally visualised by using X-rays, they may be visualised if they can be filled with a medium of different attenuation coefficient, i.e. with a suitable *contrast medium*. Contrast media may rely on a higher atomic number, e.g. barium, or a reduced density, e.g. air. Both parameters will profoundly affect the value of $(\mu_1 - \mu_2)$ in the above equation.

Patient movement

Further image unsharpness or blur may be caused by patient movement during the exposure. This can be minimised by careful immobilisation of the patient, by asking the patient to lie still and/or to hold the breath. The most effective method is to arrest that movement by the use of short exposure times, providing these are consistent with other factors governing the image quality.

Some movement of the patient can, however, provide important information. It is not physically possible to stop the patient undergoing radiation treatment from moving altogether. During simulation, therefore, it is helpful to ascertain the magnitude of that movement so that an allowance may be made for it in subsequent procedures, such as in radiation treatment planning. The rise and fall of the chest wall, for example, may be several centimetres.

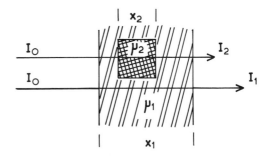

Fig. 7.5 Exponential attenuation through an inhomogeneity in an otherwise homogeneous medium (see text).

Quantum mottle

The production of X-rays is a random process involving the bombardment of a target by high speed electrons. Over a long period of time, the distribution of photons in the X-ray beam is averaged out and can be predicted with some accuracy. However, if the exposure times are very short, in order to arrest all movement, as suggested above, the averaging effect of this random process with time may be incomplete and the distribution of photons less uniform, giving rise to what is called *quantum mottle* on the radiographic film.

RADIOGRAPHIC FILM

The radiographic film is a bluish transparent polyester base approximately 0.2 mm thick, coated on both sides with a gelatine layer containing silver halide crystals in suspension. Each crystal will be a regular lattice of Ag^+ and Br^- ions made sensitive to visible light or X-ray photons by the addition of a small impurity—of silver sulphide. This adds a *sensitivity speck* to each otherwise perfect crystal of silver bromide. Now when a photon ionises a bromine ion, the negative electron is released, leaving an uncharged bromine atom behind. This electron is temporarily held by the sensitivity speck until a slower moving and positively charged silver ion drifts by and attracts the electron to itself. The electron neutralises the positive charge, leaving an uncharged atom of silver. If the exposure of photons was allowed to continue, the number of silver atoms would eventually become visible to the naked eye. However, it is normal to use a much smaller exposure to create an invisible *latent image* which can be developed later using chemicals.

Film processing

The processing of the latent image is in two stages: the *development* of the latent image by chemically accelerating the action already begun during the exposure, and the *fixation* of the developed image by the removal of the silver bromide not affected by the exposure. During both processes the emulsion swells and is easily damaged, making absolute cleanliness and careful handling essential. Automatic processing not only reduces the risk of damage through mishandling but also enables more concentrated chemicals to be used and at higher temperatures, thereby reducing the processing time to typically 90 seconds. The chemicals are not interchangeable between manual and automatic processing but the basic chemistry is common to both.

The developer is an organic reducing agent containing hydroquinone which reduces the silver halide—affected by the radiation—to the base metal silver, a process which depends on both temperature and time. For manual processing, this is typically 5 minutes at 20°C; to ensure the action of the developer is uniform over the whole surface, occasional agitation is necessary to ensure 'fresh' developer is not denied access to the emulsion by the surface build-up of bromine. With the continued use of the same solution over a period of weeks, the solution becomes diluted by the bromine and needs to be replaced by a fresh solution or replenished by the addition of a chemical high in hydroquinone and in the other alkaline elements exhausted by the process. The automatic processor injects the appropriate quantity of *replenisher* solution as required. Overdevelopment slightly increases the effective speed, the gamma and the fog level of the film.

Having developed the latent image, the image has to be fixed by removing the remaining silver halides. The fixing agent, sodium thiosulphate or ammonium thiosulphate, clears the film by dissolving the undeveloped silver halide from the emulsion. The fixer contains other chemicals to harden the emulsion to make it less prone to damage. The final but important stages in the processing of the film are the washing and the drying. The acid fixer quickly neutralises the alkaline developer but the acids need to be washed out thoroughly. Inadequate washing can result in the image turning brown and the clear film appearing greyish-white. A well-maintained automatic processor avoids many of these processing pitfalls but this does not mean careful attention to details of cleanliness can be relaxed, e.g. the use of a filtered water supply and of fresh chemicals.

The chemicals are strong and precautions are necessary to ensure the safety of the staff involved. A well-ventilated atmosphere and the use of protective clothing, goggles and gloves are essential when handling the chemicals. Those with sensitive skins or respiratory problems should be particularly careful. An eyewash bottle should be available in the darkroom for use in an emergency.

Silver recovery

The silver dissolved into the fixing solution can be recovered by electrolysis or by metal exchange. Silver can also be recovered from the processed film once the films can be released for disposal. The quantities recovered are small—0.5% by weight—but silver recovery is commercially viable and environmentally beneficial.

The darkroom

So far as the radiotherapy department is concerned the 'darkroom' should be adjacent to the simulator—a carefully positioned through-the-wall processor could dispense the processed film into the simulator control room, minimising the time the staff spend in the dark-room. It is easy to refer to this room as the 'darkroom' because it is usually darker than any other room in the department, but it is not truly dark. Some photographic material, it is true, has to be handled in total darkness, but in general radiographic film can be handled safely under subdued lighting of the appropriate colour. The film emulsion is sensitive to the green–blue–violet of the visible spectrum but relatively insensitive to the yellow–red light. Therefore, providing the darkroom is well sealed against white light entering through cracks—round the door, for example—it may be lit with safelights incorporating yellow–red filters. The precise filter requirements will be given in the film data sheets. When checking the sources of light in the darkroom, it is necessary to stay in the dark for a minimum of 10 minutes simply to let the eyes adjust to the low level of lighting before making any checks. Once accustomed, the eyes will readily identify spots of white light or of light likely to affect the emulsion on the film. Pieces of unwrapped, unexposed film can be used to check any doubtful sources of light—including the indicator lights on the processor control panel!

The so-called daylight processing is currently gaining popularity. The processes are essentially the same as those described above except that the film is transferred from the store to the cassette and from the cassette to the processor automatically, thereby making the dark-ened room unnecessary. The design of the equipment is so radically different that it is unique to the system, although some cassettes are available which may be used interchangeably.

The characteristic curve

The degree of blackness or the *optical density* of the processed film depends on the exposure received by the film, which in turn depends on the intensity of the incident beam and on the thickness and composition of the object being radiographed (Fig. 7.6). The optical density, D, is expressed mathematically as

$$D = \log_{10} (I_0/I)$$

where I_0 is the intensity of the light incident on the film and I the intensity transmitted. The instrument used to measure density is called a *densitometer*.

A graphical representation of the variation of optical density with exposure (X) is called the *characteristic curve*. At very low exposures (X), there is very little density change and the density measured is mostly that of the *fog level* of the film—the inherent density of the polyester base and the gelatine emulsion. At very high exposures (X), any further increase produces no density change and the density measured is that of the silver deposit when all the available silver halide crystals have been reduced—a situation which exists when the film has been overexposed. Between these two extremes, there is a region of *correct exposure (X)*—the relatively straight portion of the characteristic curve where the gradient is at a maximum (Fig. 7.7). The correctly exposed film will have a range of densities within this region of the curve, that is, within the range from about 0.4 to 2.0. It is important in producing a radiograph to obtain the maximum difference between points of interest. The difference in density at two points is known as the *contrast, C*, where

$$C = D_A - D_B$$

The human eye under ideal conditions can detect density differences as small as 0.02. Although contrast between two points on the film is the difference in their densities, the *film contrast* at a single point is the gradient of the characteristic curve at the point of measurement, D, in Figure 7.7A.

$$\text{Film contrast} = \frac{D_A - D_B}{\log X_A - \log X_B}$$

The slope of the straight portion of the curve is known as the *film gamma* or contrast index and represents the region of maximum contrast, usually between the densities of 1 and 3. At densities above 4, the film

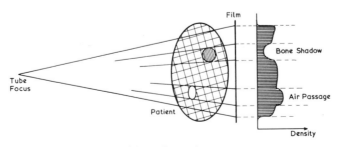

Fig. 7.6 The principle of the radiograph.

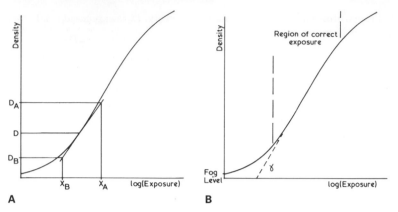

Fig. 7.7   The characteristic curve: **A** film contrast; **B** region of correct exposure.

contrast is reduced as the film becomes saturated.

In any radiograph (Fig. 7.6) a range of densities will be produced and if this range is to be accommodated within the 'straight' portion of the curve, then the exposure given will have to be carefully chosen. The gamma of the film used has to be chosen to maximise the visual contrast while accommodating the range of X-ray intensities transmitted by the patient. In general, the greater the gamma, the more critical the choice of exposure.

Another important parameter of the film is its *speed*. If only a small exposure is required to produce a given density, the film is said to be *fast*, whereas a *slow* film requires a longer exposure to produce the same degree of blackening. Unfortunately a film is made faster by increasing the size of the silver halide crystals in the emulsion, which also increases the graininess of the final image and the consequent loss of fine detail. Either a crystal is rendered 'developable' or it is not; it either turns black or it does not. The radiographic image may therefore be considered as being built-up with finite-sized black building bricks. The faster the film, the larger the building brick and the less the fine detail that results. The granular appearance can be seen under a magnifying glass. The use of intensifying screens will effectively increase the speed of the film.

Intensifying screens

The sensitive emulsion of the film is very thin and the X-ray energy absorbed is small, making the film slow to respond to the radiation. The efficiency of the latent image formation can be increased by using intensifying screens. An intensifying screen is a sheet of cardboard or plastic, the *base*, coated with a reflective layer and a layer of crystals of a luminescent material. These crystals fluoresce under irradiation with X-rays, that is they emit visible light as an immediate response to the stimulus of the X-ray photons (Fig. 7.8). (Phosphorescence or afterglow is the name given to a similar response which is delayed or persistent—an undesirable process in this context.) The brightness of the visible light is proportional to the X-ray stimulus and the wavelength of the visible light is characteristic of the screen material. The crystals are therefore carefully chosen, e.g. calcium tungstate or, more recently, compounds of the rare-earth elements of gadolinium and lanthanum, so that the wavelength of the visible light is near the peak sensitivity of the photographic emulsion of the film—in the blue–green part of the visible spectrum.

The X-ray image is therefore also formed in the intensifying screen in visible light and, providing the screen and the film are in very close contact, the light from the screen will enhance the latent image formed in the film emulsion. The crystalline structure of the screen will add to the granular appearance of the radiograph and there will be some further loss of fine detail because the fluorescent light is random in direction and not confined to the direction of the primary photon beam. The built-in reflecting layer in the screen redirects some of the light back on to the film. This loss of detail is minimised by keeping the screens scrupulously clean. Particles of dirt can prevent the light reaching the film as well as forming a space between the screen and the film, enabling the light to diffuse over a larger area of

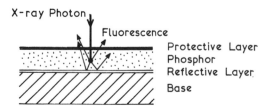

Fig. 7.8   The principle of intensifying screens.

film. Faulty cassettes can also prohibit good film–screen contact. Screens are best cleaned with a proprietary screen cleaner or a cotton cloth moistened with a mild soap solution.

Radiographic emulsion is more sensitive to visible light than to ionising radiation and therefore the exposure required is much reduced when using screens. Screens may be used singly, but more commonly in pairs to enhance the image formation in both emulsions on the film. The front screen is usually thinner than the back screen. The saving in exposure is considerable and is quoted as an *intensification factor*, IF, where

$$IF = \frac{\text{Exposure required to produce a given density when the screens are not used}}{\text{Exposure required to produce the same density when the screens are used}}$$

In practice, a pair of calcium tungstate (fast) screens have intensification factors of about 30 or 40, while rare-earth screens increase these by a further factor of four or more. Rare-earth screens will soon be in universal use in both radiodiagnosis and in treatment simulation.

Film holders

The photographic emulsion is sensitive to light and to X-rays and must be stored away from both. It also deteriorates with age, moisture and temperature. Film should therefore be stored in a cool dry place and stocks should be used in strict rotation. Film should be stored vertically to reduce the pressure on the emulsion. Adverse storage conditions result in an increased fog level on the processed film with the consequent loss of contrast.

Films may be individually *envelope-wrapped*, in which case they will be enclosed in a lightproof envelope of plasticised paper to keep out both light and moisture. There will be a loose wrap of yellow or black paper to facilitate handling and there may be a sheet of cardboard as a stiffener. Envelope-wrapped film is only used where extreme fine detail is required or where the increased radiation dose to the patient is of no consequence—intensifying screens cannot be used with envelope-wrapped film. Therapy verification film is usually envelope-wrapped.

X-ray film is otherwise supplied unwrapped. The film may still be separated by a thin sheet of paper and will be supplied packed in boxes sealed against light and moisture. The boxes must only be opened under the safe conditions of the darkroom. Unwrapped film is designed for use in a *cassette* firmly sandwiched between two intensifying screens (Fig. 7.9). For this reason the film is sometimes referred to as *screen film*, its thinner emul-

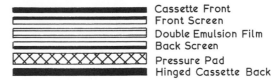

Cassette Front
Front Screen
Double Emulsion Film
Back Screen
Pressure Pad
Hinged Cassette Back

Fig. 7.9 The film cassette.

sion specially prepared to be sensitive to the fluorescence of the screens.

A cassette is essentially a lightproof container consisting of a rigid frame of aluminium or stainless steel with a hinged back and a thin aluminium, carbon fibre or plastic front through which the X-radiation enters. Carbon fibre is the preferred material for the cassette front because it provides maximum strength and minimal attenuation. Inside the front will be the front screen. A foam rubber pressure pad is sandwiched between the back screen and the back of the cassette, so that when it is closed pressure is applied evenly over the whole area of the film to ensure good film–screen contact. Care needs to be taken when loading and unloading the cassette so as to prevent the build-up of static electricity which may discharge later, emitting flashes of light and blackening the film. Poor handling can damage both the cassette and the film emulsion.

Loss of contrast

All the attention so far has been on the differential attenuation of the X-rays passing through the patient, reaching the film and causing differential blackening on the film. The contrast produced is the result of the photoelectric attenuation being dependent on the atomic number and the density of the tissues. Inevitably, Compton scatter will be present. The scattered radiation does not reflect the attenuation pattern of the primary radiation, but randomly irradiates the whole film, increasing the fog level and reducing the contrast. Fog may be reduced by:
— Lowering the tube kilovoltage to reduce the scatter generated
— Reducing the field size
— Preventing the scatter from reaching the film by using an anti-scatter grid or increasing the patient–film distance.

A *grid* (sometimes called an antiscatter grid or scatter grid) is a series of equally spaced lead strips, usually between 20 and 40 strips per centimetre, such that X-rays travelling from the tube focus can pass unhindered between the strips while scattered radiation travelling in random directions will be absorbed in the lead

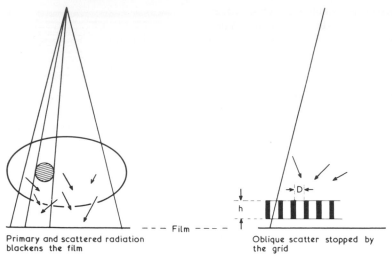

Primary and scattered radiation
blackens the film

Oblique scatter stopped by
the grid

- - - Film - - -

Fig. 7.10 The principle of the (scatter) grid.

(Fig. 7.10). For most purposes a *parallel grid* is adequate providing the *grid* ratio is not too large, the grid ratio being defined as:

$$\text{Grid ratio} = h/D$$

where h is the height and D the width of the space between the lead strips. If the grid ratio is too large, even the divergent primary radiation from the focus will be absorbed at the edges of large fields. To prevent this a *focused grid* may be used, in which the lead strips are mounted so as to lie along the rays from the focus rather than parallel to the central axis. Focused grids must be used at or close to the stated focal distance. The presence of the lead inevitably means some increase in the required exposure.

Radiographic exposure and reciprocity

Several hints have already been given as to the choice of the *exposure factors* required to produce a good radiograph, e.g. to use a low kV for maximum contrast, to adjust the total exposure to keep the range of densities within the straight portion of the characteristic curve, to use the minimum exposure time to arrest any voluntary or involuntary movement of the patient and to use a fast film–screen combination to minimise the dose to the patient. The exposure (X) at the surface of the patient is related to the exposure factors as follows:

$$X \propto (kV)^2 \times (mA) \times (s)/d^2$$

where d is the distance, kV the peak voltage of the tube, mA the tube current and s the exposure time in seconds. For a given kV and patient–film geometry, the total

exposure (X) is proportional to both the tube current and the exposure time; the film response will be the same whatever combination of these two parameters is chosen, providing their product remains constant. This is known as *reciprocity*. It is often convenient therefore to quote the exposure in mAs, leaving the final choice of tube current and exposure time to the radiographer. An effect known as *reciprocity failure* used to occur under conditions where the exposure time was very long or very short, but modern equipment usually corrects for this automatically. In general, one chooses the shortest exposure time to arrest the patient movement and therefore the maximum mA. If this necessitates a change of focal spot size—from fine to broad focus—then other factors will need to be considered.

How does the radiographer ascertain the correct mAs in the first place? In any one department, the film–screen–grid combination will be decided upon in advance and there will be little or no choice. Secondly, radiographs will have been taken many times before and satisfactory exposure factors will be available based on experience. Published 'Exposure Tables' may be used as an alternative guide, but it must be remembered that on a simulator the SSD and the FFD may be very different (by up to a factor of 3) from those used in a diagnostic department and the mAs recommended may need to be increased to obtain comparable films. It is for this reason that X-ray generators giving up to 800 mA or even 1000 mA are used on simulators. Once the mAs have proved adequate for a given examination, then patient-to-patient differences will usually be accommodated by small changes in kV.

Unlike the policy adopted in diagnostic X-ray departments, it is often said that in simulation the patient dose is unimportant, in that the dose to be given in the treatment situation will be many times greater than that from the simulator. This is true of the lesion and the surrounding tissues. However, if the patient receives an extensive radiographic examination in regions where every effort will be taken to minimise the dose received during the treatment (e.g. the lens of the eye), then the radiographic dose may be a significant fraction of the whole. Patient dose is minimised by the use of high kV and long SSD. The final choice of kV is therefore a compromise between maximum contrast and minimum patient dose.

Therapy verification films

Therapy verification film is designed for megavoltage radiations, usually envelope-wrapped and used without intensifying screens. It is very slow, requiring a dose of approximately 1 gray, it being advantageous to leave the film in the transmitted beam throughout the treatment fraction. A scatter grid is of no value in eliminating the effects of scattered radiation in that the forward scatter is of a similar photon energy as the primary beam. It is, however, advantageous to place the verification film in close contact with, but *behind,* a 1 mm (up to 6 MV) or 2 mm lead (over 8 MV) sheet. This serves two purposes. It attenuates some of the low energy scatter resulting from the multiple scattering processes, but more importantly it helps to restore the dose build-up lost in the air gaps between the exit surface of the patient and the surface of the film. The attenuation of the primary radiation in the lead is negligible and therefore the exposure is unaffected by the presence of the lead. If a 'cassette' is used to hold the (wrapped) film in close contact with the lead, ensure the radiation passes through the lead before reaching the film.

Inevitably the quality of the verification film image is very poor, relying as it does on the differential absorption in the tissues due to the Compton scattering process. This differential is dependent on the density and the electron density of the tissues and is independent of atomic number. The contrast between tissue and air is therefore much greater than between tissue and bone, as illustrated in Figure 7.1.

An alternative film is available which is about eight times faster than the verification film described above, and therefore requires a smaller incident dose. This film is used for the double exposure technique of beam verification, where the film is placed in the transmitted therapy beam and given a short exposure with the field collimators wide open, only to be followed by a second exposure with the field collimators closed down to the

planned therapy field size. This double exposure identifies the small therapy field within the context of the adjacent anatomy. Some advocates of this technique give the first exposure using a diagnostic X-ray tube mounted on the side of the therapy generator (and at a known rotation angle from the therapy beam). The rather grey low contrast therapy beam image is then seen superimposed on the diagnostic quality image of the anatomy. Whatever the technique, it is important that the patient is not allowed to move between the two exposures.

An alternative device for portal imaging is discussed on page 128.

IMAGE INTENSIFICATION

So far we have concentrated on the production of the image on film and much of what has been said is true for any other radiographic image. Following the development of the image intensifier, it was soon realised that the immediate display of a dynamic image was, in many situations, far superior to the image produced using film which, after all, needed processing. The dynamic image on the simulator not only enables the operator to watch for patient movement but also enables the simulator movements to be adjusted to the desired positions, quickly and positively.

The image intensifier tube is a highly evacuated glass envelope containing a fluorescent screen. Like the intensifying screens discussed above, the fluorescent screen or *input phosphor* is a layer of crystals (in this situation caesium iodide is preferred) which absorb some of the X-ray photons and convert the invisible X-ray image into a visible fluorescent image, albeit of low brightness. In contact with the input phosphor is a photocathode which promptly converts the visible image into an electronic image (Fig. 7.11). This input phosphor and photocathode are usually convex to the incident X-ray beam. The electrons emitted from the concave surface are accelerated by a high voltage (~ 25 kV) and focused on to a much smaller *output phosphor*. The acceleration of the electrons increases their energy, while the minification of the image concentrates the electron flux on to a smaller area, further increasing the brightness of the visible image produced in the output phosphor. (The output phosphor is made up of even smaller crystals than the input phosphor in order to maintain the fine detail of the image.) This bright image may be viewed by the naked eye, providing sufficient X-ray protective material is available to make it safe to look directly at the output phosphor which is in the primary X-ray beam. More commonly the small image is viewed through a mirror by a built-in television camera and displayed on a television

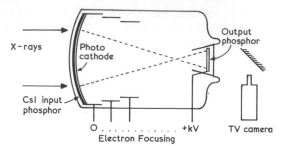

Fig. 7.11   The image intensifier.

monitor. The use of the 45° mirror enables the camera to be positioned outside the X-ray beam and reduces the overall length of the intensifier—an important factor in simulator design.

The X-ray image contained within the transmitted beam is therefore converted in turn into light, into electrons, into light again and then into the final television viewing system. At each stage there will be some loss of information and the displayed image will be of poorer quality than the original. The image may be further degraded if the X-ray beam penetrates through to the output phosphor, if there is poor focusing of the electrons (this is particularly noticeable at the edges of the image) or if there are stray light or stray magnetic fields (from MRI equipment, for example). These losses of image information are outweighed by the advantages of the visual acuity which results from being able to view the brighter image with cone vision. The gain in brightness is sufficient to allow a reduction in the X-ray beam intensity and therefore in the dose to the patient. The television can also enhance the image contrast. The viewing of the poor fluorescent image with rod vision in a darkened room after a period of dark adaptation for the eyes is now an obsolete technique.

There are several other advantages which result from the use of image intensifiers. The television screen may be viewed in any position in any location—in the case of the simulator, the television monitor will normally be located in the adjacent control room—and the image can be readily recorded on video tape. Under normal operation the dynamic image is ideal for the positive localisation of anatomical structures and, for example, the barium meal examination where the radiotherapist may be localising an oesophageal obstruction. However, in many examinations a static picture gives the operator time to absorb more of the detail displayed, which would otherwise be lost. Equipment is now available to feed the television display with a series of static pictures (as in cine photography) in place of the dynamic one. By the use of a *video disc* to record a television frame, or by the

use of a *storage display tube*, a static picture can be produced by a flash of X-rays and displayed for any length of time. A press of a button will initiate another flash of X-rays and a new picture on the screen. This updating of the picture may be triggered automatically at some prescribed frequency if required. This *flash radiography* again helps the diagnostician to reduce the patient dose and at the same time to freeze the picture he or she wishes to scrutinise at length. The real value of the immediate television display over the delayed radiographic film will become clear when the use of the simulator is discussed below, but both facilities are required if the simulator is to be used to maximum advantage. The full-sized radiograph is required for the planning of the treatment and the dynamic television picture in the initial localisation and verification procedures. Miniature multiformat pictures may be used for record keeping and follow-up purposes.

Digital imaging

A recent development in imaging technology is the use of a matrix involving a very large number of individual detectors (e.g. silicon diodes or ionisation chambers) as the image receptor. Each detector occupies a unique position in the matrix and provides a signal proportional to the incident radiation intensity. Processing these signals through a computer can electronically enhance the contrast before displaying the image on a remote video display unit. The fine detail is limited by the pixel size (of each detector) and this may restrict the use of the system to treatment verification on the therapy equipment. The dose required is greater than for a fast film but less than for a full treatment fraction, enabling the beam to be verified almost immediately. The potential of the system as an alternative to the image intensifier is enormous, but its application in diagnostic radiology will be limited for the foreseeable future to computed tomography where a linear array of detectors may be used (p. 134).

TREATMENT SIMULATOR

Having looked in some detail at the formation of the radiographic image, we must now examine the treatment simulator itself (Fig. 7.2). The simulator adds the X-ray system of a diagnostic unit to a gantry–couch system of an isocentric therapy unit and incorporates a unique beam collimating system.

The requirement of the gantry–couch system is that the simulator will have all the movements of the therapy gantry and couch and to the same accuracy or better than the therapy unit. The source–axis distance (SAD) may have to be variable if the unit is to simulate several therapy units. The couch will have to offer all the immobilisation devices used on the therapy equipment and at the same time be transparent to the diagnostic quality X-ray beam. The couch top will therefore be both light and strong in construction—carbon fibre perhaps being the best material currently available. All the movements will be available under both local and remote control.

The X-ray system will comprise a voltage generator, X-ray tube, image intensifier and television monitor. The generator may be of a simple design similar to those described earlier in Chapter 3, but a three-phase generator providing a rectified potential of 6 or 12 pulses per cycle, using six or twelve rectifiers, is more likely. The student is referred to more advanced texts for a full description, but Figure 7.12 shows the secondary circuit of a six-rectifier six-pulse three-phase generator. The secondary voltages from the three windings of the HT transformer will be 120° out of phase, each reaching its peak value in turn. Thus, in general, one voltage will be increasing when the other two are decreasing or vice versa, which means three of the rectifiers will be conducting and three will not. In the diagram, the electron flow is indicated for the instant in time, T,

when two windings are generating half their peak positive potential with respect to earth and the third is at its peak negative potential. The secondary voltage applied to the tube peaks six times during each cycle, giving an almost constant potential. The few per cent voltage ripple may be further smoothed using capacitors (not shown) as described in Chapter 3.

The diagnostic unit operates at between 50 and 125 kV but at much higher tube currents than found in therapy units. Tube currents are commonly 300 or 500 mA and may go as high as 1000 mA in the radiography mode, while in fluoroscopy mode the tube current will normally be less than 2 mA. The heat dissipation in the target during radiography is therefore some 10 times higher than in a therapy tube, albeit for very short exposure times, and dictates the design of the target. The diagnostic tube insert is usually of the rotating anode type (Fig. 7.13). The electrons from the off-axis filament strike the bevelled edge of the anode which rotates at up to 3000 r.p.m., spreading the heat dissipation over an annulus. The bevelled edge acts as a reflection target. The rate at which the target can cool is limited because the heat has to be lost by radiation from the surface, which can reach incandescence when operated close to the maximum. (There can be no convection in a vacuum and conduction has to be minimised to prevent the rotor bearings seizing up due to thermal expansion.) The anode will be permanently damaged if repeated exposures are made too frequently. The recommended tube rating and duty cycle should never be exceeded. The target is usually tungsten mounted on a molybdenum disc and stem.

The anode is mounted on the rotor of an induction motor within the evacuated glass envelope. The stator coils are outside the tube insert and, using the three-phase supply, cause a magnetic field to move round the tube at high speed. Fields are induced in the copper cylinder, the rotor, causing it to rotate. The rotation of the anode should be heard to start as soon as the exposure button is pressed to the 'prep' (preparation) position. The recommended pause at 'prep' is to allow the anode rotation to reach its maximum speed before the exposure is made. The rotation continues for several

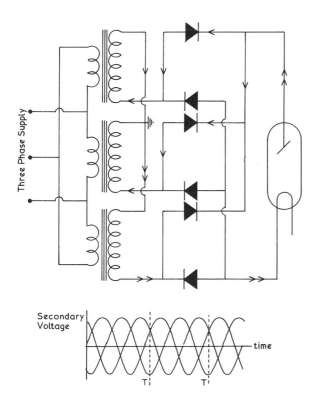

Fig. 7.12   A three-phase, six pulse, six rectifier X-ray generator circuit.

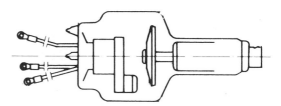

Fig. 7.13   A rotating anode diagnostic tube insert. (Courtesy of Philips Medical Systems Ltd.)

minutes after the exposure has been completed. This free running of the anode confirms the rotor and its bearings are in good condition.

The diaphragm system is unique to the treatment simulator (Fig. 7.14). In addition to the beam limiting diaphragms—similar to those on a diagnostic unit—there are field defining wire diaphragms. The latter are designed to give an accurate indication of the edges of the therapy beam being simulated and to allow the anatomy outside the therapy beam to be visualised. The beam limiting diaphragms are used to control the amount of tissue irradiated outside the therapy beam size and to minimise the production of image degrading scatter. Under computer control these diaphragms can limit the maximum beam to the area covered by the image intensifier or radiographic film and automatically reduce it to a size only slightly greater than that delineated by the wires. This automatic linking of the two systems is desirable because, without it, eight independent diaphragm controls would be required to define the field size in the asymmetric mode, with a further one to rotate the system.

Treatment simulation is primarily the simulation of the therapy beam edges. The correct and reproducible alignment of the wire delineators over the whole range of field sizes is of paramount importance. It is unavoidable that the imaging parameters for the wire delineators are not ideal (Fig. 7.4), with the result that they are not sharply imaged on the image receptor. Their magnification factor is large. Their diameter is small compared with the focal spot, giving rise to considerable image unsharpness. However, providing measurements are taken to the centre of their visible image then errors will be small.

The choice of image receptor on the simulator is commonly radiographic film (43×35 cm² or 35×35 cm²) and an image intensifier of 9 inch (23 cm) or 12 inch (30 cm) diameter. Neither will image the maximum available field size at the isocentre in its entirety. To do so would be unwieldy and impracticable. The very presence of an image receptor identifies the simulator as different from the therapy unit it seeks to mimic and, the more bulky the receptor, the more it restricts the movement of the simulator. A typically difficult situation is illustrated in Figure 7.15. A compromise therefore has to be reached between the physical size of the image receptor and the versatility of the simulator. The XY scanning movement of the image intensifier enables it to track round the edges of a large field in most situations.

Within these restrictions, then, the simulator can provide images in planes parallel or slightly inclined to the long axis of the patient with considerable accuracy and thereby localise the tissues targeted for radiotherapy and verify the proposed treatment plan.

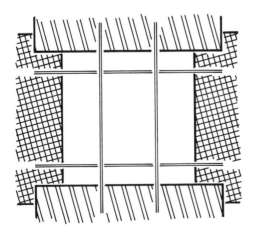

Fig. 7.14 The beam limiting and field defining diaphragm system.

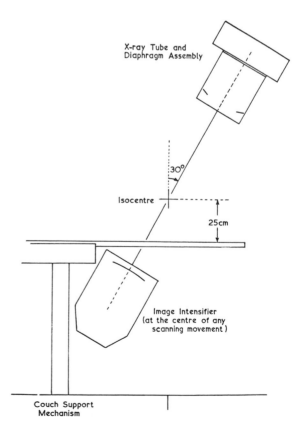

Fig. 7.15 The image intensifier can restrict the movement of the simulator.

Role of the simulator in treatment planning

The treatment simulator is a sophisticated diagnostic X-ray unit and has two principal roles in radiotherapy—the localisation of the target tissues and the verification of the treatment plan. It is not intended as an aid to diagnosis. The diagnosis of the disease and its extent is more readily achieved using the facilities in the departments of Diagnostic X-ray, Nuclear Medicine, Ultrasound and of Magnetic Resonance. The results of such tests should be available at the first simulation of the patient. Similarly, if the patient is expected to require an immobilisation mould/shell, that too should be made and brought to the first simulation where the sole aim is to localise the target tissues within the patient in relation to external markers attached to the patient or the shell. During simulation, the patient must adopt the position to be adopted during treatment. After placing the midpoint of the target volume at the isocentre and indicating the cephalo-caudal dimension with the field defining wires, two orthogonal films are taken of known magnification. These AP and lateral films will provide the localisation information on which the treatment plan will be based. Where possible, the simulator scale readings as well as the exposure factors should be recorded for future reference.

The patient contours should perferably be taken whilst the patient remains in the same position on the simulator couch so that the contours relate uniquely to the information recorded on the localisation films. Alternatively the patient contours could be taken from the patient's shell afterwards, providing the shell is not distorted by the weight of the patient. Patient contouring devices were described in Chapter 6. The orthogonal films do not have to be AP and lateral, any orthogonal pair may be used providing they can be uniquely related to the contour.

The patient's second visit to the simulator will be to verify the treatment plan prior to the commencement of treatment. The most accurate means is to set the patient up on the simulator as planned for the treatment and then to set up each proposed treatment beam in turn—in position, size, direction, etc.—and to confirm that the included and excluded tissues are exactly as required. In some instances the small oblique projection of the anatomy displayed on the screen will not be sufficiently familiar to provide this confirmation, and alternative verifications will have to be devised. On the other hand, the actual visualisation of each beam in turn may be the only means of verifying the beam edges are placed correctly in relation to excluded sensitive tissues. Where tailor-made shielding blocks are required, it is essential that each beam is accurately simulated, so that the film can be marked up to show the shapes required in relation to the principal axes of the field. Such films are not required where the local shielding will be achieved by selecting blocks from a standard set. In this event the position of the blocks may be indicated by skin marks and recorded by attaching wires (or lead solder) to the skin marks whilst films are taken.

Localisation from films

In the following analysis the films will be referred to as AP (suffix 1) and Lateral (suffix 2) although any pair of orthogonal films could be considered (Fig. 7.16).

Under screening conditions, the midpoint of the target tissues is placed at the isocentre and the film–axis distance for each film, F_1O and F_2O, are noted; they may be the same or different. The magnification factors for the target tissues imaged on the two films are therefore:

$$M_{\text{Lat}} = \frac{S_2F_2}{S_2O} = \frac{S_2O + F_2O}{S_2O}$$

and

$$M_{\text{AP}} = \frac{S_1F_1}{S_1O} = \frac{S_1O + F_1O}{S_1O}$$

where S_1O and S_2O are the source–object distances, say 100 cm.

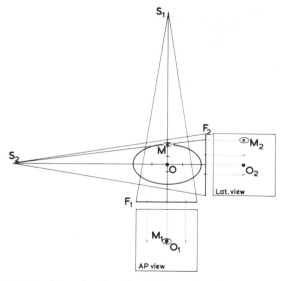

Fig. 7.16 The principle of localisation using orthogonal films.

The principal axes of the target volume can therefore be measured off the films and reduced to their actual size by dividing by the appropriate magnification factor. The cephalo-caudal dimension can be obtained from either film. Similarly, the depth of the target centre, O, below the marker, M, can be measured on the lateral film and demagnified. Regular quality assurance will ensure that the patient contouring device reproduces the correct size of contour.

Some centres prefer to use a ring of known outer diameter, d (say 5 cm), as a marker and determine magnification factors from that instead of having to record F_1O and F_2O. The image of the ring will be permanently recorded on each film, and being a ring, the *maximum* diameter of the image divided by the known diameter gives the magnification of the *ring* (Fig. 7.17).

For the lateral film in Figure 7.17, the magnification factor is required at the midline and will be that of the ring: $M_{Lat} = d_2/d$. On the AP film, however, the ring is at a different distance from the focus than the target tissues and therefore d_1/d cannot be applied without modification (Fig. 7.16):

$$M_{AP} = \frac{S_1F_1}{S_1O} = \frac{S_1M \times d_1/d}{S_1O}$$

S_1M is unknown but S_1O is known and MO can be calculated from the lateral film and therefore:

$$M_{AP} = \frac{(S_1O - MO)\, d_1/d}{S_1O}$$

In some circumstances, it is more convenient to place the marker M at the isocentre, in which case the relevant magnification factors derived from the diameter of the ring placed at M become:

$$M_{Lat} = d_2/d \text{ and } M_{AP} = \frac{S_1M \times (d_1/d)}{S_1M \times MO}$$

The use of the ring is particularly valuable when the planning/simulator films are likely to be archived in a miniature format—the relevant magnification data will remain without addition.

Localisation of sealed sources

The use of the simulator is not confined to external beam therapy. It provides an accurate means of localising any internal structures, including implanted sealed sources or 'dummy' sources, if the activity is to be afterloaded either under manual or remote control. It will become evident in the next chapter that the dose distribution around any implant containing more than one sealed source is critically dependent on the relative positions of those sources. Since the sources are metallic or enclosed in a metallic sheath they will show up clearly on a radiograph or image intensifier.

Under screening conditions, the accuracy of the implant can be examined in detail before the localisation films are taken. For example, a single plane implant can be screened and the X-ray beam positioned to give the 'best' edge-on view of the implanted plane. If the calculation is to be done manually using Paterson–Parker tables (p. 144), then a film taken in a direction perpendicular to the edge-on view will give a true projection of the plane, thereby simplifying the calculation. If the calculation is to be done on a computer then two orthogonal films at (say) 45° to the edge-on view will enable the two ends of each source to be readily identified, thus simplifying the data input to the computer. The computer program may accept data from two non-orthogonal films providing some other correlation of the films is available. (Note. Some computer programs have a facility of matching the two sets of end coordinates automatically, but the results must be checked very carefully.) Where sealed source implants are done regularly, a small operating theatre adjacent to the

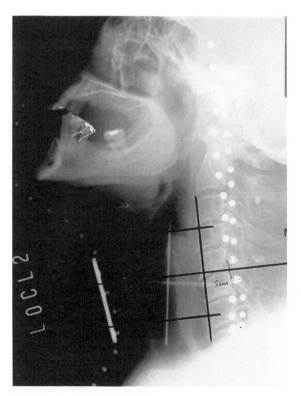

Fig. 7.17 A typical localisation film showing the markers and ring.

simulator can be very useful. If the implanted sources are checked immediately on completion, any deviations from the planned insertion can be corrected without delay.

Electron treatment simulation

There is little experience to date in the simulation of electron treatment. It is advantageous if the electron applicators can be attached to the simulator. The positioning of the rather bulky applicator to treat the more difficult site can then be sorted out in the simulator room rather than in the treatment room. Once the position has been determined, the profile of the field shaping cut-out (to fit the end of the applicator) can be marked and made ready for casting in low melting point alloy. Electron treatment simulation is largely mechanical and does not involve the X-ray imaging facilities unless a verification film is required through the field shaping cut-out.

Where mixed modality treatments, involving both X-ray and electron fields, or two or more electron fields, are planned, then the accuracy of the beam edges becomes critical and simulation is important. It must be remembered, however, that neither the light beam diaphragm nor the diagnostic beam will adequately simulate the penumbra and divergence of the electron therapy beam. Sophisticated computer planning systems are required to ensure the overlap of divergent beams does not lead to gross over- or underdosage of the target, or healthy tissues.

Quality assurance

The quality assurance programme for the treatment simulator will follow a similar pattern to the one used for the linear accelerator in so far as the mechanical alignment and the X-ray/optical beam coincidence is concerned. The latter needs to be repeated under both fine and broad focus conditions. The geometry of the simulator needs to be at least as accurate as the treatment units in every respect.

The radiographic and fluoroscopic image quality on the simulator may not be as good as on the diagnostic

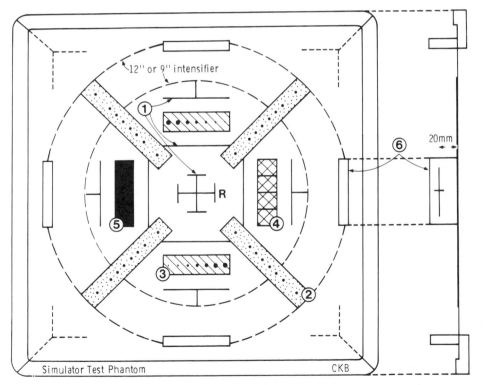

Fig. 7.18 A test phantom to fit in the film holder for regular checks on the simulator to check a variety of parameters including: (1) field sizes and SSD; (2) uniformity of the image; (3) image resolution; (4) beam quality; (5) image brightness; (6) isocentre projectors and many others. (The *R* is simply to aid the correlation of the image with the test object.)

X-ray unit, where all the parameters can be optimised to that one end. Image quality is, however, important and steps must be taken to ensure that quality is the best possible. The regular use of a test phantom, such as that shown in Figure 7.18, enables most of the geometrical and radiographic parameters to be checked on a daily basis. A check against the previous record will draw attention to any dramatic change, whereas a careful study of the records will highlight any gradual deterioration of performance.

CT SCANNER

The computed tomographic (CT) image is a reconstruction in the plane of the scan portrayed by the attenuation coefficients of the tissues. Therefore the CT image identifies the tissues in terms of atomic number and density and they will only be differentiated providing there are differences in either or both of these parameters, as in any diagnostic X-ray procedure. (In contrast, an image produced by magnetic resonance shows the tissues in terms of their hydrogen content, making, for example, bone appear black in an MR image, but white in a CT image.)

The CT scanner is primarily an annulus of 600 or more individually collimated detectors, with the patient along the axis (Fig. 7.19). Each detector is calibrated and measures the intensity of the transmitted X-ray beam. The patient is irradiated by a fan beam from a small focus X-ray tube as the tube rotates, preferably in a few seconds, through about 360°. The radiation is usually pulsed at a rate of (say) 100 pulses per second, each pulse lasting a few milliseconds. During the scan, therefore, some 100 000 measurements are made by the detectors and recorded in the computer.

The detectors need to be very reliable and stable in operation, linear in response and above all sensitive and responding very quickly while being of small physical size. Thallium-doped caesium iodide crystals—as used in image intensifiers—have been used in conjunction with good quality silicon photodiodes, which together have the added advantage of not requiring a high voltage power supply. The alternative is to use sealed ionisation chambers. Normally ionisation chambers require large volumes to improve their sensitivity, but increasing the contained air mass by using high atomic number gases under pressure can increase their sensitivity while keeping the volume small. Under saturation conditions, ionisation chambers can be very stable. Whatever the detector system, regular calibration is vital and is often carried out automatically using the edge of the fan beam.

The number and spacing of the detectors is fundamental to the detail in the computed image—the larger

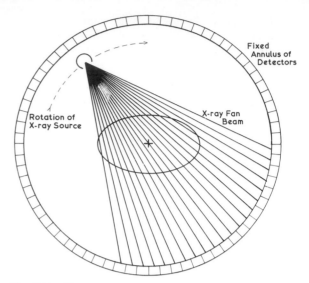

Fig. 7.19 The principal components of the CT scanner.

the number of measurements recorded the smaller the pixel size. The thickness of the fan beam determines the thickness of the slice of tissue irradiated, which may be varied up to, say, 15 mm (Fig. 7.20). (The pixel is the two dimensional picture element derived from the average X-ray attenuation in the voxel or volume element within the patient.) The image may be degraded by the scattered radiation generated in the thicker slice, or by using fewer (larger) detectors. On the other hand the thinner the slice and the more (smaller) detectors used, the smaller the signal-to-noise ratio. (Noise, in this context, is the unwanted signal generated in the electronics of the detector system and is present irrespective of the radiation incident on the detectors. The smaller the signal generated by the radiation, the greater the significance of the noise.) These factors have to be carefully balanced to obtain the optimum image quality.

The X-ray tube requires a small focal spot, say 0.6 mm, and a high output so, although the applied voltage is pulsed, the target cooling may limit the frequency of the scans. The tube is operated at no more than 120 kV, for above that the Compton scattering interactions begin to dominate, reducing the differential absorption in the tissues, and the radiation is less effectively absorbed in the detectors. So although the radiation is more penetrating—reducing the dose to the patient—the image quality deteriorates to an unacceptable level. (In comparison with other diagnostic X-ray examinations, the CT patient dose is very high.)

A variety of mathematical algorithms have been used to reconstruct the two-dimensional image from the measured transmission profiles, but in the main these

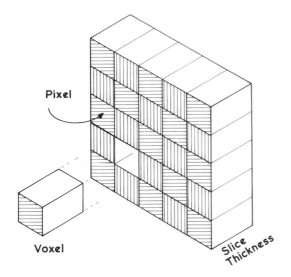

Fig. 7.20 The pixel and the voxel.

are beyond the scope of this book. Let two examples suffice. If the pixels in a square array produce the two transmitted beam profiles shown in Figure 7.21A, then immediately we can expect the centre to produce more attenuation than the periphery because both profiles dip in the centre. If we now use the method of *back projection* and add the profiles together row by row and column by column, the matrix fills, as in Figure 7.21B, confirming the greater attenuation in the centre. Although this illustrates the technique the actual computation is far more complex!

A second method is known as the *iterative* method where a guess is made and then modified repeatedly until the model fits the measured data. This method is perhaps best illustrated by the party puzzle where one is asked to place the numbers 1 to 25 into a five by five matrix in such a way that each row, column and diagonal adds up to the same value, namely 65. Although there is a logical approach to such a problem, most party-goers use the purely iterative approach.

Whatever method is used to reconstruct the image, a CT number is allocated to each pixel as a measure of its attenuation coefficient relative to water. The numbers vary between −1000 for air to +1000 for the densest bone, and these numbers are used to determine the degree of blackness in the final picture. The average video display system can only display about 10 different levels of grey between black and white, but fortunately the operator can select the range of CT numbers to be displayed—a wide *window* portrays the tissues with grossly different attenuation coefficients and is ideal for obtaining patient contours and principal anatomy, for example. A narrow window enables tissues only marginally different in attenuation coefficient to be displayed in different shades of grey. A window width of 1 enables the CT number of individual pixels to be identified. Unfortunately it does not follow that one can distinguish malignant tissue from healthy tissue.

Role of CT in treatment planning

The CT scanner has two distinct roles in radiotherapy—as an aid to diagnosis and as an aid to treatment planning—and in general the patient will be referred to the diagnostic X-ray department for the first in the usual way. A second visit, for treatment planning, will require a much longer appointment (up to an hour perhaps) and with the attendance of staff from Medical Physics, Therapy Radiography and, preferably, the Radiotherapist.

A flat-topped couch insert will be required with the appropriate facilities to enable head-rests and other patient immobilisation devices to be fitted. It may be advantageous to incorporate markers into the couch insert to facilitate localisation and/or magnification factors to be determined from the CT image. Metals, however, must be avoided as these cause artefacts in the image. All markers must be of a lower contrast medium to give a clear mark with the minimum of artefacts—nylon tubing filled with a mixture of barium and silicon cream, for example. They must be continuous line markers and positioned to intersect the scan plane if they are to be recorded on the image. Two parallel lines of known separation laid into the couch top will provide a record of the magnification factor, whereas two divergent straight lines enable the distances between slices to be recorded and measured; a large capital N provides both magnification and slice separation.

Before the patient is subjected to CT scanning for

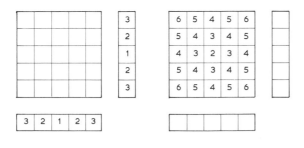

A Measured profiles   **B** Reconstructed image

Fig. 7.21 The principle of back projection.

treatment planning it is essential to have a clear idea of the information required from the scan and how it is likely to be used to aid the treatment plan. A single scan through the midplane of the proposed treatment will present the patient contour and internal anatomy in the transverse plane, to which the planning computer can add the two-dimensional isodose curves. By assigning correction factors to particular internal contours within the patient, e.g. lungs, the isodose distribution can be corrected for the specified inhomogeneities (Fig. 5.23). Unfortunately, the CT numbers cannot be used as correction factors because of the energy dependence of the absorption coefficient.

Superior and inferior borders of the treatment fields together with an off-axis planning program will enable the distribution at these two levels to be similarly computed, providing one principal axis of the treatment field is parallel to the principal axis of the patient, i.e. provided the treatment does not require a diaphragm or couch rotation (Fig. 7.22A). Once a diaphragm or couch rotation is introduced it implies the treatment plane is not truly transverse and the axis of the target volume is not parallel to the axis of the scanner or to the gantry rotation axis of the therapy unit. In other words, the charted isodose data are neither coincident with nor parallel to the anatomical data depicted on the transverse CT scan (Fig. 7.22B). Furthermore the beam entry and exit points and other data are not readily transferred from one CT slice to another. The means by which some of these problems may be overcome is to take a larger number of CT slices close together so that further CT images can be constructed, by interpolation, in planes at right angles to the axis of the inclined target volume (Fig. 7.22C). There is one special case where this may not be required and that is where the treatment fields are laterally parallel opposed and the diaphragm rotation is small and within the range of tilt available on the scanner (Fig. 7.22D), but remember the movement of the couch used is no longer at right angles to the scan plane. (This is probably the only use for the CT tilt facility in radiotherapy.)

In all these cases the treatment planning is very much more complex than in the traditional two-dimensional techniques and, quite apart from requiring a comprehensive treatment planning computer system, it needs to be very carefully thought through, before, during and after the session on the scanner with the patient. The benefits have yet to be proven.

One further benefit which can be derived from a CT planning package is known as the *beam's eye view*. All the CT data derived so far have been in parallel transverse planes, although sagittal and coronal planes can often be displayed. In radiotherapy, however, the

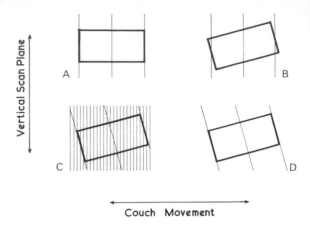

Fig. 7.22 Potential sources of error in CT planning: **A** the scan plane parallel to the upper and lower borders of the treatment field; **B** rotation of the diaphragms or couch: **C** a skew beam makes data transfer from one slice to another difficult and **D** the limited value of tilting the CT scanner.

tissues are irradiated by a divergent beam. The beam's eye view facility not only allows the anatomy at different distances to be visualised as from the target of the therapy beam, but also to be seen with the isodose distribution superimposed. This is particularly valuable where critical organs are likely to be exposed to a dose close to their tolerance dose.

CT on the simulator

Several attempts have been made to enable the rotation of the simulator to be used to produce the same transverse data as the CT scanner. There are several good reasons for wanting such a dual modality simulator. The restricted aperture of the CT scanner (approximately 70 cm diameter) prevents some radiotherapy treatment positions being adopted by the patient. Most radiotherapy departments cannot justify the expense of having their own CT scanner and can only get restricted access to one in another department. The CT scanner is seen to complement the simulator and not as an alternative. From the point of view of both the patient and the staff, it would be more convenient and economic if the two procedures could be carried out at the same session and on one machine. Current technology (Fig. 7.23), however, is insufficient to produce the same quality CT image without compromising the simulator specification but the technology is continually improving.

MEDICAL ULTRASOUND

Ultrasound is a major diagnostic tool in medicine. It

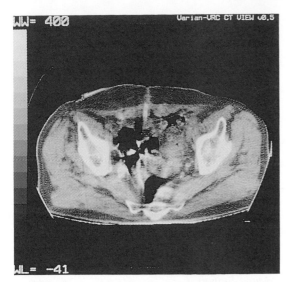

Fig. 7.23 A simulator CT scan. (Courtesy of Varian-TEM Ltd.)

can provide information about the structure of organs, particularly soft tissue, and about the function of the cardiovascular system.

Physical properties of ultrasound

Sound is a form of energy resulting from the transmission of mechanical vibrations through a medium. Ultrasound is sound having a frequency exceeding that which can be detected by the human ear. Frequencies in the range 1–20 MHz are used in medicine, compared to the audio range of 20 Hz to 20 kHz. Ultrasound energy travels through a medium in the form of a compression wave (Fig. 1.7). However, unlike electromagnetic waves, sound waves cannot travel through a vacuum as they need the medium to carry the vibrations. A typical source of the mechanical vibrations (called a 'transducer') is a piezoelectric crystal. These crystals change in thickness, or vibrate, when an electric voltage pulse is applied, and conversely mechanical deformation, or vibration, of the crystal produces a voltage pulse across it. The same crystal can therefore be used to both transmit and receive ultrasound waves. If the transducer is placed in contact with the outside surface of the medium and a pulse of ultrasound transmitted, then the surface particles of the medium begin to vibrate backwards and forwards about their mean position, the net force on their neighbouring particles alters and they also begin to vibrate. The amplitude of the vibrations is very small, being measured in nanometres. In this way energy is quickly transferred through the medium.

A sound wave can be described in terms of its wavelength (λ), its frequency (f) (in ultrasound, the symbol (f) is used in preference to ν to denote frequency) and its velocity (c). These are related by the following equation:

$$\lambda = c/f$$

The frequency is the number of oscillations per second performed by the particles of the medium, the unit of frequency being the hertz (Hz). Velocity is the speed at which a wavefront moves through a medium. Since the propagation of the sound wave requires the medium through which it passes to vibrate, the velocity of ultrasound in biological tissue is dependent on the physical properties of the tissue, such as density and elasticity. Table 7.1 lists the velocity of ultrasound in a range of materials.

Reflection and acoustic impedance

When sound strikes the boundary between two tissues of different acoustic properties some of the sound will be transmitted through the boundary and some will be reflected back towards the transducer. The fraction of total energy reflected depends on the difference in acoustic impedance of the tissues on either side of the boundary. The acoustic impedance Z of a tissue type is equal to the product of the density of the tissue, ρ, and the velocity of water propagation in the tissue:

$$Z = \rho c$$

The acoustic impedance of various materials is given in column three of Table 7.1. A large difference in impedance, as at a bone–soft tissue interface, leads to a high degree of reflection, while interfaces between different soft tissues, such as fat and muscle, result in very small reflections or echoes. An air–tissue interface reflects nearly all the incident energy and it is for this reason that the transducer must make good contact with the patient's skin. This is achieved by the use of a special coupling oil or gel. If the ultrasound beam is incident on a rough surface, or a small object such as a

Table 7.1 Velocity and acoustic impedance of sound in various materials

Material	Velocity (m s^{-1})	Density (kg m^{-3})	Impedance (kg m^{-2} s^{-1})
Air	330	1.2	0.0004×10^6
Blood	1570	1025	1.61×10^6
Muscle	1580	1075	1.70×10^6
Fat	1450	952	1.38×10^5
Bone	3500	2230	7.80×10^6
Soft tissue	1540	1060	1.63×10^6
Lung	1160	400	0.46×10^6

red blood cell, then the ultrasound will be scattered in all directions rather than reflected.

Attenuation

As ultrasound passes through the tissues it is attenuated (reduced in intensity). This is due to a number of factors: reflection, refraction and scattering of the beam at acoustic interfaces; absorption, mainly by conversion of the mechanical vibrations into heat; and wave front divergence. The attenuation of ultrasound energy varies from tissue to tissue (e.g. muscle attenuates more than fat) and is approximately proportional to transmission frequency. The choice of ultrasound frequency is therefore a compromise between adequate penetration, which requires low frequencies, and good resolution which is best achieved with higher frequencies. Typically transducers operating at frequencies in the range 2–4 MHz are used to investigate organs in the abdomen and pelvis, whereas superficial structures such as peripheral blood vessels and the thyroid gland will be examined using frequencies of 7-10 MHz. In general terms, the highest frequency compatible with the depth produces the greatest detail.

Image production

An ultrasound transducer transmits and receives signals along a narrow beam. Typically the transducer emits a 1 µs pulse of ultrasound every 0.1 ms and this is reflected back to the transducer from the tissue interfaces. The time of arrival of the reflected pulse is dependent upon the depth of the reflecting interface. The amplitude of the reflected pulse (echo) is dependent upon the physical composition of the reflector. This information can be used to set both the position and brightness of a dot on a cathode ray tube.

Imaging modes

A-scan

The simplest technique is the A-scan. A stationary transducer is pointed in the direction of interest and echoes are received from interfaces that intersect the single beam. These are displayed on a cathode ray tube as a graph of amplitude versus time (Fig. 7.24). On the left of the screen is a vertical pulse corresponding to the transmission of the ultrasound signal, while the echo pulses follow some time later, the time delay being measured as a horizontal deflection. The A-scan provides information as a one-dimensional picture since only those interfaces lying within the single beam are recorded.

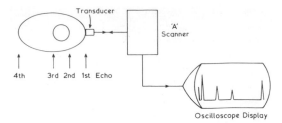

Fig. 7.24 An A-scan display.

The A-scan is not widely used, but it is simple to operate and can be used for examining structures such as the midline of the brain, the bulb of the eye and the penetration of the eye by choroidal malignant melanomas, or the thickness of the chest wall in preparation for post-mastectomy electron beam therapy.

Real-time B-scan

Real-time B-scans present real-time two-dimensional pictures of structures. This is accomplished by rapidly scanning the ultrasound beam through the tissue using either a mechanically rotating transducer encased in an oil-filled cylinder (Fig. 7.25), or a multielement transducer in which the beam is steered electronically.

The echo signals received from each beam position are displayed as spots on the display unit, the brightness indicating the amplitude of the echo. The position of the spots are determined by the time of arrival of the echoes and the orientation of the beam. Thus a grey scale image is built up of a slice through the tissues. Images are produced at a rate of 25–30 frames per second. This means that the motion of organs, such as the heart, or

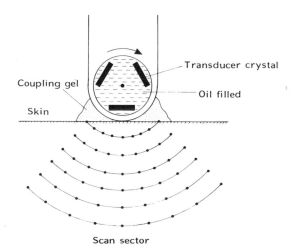

Fig. 7.25 Schematic diagram of a mechanical rotating transducer.

the movement of the fetus can be observed, and, of equal importance, it enables rapid alteration of the scan plane allowing the operator to search through the anatomy.

B-mode scanning is invaluable for the imaging of soft tissues. It plays an important role in: the management of both normal and complicated pregnancies; the investigation of abdominal organs such as the liver for assessment of size and focal disorders—primary and secondary malignancies, diffuse diseases, and therapeutic outcome; and the differentiation of cysts and tumours in superficial organs like the thyroid and breast. Figure 7.26 shows a grey scale image of a fetus in utero.

Doppler

Movement of reflectors or scatterers in the ultrasound beam changes the frequency of the reflected or back scattered echo. This event is known as the Doppler effect. The magnitude of the frequency change, or Doppler shift (Δf), is proportional to the velocity (v), and direction of the movement ($\cos \theta$) relative to the transducer and is given by:

$$\Delta f = 2f_0 v \cos \theta / c$$

where f_0 is the transmission frequency and c is the velocity of sound in the tissue (Fig. 7.27).

Doppler ultrasound can be used to investigate the cyclical variation of blood flow in the arteries and veins. After frequency analysis these changes can be displayed graphically (Fig. 7.28).

Duplex

The Duplex concept combines real-time B-mode imag-

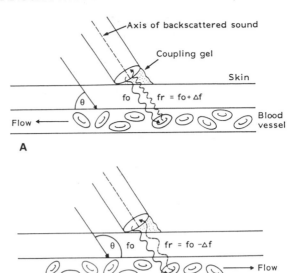

Fig. 7.27   Doppler shift produced by moving red cells: a red cell moving towards the transducer gives a shift incidence frequency of $+\Delta f$ (**A**) and away from the transducer of $-\Delta f$ (**B**).

ing with Doppler flow measurements. The walls of a blood vessel, or heart chamber, are defined by the real-time B-mode scanner. The image is then used as a 'map' to place the sample volume of a pulsed Doppler flow-meter at various sites within the vessel. The flow patterns at these sites are then evaluated (Fig. 7.29).

Colour flow Doppler

Colour flow Doppler adds a third capability to the ultrasound image. These machines integrate the real-time B-scan and the Doppler information still further by superimposing the image of moving blood, in colour, on to the real-time grey scale image. By appropriate colour coding, direction of flow, velocity of flow and regions of disturbed flow can be easily visualised (Plate 2). These techniques can be used to investigate: the flow through the valves and within the chambers of the heart, and the blood flow in normal and diseased tissue. Plate 3 shows the blood supply to an occular tumour.

Advantages and disadvantages

The major advantages of diagnostic ultrasound techniques over alternative procedures are:

— No harmful side-effects, either immediate or long term, have been shown to be associated with diagnostic ultrasound.
— It is non-invasive and causes no discomfort to the

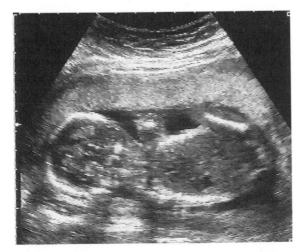

Fig. 7.26   Real-time B-mode grey scale image of a fetus in utero.

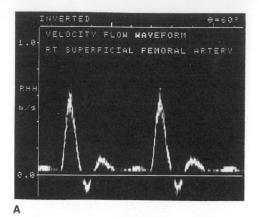

A

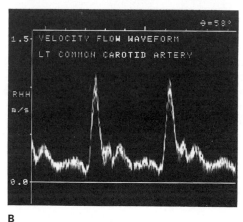

B

Fig. 7.28   Doppler shift frequency spectrum from **A** a superficial femoral artery and **B** a common carotid artery.

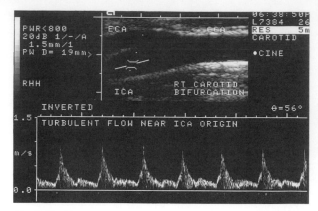

Fig. 7.29   Duplex scan display: grey scale image of the carotid artery (above) and blood velocity waveform (below).

— Information about tissue type can be ascertained.
— Quantitative measurements of structures within the body can be made, for example the biparietal diameter of the fetal head.
— Blood flow can be visualised and flow dynamics investigated.

There are of course some disadvantages with the technique. These include: difficulty in image interpretation; imaging problems in the presence of bone and gas; and difficulties in actually locating and accessing some structures of interest.

patient, enabling repeated examinations to be performed.
— It is relatively cheap.
— Tissue structure and movement can be imaged in detail.

8. Brachytherapy

INTRODUCTION

Radioactive materials are used in a wide variety of ways in medical practice. Chapter 3 has dealt with the use of isotopes for the production of gamma ray beams for radiotherapy. Chapters 9 and 10 deal with the use of unsealed radioactive materials, i.e. liquids, gases, etc. The present chapter will describe the physical aspects of the use of small quantities of radioactive material in the form of *sealed sources* where the active material is contained in a metal capsule. Their use for producing gamma ray effects in limited regions of tissue is one of the oldest established practices of radiotherapy. Both radium-226 and radon-222 have been used for this purpose. They are alpha emitters but within their common decay scheme are the daughter products radium B (lead-214) and radium C (bismuth-214). Radium B and C are radioactive solids emitting gamma ray photons with energies in the range 0.2–2.4 MeV. With an effective photon energy of approximately 1.0 MeV and a half-life of 1640 years, radium was ideal as a small gamma ray source, but the higher energy photons in its spectrum made radiation protection difficult and its first daughter product, the inert gas radon, was a constant additional hazard.

More recently, caesium-137 has largely replaced radium as the nuclide of choice. It has a lower photon energy of 662 keV and a half-life of 30 years. Caesium-137 is a by-product of nuclear fuel reprocessing. It is an alkaline metal but as a compound of chloride or sulphate it is chemically stable. These salts are soluble and therefore for clinical sources the caesium is incorporated into glass for high activity sources or into zirconium phosphate for needles and tubes. In both these forms the caesium is relatively insoluble. Caesium sources are doubly encapsulated and carry a recommended working life of 10 years, during which their activity falls by approximately 20%. Other nuclides are also in use in selected applications, but each one has the disadvantage of a shorter half-life, requiring some correction to be

Table 8.1 Isotopes used in brachytherapy

Isotope	Half-life	Photon energy (MeV)	Air kerma rate per GBq at 1 m (mGy h^{-1})	Sources available
Caesium-137	30 years	0.662	0.078	Needles and tubes; beads for afterloading
Cobalt-60	5.26 years	1.17,1.33	0.307	Needles and tubes; beads and pellets for high dose rate afterloading
Gold-198	2.7 days	0.41	0.055	Grains for permanent implantation
Iridium-192	74 days	0.3–0.6	0.113	Wire and pins for manual afterloading; pellets for remote afterloading
Iodine-125	60 days	0.027–0.036	0.034	Seeds for permanent implantation
Radium-226	1640 years	0.2–2.4	0.195	Needles and tubes

made for radioactive decay either before or during the treatment. Their advantage is a lower photon energy, making radiation protection somewhat easier, and in every case the absence of gaseous daughter products. Essential data on these alternatives to radium are summarised in Table 8.1. Each source will have a recommended working life beyond which the manufacturer will not guarantee the integrity of the source.

This use of small sealed gamma ray sources to irradiate the tissues is usually referred to as *brachytherapy* and it falls into three distinct applications. Interstitial therapy is where the sources are implanted directly into the diseased tissues. Intracavitary therapy is where the sources are arranged in a suitable applicator to irradiate the walls of a body cavity from inside. The use of surface applicators is where an external surface of the patient is treated by locally applied sources arranged on an appropriately shaped applicator. (This latter application has been largely replaced by the use of electron beams.)

Before considering complex arrays of sources, consider the simplest source of all—an isolated point source. Gamma rays are emitted isotropically. It follows, therefore, that the intensity of radiation will decrease with the inverse square of the distance from the source (p. 60) and the intensity will be uniform over a spherical surface centred on the point source. The dose rate will therefore be proportional to the activity of the source (the number of photons emitted per unit time) and to the inverse square of the distance from the source. Figure 8.1 represents a line of five equally spaced point sources, each emitting gamma rays in all directions and producing a complex pattern of isodose lines, but each line representing the cumulative effect of the inverse square law applied to each source. From this one figure several important conclusions may be drawn.

1. Despite the complex nature of the isodose lines

shown, each one will be circular in cross-section, i.e. when viewed from one end of the line of sources as axis.

2. At points close to any one source the isodose surface will be essentially spherical, the influence of the neighbouring sources being negligible.

3. The dose distribution along a line close to and parallel to the line of sources will be very uneven: high close to each source and low between adjacent sources.

4. Each low point could be raised by inserting a further source halfway between each existing source, making the distribution more uniform.

5. As the distance between the line of interest and the line of sources is increased, the uniformity of dose improves until the isodose line becomes the arc of a circle with the middle source as centre and the separation of the sources insignificant.

6. Keeping the distance between the line of interest and the line of sources the same and bringing the sources closer together has the same effect as in (5).

The student will appreciate that the extension of (4) is to make a continuous line source and the extension of (5) and (6) is that the five sources become effectively a single point source. The corollary of (1) is that the distribution shown is essentially that of a section through five parallel line sources viewed end-on. The three valuable consequences drawn from the above analysis are:

1. The uniformity of dose achieved is dependent on both the distance from the plane containing the sources and the spacing of those sources.

2. A line source may be thought of as a line of closely spaced point sources and vice versa.

3. The uniformity of dose is further improved by increasing the activity of the sources at the end of the line.

NEEDLES AND TUBES

Figure 8.2 shows the isodose distribution surrounding an interstitial needle and its construction. The radioactive content (usually caesium-137) is packed in several individual cells down the length of a tube. The tube is closed at one end by an eyelet (the eye of the needle) and by a trocar point at the other. The cell loading not only ensures the activity is distributed uniformly down the length of the needle but also minimises the spillage of active content should the needle become damaged. It also offers the possibility of manufacturing needles with a more active cell at one or at both ends—referred to as *indian club* or *dumb-bell loaded* needles respectively. A variety of metals have been used for the outer casing of the needle (platinum–iridium alloy, silver, stainless

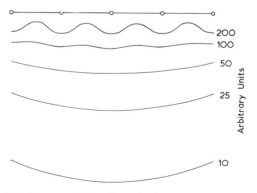

Fig. 8.1 The complex isodose distribution from a line of five point sources.

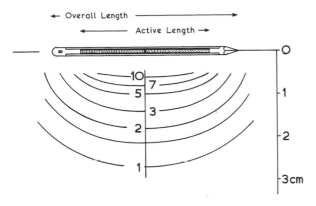

Fig. 8.2 The construction and isodose distribution for an interstitial needle.

steel, etc.), the principal properties required being physical strength to withstand damage in normal wear and tear, non-toxicity and inertness in the presence of body fluids and the ability to absorb the associated beta emissions. The platinum–iridium alloy was preferred because its high atomic number ($Z = 78$) and high density ($21.5\ \mathrm{g\ cm^{-3}}$) ensured absorption of the unwanted alpha and beta emissions and its high melting point ($1769°C$) prevented damage in the event of accidental loss and incineration! When needles are used it is important to know the difference between the overall length (as visualised on the radiograph) and the active length (as required for dosimetry purposes)—the 'inactive ends' are of equal length.

The sources for intracavitary therapy are of the same basic construction but with square ends. They are usually of greater diameter and greater activity but shorter in length (Fig. 8.15).

Each needle and tube will have an identification number or code engraved on it. This is necessary not only for identification purposes but also for the routine tests that are carried out periodically (especially the 'leakage test', p. 158). Detailed records must be kept of every individual radioactive source with a half-life of more than a few days. Gold-198, ($T_{1/2} = 2.7$ days) is the only radionuclide excluded in practice from these records.

Gold grains

The necessary rigidity of needles implanted for up to a week can be the cause of considerable discomfort and inconvenience to the patient despite the fact that this rigidity simplifies the dosimetry. An alternative is to use small individual grains (usually of gold-198). Gold grains are 2.2 mm lengths cut from 0.5 mm diameter gold wire and covered with 0.15 mm platinum to ab-

sorb the beta particle emission, bringing their overall size to 2.5 mm long by 0.8 mm diameter. The platinum coating will be slightly radioactive which means the grains are technically unsealed sources and must be handled with care. Being so small, once inserted into muscle tissue they cannot be removed but constitute a permanent implant—unless the body excretes them as foreign bodies in the normal course of events. The short half-life of 2.7 days means that only 12.5% of the implanted activity remains after 8.1 days (three half-lives), or to put it another way, 87.5% of the final dose is delivered in the first 8.1 days, or 97% in 14 days. This complicates the dosimetry calculations because the dose rate is not constant. However it can be shown that the total dose delivered in an infinite time is numerically equal to that delivered in a time equal to $1/\lambda$ if the dose rate is assumed to remain constant from the time of implant. $1/\lambda$ is called the mean life and, for gold-198, equals 2.7 d/0.693 or 93.5 h. It can be shown (p. 145) that 1 GBq gold-198 produces the same air kerma rate as 7.6 mg radium-226 (it is said to be 7.6 mg radium equivalent) and therefore 1 GBq gold-198 permanently implanted will deliver the same total dose as 7.6 mg radium implanted for 93.5 h or 710 mgh. (The mgh is explained on p. 145).

The grains supplied for interstitial therapy are supplied in magazines of 14 grains in tandem. The magazine is 'loaded' into the barrel of an implantation 'gun' (Fig. 8.3); the stilette then transfers the grains to the end of the 'barrel'—one of a selection of hollow needles, usually graduated in centimetres on the outside. The needle penetrates the tissues to the maximum depth required and operating the trigger deposits one grain at the tip; partially withdrawing the needle enables further grains to be deposited at measured intervals.

A further advantage of the short half-life is that the patient can be allowed home—other considerations permitting—when the total implanted activity of gold has decayed to less than 1 GBq.

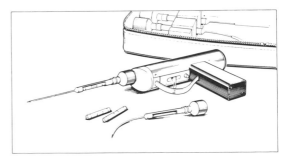

Fig. 8.3 The implantation gun for gold grains. (Courtesy of Amersham International plc.)

Gold-198 is produced by neutron bombardment of pure gold in a reactor and decays to mercury-198 with a beta particle and a gamma ray photon of 0.41 MeV—an ideal photon energy for brachytherapy.

Paterson–Parker system

The Paterson–Parker system (sometimes called the Manchester system) sets out rules relating to the distribution of sources in various geometric configurations to deliver a uniform dose to the prescribed plane or volume and provides data for the calculation of this dose based on the activity used. The rules envisage five different applications: linear sources to irradiate a concentric cylindrical surface, surface applicators to irradiate an external skin surface, planar implants to irradiate the adjacent tissues, multiple plane or volume implants to irradiate a thicker block of tissue, and a cylindrical implant to irradiate the enclosed tissues. In radiotherapy today only two applications are in widespread use, and the rules for these will be outlined below. They may be used with caesium tubes and needles or with gold grains, providing the source activity is quoted in milligrams radium equivalent. Where the sources are mounted in applicators for intracavitary use or on applicators for surface use, the material used to make the applicator is relatively unimportant, providing there is no significant absorption of the radiation. Several layers of vacuum-formed plastic (p. 108) are ideal. In brachytherapy the dose distribution is primarily determined by distance.

Rules for planar implants

In general, a planar array of sources will be circular or rectangular with elliptical areas being approximated to either according to their eccentricity. Implants are more conveniently made with needles arranged as a rectangle and surface applicators with small discrete 'point' sources arranged in a circle. The same rules can be applied to both surface applicators and planar implants. The implanted plane is designed to treat a volume of tissue of the same area to a thickness of 5 mm on either side.

Sources used end-to-end to make up a line source should be sufficient in number to ensure that the gap between adjacent active ends does not exceed the treatment distance, h, i.e. the length of the normal between the active plane and the treated surface. If the surface applicator is applied to a curved surface—the rules may be applied up to hemispherical or hemicylindrical surfaces—the activity will be calculated on

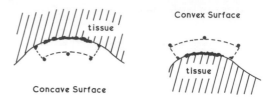

Fig. 8.4 Concave and convex surface applicators.

the basis of the *smaller* area in each case. It will be distributed over the larger area where the treated surface is convex (Fig. 8.4), but over the smaller area where the treated surface is concave.

Circles. Normally surface applicators are of such a diameter, D, that the ratio D/h lies between 3 and 6 and they require the activity to be distributed so that 5% lies in the centre and 95% round the periphery. If the ratio D/h is less than 3, all the activity is placed round the periphery, the 'ideal' distribution being obtained when $D/h = 2.83$. If D/h is 6 or larger, then an 'inner circle' of half the diameter is added and the activity apportioned as in Table 8.2. A minimum of six sources is required to define a circle.

Table 8.2 Distribution of activity when $D/h > 6$

	D/h		
	6	7.5	10
Periphery (%)	80	75	70
Inner circle (%)	17	22	27
Centre spot (%)	3	3	3

Rectangles. For square distributions, the activity is distributed uniformly around the periphery and then the area divided into strips of width not greater than $2\,h$. If one extra line is required, a half strength needle is used; for more than one extra line then two-third strength needles are required. In the case of rectangles the added lines are parallel to the longer sides and their activity is relative to that of the longer sides. Where the rectangle has sides in the ratio of 2, 3 or 4, the overall activity should be increased by 5, 9 and 12% respectively. If it is not possible to 'cross' the ends of the rectangle, the area treated is effectively reduced by 10% for each uncrossed end unless 'indian club' or 'dumb-bell' loaded needles are used.

The calculation. The Paterson–Parker system of rules included data for dosimetry based on the use of radium. The data may be used for other nuclides providing their photon energy is similar and their activity, A, is converted to milligrams-radium-equivalent by multiplying by the ratio of the air kerma rates. The mg Ra equivalence of another isotope is given by

$$\frac{A(\text{MBq}) \times K}{37 \times 195} \text{ mg}$$

where K and the 195 are air kerma rates (in nGy h^{-1} per MBq at 1 m, Table 8.1) for the new isotope and radium respectively; the 37 converts MBq to mg. Once this has been calculated and provided the decay during the proposed treatment is negligible, all the radium data referred to above may be used. (All radium sources are assumed to be filtered by 0.5 mm Pt, unless otherwise stated.)

The dose calculation using the Paterson–Parker system usually falls into two parts. Stage 1 is a theoretical calculation of the ideal and stage 2 is a practical calculation based on the available sources. In both, a clear understanding of the milligram-hour concept is all that is required. At its simplest, the 'mgh' is a measure of 'dose' under a given geometry, the geometry determining the intensity of radiation from 1 mg radium. Paterson and Parker produced tables and graphs which give the milligram-hours of radium filtered by 0.5 mm Pt required to deliver 1 Gy to a particular geometrical situation. Figure 8.5 illustrates the typical source arrays and provides the data for planar implants and surface applicators. From this point on all we have to do is to find two numbers (the milligrams and the hours) whose product is the figure derived from the graph.

For example, a prescription may read 'A needle implant is required to cover an area of $3 \times 4.5 \text{ cm}^2$ and deliver 6 Gy to a plane at 0.5 cm distance in 5 days.'

Stage 1 To calculate the required activity for the prescribed treatment.

Area of implant = $3 \times 4.5 \text{ cm}^2 = 13.5 \text{ cm}^2$

To deliver 1 Gy at 0.5 cm distance requires 30 mgh (Fig. 8.5)
To deliver 60 Gy at 0.5 cm distance requires 30×60 mgh
To deliver 60 Gy in 5 days ($\times$ 24 hours) requires

$$\frac{30 \times 60}{5 \times 24} = 15 \text{ mg}$$

Stage 2 To calculate the actual treatment time using the practical sources. We shall need to add extra lines parallel to the longer side to divide the 3 cm width into strips not greater than 2×0.5 cm. We shall, therefore, require two extra lines each containing two-thirds the activity of the longer side.

We must use the layout of needles illustrated in Figure 8.6, each with a linear density of 0.66 mg cm^{-1}.

Periphery $2 \times 3 \text{ mg} + 2 \times 2 \text{ mg}$ = 10 mg
Extra lines $2 \times 2 \times 1 \text{ mg}$ = 4 mg
Total activity used = 14 mg

The dose of 60 Gy at 0.5 cm distance requires 30×60 mgh and therefore the

$$\text{Revised treatment time} = \frac{30 \times 60}{14} = 128.5 \text{ h}$$

The dose rate per mg is the reciprocal of the mgh per Gy. In the above example, where 30 mgh were required to give 1 gray, the dose rate is 1/30 Gy h^{-1} per mg, or 0.467 Gy h^{-1} per 14 mg.

Because of the inherent non-uniformity of dose in the implant situation, a relaxation of the above rules is permitted, namely to implant a fraction of the total activity round the periphery and to distribute the

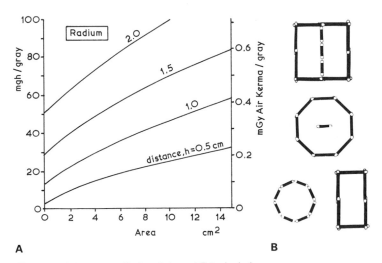

Fig. 8.5 **A** Paterson–Parker data and **B** typical planar source arrays.

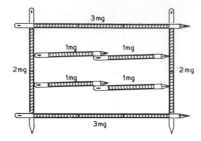

Fig. 8.6   A typical needle implant.

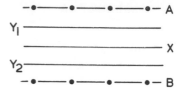

Fig. 8.7   A two plane implant.

Two plane implants

The single plane implant can effectively treat a volume of tissue of the same area and 1 cm thick, i.e. 0.5 cm either side of the implanted activity. The same volume could be treated with a two plane implant, providing the same total activity is divided equally between the two planes 1 cm apart. Where the implanted planes are separated by more than 1 cm, then the dose in the central plane will be low—at separations greater than about 2 cm, unacceptably low. The dose calculation may be carried out as above or by considering the contribution of each plane to the total dose rate as in the example below.

Consider a two plane implant, each plane of equal area and 2 cm apart. Let the implanted planes be A and B and consider the dose at the midplane X and 0.5 cm either side of the midplane at Y_1 and Y_2 (Fig. 8.7). The implanted area is 15 cm². The calculation of dose rate shown in Table 8.3 demonstrates the midplane dose is lower by 20% than the dose to the other two planes. If the implanted planes are of different areas or of different activities, the same principle can be followed, but in either case the doses or dose rates to Y_1 and Y_2 will also be different. Where the target volume is thicker than 2 cm then external beam therapy is likely to be the treatment of choice.

Rules for linear sources

Line sources may be made up of several collinear tubes

remainder as evenly as possible over the enclosed area. The peripheral fraction for areas less than 25 cm² is two-thirds of the total, one-half for areas between 25 cm² and 100 cm² and one-third for areas greater than 100 cm². Using this approximation in the above calculation would have led to the same 10 mg round the periphery and 5 mg over the enclosed area and precisely the prescribed treatment time of 120 h.

In practice, the precise layout of needles will not always be achieved, in which case the calculation is repeated a third time using the implanted area— estimated from radiographs (p. 132)—and the implanted activity to determine the actual treatment dose rate.

Recent recommendations from the International Commission on Radiation Units and Measurements (ICRU) suggest that one parameter in the recording of any brachytherapy treatment should be the *total reference air kerma*, that is the sum of the air kerma rate at 1 metre multiplied by the insertion time for each individual source. Since the air kerma rate at 1 metre from 1 mg radium (filtered by 0.5 mm Pt) is 7.2 µGy h⁻¹, the total reference air kerma for 1 mgh is 7.2 µGy and for the implant described above, it is $30 \times 60 \times 7.2$ µGy or 13.0 mGy. In practice, this approximates to the total dose delivered at a point 1 metre from the implant over the duration of the implant.

Table 8.3   Calculation of dose rate in a two plane implant

		For dose planes		
		Y_1	X	Y_2
From plane A, the treating distance (cm)	=	0.5	1.0	1.5
the activity required (mgh Gy⁻¹)	=	32.6	58.9	85.2
and the dose rate per mg (Gy h⁻¹)	=	0.0307	0.0170	0.0117
From plane B, the treating distance (cm)	=	1.5	1.0	0.5
the activity required (mgh Gy⁻¹)	=	85.2	58.9	32.6
and the dose rate per mg (Gy h⁻¹)	=	0.0117	0.0170	0.0307
Total dose rate from *10 mg* in each plane (Gy h⁻¹)	=	0.424	0.340	0.424
Giving in 24 h a dose (Gy)	=	10.2	8.2	10.2

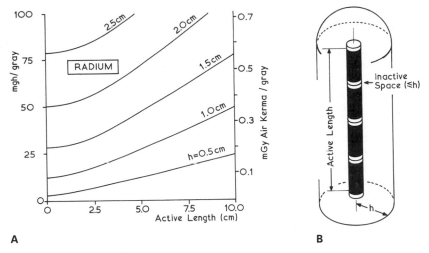

Fig. 8.8 **A** Paterson–Parker data and **B** a typical line source applicator.

mounted in some form of applicator (e.g. Perspex) or outer tube and can be used for treating the inner surface of certain body cavities, e.g. the uterus. There are just two rules for this simple applicator. First, the active length is defined as the distance between the active ends of the whole composite source. (This will be greater than the sum of the active lengths of the individual sources.) Secondly, the inactive space between the active ends of adjoining sources should not exceed the source–surface distance, h. The irradiated cylindrical surface is that defined by the radius, h, and the active length of the source. The uniformity of dose will be ± 10% (Fig. 8.8).

The method of dose calculation is exactly the same as in the previous example, but using the data appropriate to line sources as in Figure 8.8.

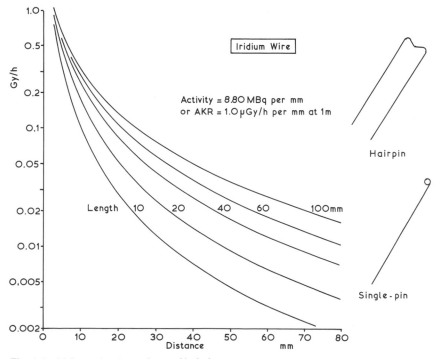

Fig. 8.9 Iridium wire data, pins and hairpins.

IRIDIUM WIRE

The Paterson–Parker system is ideal where sources of appropriate loading and length are available to satisfy both the requirements of the rules and the planned implant, as in the worked example above. However there are many situations where an alternative system is required to take advantage of the newer sources like iridium-192 (Fig. 8.9). Iridium is available with a wide variety of activities per unit length either as pins (0.6 mm diameter × 60 mm maximum) or as wire (0.3 mm diameter × 500 mm maximum). Non-uniform loadings are not available. With a 74 day half-life, the activity of the iridium should be quoted about midway through the planned treatment time, but otherwise the decay during the few days of treatment may be ignored. The iridium pins and wire are coated with 0.1 mm Pt to absorb the associated beta emission, but since both pins and wire can be cut to the length required at the time of the implant, iridium is technically not a sealed source—small fragments can be left on the cutting device for example, making regular monitoring for contamination essential. Iridium-192 is activated in the reactor by the neutron bombardment of an alloy of platinum and iridium-191 and decays to platinum-192. The spectrum from iridium is complex covering a range from 0.3 to 0.6 MeV.

With the remote afterloading techniques now available iridium implants are often larger than the needle implants of recent years—radium needle implants of the chest wall would now be unacceptable from the radiation hazard point of view, whereas with afterloading of iridium wire and the lower photon energy the hazards are much reduced.

The use of iridium wire and iridium hairpins is usually a manual afterloading technique. The use of wire involves the implantation of nylon tubes into the superficial tissues, the tubes being secured at both ends with nylon balls. The position of these tubes can then be checked radiographically by inserting inactive 'fuse' wire into the tubes. The iridium wire is cut to the required length and inserted into a second nylon tube of a smaller diameter than the first. This tube is then threaded through the implanted tubes (preferably leaving at least 5 mm between the end of the wire and the skin) and secured by crimping lead discs outside each nylon ball as shown in Figure 8.10. After the required treatment time, one lead disc is cut off each source assembly and the other is used to withdraw it.

An alternative technique is to insert rigid steel guide needles in to the tissues through a template to enable the spacing to be accurately controlled, and through a second template where the guides exit from the tissues, if possible. This rigid framework not only provides an 'ideal' arrangement of sources, but maintains the configuration throughout the duration of the treatment and allows some compression of the tissues. This technique is often used in the treatment of the breast (Fig. 8.11).

Where the implant is not superficial, rigid slotted steel guide needles can be inserted and their position checked prior to inserting iridium (single) pins or (double) 'hairpins'. The guide needles can then be removed; the bridge of the hairpin and the loop of the single pin slide down the slot in the guide.

Paris system

The Paris system of dosimetry accepts equally spaced straight sources distributed over one or two planes, each source of the same activity per unit length, but of a length primarily determined by the target size. The volume treated to the prescribed dose is some 30% less than the length of the sources, in the absence of 'crossed ends', while the thickness depends on the separation of the sources—approximately 60% of the source separation for a single plane implant and 120% for a two plane. The equal spacing of identical sources in a plane means that the treatment volume or isodose surface is more ellipsoidal than rectangular, as with the Paterson–Parker system.

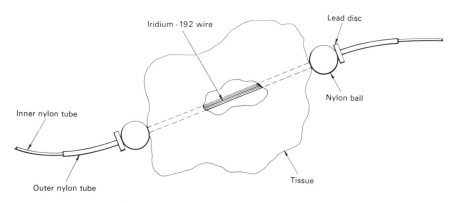

Fig. 8.10 A typical assembly of the Pierquin/Paine afterloading technique for iridium wire. (Courtesy of Amersham International plc.)

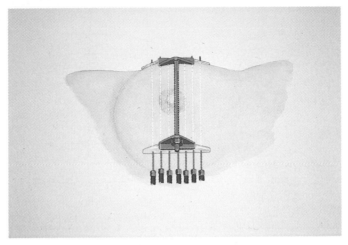

Fig. 8.11 Interstitial therapy of the breast using a remote afterloading technique. (Courtesy of Nucletron Trading Co., Chester.)

The isodose distribution for a straight iridium wire will be similar to that shown in Figure 8.2. It should be remembered that along a line bisecting the length of the source the dose rate does not follow the inverse square law until the distance from the source is large compared with its length. In the Paris system, these data are tabulated or presented as graphs (Fig. 8.9) and form the basis of the dose calculation. The data for pins will be different from those for wire, taking into account their greater diameter and therefore greater self-filtration.

The space between any two adjacent sources is referred to as a 'corridor', and the basal dose rate is calculated as the mean of the dose rates at the centre of each corridor. These are determined by measuring or calculating the distance from each source, summing the dose rates given in the tables/graphs at these distances and correcting for the activity per unit length. The treatment is prescribed to 85% of the basal dose rate. The choice of 85% is not entirely arbitrary, but produces an isodose surface closely approximating that described in the Paterson–Parker system by the distance, h. As an alternative, the dose rate at any prescribed point can be calculated in a similar fashion.

Faced with the same prescription as before (p. 145), three 60 mm iridium wires are required, separated by 15 mm. The basal dose rate would be calculated as in Table 8.4 where the three wires are identified as ABC and the centre of each corridor as X and Y; the dose rate figures are taken from Figure 8.9. The mean basal dose rate calculated in the table is 0.837 Gy h^{-1} and 85% of this is 0.711 Gy h^{-1} (using sources of 8.8 MBq mm^{-1}). The prescription requires a dose rate of only 60 Gy in 5 days, or 0.50 Gy h^{-1}. The source activity required is therefore $8.80 \times 0.50/0.711 = 6.19$ MBq mm^{-1}. Point Z in the table is 5 mm from point Y in a direction perpendicular to the implanted plane and serves to compare this technique with that outlined previously (p. 145). The calculated dose rate at point Z is 0.695 Gy h^{-1} or 83% of the basal dose rate, confirming the use of the apparently arbitrary 85% figure above. Using three 60 mm wires of 6.19 MBq mm^{-1} means the total implanted activity is $3 \times 60 \times 6.19 = 1114$ MBq. Given that the air kerma rate at 1 m for iridium is 0.113 mGy h^{-1} per GBq and the treatment is 120 h, the total reference air kerma is 15 mGy.

Figure 8.12 shows the dose distribution around four 60 mm iridium wires implanted at the corners of a 2 cm square. The basal dose rate is calculated at the centre of the square by summing the dose rates from each of the wires. In this example all the wires are the same length and equidistant from the centre, i.e. at 1.4 cm distance. Figure 8.8 gives the dose rate at 1.4 cm from a 60 mm source as 0.2 Gy h^{-1}. The basal dose rate is therefore $4 \times 0.2 = 0.8$ Gy h^{-1} when the activity is 8.8 MBq mm^{-1}. Prescribing to the 85% isodose gives a dose rate of 0.68 Gy h^{-1}. Thus a typical

Table 8.4 Calculation of iridium wire implant

	Point X		Point Y		Point Z	
	d (cm)	Gy h^{-1}	d (cm)	Gy h^{-1}	d (cm)	Gy h^{-1}
Source A	0.75	0.373	2.25	0.091	2.30	0.087
Source B	0.75	0.373	0.75	0.373	0.90	0.304
Source C	2.25	0.091	0.75	0.373	0.90	0.304
Total dose rates		0.837		0.837		0.695

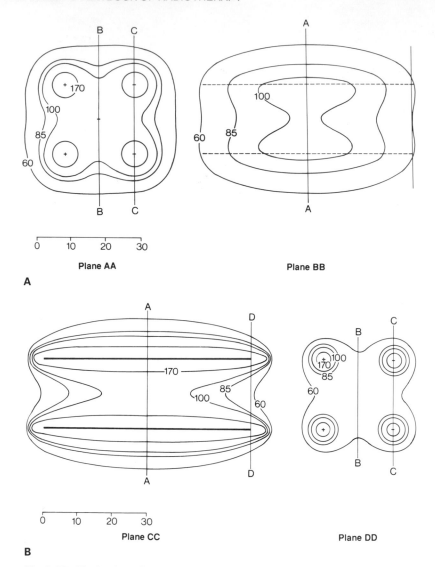

Fig. 8.12 The isodose distribution from four iridium pins: **A** midplanes and **B** peripheral planes.

prescription of 10 Gy per 24 h (0.417 Gy h⁻¹), requires a linear activity of the sources of 8.8 × 0.417/0.68 = 5.4 MBq mm⁻¹. In the figure, the 170% isodose curves are shown enclosing each source and indicate the volume of tissue irradiated to twice the prescribed dose.

The absence of 'inactive ends' simplifies reading the radiographs. Where the wires are not straight, the computer will accept their sub-division into several shorter (approximately straight) lengths.

SEEDS

Several applications have been suggested for the use of seeds containing the isotope iodine-125. Iodine-125 has two primary photon energies of 27 and 36 keV, considerably lower than any other brachytherapy source, and within the photoelectric absorption dominated region in soft tissue. It is the daughter product of xenon-125 ($T_{1/2}$ = 18 h) which is produced by neutron bombardment of xenon-124. Iodine-125 decays by electron capture to tellurium-125 with a half-life of 60 days. Two designs of seed are available, one contains two spherical resin beads impregnated with iodine-125 separated by a gold sphere, each of 0.6 mm diameter, within a titanium tube crimped and welded at each end. The second (Fig. 8.13) has the iodine-125

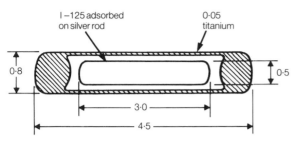

Fig. 8.13 Iodine-125 seeds. (Courtesy of Amersham International plc.)

adsorbed on a silver rod encapsulated in 0.05 mm titanium. In both cases, the overall length is 4.5 mm. The gold sphere and the silver rod provide an X-ray marker to locate the seed in radiography. The low photon energy makes the assay of the seeds difficult, the emission anisotropic and the dose deposition local. Iodine-125 seeds have been used both for permanent implant (e.g. in the pituitary) and for surface applicators (e.g. to treat the cornea). The low energy photons are readily attenuated and only thin lead shielding (0.10 to 0.35 mm lead equivalent) will be required to protect staff from the stray radiation emanating from the patient.

TREATMENT OF THE CERVIX

Perhaps the most common use of sealed sources has been in the treatment of cancer of the cervix and for many decades the technique has involved inserting preloaded sources into the uterine canal and vagina in theatre. More recently remote afterloading techniques have been widely adopted; these will be discussed in the next section. Radium tubes were used originally but these were replaced with caesium tubes in the late 1960s. The tubes were loaded into applicators designed to fit the uterine canal and the lateral fornices of the vagina—with a limited range of sizes of each. Three lengths of uterine applicator were used, incorporating one, two or three tubes in tandem, the uppermost source being of higher activity. Two vaginal applicators were used, again in three sizes with one tube in each. The Manchester 'ovoids' were designed so that the dose rate was uniform over the whole surface—the ovoid was therefore circular with the tube at the centre and approximately elliptical in the orthogonal plane. The vagina was slightly distended by placing a 'spacer' or 'washer' between the ovoids and the vagina packed to push the ovoids away from the rectum and to hold them in situ (Fig. 8.14A). The Sheffield kidney-shaped vaginal applicator contains two caesium tubes, but being

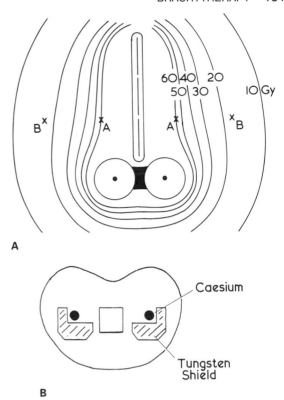

Fig. 8.14 **A** The source array and dose distribution for the treatment of the cervix. **B** The Sheffield vaginal applicator.

firmly supported from a perineal bar the vagina does not require packing and the rectal dose is reduced by the two built-in tungsten shields (Fig. 8.14B).

Despite the possible variations, the basic shape of the dose distribution remains essentially pear-shaped (Fig. 8.14) and the duration of the insertion is based on the dose rate to two defined points, namely point A and point B. These are not anatomical landmarks. Point A is simply a reference point defined as 2 cm lateral to the uterine canal and at a level 2 cm above its external os or above the level of the lateral vaginal fornices. Being so close to the sources, the dose gradient at point A approaches 10% per mm. Point B is taken at the same level but on the pelvic wall—taken to be 5 cm lateral to the midline. The dose gradient at point B is much lower. If the uterus is not midline then the distance between points A and B will not be 3 cm. However the dose rates at these two points may be tabulated for a range of *standard insertions* and used as an alternative to calculating each individual case. Where individual calculations of dose rate are required, then it is necessary to determine the dose rate each tube contributes to each point. In most cases the inverse square law

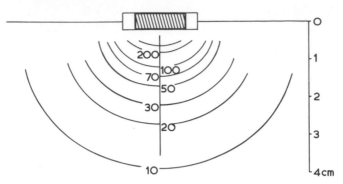

Fig. 8.15 The isodose distribution from an intracavitary tube.

approximation may be applied for point B as its distance from each individual tube is large with respect to the active length. For point A, however, it is necessary to determine the precise position of the point in relation to each tube and its dose rate contribution using isodose charts (e.g. Fig. 8.15) or a mathematical approach such as the *Sievert integral* or *Young and Batho tables* (see more advanced texts). For a more complete and accurate estimation of the dose distribution, the calculation is most conveniently done on a computer, using the accurate localisation films from the treatment simulator to provide the patient input data.

Although the quotation of the dose at points A and B has sufficed for several decades, other dose points have been regularly calculated to estimate the dose to other organs at risk. These have included the bladder and the rectum in particular and the sigmoid colon and ureters. The estimations have often been based on direct measurements using special rectal probe dosimeters, but clearly the results of such measurements are very dependent on the position of the probe and the relative anatomy at the time of measurement; and in the steep dose gradients surrounding intracavitary sources the errors may be gross. More recently specific recommendations have been laid down on how these points should be defined on lateral and AP radiographs so that the computer can calculate the dose to each organ at risk.

In addition to the quotation of the dose at each of those organs, it is recommended that the treatment specification should include the *total reference air kerma*, i.e. the summation of the products of the air kerma rate (at 1 m) and the total insertion time for each source. Typically this will be in the range 40–60 mGy. (The reader will note that the concept of the total reference air kerma is very reminiscent of the concept of milligram-hours used in the days of radium.) And finally the length of the three principal axes of the

pear-shaped 60 Gy isodose surface is to be recorded, the principal axes being along the intrauterine source and orthogonal to it at the widest point of the surface. In calculating the 60 Gy isodose the subsequent external beam therapy (if any) should be taken into account. This precise specification is not intended to replace the locally determined treatment schedules, but primarily to justify multicentre intercomparisons.

Remote afterloading systems

The manual insertion of preloaded sources into the cervix is the one medical application which gives rise to the highest radiation exposure to staff—in the operating theatre, in the transfer to the ward and to all those attending the patient in the ward during the subsequent treatment time of some 48 hours. While non-essential procedures (e.g. mopping the floor) can be deferred until the sources have been removed, and essential procedures performed from behind lead bedside shields (Plate 5) the exposure to staff is considered unacceptable and contrary to the ALARA principle (Ch. 12). The preferred alternative is to use a remote afterloading system.

Remote afterloading systems have three essential advantages over the manual insertion of preloaded sources:

1. The elimination of exposure in transporting the patient and minimising the exposure to theatre and ward staff.
2. Maximising the time available to improve the geometrical arrangement of the source catheters.
3. The opportunity to increase the activity used and thereby reduce the treatment time.

The technique, then, is to introduce catheters into the uterine canal and the vaginal vault using appropriate applicators. The catheters may be rigid or bendable.

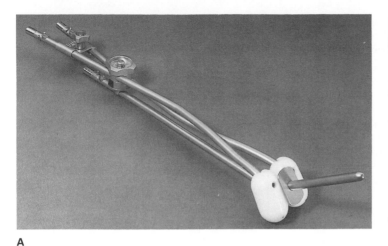
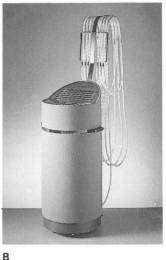

Fig. 8.16 **A** Vaginal and uterine catheters used with the remote afterloading equipment shown in **B**. (Courtesy of Nucletron Trading Co., Chester.)

The degree of flexibility that is acceptable depends on the system to be used. The catheters are then locked into place. If appropriate at this stage, very low activity sources may be temporarily inserted into the catheters to allow a measurement of the rectal dose rate to be made; the measured value will then be increased by the ratio of the source strengths to give the true value.

Again, if appropriate, the patient may be sent to the treatment simulator or to the diagnostic X-ray department for localisation films to be taken. A treatment planning programme will be used to plan the treatment according to the required prescription. For treatment using low or medium dose rate regimes, the patient is returned to the specially equipped single-bedded side ward before the catheters are connected through flexible tubes to the remote afterloading machine (Fig. 8.16). Only after all the staff have left the room will the prepared source trains be transferred from the machine to the patient and the treatment started. As with external beam therapy, the treatment may be interrupted at any time, i.e. the sources may be remotely transferred from the patient to the safe within the machine whenever the patient needs the staff or visitors to enter the room. The treatment can only be resumed from the control outside the room after they have left.

With the preloaded source technique, the range of available sources is very limited, but with remote afterloading systems, the variety is very much greater and in many cases can be tailored to the exact requirements of the patient. The treatment planning programme will therefore take these requirements into account and specify the source array and treatment time for each catheter. The sources may be beads or spheres, usually of caesium-137 for low dose rate systems or cobalt-60 for high dose rate systems. In low dose rate systems the irradiation time is usually 15 to 50 hours, depending on source activity (Table 8.5). The high dose rate systems will reduce the time to less than 1 hour, and will be accommodated in or adjacent to the operating theatre in an area not dissimilar to a gamma ray beam therapy room.

Alternatively a single source pellet (of, say, 400 GBq iridium-192) may be programmed to 'dwell' at different points in turn down the length of each catheter, and by adjusting the dwell time at each point almost any conceivable dose distribution can be achieved. The dwell times should be kept short and the programmed cycle repeated many times to average out the rate at which the dose is delivered to the adjacent tissues. This equipment may be used to simulate a low/medium dose rate treatment by repeating the programmed cycle but with a prescribed time interval between each cycle.

Remote afterloading equipment is regarded as a

Table 8.5 Dose rates in brachytherapy

Low dose rate	0.4–2.0 Gy h⁻¹	2 fractions
Medium dose rate	2.0–12 Gy h⁻¹	2 fractions
High dose rate	12–60 Gy h⁻¹	>6 fractions

Note. On the experience gained at low dose rates, the total prescribed dose may need to be modified once the dose rate exceeds about 1 Gy h⁻¹. The number of fractions refers to the brachytherapy component only of the treatment of the cervix.

gamma ray beam unit for radiation protection purposes, and requires all the associated facilities: independent gamma alarm, regular 'wipe' tests, door interlocks and warning lights, patient intercom and viewing systems, etc. An infrared CCTV may be preferred where treatments may continue through the night. The unit itself will contain a large single source or a number of radioactive sources and will therefore incorporate a secure protected safe with leakage radiation levels below the required limits. The wipe tests are usually effected by monitoring the catheters on a regular basis, and where these are disposable they should be checked immediately prior to disposal. A more detailed wipe test should be carried out on each source during inspection, but the technique will be very dependent on the remote afterloading system in use and the guidance in the manufacturer's instructions should be followed. A strict quality assurance protocol must be followed whenever the sources are replaced to ensure the integrity of each source and its activity. (Note. Where iridium-192 sources are used, they will need replacing every 3 months.) Similarly where the source trains are made up to meet the individual requirements of each patient, some checks should be carried out to confirm that the total activity and its distribution are correct before the treatment is commenced. Autoradiographs of each source train superimposed upon a scaled image of the catheter is one simple means of confirming the source array.

These systems are not confined to the treatment of the cervix. They have been used to treat the oesophagus and, where extra fine sources and catheters are available, they can be used for interstitial therapy (p. 149).

Manual afterloading systems

Where remote afterloading equipment is not available manual afterloading may be used. The same procedure is followed but laboratory-prepared source trains (Fig. 8.17) are loaded into the catheters manually, using appropriate forceps, etc., on arrival in the ward. It is not practical however to unload and reload the source trains for each interruption for essential nursing and therefore the same ward procedures have to be followed as for preloaded sources. The advantage lies in the improved geometry and reduced exposure to theatre staff. (The manual afterloading of interstitial iridium was discussed on page 148.)

OPHTHALMIC APPLICATORS

Strontium-90 ($T_{1/2}$ = 28 years) has been used for oph-

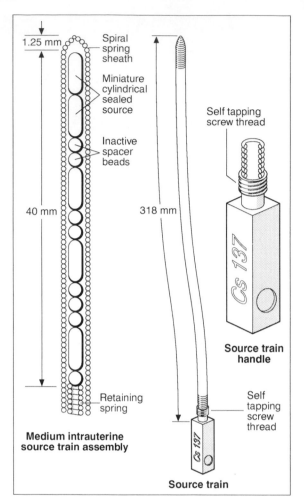

Fig. 8.17 Source trains for manual afterloading. (Courtesy of Amersham International plc.)

thalmic applicators. The strontium-90 compound is incorporated in a rolled silver foil bonded into the silver applicator and formed so that it presents an active concave surface of 15 mm radius to the cornea, with a surface filtration of 0.1 mm silver. Strontium is only useful when in (secular radioactive) equilibrium with its daughter product, namely yttrium-90 ($T_{1/2}$ = 2.7 days). The 0.1 mm Ag filter is designed to absorb the low energy beta particles from the strontium decay (0.54 MeV max) while transmitting the higher energy beta particles from the yttrium-90 (2.27 MeV max). The back of the applicator is finished with a much thicker (0.9 mm) layer of silver to reduce the transmitted dose rate to a safe level.

The measurement of the beta dose rate is complex and involves the comparison of the dose rate of the ophthalmic applicator and that of a plane strontium-90

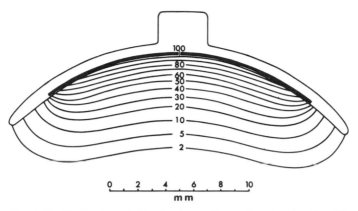

Fig. 8.18 The isodose distribution for an 18 mm diameter strontium-90 ophthalmic applicator. (Courtesy of Amersham International plc.)

plaque which has been measured using a special ionisation chamber known as an *extrapolation* chamber. This enables the dose rate at a surface to be extrapolated from a series of readings of the ionisation at different distances from the surface. A variety of plaques are available. The activity may be circular and central to treat the whole of the cornea (Fig. 8.18), eccentric to treat only a segment or annular to treat the periphery. Each is designed to give a useful dose rate of approximately 1 Gy min^{-1} at the surface, reducing to 50% at 2 mm, with 7% at 5 mm.

Ruthenium-106 (T$_{1/2}$ = 369 days) is a fission product of uranium and decays with a low energy beta emission to rhodium-106 (T$_{1/2}$ = 30 s) which has a higher energy beta emission than strontium-90, namely 3.54 MeV max. The ruthenium applicator is made of silver with a window thickness of 0.1 mm Ag and a thicker protective layer of 0.9 mm Ag on the back. The spherical radius of the window is 12 mm. The applicator is designed for suturing to the sclera for 7–10 days. The useful dose rate is typically 0.1 Gy min^{-1} at the surface, giving approximately 50% at 2.7 mm and 22% at 5 mm.

Treatments of retinoblastoma have been effected using cobalt-60 ophthalmic applicators of similar construction. Their longer half-life was an advantage, but the high energy gamma radiation gave higher doses to other vital structures, e.g. the lens, macula and optic nerve, than anticipated with the ruthenium beta particle radiations. The cobalt-60 applicators had a useful dose rate of typically 0.06 Gy min^{-1}, 50% at 2 mm and 17% at 5 mm deep.

The theatre procedures should be rehearsed using non-active applicators to ensure the radiation dose to the operator is minimal when the active applicator is employed. In fact, if an accurate 'dummy' is available, the sutures can be positioned using the dummy, making the attachment of the active applicator a very swift and safe procedure. A 15 mm acrylic visor is recommended to protect the eyes of the operator when using the ruthenium applicators. All ophthalmic applicators should be handled using rubber-tipped forceps to protect the very thin active 'window' from damage.

RADIATION PROTECTION IN BRACHYTHERAPY

Design of brachytherapy rooms

Brachytherapy sources will be accommodated in secure protected safes and used in specially prepared rooms. In many respects, a laboratory used for the storage and preparation of brachytherapy sources and the wards for brachytherapy patients require many of the same facilities as those described in Chapter 3 for beam therapy equipment, and as described in Chapter 9 for unsealed sources, including the radiation trefoil and controlled area sign. Where low usage is anticipated, it may be agreed to make the room a temporary controlled area, from the time of the arrival of the sources until the sources are removed from the room. There is no 'useful beam' or primary beam of radiation and it must be assumed that the ceiling, floor and walls will be irradiated isotropically by the maximum possible exposed activity, ignoring attenuation within the patient.

The calculation of the protective barriers is based on the air kerma rate for the isotope in question (Table 8.1). For example, a remote afterloading unit has the capacity for 48 caesium sources, each of 1.6 GBq activity. Assuming the sources will be at the centre of a room 3 m square, typical of a single-bedded room, and the nearest occupied area outside the room is 2 m from the sources, then:

$$\text{Air kerma rate at } 2\text{ m distance} = \frac{48 \times 1.6 \times 0.078}{4} \text{ mGy h}^{-1}$$

If the dose limit applicable to the adjacent area is 1 mSv y^{-1} (1 mGy y^{-1}) and the occupancy is unlikely to exceed 5 days per week and 8 hours per day then the annual total air kerma will be

$$\frac{48 \times 1.6 \times 0.078 \times 8 \times 5 \times 52}{4} \approx 3000 \text{ mGy}$$

thus the attenuation required in the wall will be

$$1 \text{ mGy}/3000 \text{ mGy} = 10^{-3}/3 = 3.3 \times 10^{-4}$$

or approximately 3.5 TVL. This requires 580 mm concrete based on the TVL for caesium being 165 mm (Table 12.4).

The other facilities for an afterloading suite will include a maze entrance with an interlocked barrier, a means of observing the patient, an intercom and an independently powered gamma alarm as for a gamma ray beam unit. Facilities will also be required—and readily available—for measuring and checking the make-up of source trains and for monitoring the patient and the empty catheters for radioactive contamination on completion of each treatment.

Storage

Normally all brachytherapy procedures will be carried out in specially designed accommodation, and where facilities other than remote afterloading are required, then one room should be set aside solely for the purpose of storing and processing the sources. The central safe for the storage of these sources will be designed so that sources may be divided into individually protected drawers, each drawer being fitted to accommodate a specific type and number of sources in an orderly fashion (Fig. 8.19). It should be possible to check the number and type of source in each drawer at a glance. Wherever radium is held in stock, the store should be ventilated to the open air by a fan operated both before and during the transfer of sources to and from the safe. Every transfer must be accompanied by an entry in the record book and the signature of a responsible individual. The safe should be kept locked whenever it is not being used. Both the room and the safe should be marked with the black and yellow warning trefoil to indicate the presence (or potential presence) of ionising radiations. The room should not be used for any other purpose, and will be designated a 'Controlled Area—Gamma Rays'.

Handling

The principal hazard of small sealed sources is that of their beta or gamma radiation and from the fact that gamma rays have considerable penetrating power. There is not the additional hazard of contamination as exists with unsealed sources unless the sealed source is damaged. (Iridium is technically an unsealed source in that fragments of active material may be left behind on the cutting jig, etc.) The sources must always be handled using forceps—for threading needles, implanting sources into patients and then cleaning and preparing them for the next patient. In some larger departments some of these operations will be done using slave manipulators (Fig. 8.20).

In general, there are three methods of reducing the radiation hazard. The first is to reduce the *time* spent in manipulation, the second is to increase the *distance* between the source and the operator and the third is

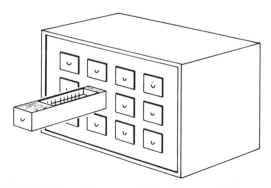

Fig. 8.19 The multidrawer protected storage safe for sealed sources.

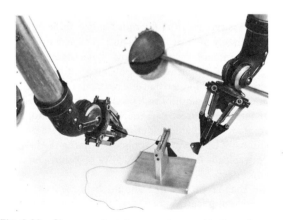

Fig. 8.20 Slave manipulators may be used to thread interstitial needles. Note the use of a needle threader in the fingers on the right.

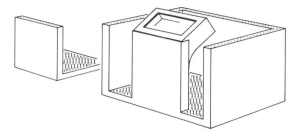

Fig. 8.21 Protected lead benches for the small sealed source laboratory.

to use *protective barriers* or screens. To some extent these three measures work against each other. For example, the time spent manipulating the source may be increased by either increasing the distance or by the use of protective screens. Invariably a compromise has to be reached.

A simple lead bench is shown in Figure 8.21; it consists of two pieces of lead approximately 35 × 35 × 5 cm³ firmly secured together. Its surfaces may be finished with a plastic laminate. The lead bench can rest on a laboratory bench so that the operator can sit or stand behind it with only the head and arms exposed to the sources being manipulated on the horizontal section. Such a simple bench is adequate for manipulating small activities. The alternative is to use a specially constructed bench where the protective material is built up all round and incorporates a protected observation window. Such a system is better where high activities are being handled or where the manipulation may take a long time. A selection of long-handled forceps should always be available.

Care must be taken in the detailed manipulation of sealed sources to avoid excessive irradiation to the fingers. Under no circumstances should the operator pick up the sources in the fingers. Where the manipulation requires skill, the procedure should be practised using inactive dummy sources made to the same

dimensions. The threading of needles prior to their use in theatre is a good example of this, in that considerable exposure could be accumulated if the task were not practised following the correct procedure. A simple device (Fig. 8.22) can be made to reduce the hazard involved and to hold the needles securely during the procedure. The lead block has a series of holes bored vertically to hold the needles so that only the eye of each needle protrudes through the top of the block. The horizontal pin is inserted into the hole appropriate to the length of the needle. Attached to the bottom of the block is a notched rubber sheet to hold the threads and to prevent them getting tangled. The use of a needle threader is to be recommended (one is shown in the tongs of the slave manipulator in Figure 8.20). Once threaded, the thread is knotted 5 to 10 mm from the needle's eye so that the clinician can still get hold of the needle with the needle forceps without damaging the thread and to enable the thread to be easily cut away prior to the cleaning of the needle after use.

Sterilisation

Sterilisation of sealed sources may be achieved by a variety of means: ethylene oxide gas sterilisation, immersion in cold sterilising liquid, boiling in water, etc. In any case, care must be taken to reduce the risk of damage to the source or corrosion of the surface. Where heat is used (as in boiling) care must be taken to ensure that in the event of failure (e.g. boiling dry) the temperature cannot rise above 180°C. (Radium sources present a greater risk than the radium substitutes.) Sources should be examined for any defects before any sterilising procedure is undertaken and any source thought to be defective should be taken out of use until it has been thoroughly examined and tested. Sources used for remote afterloading do not require sterilising because they do not come into contact with the patient— the catheters used can be sterilised in the usual way.

Nursing

It has already been indicated that a patient undergoing treatment with sealed sources will have them in situ for 2–7 days. Single ward accommodation is essential and the door should carry a radiation trefoil warning sign with the words 'Controlled Area—Gamma Rays' (Plate 4). Unless remote afterloading equipment is being used, mobile lead bed shields (Plate 5) should be placed by the bed so that the staff are protected whilst carrying out the essential nursing procedures, non-essential procedures being postponed until after

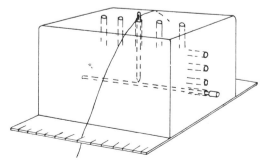

Fig. 8.22 A lead block for supporting needles whilst threading.

the removal of the sources. Staff should not remain unnecessarily in the vicinity of the patient. The Radiation Protection Supervisor (RPS) will assess the hazard presented by each patient with sources in situ and may restrict the time spent by the staff nursing the patient. Routine procedures should be shared by using a rota system in order to minimise the exposure to individual members of staff. The RPS will also restrict the patient's visitors.

The basic principles of speed and distance and the use of protective barriers must be followed during the actual insertion of the sources in theatre and during their removal. The use of protective barriers in the recovery area should not be overlooked. (Where remote afterloading equipment is being used, the sources can be temporarily removed to allow essential nursing and other procedures to be carried out in a radiation-free environment. The warning signs will still be required, but not the lead screens.)

Cleaning

Cleaning can contribute significantly to the exposure of the fingers unless some automatic devices are used and a rigid procedure followed. For example, the immersion of the sources in hydrogen peroxide solution or normal saline solution immediately after their removal from the patient will ensure that any blood adhering to the sources does not harden and become caked to the surface. The use of a low power ultrasonic cleaning bath (suitably surrounded with lead) reduces the handling of the sources to a minimum. The replacement of Perspex applicators before they become roughened or cracked will reduce the time required to clean them. Abrasive substances should never be used for cleaning.

Movement

Movement of sources both within the hospital premises and outside must be fully documented so that, in the event of fire or the suspected loss of a source, the exact location of each source can be readily identified. Movements outside the hospital complex should be kept to a minimum and in any case conform to the current regulations or codes of practice relating to the mode of transport to be used and outlined in Chapter 9. Regular movements within the hospital should follow specified routes which should be the shortest or the easiest. The design of new departments should be drawn up with this in mind; for example, if the main store and laboratory are adjacent to the theatre to be used, the sources can be transferred via a pass-through safe in the dividing

wall. Other movements of the sources should be in long-handled containers specially designed for the purpose, that is providing adequate protection, appropriate labelling and minimising the risk of loss or damage. Patients with sealed sources in situ should not be allowed to leave their ward without permission and that should only be granted if there is good reason and the radiation safety of others can be guaranteed.

The use of permanently installed gamma alarms at strategic points along the corridors and at doorways to detect the passage of any source is to be recommended. They may also be usefully situated at sluices. Such installations need to be checked regularly.

Records

It is normal practice to appoint a custodian to take the overall responsibility for the safety of sealed sources in the hospital. It will be his or her responsibility to ensure adequate records are kept. These should include:

1. A register of stock of all sealed sources having a half-life greater than a few days (which means, in practice, the only isotope likely to be excluded is gold-198). This register will contain the detailed specification of each individual source, its identification marks, its serial number, both the certificated and the locally measured activity and the reports of leakage tests and repairs. In addition the record will contain the date and mode of disposal of the source.

2. A record of all sealed sources issued from and returned to the main store and the signature of the responsible person making the transfer. This record may be accompanied by some visual display system to indicate what is in the store and available for issue.

3. A record of the administration of radioactive sources and of the removal of temporary implants.

4. An annual audit of the total stock must be made by an independent observer.

Leakage (wipe) tests

All sealed sources should be checked for free activity at least annually and whenever there is any suspicion of damage to the source. Any source is capable of being damaged, but needles are the most vulnerable as they may be bent by mishandling, by being dropped or by being pushed against a bone during insertion into the patient. They may be easily checked for straightness by rolling them on a hard flat surface—a piece of plate glass is ideal.

The leakage (wipe) test is readily carried out by passing the source—using forceps—through a foam pad moistened with ethanol. The activity on the pad should then be measured in a calibrated well counter. A bubble test may be performed by immersing the source in water and reducing the pressure to 100 mmHg (13 kPa)—no bubble must be observed. A third alternative is to immerse the source in warm (50°C) water for 4 hours and then measure the activity of the water.

If any test shows a free activity greater than 200 Bq the source must be regarded as leaking and steps taken to get it examined and repaired accordingly. Any source suspected to be leaking must be sealed in an airtight (preferably glass) container pending its repair or disposal, by a competent authority.

Suspected loss

Every effort must be taken to prevent the loss of sealed sources; although the records keep a check on the movement of sources, it is still possible for sources to get mislaid in transit or lost from a patient. In the event of a source being suspected lost, a routine such as the following should be adhered to closely. Notices outlining the procedure should be posted in all areas where sealed sources are routinely used.

1. All avenues by which the source may have been removed from its last known vicinity must be closed immediately. There should be no flushing of toilets or sluices, no removal of dirty dressings, laundry or rubbish of any sort, no sweeping of floors, no movement of patients, staff or perhaps even visitors. No further material should be placed in the hospital incinerator.

2. The persons responsible for the radiation safety in the department or ward and in the hospital as a whole must be notified as soon as possible.

3. A search for the source must be initiated as soon as possible, bearing in mind that other sources known to be in the vicinity will also be detected by the monitor used in the search. If at any stage the search suggests the lost source is damaged, then the further precautionary measures relating to unsealed sources (p. 175) should be observed.

4. If the initial search is unsuccessful, consideration must be given to calling in assistance from outside.

Discharge of the patient

A patient undergoing treatment with long-lived sealed sources must not be discharged until all the sources have been removed. In the interests of safety—of other people and of the sources—a patient determined to discharge him- or herself must be detained long enough to recover the sources. Where the isotope is of shorter half-life and not removable (e.g. gold grains), then the patient must be detained so long as the total implanted activity exceeds the limits laid down. The limit for discharge of the patient is dependent on the isotope, its form, the mode of transport and the duration of the journey. For gold grains and a journey not exceeding 1 hour by private transport the limit is 2 GBq, or by public transport (including ambulances and taxis) 1 GBq. The decision to discharge such a patient should also take into account the home circumstances to which the patient is returning, particularly if there are young children or pregnant women in the home. The patient must be given written instructions about any necessary restrictions to be observed, e.g. about nursing young children, returning to work, etc., and the date from which these restrictions can be relaxed.

Death of the patient

It is unlikely that the radiation sources contributed to the death of the patient, and all sealed sources of a half-life more than a few days must be removed immediately. If this is not possible (e.g. in the case of a permanent implant), then the Radiation Protection Adviser must be called upon to advise on the precautions to be taken in recovering the sources at post mortem and on the disposal of the body.

The above principles of safe operation are based on the recommendations laid down but the student is referred to the Regulations themselves and to Chapter 12 for a fuller account of the requirements.

Disposal of sources

With the increasing use of short-lived radium substitutes, the disposal of 'spent' sources has to be arranged, at least from time to time. Long-lived isotopes (e.g. caesium) with half-lives of several years will need to be sent to an approved organisation for disposal. If the sources are being replaced, the supplier may be willing to take the spent sources for disposal. The alternative is to employ the services of a specialist disposal company. Under no circumstances must the sources be allowed into inexperienced hands, either deliberately or accidentally. Where the isotopes have half-lives of less than a few months, the spent sources should be stored in lead pots, either until they can be disposed of as inactive waste or until sufficient have been accumulated to justify their disposal as outlined above. Full details of each source sent for disposal must be recorded, together with the date, activity and method of disposal. These records must be kept for a specified number of years.

9. Nuclear medicine: technical aspects

ASSAY OF RADIOACTIVE MATERIALS

Radioactive materials which emit gamma rays may, if the gamma ray intensity is high enough, be detected and measured by the ionisation techniques or other methods described in Chapter 5. Occasionally, even beta emitting materials, if sufficiently active, can be detected and measured by the 'bremsstrahlung' type of X-radiation produced by the stopping of the beta particles in the containing medium. In general, however, beta particle emitters are detectable by ionisation chamber devices only if they can penetrate the thin window of the chamber and give a sufficiently high radiation intensity.

Unsealed radioactive materials are, however, generally used in amounts which are too small to make simple ionisation chamber methods very satisfactory and much more sensitive devices are available. The most common of these devices are the *Geiger counter* and the *scintillation counter*. These are very sensitive systems in which individual ionising particles or individual photons from the radioactive emitter can be detected. Each beta particle or photon gives rise to a pulse of electrical charge at the output of the detector. The recording system usually records the total number of individual pulses produced in the detector. Hence the use of the word 'counter' in this connection. A detector of this type therefore measures pulses and counts them. The number of pulses recorded per unit time is a measure of the rate at which particles or photons arrive at the detector and this is proportional to the disintegration rate of a radioactive material situated in the vicinity of the detector.

The Geiger counter

The Geiger counter (sometimes referred to as the Geiger–Müller counter after its co-inventors) is essentially a simple ionisation chamber in which the ionisation produced by a single charged particle takes place in a gas at very low pressure and under an electric field high enough to cause multiple secondary ionisation in the

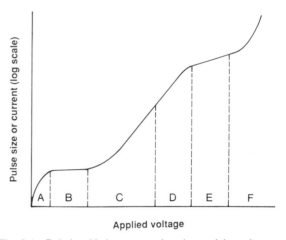

Fig. 9.1 Relationship between pulse size and the voltage applied between the anode and cathode. A, Recombination; B, ionisation chamber; C, proportional counter; D, transition range; E, Geiger counter; F, discharge.

gas. In this case, unlike the thimble chamber described in Chapter 5, the current produced is not only saturated but also undergoes an enormous amplification. Figure 9.1 shows the graphical relationship between the current or count rate through the ion chamber or Geiger counter and the voltage applied between the anode and the cathode in a constant radiation field. At low voltages, when the counter is placed in a radiation field, the pulse size increases as the voltage increases until the region of saturation is reached. At this stage the count rate is independent of applied voltage and all the ions produced in the gas are collected (ion chamber operation). As the applied voltage is increased above the saturation region the ions are given enough energy to produce further ionisation by collision and the pulse size increases as the applied voltage increases. This is known as the proportional region because the pulse size is proportional to the energy liberated by the initial interaction. If the applied voltage is increased still further, a plateau, known as the Geiger region, is reached. In this region the pulse size is

161

almost independent of applied voltage, the maximum possible amplification takes place and all ionising events produce pulses of the same magnitude. Thus a heavily ionising alpha particle or a lightly ionising beta particle produces a pulse of the same size. At voltages above the Geiger region, the intensity of the electric field is itself sufficient to ionise the gas atoms and produce continuous unwanted multiplication. The tube will then break into continuous discharge.

The Geiger counter normally consists of a cylindrical conductor, the cathode, along the axis of which is stretched a fine wire acting as the positive electrode, the anode. This electrode system is often placed in a glass container filled with a gas at a pressure of 10 cmHg (1.3 kPa) (Fig. 9.2). However, the outer electrode may itself be the container for the gas. Typically the gas is 90% argon and 10% ethanol or 99.9% neon and 0.1% chlorine. These are known as organic or halogen quenched tubes respectively. A high voltage of between 500 and 1000 volts is applied across the electrodes producing a high electric field around the central wire.

The ions originally produced by the fast charged particle are, under the influence of the high electric field, attracted towards the collecting electrodes. The positive ions move towards the cathode and the negative ions (electrons) towards the anode. Because of the high electric field and the low gas pressure, the path length between each successive collision of the electrons and the un-ionised molecules surrounding them is long enough for the electrons to acquire sufficient energy to ionise these molecules. The secondary electrons so produced are also accelerated to an energy level where they too cause ionisation. A cascade process is thus produced which gives rise to an avalanche of charged particles being swept to the collecting electrode, giving an amplification of the initial ionisation of several million and a very high charge pulse on the electrode system. Any ionising radiation, therefore, which produces ions in the sensitive region triggers off the counter. Such radiation may be, for example, a beta particle which can penetrate the walls of the counter or a fast secondary electron arising from the absorption of a gamma or X-ray photon in the gas of the tube or more likely in the walls of the tube. The avalanche process involves only the light electrons. It takes only a few microseconds for the avalanche effect to take place and for the electrons to reach the anode. The heavy positive ions, however, migrate more slowly towards the cathode, where upon arrival they may initiate a further discharge. These spurious discharges will be quenched by dissociation, rather than ionisation, of the molecules of ethanol or halogens in the gas.

Until they have been neutralised at the cathode the presence of the slowly moving positive ions disables the counter from further detection. This may take several hundred microseconds and is known as the *dead time*. The Geiger counter, therefore, will miss some particles if it is exposed to a radiation field of high intensity. Counting rates of 250 per second, for example, will miss about 5% of the received ionising particles.

Three properties of the Geiger counter are important for its use as a sensitive detector for radiations from radioactive material or X-rays.

1. The pulse size is dependent only on the number of ions initiating the discharge. It cannot therefore be used to distinguish, say, an alpha particle from a beta particle, or between photons of different energy. It is in fact a 'trigger' device.

2. The detection efficiency for beta particles can be very high, but for X or gamma rays is low. The response of the counter to X or gamma rays depends mainly on the interaction of the photons in the walls of the detector and is therefore dependent on the atomic number of the wall material and the energy of the photon. In some Geiger tubes a cathode of very high atomic number, lead for example, is introduced deliberately to enhance the sensitivity for high energy gamma rays. Even so, the efficiency of Geiger counters to gamma rays is only 1–2%. The Geiger counter therefore is unsuitable for accurate measurement of X- or gamma rays but very suitable for detecting and estimating low intensities of these radiations.

3. When the voltage applied to a Geiger tube is too low the cascade process does not work and if it is too high

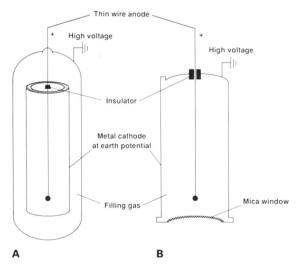

Fig. 9.2 Schematic diagram of two types of Geiger counter: **A** gamma counter; **B** end window beta counter.

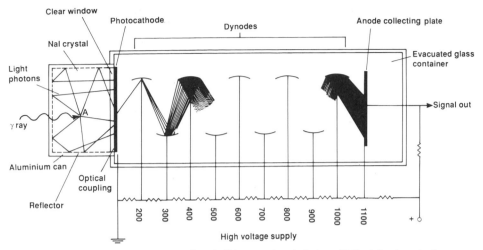

Fig. 9.3 A scintillation counter — sodium iodide crystal and photomultiplier tube (see text).

a continuous discharge is set up which damages the electrodes. However, over an intermediate range, the plateau, the counting rate is nearly independent of the voltage for a constant radiation intensity. Under good working conditions, therefore, the counter is relatively insensitive to fluctuations in the voltage supply. It thus becomes a simple and fairly rugged instrument of high sensitivity easily made in a portable form.

The scintillation counter

The scintillation detector makes use of the light flashes produced in a suitable crystal when it absorbs photons. The device consists of a crystal sealed in a container, usually made of aluminium, which is light tight except on one face. This face is optically coupled by the use of silicone grease, or in some cases a specially constructed light pipe, to the photocathode of a photomultiplier (Fig. 9.3).

The crystal material most commonly used is sodium iodide activated by the addition of a small amount, 0.1–0.5%, of the element thallium. The addition of the thallium greatly increases the light output. When a photon is absorbed in the crystal by means of either the photoelectric or Compton process its energy is transferred to an electron, point A in Figure 9.3. As the secondary electron moves around the crystal it excites the atoms and electrons of the crystal. This produces many photons of light which emerge in all directions and are reflected back towards the photomultiplier by the diffuse reflector, titanium dioxide or magnesium oxide, which lines the container (dashed lines Fig. 9.3).

The *photomultiplier* (PM) tube converts the light photons from the crystal into an electrical pulse. The tube consists of a photocathode, a series of dynodes and an anode all sealed in an evacuated glass envelope (Fig. 9.3). When light strikes the photoemissive surface of the photocathode, low energy photoelectrons are ejected, about one electron for every eight light photons. A voltage of approximately +200 volts is applied between the photocathode and the first dynode, and then 100 volts between the first and the second dynodes, between the second and third dynodes and so on along the dynode chain. Each electron leaving the photocathode is focused and accelerated towards the first dynode with sufficient energy to release additional electrons, typically about four. These four secondary electrons are in turn accelerated towards the second dynode where each one releases four more electrons. This acceleration and multiplication process takes place along the length of the photomultiplier tube. For a 10-dynode tube releasing four electrons for each incident electron then the *electron gain* or *multiplication* is 4^{10}. That is, for each electron released by the photocathode there will be over one million electrons arriving at the anode, producing a pulse of electricity of a few microvolts. The average number of electrons released at the dynodes depends on the accelerating voltage applied, and on the material coating the dynode. Increasing the applied voltage increases the number of electrons released and hence increases the gain of the PM tube.

The most important feature of a scintillation detector is the relationship between the energy of the incident gamma ray and the size of the electrical pulse coming from the detector. If the incident gamma ray is completely absorbed within the sodium iodide crystal then the average quantity of light produced in the crystal is proportional to the energy of the incident gamma ray.

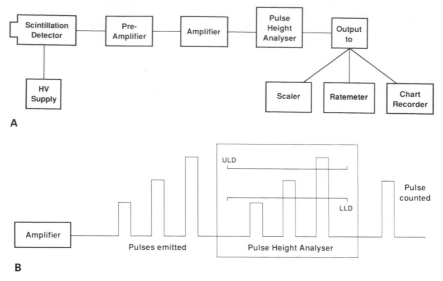

Fig. 9.4 **A** The components of a scintillation spectrometer and **B** pulse height processing.

The average number of electrons ejected from the photocathode is proportional to the amount of light reaching it, and the size of the pulse arriving at the anode is the gain factor of the PM tube times the number of electrons released at the photocathode. Thus the size of the electrical signal emerging from the detector is, on average, proportional to the energy of the gamma ray absorbed in the crystal. A 300 keV gamma ray would thus produce a pulse twice the height of that from a 150 keV gamma ray.

This proportionality property of the scintillation counter can be used to determine the spectrum of the pulses deposited in the crystal when photons are absorbed and hence the energy spectrum of the photon field itself can be explored.

The components that make up the spectrometer system are shown in Figure 9.4A. The pre-amplifier is usually attached directly to the PM tube. It serves to match the electrical impedance of the PM tube and the amplifier. This is necessary in order to avoid distortion and loss of the signal during its transit along the cable. The amplifier amplifies the signal from one of a few microvolts in size to one of a few volts. The pulse height analyser (PHA) makes it possible to select for counting only those pulses which have a predetermined size. Pulses may therefore be selected corresponding to particular values of the amount of energy transferred to the crystal in the absorption process.

Pulses from the pulse height analyser are recorded either in the form of counts, in a given time or count rate. A scaler is a digital counter which totals the number of accepted pulses for a selected length of time. A ratemeter continuously displays an estimate of counts per unit time.

The PHA consists of an electronic circuit containing a lower level energy discriminator (LLD), which only allows inclusion of pulses greater than a given size, and an upper level energy discriminator (ULD), which rejects signals greater than a predetermined size. Thus the only pulses counted are those which fall within the 'window' between the upper and lower discriminator settings. This is shown diagrammatically in Figure 9.4B. By adjusting the position of the window the scintillation spectrometer can be made to respond only to photons from one specific isotope, ignoring photons of different energy, since pulses which are initiated by photoelectric absorption in the crystal of a line spectrum of gamma rays from a particular isotope will all have a size representative of the photon energy of the radiation concerned. Similarly it is possible to reject pulses which arise from general background radiation, so that pulse selection in this way makes possible a much improved ratio of source to background count. By varying the pulse magnitude selected for counting, the energy spectrum of a gamma ray source may be explored and the assay of two or more gamma emitting isotopes in one sample becomes possible.

It will be remembered that in the case of the Geiger counter the pulse size was independent of photon energy. A further characteristic of scintillation counting is important. In a crystal any photon absorption results in a detectable event. A large mass of crystal may therefore be used to detect photons, as long as it is a single optically transparent crystal so that light pulses produced anywhere inside it can reach the photocathode of the multiplier. This makes the scintillation counter very sensitive compared to the Geiger counter in which gamma ray photon detection is possible only because of secondary electrons which arise either on the inner surface of the cathode or from the gas content of the tube.

Gamma spectrometry

Each gamma emitting radionuclide has a characteristic spectrum, and unlike beta particle emission the energies are discrete and discontinuous. A few radionuclides produce photons of only one energy while others produce photons at several energies. For example caesium-137 emits photons at a single energy of 662 keV, but iodine-131 emits photons with five principal energies: 80 keV; 284 keV; 364 keV; 638 keV and 724 keV. As shown in Figure 9.5A and B, the true emission spectrum is a series of lines. In the case of iodine-131, 80% of the gamma rays emitted have an energy of 364 keV.

When a radionuclide is counted with a scintillation spectrometer and the count rate plotted against energy, a pulse height spectrum is produced as shown in Figure 9.5C and D. Instead of a series of discrete lines we find a series of humps. This distortion is caused by a number of factors.

A monoenergetic photon gives rise to pulses of slightly different sizes because of statistical variations within the crystal and the photomultiplier. Firstly, not all the photon's energy appears as light, a variable fraction is turned into heat. Moreover there is a variable loss in light before reaching the photocathode. Secondly, the photocathode is not completely uniform in its sensitivity to light and its photoelectron production. Finally, there is variable efficiency of multiplication in succeeding dynodes. All of these effects combine to produce a distribution of pulses about the mean value.

Gamma rays interact with the crystal by both the photoelectric and Compton effects. The photoelectric effect gives rise to the bell-shaped total absorption peak centred around the photon energy. If a Compton interaction takes place the scattered photon may escape from the crystal. The recoil electron will be absorbed and the energy of the light flash will be proportional to the energy of the recoil electron, not the energy of the initiating photon. As we saw in Chapter 4 the recoil electron can have a range of energies depending on the scattering angle. In addition, multiple Compton collisions may occur and the resultant pulse height represents the total energy lost. These events give rise to the region known as the Compton continuum (Fig. 9.5C). Multiple Compton interactions may culminate with a photoelectric interaction and hence total absorption of the photon energy. The pulse from these combined

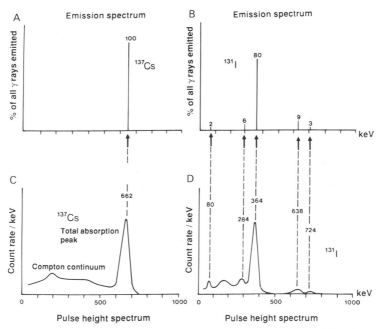

Fig. 9.5 Emission spectra and pulse height spectra for caesium-137 and [^{131}I] — sodium iodide crystal, 3″ × 3″, source in small bottle.

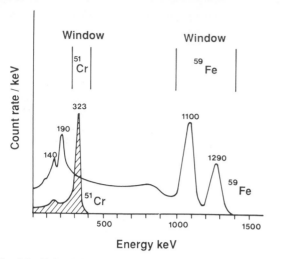

Fig. 9.6 Pulse height spectra and window positions for chromium-51 and iron-59.

scintillations will appear in the total absorption peak of the pulse height spectrum.

Other extraneous events, such as photon scattering within the patient, annihilation radiation following pair production, and characteristic X-radiation from interactions within the lead collimators, can all add to the features of the pulse height spectrum.

Multiple nuclide detection

When two radionuclides are present in the same sample or patient then careful use of the spectrometer window will enable simultaneous measurement of the two nuclides. Each nuclide will have one or more total absorption peaks as shown in Figure 9.6 where the pulse height spectra for chromium-51 and iron-59, two nuclides frequently used together in haematological studies, are plotted. Two pulse height analysers are set, one to encompass the two high energy absorption peaks from the iron-59, and the other to encompass the lower energy peak from the chromium-51. It will be seen that the iron-59 can be detected free from contamination by the chromium-51, but that the chromium-51 window includes counts, or cross-talk, from the Compton continuum of the iron-59. Corrections can be made for this cross-talk to give true chromium-51 counts.

MEASUREMENT OF ACTIVITY IN SAMPLES

The measurement of the radioactive content of fluid samples such as blood or urine is necessary in many procedures involving the use of unsealed sources for therapy, diagnosis and radioimmunoassay. The level of activity of the samples is usually very low, less than a kilobequerel, so the sensitivity of the detector needs to be high. For gamma emitters this is achieved by using a *well counter*. A well counter is a scintillation counter with a sodium iodide crystal 5 to 7.5 cm in diameter and 5 to 7.5 cm deep into which has been drilled a cylindrical hole. The crystal and photomultiplier tube are mounted inside a substantial lead shield to reduce background radiation, and a small bottle containing the sample to be assayed is placed inside the well.

Some isotopes used in clinical work are pure beta emitters. Beta particles can only penetrate the walls of the counting system with very low efficiency and in the case of low energy beta particles, such as those from carbon-14 and hydrogen-3, do not penetrate even the thinnest walls. These isotopes are assayed by *liquid scintillation counting*. The sample is dissolved in a solution containing a solvent such as toluene and a scintillating solute, usually a sensitive organic phosphor. The sample and liquid scintillating cocktail are contained in a transparent counting vial which is placed between two photomultiplier tubes. The intimate contact of beta particle emitter and scintillator results in efficient energy transfer.

DETECTION AND MEASUREMENT OF RADIOACTIVITY IN THE BODY

Diagnostic procedures and the control of therapy with radioactive agents both involve accurate measurements of radioactivity in the patient. In vivo measurements are almost always made with scintillation detectors. In the simplest form a detector of this type is used to measure the activity in some particular organ of the body. In the thyroid gland, for instance, the total radioiodine content is required for thyroid function tests (p. 184) and a simple detector system can be used. Much more complex detecting systems are required for studies of the distribution of activity in various organs of the body.

Simple collimator systems

For measurements such as that of the radioactive content of a single small organ, the sodium iodide crystal is mounted on the cathode face of a photomultiplier and surrounded by a lead shield which reduces the natural background radiation to a reasonable level and at the same time forms a 'collimator' so that the crystal may receive photons from a limited portion of the body only. Cylindrical crystals having a diameter of 2 to 5 cm with thickness of about 2.5 cm are used in these detectors. As an example, Figure 9.7 shows a diagram of an inter-

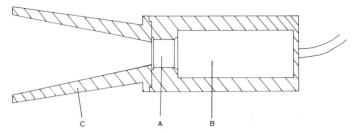

Fig. 9.7 Standard detector system for thyroid uptake measurements. A, Crystal detector; B, photomultiplier; C, collimator and shielding in lead.

nationally recognised standard collimator system for measuring the uptake of iodine-131 in the thyroid gland. The collimator will allow radiation from an area of about 13.5 cm diameter to reach the crystal at a working distance of 25 cm. The lateral shielding round the crystal reduces both the natural background and the back-ground due to circulating activity in the tissues outside the thyroid gland.

Variations of this basic design of detector mounting are made to suit the size of the organ in which the activity is to be measured, and to suit the isotope involved. The shielding thickness of a collimator for use with, for example, technetium-99m with a 140 keV gamma ray emission can be much thinner than one designed for use with iodine-131 which has its main gamma ray energy at 364 keV.

Accurate measurement of the radioactive content of an organ is difficult. Many precautions must be taken, such as a correction for attenuation in the tissues and the elimination of scattered radiation in the measurement field of the collimator. In practice, for thyroid uptake measurements a calibration procedure is adopted to check the sensitivity and the accuracy of the counting system. This is normally done by using a simple model of the neck in the form of a cylinder of Perspex filled with water and containing, in an appropriate hole, a small bottle holding a known quantity of the isotope to be measured, generally iodine-131.

Such simple collimator systems may be connected to a scaler-timer unit so that the count rate is simply deduced and this gives a figure proportional to the activity in the organ. Alternatively the system may be connected to a ratemeter and a chart recorder so that a direct display can be obtained of the time variation of activity in the organ.

Whole body counting

One further use of scintillation counting is the measurement of the total radioactive content of the body.

This is of value in the estimation of body radioactivity following the accidental intake of radioactive material, and in some clinical studies, particularly of absorption problems. In this latter case the fate of an administered isotopic label in the body can be followed without the necessity of measurements of faecal or urinary excretion of the active material.

It is of course possible to get an estimate of the total radioactive content of the body by relatively simple detecting equipment if enough activity is present to give readings much larger than the natural background. However, most whole body counters are very sensitive devices in which the patient and the detector are enclosed in a thick attenuating shield inside which a low background count is obtained. In this case very high sensitivities can be achieved, and for the common isotopes activities of the order of tens of becquerels can be detected. This means that a radioactive content of the body well below the maximum permissible body burden can be measured, and in some equipment the natural potassium-40 content of the body (and therefore the total body potassium) can be accurately estimated.

A typical arrangement of a whole body counter is illustrated in Figure 9.8. Here an array of four large crystals each 5″ (12.5 cm) diameter is arranged around the patient inside a low background enclosure. Many

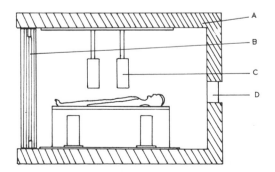

Fig. 9.8 Whole body counter. A, Steel enclosure; B, thick door; C, crystal photomultiplier detectors; D, window.

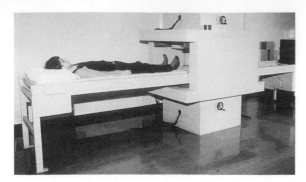

Fig. 9.9   A shadow shield whole body counter.

variations of detector and shielding arrangements of whole body counters are in use. In particular, in one arrangement the patient, lying on a couch, is passed slowly between two sets of highly shielded sensitive detectors (Fig. 9.9). This device, called a *shadow shield counter*, is cheaper than more elaborate systems but still serves some valuable clinical purposes.

Whole body counting is a very specialised use of scintillation counting and involves complicated procedures for background assessment, analysis of multiple isotope content of the body and calibration of the counter sensitivity for patients of different weights. Details are beyond the scope of this book.

Gamma cameras

A further very important use of a scintillation detector is to observe the distribution of an isotope in an organ, or in a part of the body. Such information can be obtained by use of a gamma camera. In this device a very large diameter crystal, 50 cm diameter by 1 to 1.3 cm thick, receives the gamma ray photons from the patient through a grid of thousands of holes drilled parallel to each other in a 5 cm thick lead plate. If this multihole collimator is placed near the patient a distribution of scintillations is produced in the crystal which correspond to the distribution of isotope in the field of view covered by the crystal and collimator. The scintillations in the crystal are detected by an array of between 37 and 75 photomultiplier tubes, depending upon the size and shape of the crystal. The output pulse from each multiplier corresponding to a particular single flash in the crystal depends on the position of the flash relative to the multiplier. The relative pulse heights from the photomultiplier tubes are compared by pulse arithmetic circuits to give, as an X, Y co-ordinate, the spatial location of the scintillation. By summing the outputs from all the PM tubes a Z pulse is obtained whose amplitude corresponds to the total energy deposited in the crystal by the gamma ray photon. Provided the Z

pulse is accepted by the pulse height analyser then the X and Y signals are applied to the deflection plates of a cathode ray tube (CRT); the electron beam is switched on and produces a brief flash of light on the face of the cathode ray tube. The position of this flash corresponds to the position of the scintillation in the gamma camera crystal and in turn to the position within the patient from which the detected gamma ray originated. Thus a distribution of thousands of dots is built up on the CRT screen corresponding to the activity distribution in the field of view. The eye sees these dots as forming a picture. The more dots there are present (i.e. the greater the number of gamma rays) the better the quality of the picture. The image can be reproduced on to film by photographing the CRT screen.

Figure 9.10 shows a diagram of the detector head of a gamma camera. The crystal, collimator and photomultiplier array are mounted inside a substantial lead shield of considerable weight, which is itself mounted on a stand so that the face of the collimator can be adjusted into any suitable position relative to the patient under investigation.

Performance characteristics

The performance of a gamma camera is characterised by six interrelated parameters:

— Spatial resolution
— Sensitivity
— Uniformity
— Spatial distortion and linearity
— Energy resolution
— Field size.

Spatial resolution. This is the ability to distinguish an object from its surroundings and is a measure of the

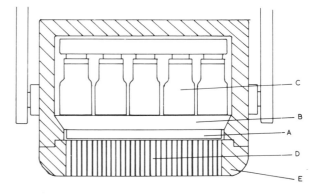

Fig. 9.10   Gamma camera head. A, Crystal detector; B, light guide; C, photomultipliers; D, parallel-hole collimator; E, lead shield.

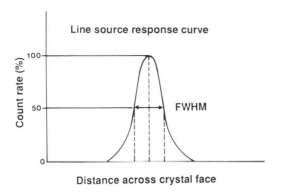

Fig. 9.11 Line source response function and the calculation of full width at half maximum (FWHM).

sharpness of the image. It is affected by: the collimator, the energy resolution, and the electronic positioning circuitry. It is often specified as the *Full Width at Half the Maximum* count rate (FWHM) of the counting profile obtained from a single line source. This is shown diagrammatically in Figure 9.11. Two types of spatial resolution are specified: the intrinsic resolution, which is the fundamental resolution of the crystal photo-multiplier electronics assembly without a collimator applied, and the system resolution, which includes the collimator. The intrinsic resolution of a modern gamma camera is about 3 mm.

Sensitivity. This term relates to the counting efficiency of the gamma camera. It is normally quoted as counts per second per megabecquerel. The thickness of the crystal, the width of the pulse height analyser window and the type of collimator in use are all factors which affect sensitivity.

Uniformity. This refers to the variations in count rate across the field of view when the detector is exposed to a uniform source of a gamma ray emitting radionuclide. Variations are caused by such factors as: deviations in the sensitivity across the crystal, variability in the responses of the photomultiplier tubes, and mechanical imperfections in the collimator.

Spatial distortion and linearity. These refer to the ability of the gamma camera to translate and accurately reproduce both the spatial and geometric relations of a radioactive distribution beneath the detector and so reproduce a linear activity source as a linear image. Factors influencing distortion include errors in the calculation of the point of interaction within the crystal of the gamma ray and the thickness of the crystal.

Energy resolution. As we saw earlier in this chapter, statistical variations in the detection of gamma rays by the crystal photomultiplier assembly result in a charac-teristic broadening of the total absorption peak of the energy spectrum. The energy resolution is expressed as the width of the absorption peak at half the maximum count rate observed at the peak. This is analogous with the FWHM concept discussed previously in connection with spatial resolution. Poor energy resolution has an adverse effect upon spatial resolution, sensitivity and uniformity.

Field size. This refers to the maximum field of view of the camera. Field sizes vary from 25 to 50 cm.

With the aid of digital microcomputer technology corrections can be made to overcome some of the non-random defects in camera performance mentioned above. These include corrections for intrinsic non-uniformity and non-linearity.

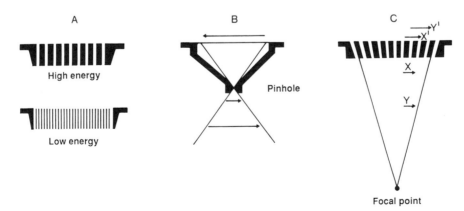

Fig. 9.12 Examples of collimators for a gamma camera. **A** Multihole parallel — high energy having thicker septa than the low energy; **B** pin-hole — objects closest to the hole are imaged with greatest magnification; **C** converging — objects X and Y are displaced and appear as different sizes on the image.

Collimators

The function of a gamma camera collimator is to project an image of the radioactive distribution beneath the camera face on to the scintillator. This is achieved by stopping gamma rays from entering the crystal by any route other than via the holes in the collimator. Three principal types of collimator are in use, parallel-hole, pin-hole and converging. These are shown schematically in Figure 9.12.

Parallel-hole collimators. These are the most commonly used and consist of a thick lead plate with several thousand small parallel-sided holes penetrating the lead perpendicular to the plane of the plate. For this type of collimator there is a 1:1 relationship between the object and its projection on to the crystal. Thus the size of the image is independent of the distance from the subject to the detector face. Similarly, provided the object is completely in the field of view, the sensitivity of the collimator or the count rate remains essentially the same irrespective of the distance in air between the subject and the collimator face. However the image resolution is best when the subject is close to the collimator face.

Various factors affect the performance of a parallel-hole collimator. These include hole diameter, hole length and septal thickness. Sensitivity and resolution are intimately linked and improvements in one almost inevitably lead to deterioration in the other, as shown in Table 9.1. For example, improving the resolution by a factor of two by increasing hole length will decrease the sensitivity by a factor of four.

A low energy collimator has thin septa. If this were to be used with high energy gamma rays the gamma rays would pass through the septal walls and impinge on the crystal from directions other than those defined by the holes, thus degrading the image. On the other hand a high energy collimator has thick septal walls and would appear to be suitable for all gamma ray energies. However, in this case one is unnecessarily sacrificing sensitivity. In practice there is a range of collimators available, as shown in Table 9.2, low medium and high

energy, high resolution-low sensitivity, medium energy-medium sensitivity, and low energy-high sensitivity.

Pin-hole collimators. The pin-hole collimator works in an analogous way to the optical pin-hole camera. It consists of a lead cone with a small hole, a few millimetres in diameter, at the tip of the cone (Fig. 9.12B). Its main use is to give an enlarged image of a small superficial organ such as the thyroid gland. For objects close to the aperture this type of collimator provides the best effective resolution, being close to the inherent resolution of the camera. However it is very insensitive and, in addition, sensitivity falls off with distance in accordance with the inverse square law. Objects close to the collimator are magnified more than objects further away and objects located off the central axis or at a different depth are imaged obliquely. These factors cause image distortion.

Converging collimators. The converging collimator is a half-way house between the parallel-hole collimator which has good sensitivity and the pin-hole collimator which has good resolution. It is a multihole collimator with the holes converging on a focal spot several centimetres in front of the collimator face (Fig. 9.12C). The resolution improves with distance from the collimator face until the focus is reached. Sensitivity also increases with distance since a larger number of photons from each point within the object can pass through the holes in the collimator. Unfortunately the image is distorted, the back of the object being magnified to a greater extent than the front and the side of the object being seen at a more oblique angle than the centre. The main use of this type of collimator is brain imaging.

Table 9.1 Factors affecting the performance of parallel-hole collimators

Parameter increases	Resolution	Sensitivity
Hole diameter	Deteriorates	Improves
Hole length	Improves	Deteriorates
Septal thickness	No change	Deteriorates
Object distance	Deteriorates	No change

Table 9.2 Examples of types of collimator and their characteristics

Type	Energy limit (keV)	Number of holes	Length (mm)	Size (mm)	Resolution at 10 cm (mm)	Absolute sensitivity (cps MBq^{-1})
Low energy – high sensitivity	160	20000	22.5	2.5	15.5	405
Low energy – general purpose	170	50000	22.5	1.5	9.5	158
Low energy – high resolution	190	55000	27.5	1.5	7.5	101
Medium energy – general purpose	300	10000	27.5	2.5	14.0	180
High energy – general purpose	400	4200	57.0	4.5	15.6	180
Pin-hole	400	1	213	3.0	4.8	45

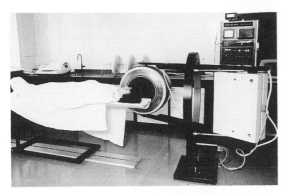

Fig. 9.13   A gamma camera capable of SPECT imaging.

Tomographic gamma cameras

There are two major types of tomography using gamma cameras, single photon emission computed tomography (SPECT) and positron emission tomography (PET). The first uses a conventional gamma camera with the detector head mounted in such a way that it can rotate around the patient. A photograph of such a system is shown in Figure 9.13.

A series of two-dimensional images, typically 64, are taken and stored on computer as the camera rotates. The data can then be manipulated to produce tomographic sections. PET scanning uses a special kind of gamma camera which is able to detect the coincidence photons from the annihilation of the positrons emitted from radionuclides such as carbon-11. The theory of emission tomography is discussed in detail elsewhere (see Bibliography) and is beyond the scope of this book.

RADIATION PROTECTION IN NUCLEAR MEDICINE

There is a great deal of legislation governing the use of radioactive materials, and the protection of persons against ionising radiations arising from their medical use. In general, in the following pages the United Kingdom regulations have been quoted. However, these are based on the recommendations of the International Commission on Radiological Protection (ICRP Publications 25, 26, and 35), the International Atomic Energy Agency (IAEA) Regulations, and the relevant Directives of the Council of the European Communities. (Regulatory documents are listed in the bibliography.)

Supply of unsealed sources

The use of radionuclides in liquid form for either therapy or diagnosis involves a number of procedures which are different from those in other hospital departments, and which arise from the radioactivity of the material used. Arrangements must be established for the regular receipt of supplies from a company manufacturing radiopharmaceuticals. For radioactive materials of rather long physical half-life, such as chromium-51 ($T_{1/2}$ 27.8 days), no great problem is encountered in dealing with the day to day diagnostic programme using supplies stored in the hospital dispensary. Other isotopes with a shorter half-life, such as thallium-201 ($T_{1/2}$ 73.1 h), must be ordered regularly so that the delivery matches a carefully designed programme of diagnostic procedures. A third group of radioisotopes consists of those in which the half-life is so short that they are generally only available by production in the hospital from relatively longer-lived generator columns (p. 29). The most common example is technetium-99m ($T_{1/2}$ 6 h) produced from a molybdenum-99 column ($T_{1/2}$ 67 h). Weekly purchase of a new generator column is necessary in this case.

Transport

A second consideration regarding supplies of radioactive materials is that they must be transported and stored under conditions such that they are secure and that the leakage radiation from the container presents no hazard either to any worker or to a member of the general public. The transport of a pure beta emitter such as phosphorus-32 is generally an easy matter, but for isotopes with penetrating gamma radiation such as sodium-24 the protection during transit is more difficult and involves large and heavy shielded containers.

The transport of radioactive materials falls into two categories: transport outside the hospital by means of road, sea and air; and transport and movement within the hospital. There are national and international regulations governing the transport of radioactive materials which take care of the leakage of ionising radiation from the intact container and also prescribe packaging methods so that, in the event of an accident, leakage of the contents, and therefore the spread of contamination, are most unlikely. The source document for all these regulations is the IAEA Regulations for the Safe Transport of Radioactive Material.

Packaging

Three types of packaging are defined by the IAEA: *excepted, type A* and *type B*. Table 9.3 lists the maximum activities of radionuclides in common hospital use which may be transported with type A packaging. It can be seen that, in general, type A packaging is adequate for hospital users of unsealed radionuclides. All packaging is designed to withstand minor accidents.

Table 9.3 The maximum activities, for various radionuclides, which may be transported with type A packaging

Radionuclide	Max. activity (TBq)
^{198}Au	0.5
^{51}Cr	30
^{57}Ga	6
^{131}I	0.5
^{99}Mo	0.5
^{24}Na	0.2
^{32}P	0.3
^{201}Tl	10
^{90}Y	0.2

Labelling

An internationally recognised design of warning label, known as white and yellow labels, specifying a transport category between I and III must be affixed to the package. The label must identify the contents of the package, the activity of the radionuclide and, by use of the category rating and the transport index, give an indication of radiation dose rate on the external surface of the package and at 1 m from it. The transport index is defined as this latter quantity measured in $mSv\ h^{-1}$ multiplied by 100. Table 9.4 lists the surface dose rate for each transport category and the transport index.

A package may contain so little radioactive material or the material may be in such a dilute form that the risk of contamination is negligible. In this case provided the surface dose rate is less than $5\ \mu Sv\ h^{-1}$ the package can be excepted from most of the packaging and labelling requirements. For example, 800 MBq of technetium-99m or 50 MBq of iodine-131 per package could be transported as excepted packages. Nevertheless the contents of the package must be described in the accompanying paper work.

Movement of radioactive sources within the hospital are not subject to the various transport regulations. However these movements are subject in the UK to the Ionising Radiation Regulations (IRR-85 Reg. 21). General principles for internal movement include:

1. The material must be securely contained in a

Table 9.4 The surface dose rate for each transport category

Category	Max. surface dose rate	Max. transport index
I (white)	$<5\ \mu Sv\ h^{-1}$	—
II (yellow)	$<500\ \mu Sv\ h^{-1}$	1.0
III (yellow)	$<2\ mSv\ h^{-1}$	10.0

double container. The outer container should be rigid and capable of leakage containment should the inner container break.
2. Both inner and outer containers must be clearly labelled with the radionuclide, its chemical form and the activity at a specified time.
3. The radioactive material must not be left unattended during transit.
4. Adequate shielding must be provided to protect the person carrying or accompanying the radionuclide.

Custody and storage

On arrival at the hospital a suitable place for the receipt of the containers must be arranged and the sources themselves must be placed when unloaded in a suitable shielded store. Small cupboards with 1–2" (2.5–5 cm) of lead wall are convenient for many of these sources. Any container holding a radionuclide should be marked with the radiation symbol.

Regulations 19 and 20 of the IRR-85 relate to accounting for and keeping of radioactive substances. Accounting procedures are essential to ensure that all radioactive sources are traceable and that losses of significant quantities are identified as quickly as possible. The records to be kept of each substance should include:

— A means of identification of the radionuclide by name and by batch
— The date of receipt
— The activity of the radionuclide at a specified time and date
— Any activity used and date and time of use
— The location of storage
— The date and manner of disposal.

These records must be kept for at least 2 years from the date of disposal. Inevitably some radionuclides will have undergone significant radioactive decay before disposal and this must be allowed for in the accounting procedure.

Design of facilities

The facilities in a nuclear medicine department are designed to minimise the hazard from (1) external radiation arising from the radioactive materials or from the patient following injection of a radiopharmaceutical, (2) surface contamination, and (3) ingestion, inhalation, or skin absorption of a radioactive material.

Shielding from gamma radiation is in general a problem very similar to that encountered in dealing with small sealed radioactive sources (Ch. 8). The gamma ray exposure rates normally met are, however, smaller than when working with sealed sources so that quite simple shielding arrangements, such as small lead bench shields, are adequate.

All surfaces should be smooth and impervious, with the main aim being to prevent retention of surface contamination in the event of a spill. Bench tops and floors are always covered with a continuous non-absorbent surface such as plastic laminate and seam welded linoleum. Walls and ceilings are covered with good quality gloss paint which can be cleaned easily. Covings should be used where the walls meet floor and ceiling and at the rear of laboratory benches.

Hand-washing facilities, with elbow or foot operated taps, must be provided in rooms where unsealed radioactive sources are handled. Drainage from sinks and wash basins should pass directly to a main sewer in order to avoid accumulation of radioactive waste and to allow rapid dilution by non-active waste.

Some radioactive materials may have to be handled in conditions under which active products may escape into the atmosphere as volatile products from the surface of a solution, as dust from dry preparations or as gaseous products. To prevent ingestion or inhalation from any of these products work of this type must be conducted in a fume cupboard. To give adequate containment of escaping products the fume cupboard requires an exhaust system which provides an air flow inwards across the whole of the open working window at a rate of at least 0.5 metres per second.

Controlled and supervised areas

Different areas within the nuclear medicine department may be classified as *controlled* or *supervised* (Ch. 12) depending upon the total activity present. Entrances to all rooms in which radioactivity is used must display appropriate warning signs bearing the international radiation warning symbol (trefoil, see Plate 4) and an indication of the classification of the area and the nature of the hazard, e.g. 'Supervised area. Unsealed Radioactive Sources'.

Examples of controlled areas might be the radiopharmacy or the room of a patient undergoing iodine-131 thyroid ablation therapy. A waiting room may be designated as a controlled area. However, schedule 6 of IRR-85 provides for an exception where the product of activity and gamma energy in the area does not exceed 150 MBq MeV. This limit will not be exceeded for any single routine diagnostic procedures, but when several patients are present the limit may well be exceeded.

Monitoring

Suitable monitoring equipment must be available to sensitively detect all radionuclides in use in the department. The calibration of such monitors should be traceable to national standards.

The IRR-85 requires that levels of ionising radiation are adequately monitored for any area where unsealed radioactive materials are in use or stored. Monitoring is an important means of ascertaining the efficacy of techniques in use and in restricting exposure.

Hands, clothing and work surfaces should be monitored at the end of each working period and the results recorded. If the monitoring shows levels of contamination greater than those given in Table 9.5 then decontamination procedures should be followed (p. 175).

Safe administration

The administration of radionuclides for diagnostic or therapeutic purposes requires great care, to ensure that

Table 9.5 Maximum permissible contamination levels

Category	Surface	Level of contamination that should not be exceeded (Bq cm^{-2})		
		Class III	Class IV	Class V
B	Surfaces in controlled areas including any equipment therein	30	300	3000
C	Surfaces of the body	3	30	300
D	Supervised and public areas, clothing, hospital bedding	3	30	300

Classification of radionuclides in common use in hospitals (for surface contamination purposes only): class III, ^{32}P, ^{111}In, ^{59}Fe, ^{90}Y, ^{131}I; class IV, ^{123}I, ^{125}I, ^{99m}Tc, ^{67}Ga, ^{201}Tl; class V, ^{51}Cr.

the patient receives the correct isotope and dose, any possible spillage is contained, and that exposure to personnel is kept to a minimum. All staff involved in this type of work must receive appropriate training (IRR-88).

Staff administering radiopharmaceuticals will be exposed to radiation during the administration and when it is inside the patient. To minimise the risk of ingestion, eating, drinking, smoking and the application of cosmetics are strictly forbidden in the presence of radioactive materials. Similarly, to prevent personal contamination, staff should wear protective clothing such as disposable gloves, a lab coat or overall buttoned up, and possibly a plastic apron, so that any spilt radioactive solution will not contact the skin. The hands should always be washed after handling radioactive materials. Examples of potential ingestion and contamination hazards to staff from diagnostic and therapeutic procedures are found in ventilation lung scanning where radioactive gases or aerosols may leak into the air and subsequently be inhaled, and in the oral administration of liquid iodine-131 where a risk of contamination exists. The availability of therapeutic doses of iodine-131 in capsule form has greatly reduced this latter risk, as well as being a simpler and quicker method of administration.

There are three principal factors which staff can use to help reduce their external radiation exposure. These are distance (inverse square law), shielding and time. Good radionuclide working practice includes the use of long-handled forceps, syringe shields, protective screens and swift yet careful working practices commensurate with the adequate and safe administration of the radionuclide.

The majority of radiopharmaceuticals are administered by intravenous injection. Equipment required for this purpose includes a shielded container in which the radiopharmaceutical can be transferred from the dispensary to the injection area, a tray over which any transfer of radioactive solutions can take place, and an impermeable shielded receptacle for discarded materials.

For sources to be dispensed or administered using a syringe, a syringe shield made of a suitable shielding material with a window in the side so that the contents are visible can be fitted over the barrel of the syringe (Fig. 9.14). The use of syringe shields must be considered in order to minimise the exposure to the fingers and hands. These shields, which are designed to absorb the majority of the beta particles, as well as to attenuate the gamma ray photons, are typically made of high atomic number metals such as tungsten, or thick cylinders of transparent Perspex. There are, however, further considerations in the use of each type. Metallic syringe shields are used for the majority of radionuclides,

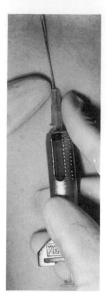

Fig. 9.14 Intravenous injection of a radioactive material using a shielded syringe.

but they are not ideal for pure beta emitters as bremsstrahlung radiation can contribute significantly to the finger and hand dose. Perspex syringe shields, which can be 7 to 15 mm in diameter, are used for this purpose.

Precautions following therapeutic administration

Special precautions are required when dealing with patients undergoing unsealed source therapy with high levels of activity. The following action should be taken:

1. The patient must be confined to his or her own room.
2. The patient must use a designated toilet en suite adjacent to the room and will have exclusive use of the bathroom facilities.
3. All body fluids including perspiration and saliva may be contaminated with radioactivity; staff must wear protective clothing when handling the patient or any articles which may be contaminated.
4. All nursing procedures should be carried out in the minimum time compatible with good nursing care.
5. Bed linen, towels and clothing must be monitored for contamination before being sent to the laundry (see maximum permissible contamination limits in Table 9.5).
6. Wherever possible utensils such as cutlery and crockery should be disposable and must be collected and retained in the room together with other contaminated material, such as disposable

Table 9.6 Maximum activity levels of unsealed therapeutic radionuclides for discharging patients from hospital

Radionuclide	<10 MBq MeV No restrictions	<50 MBq MeV No transport restrictions*	<150 MBq MeV Travel by public transport	<300 MBq MeV Travel by private transport
^{131}I	30 MBq	150 MBq	400 MBq	800 MBq
^{32}P	300 MBq	1.5 GBq	4.5 GBq	9 GBq
^{90}Y	100 MBq	500 MBq	1.5 GBq	3 GBq
^{198}Au	30 MBq	150 MBq	400 MBq	800 MBq

* Continue to avoid close contact with children and pregnant women.

handkerchiefs, until dealt with by authorised personnel.

7. Visiting by adults should be discouraged for the first 24 hours and restricted thereafter; visiting by children and pregnant women is forbidden.
8. The patient may not be discharged home until the level of activity has fallen below a certain limit (Table 9.6).
9. Following patient discharge, the room may not be reused until it has been monitored and if necessary decontaminated.

Discharge of patient

Patients who have received radionuclide therapy present a radiation hazard to persons with whom they come into contact. Table 9.6 lists the activity levels at which the patient may be discharged and any restrictions on the mode of transport used following discharge.

All patients who exceed the '50 MBq MeV' activity level at the time of discharge should be given written instructions about precautions to be taken on leaving hospital. This may take the form of a card, as shown in Figure 9.15.

Spillage and decontamination

In spite of every care and in spite of attention to technique, accidental spillage of radioactive materials does occur and a clinical unit which handles unsealed radioactive sources should have fully documented procedures and equipment for dealing with emergency

RADIONUCLIDE INSTRUCTION CARD

Name:

Address:

Hospital No:

Department:

Address:

Consultant:

It is important that you carry this card with you at all times and observe the following instructions until ....

a) Avoid journeys on public transport until ....

b) Avoid going to places of entertainment until ....

c) Do not return to work until ....

d) Avoid prolonged personal contact at home until .... and observe the verbal instructions given to you before leaving hospital.

e) other ....

Signed .... On............

Radionuclide administered:.............

Activity:..............

On:...............

If an accident occurs or you have any difficulty, please telephone:
....

Ask for: ....

Extension:.................

Fig. 9.15 Radionuclide instruction card for patients leaving hospital with significant residual activity. (The card should be of a distinctive colour, preferably yellow.)

spills. Staff should also be trained to deal with spills as required by Reg. 12 IRR-85. In the clinical situation there are various ways in which the spill of a radionuclide can occur. These include accidental spillage in dispensing or administration, and contamination resulting from urinary incontinence or the patient vomiting following the oral administration of a radioactive material. For diagnostic procedures radioactive urine presents the main contamination hazard. This is particularly so in patients having bone scans, where a high proportion of the injected radiopharmaceutical is excreted in the urine and patients are required to empty their bladder before imaging commences.

Decontamination

Two principal criteria pertain when implementing decontamination procedures. Firstly, the safety of the individual is paramount. Secondly, it is essential to contain the spill and avoid spread. In the event of a major spill, e.g. 30 MBq of iodine-131, the following action should be taken:

1. Take immediate action to contain the contamination; all persons not contaminated and not involved in the incident should leave the area.
2. Notify the radiation protection supervisor and obtain appropriate assistance.
3. Give priority to the treatment of injured persons rather than decontamination procedures.
4. Decontaminate personnel.
5. Decontaminate the room.
6. Prepare an incident report and report the incident to the radiation protection adviser.

Personnel decontamination. Any person who is contaminated with radioactive material must be decontaminated as quickly as possible. The aim is to prevent absorption through the skin, ingestion, and spread of the contamination. The following steps should be carried out:

1. Obtain contamination measuring instrument and assess the extent of contamination.
2. Remove all contaminated clothing.
3. Wash the contaminated area with soap and water; avoid the use of abrasives.
4. If the contamination is extensive and a shower is required then this should be taken after the decontamination of any localised high activity contamination.
5. Take special care when decontaminating the face to avoid spread into the eyes or mouth.
6. If the eyes or open wounds are contaminated irrigate with copious amounts of water.

7. Decontamination should continue until the activity level is less than that contained in Table 9.5; a designated commercial decontaminant such as 2% Decon-90 may be used if soap and water has failed.

Room decontamination. A 'spill kit' containing appropriate tools and equipment to deal with a radioactive spill should be available within the nuclear medicine department. This kit might include overshoes and protective clothing, plastic bags, radioactive warning tape, pens, appropriate decontamination materials, tools for handling contaminated articles, and portable monitoring equipment. To decontaminate the room the following steps should be carried out:

1. Persons not involved in the decontamination procedure should leave the area.
2. Wear the appropriate protective clothing, e.g. gloves, lab coat, overshoes.
3. Mark the edges of the area of contamination.
4. Mop up the spill with an absorbent material such as paper towels.
5. Working from the outer edge of the contaminated area towards the centre, scrub the surface with soap and water, a detergent or a decontaminant.
6. Monitor the area to check activity has been reduced to an acceptable level (Table 9.5); if radioactivity above these levels persists, cover the contaminated area and post a warning sign.
7. Remove all radioactive waste materials for appropriate disposal.

Waste disposal

Radioactive waste arises from: the excreta of patients undergoing diagnostic and therapeutic nuclear medicine procedures; the syringes, swabs, paper tissues, etc. used in the preparation and administration of the radiopharmaceutical; expired stock solutions; and the waste from decontamination following spills. Waste products therefore fall into two main categories—liquid and solid—although a third category, gaseous waste, will be encountered from fume cupboards, lung ventilation scanning, and the chimney-stack of incinerators where contaminated refuse may be burnt.

The disposal of radioactive waste from a hospital unit must be thoroughly organised and carefully controlled and documented in compliance, in the UK, with the Radioactive Substances Act 1960, not only to avoid hazard to staff and patients in the hospital, but also to avoid any hazard to the general public. The disposal of radioactive waste is subject to legislation which varies from country to country. In the UK, Her Majesty's

Inspectorate of Pollution, Department of the Environment, ensures compliance with the relevant legislation.

Liquid waste

In most cases the disposal of radioactive excreta from patients is best dealt with by discharging to the sewage treatment system. In this way, hazard to staff involved in collection and disposal is avoided. It is permitted to do this because a very high dilution of the active material quickly reduces the waste to low concentration levels in the routine effluent of a hospital. It is important, however, to ensure that there is adequate inactive effluent flow and that the toilets reserved for radioactive waste are connected directly to the main drainage system of the hospital. Similar conditions must also be applied in disposing of radioactive liquid waste from the laboratories. The waste-pipes between the ward/laboratory and the main sewer should be labelled as potentially radioactive. Some storage facilities are, however, always required for samples, sometimes excreta, needed for measurement purposes or for highly concentrated residues of radioactive stock solutions. Such storage facilities must be adequately shielded and designed to prevent risk of escape of material.

Solid waste

Solid waste from the nuclear medicine department, such as used swabs and syringes, is usually of low activity and may be collected separately in a special container. If the contaminating radionuclide is one with a short half-life, such as technetium-99m, this material can be stored for a couple of days until the isotope activity has decayed away. Dustbin disposal level waste is limited to 400 kBq in 0.1 m³ of waste material with no single item containing more than 40 kBq of isotope activity.

Solid waste may also be disposed of in the hospital incinerator where, depending upon the chemical form, the radioactivity will either be dispersed into the air, left behind in the ash or collected by the gas cleaning system. Limits are set on the level of activity which may be disposed of in this way, dependent on environmental impact.

For the disposal of somewhat higher levels of activity of long-lived radionuclides, special burial to a specified depth at a suitably controlled refuse tip may be appropriate, but once again strict activity limits are imposed.

Detailed records must be kept of the disposal of radioactive materials irrespective of which route of disposal has been used. These records should include the type of radionuclide, its activity at disposal, the route of disposal and the date of disposal.

Safety of the patient

The administration of any radioactive material to the patient has an associated risk factor. Any member of staff concerned with carrying out nuclear medicine procedures on patients has a responsibility to ensure that the techniques used are appropriate for their purpose, and that the radiation dose to the patient is no higher than is absolutely necessary to achieve this purpose and that the benefits of carrying out the test outweigh the risks. Effective dose equivalents for some common nuclear medicine procedures, together with average values for some common radiographic procedures, are given in Table 9.7. It is essential that each investigation is justified on clinical grounds and that there is no lower risk alternative.

ARSAC requirements

It is a legal requirement under the Medicines (Administration of Radioactive Substances) Regulations (1978) and IRR-88 that all administrations of radiopharmaceuticals are carried out under the direction of a medical practitioner who holds an appropriate certificate from the Administration of Radioactive Substances Advisory Committee (ARSAC). The authorisation certificate

Table 9.7 Effective dose equivalent (EDE) from some common investigations using (1) radiopharmaceuticals and (2) radiology

Radiopharmaceutical	Activity (MBq)	EDE (mSv)	Radiological examination	EDE per examination (mSv)
[^{99m}Tc] Pertechnetate	500	7	Chest	0.05
[^{99m}Tc] MAA	80	1	Abdomen	1.4
[^{99m}Tc] Phosphonate	600	5	Pelvis	1.2
[^{57}Co] Vitamin B$_{12}$	0.04	0.2	Barium meal	3.8
[^{131}I] Iodide	0.2	3	Barium enema	7.7
[^{201}Tl] Thallous ion	80	25		
[^{67}Ga] Gallium citrate	150	15		

Data extracted from ARSAC (1988) and Shrimpton et al (1986).

details: the radionuclide; its chemical form; the purpose for which authorisation is allowed; the route of administration; the maximum isotope activity; and the institution where the procedure can be undertaken.

Special conditions

Pregnant patients. The greatest care must be exercised when carrying out procedures on women of child bearing age as there is increased risk to the unborn child of mental retardation and carcinogenesis. It is essential to determine by appropriate questioning whether the woman is or may be pregnant. If the answer is yes, then the clinician requesting the investigation must balance the risks against the benefits, and the minimum activity possible must be administered, commensurate with obtaining a diagnostic result.

Lactating mothers. If a radionuclide is administered to a lactating mother then radioactivity may be secreted in the mother's milk. A breast-fed infant will receive a radiation dose from ingested radioactivity. The magnitude of this problem depends upon the radiopharmaceutical administered, but may require an interruption to, or even cessation of, breast-feeding. In addition a child may be exposed to radiation from retained activity within the mother. For an appropriate time period following administration of the radionuclide non-essential close contact with infants should be discouraged. This is generally not longer than 24 hours.

Children. There is an increased risk of carcinogenesis in children and the amounts of radioactivity administered should always be reduced compared to the normal adult dosage. The administered dose is normally reduced in proportion to the child's body weight or body surface area relative to that of the average adult.

10. Nuclear medicine: diagnostic and therapeutic procedures

INTRODUCTION

It has been shown in Chapter 2 that radioactive isotopes of practically all elements can be produced. Nuclear medicine is the science and clinical application of unsealed radiopharmaceuticals for diagnostic, therapeutic and investigative purposes. By combining a suitable radionuclide with a pharmaceutical we are able to monitor the behaviour of the pharmaceutical by measuring the distribution of the radioactivity. The procedures routinely performed in nuclear medicine departments can be broken down into four main categories; (1) imaging procedures, (2) in vivo function studies, (3) in vitro tests and (4) therapeutic applications.

Imaging procedures provide diagnostic information about organs or body systems based upon the accumulation or selective exclusion of the radiopharmaceutical. The images are only clinically useful if the disease state under investigation causes the localisation of the tracer in a different manner to normal. Measurement is usually made with a gamma camera.

In vivo function studies measure the function of a given organ based upon the concentration, dilution, absorption or excretion of a radiopharmaceutical. They do not require an image of the distribution of the radiopharmaceutical but an accurate measurement of the activity present within an organ or body fluid sample.

In vitro studies are made on samples such as blood, urine and faeces taken from the patient. They do not involve the administration of a radioactive material to the patient. The sample is subjected to procedures such as radioimmunoassay and becomes radioactive outside the patient.

In all cases the diagnostic information is provided by the pharmaceutical; the radionuclide simply acts as a detectable 'marker'. Our aim should always be to use the smallest activity practicable and hence minimise any potential radiation hazard to the patient or the radiation worker.

Therapeutic applications involve the administration of a radiopharmaceutical with the intent of selectively destroying diseased tissue. The biological effects of the emitted ionising radiations are maximised to produce local therapeutic results in the tissues in which the radionuclide is deposited.

The required properties of the radiopharmaceutical vary according to the category of work being performed and are discussed below.

RADIOPHARMACEUTICALS

A wide range of radiopharmaceuticals are available to meet the varied needs of the different procedures. The primary route of administration is intravenous, but oral, intramuscular, intracavity and intrathecal routes may also be used. When deciding upon the efficacy of a given radiopharmaceutical, the physical and chemical properties of the radionuclide, together with biochemical, physiological and pharmacological properties of the pharmaceutical, must be considered.

The radionuclide

The various properties which need to be considered when choosing a suitable radionuclide are listed below.

1. Type of radiation emitted
   a. Energy
   b. Abundance
2. Half-life
3. Specific activity
4. Radionuclide purity
5. Chemical properties.

It is apparent from the introduction that the desirable requirements of the radionuclide will vary depending upon the type of study being performed. We will consider each of the properties listed above, firstly as they apply to diagnostic imaging, then as they may be modified for other diagnostic procedures and finally as they apply to therapeutic applications.

Type of radiation

Diagnostic imaging involves external detection of the isotope. The favourable physical characteristics therefore should include the emission of gamma or X-radiation.

The photon energy should be high enough to avoid serious attenuation in tissue, but low enough to allow the photon to be stopped by and interact with the detector and for the detector to be shielded and collimated without using excessive thicknesses of lead. The design characteristics of a standard gamma camera mean that gamma rays with energies between 75 keV and 300 keV are preferred. Positron emission tomography (PET) cameras, by definition, detect the 511 keV photons released during positron annihilation.

It is also an advantage if the gamma rays are monoenergetic. If more than one gamma ray is emitted then the detector must be collimated against the higher energy photon, even though it may not be being used for the imaging. Septal penetration by the higher energy photon results in a loss of image resolution, but increasing the septal thickness to accommodate the high energy photon reduces the sensitivity of the detector (p. 170).

A primary aim in diagnostic nuclear medicine is to keep the absorbed radiation dose as low as reasonably achievable (ALARA) while obtaining the required information. It is therefore advantageous if the isotope used is one which gives no significant particulate emissions. This can be accomplished by using radionuclides which decay by isomeric transition or electron capture. Particles will still be emitted (Auger and conversion electrons) but at a much lower rate than from radionuclides decaying by beta or alpha particle emission (Ch. 2).

Radiation dose can also be limited by using radionuclides of high abundance. These are radioactive materials where a high gamma ray yield accompanies the disintegrations. Thus iron-52, which emits 99 photons of 169 keV for every 100 disintegrations, has a higher abundance than chromium-51, which emits only nine photons of 320 keV per 100 disintegrations. In the case of chromium-51, 91 of the disintegrations produce no useful externally detectable gamma ray, but they increase the radiation burden.

Physical half-life

In addition to having an abundant supply of photons of suitable energy the half-life of the radionuclide must be sufficiently long to allow for production, administration, localisation and imaging of the radiopharmaceutical within the organ of interest. At the same time it should be remembered that the radiation dose to the patient is proportional to the half-life of the isotope and the half-life therefore should be as short as possible. In practice it is advantageous to use radionuclides with half-lives about the same as the time over which the test is to be conducted.

Biological half-life

The removal of a radioactive material from a site in the body is determined not only by the physical decay of the radioisotope but also by the metabolic processes to which the isotope, as a chemical material, is subjected. The metabolic activity may result in the elimination of the material at a fast rate or, if the element is absorbed in some particular tissue, it may disappear from the body only slowly. A *biological half-life* can be defined which is the time during which the amount of an element in an organ or in the body falls to half its value by metabolic processes. The biological half-life of a given element is the same for all isotopes of that element no matter what the radioactive physical half-life might be, but it does depend on the chemical state of the element in the body.

In some circumstances the biological half-life of an administered isotope is very important, an example being the biological half-life of iodine in the thyroid gland (p. 185). In problems of dosimetry and radiation hazard the real or effective rate at which radioactivity disappears from a particular site is a critical factor. The *effective half-life* is a combination of the physical and biological half-lives and is given by the formula

$$\frac{1}{T_{\text{eff}}} = \frac{1}{T_{\text{biol}}} + \frac{1}{T_{\text{phys}}}$$

where T_{eff}, T_{biol} and T_{phys} are respectively the effective, biological and physical half-lives. Occasionally it is possible to use for human administration isotopes of long physical half-life because in the chemical form used the biological half-life is very short.

Specific activity

The specific activity, that is the ratio per unit mass of radioactive to non-radioactive atoms in the element, should be as high as possible. This will allow very small quantities of the agent to be used and will ensure that the radiolabel does not significantly alter the chemical or biological properties of the pharmaceutical. This is of particular importance when measuring physiological function.

Radionuclide purity

In order to maintain a low radiation dose to the patient and to prevent degradation of the image it is important to control radionuclide purity. Impurities can arise from the manufacturing process (Ch. 2), from daughter radionuclides or from parent radionuclides.

Chemical properties

The chemistry involved in the production of a radio-pharmaceutical is very important. Even if the radio-nuclide has ideal physical properties, it is of little value if it cannot be efficiently attached in an appropriate chemical form to a suitable pharmaceutical to give organ/disease specificity. Chemical toxicity is normally not a matter of major concern as radiopharmaceuticals are administered in extremely small quantities. For example a diagnostic dose of 400 kBq of $[^{131}I]$ sodium iodide contains approximately 8×10^{-11} g of iodine. This is only about 1 or 2×10^{-6} of the normal dietary intake of iodine. This amount of the element is well below the amount detectable by normal chemical analytical procedures and also well below the level which can produce physiological effects on the thyroid gland. It is very uncommon for the administration of a radioactive material to a patient to cause any interference with the physiological effects being investigated and it never happens if carrier-free isotopes are used.

A chemically ideal nuclide would be an isotope of one of the main biological elements, carbon, nitrogen or oxygen. Unfortunately the only radioisotopes of these elements which emit suitable gamma radiation are carbon-11, nitrogen-13 and oxygen-15. They are all cyclotron products decaying by positron emission with half-lives of 20.3, 10.0 and 2.1 minutes and are only practicable when used with a PET gamma camera situated adjacent to the cyclotron.

The ideal radionuclide for imaging

To summarise, the ideal radionuclide for routine nuclear medicine imaging using a standard gamma camera will be a high abundancy monoenergetic gamma emitter of energy 75–300 keV. It will decay with a half-life similar to the length of investigation by isomeric transition or electron capture, have low internal conversion and no radioactive daughter products. Technetium-99m comes close to meeting these requirements. It emits a 140 keV photon in 88% of its disintegrations. It decays by isomeric transition with a half-life of 6 hours and is readily 'attached' to a range of pharmaceuticals.

Nevertheless radionuclides which decay by beta particle emission and have a high gamma ray yield can be used for radiopharmaceutical preparation if their chemical and biological properties outweigh any undesirable physical properties. A good example of such a nuclide is iodine-131 which decays by beta particle emission, emits a relatively high energy photon of 364 keV in 82% of disintegrations and has a half-life of 8.1 days. The various radioisotopes of iodine are of physiological importance in thyroid work and are very chemically reactive, allowing them to be attached to many different chemical molecules. This makes them valuable radionuclides in nuclear medicine.

In vivo function studies

In these types of study the radiopharmaceutical must be a true physiological tracer. It is therefore essential that labelling the compound does not interfere with or significantly alter the chemical and biological properties of the compound. Radionuclides iodine-131, or iodine-123 will mimic stable dietary iodide in thyroid function studies. Similarly radioactive cobalt-57 or cobalt-58 can be directly substituted for stable cobalt-59 in cyanocobalamin to study the absorption and excretion of vitamin B_{12}.

The radionuclide properties required are similar to those for imaging as external detection of the uptake or absorption is desired. However the detector resolution necessary for good image definition is no longer required. The detectors are more sensitive over a wider range of photon energies. Lower activity levels are used, kilobecquerels rather than megabecquerels, hence the radionuclide requirements are less stringent and the need for a non-particulate emitter is reduced. The half-life must be similar to the length of the investigation. For investigations involving the absorption, utilisation and retention of an element this may be a period of several weeks.

In vitro studies

In vitro studies, unlike all other nuclear medicine procedures, do not involve the administration of a radionuclide to the patient. Therefore all the requirements relating to radiation absorbed dose and external gamma ray detection no longer apply.

Techniques such as saturation analysis and radio-immunoassay, used to measure the concentration of a hormone or chemical in a small sample of blood or urine, require very low levels, becquerels, of activity. The nuclide may be a pure beta emitter, such as carbon-14 which is easily incorporated into many compounds and has a half-life of 5760 years, or it may be a photon emitter such as iodine-125 with X- and gamma radiations of 27 and 36 keV and a half-life of 60 days.

Therapeutic applications

The aim of radionuclide therapy is to maximise the radiation dose to the treatment zone while minimising the dose to normal tissue. It is clearly advantageous to have a radionuclide where a large proportion of the energy emitted per disintegration is in the form of beta particles. Beta particle radiation is completely absorbed by the tissue in which it is lodged and delivers a high localised radiation dose.

A physical half-life of 1 or 2 weeks is desirable. Shorter half-life radionuclides require the administration of high levels of activity to achieve the required dose. Longer half-life nuclides produce a radiation hazard and cause problems with radiation protection.

The pharmaceutical

The desirable factors involved in the choice of pharmaceutical include: a high target to background ratio; no adverse reactions or unwanted pharmacological responses; and ease of preparation. To image an organ, or to measure the physiological function of an organ or body system, the administered radiopharmaceutical should localise in the target organ with little localisation in other organs or tissues, giving a high target to background ratio. A variety of mechanisms affect the localisation and behaviour of the different radiopharmaceuticals available, and some of these are listed below.

— Metabolic accumulation
— Synthesised compounds
— Capillary blockage
— Exclusion
— Drug analogy
— Excretion and secretion
— Compartment localisation
— Antibody antigen reactions.

Metabolic accumulation

Two elements studied in this way are iodine and iron.

Iodine is an element incorporated into the hormones produced by the thyroid gland and a study of the metabolic behaviour of iodine in the body gives valuable diagnostic evidence of thyroid function. Radioactive iodine introduced into the body therefore enables iodine metabolism to be studied easily. The concentration of iodine in the thyroid gland also means that therapeutic

doses of ionising radiation can be given to the gland from deposited radioactive beta emitters. There are a number of possible iodine isotopes which can be used in these procedures. These include iodine-131 ($T_{1/2}$ 8 days; ß γ emitter), iodine-125 ($T_{1/2}$ 60 days; γ emitter), and iodine-123 ($T_{1/2}$ 13 h; γ emitter). In every case, however, the radioactive iodine is supplied and administered as a solution of sodium iodide, though in the body the radioactive iodide ion is the entity whose behaviour is of importance.

A study of the metabolism of the element iron is of importance in the clinical diagnosis of blood disorders. The element, again in its ionic form, is built into the haemoglobin of red cells following its absorption from the bloodstream, to which it may be introduced directly or through the processing of food in the alimentary canal. The most useful isotope is iron-59 ($T_{1/2}$ 45 days; ß γ emitter) and it is administered in the form of a simple iron salt, often ferric citrate, though the precise compound used will depend on the nature of the particular test.

Synthesised compounds

A large number of medically and biologically important compounds are available where a non-radioactive component atom of the molecule has been replaced by a radioactive atom of the same element. These are *synthesised radioactive compounds*. Two examples of clinical interest are vitamin B_{12} and water.

Vitamin B_{12}, of great importance in the study of anaemias, is a compound (cyanocobalamin) containing an atom of cobalt. The compound is synthesised on a large scale by biological processes in which radioactive cobalt is built into the molecule. The most commonly used isotopes are cobalt-57 ($T_{1/2}$ 270 days; γ emitter) and cobalt-58 ($T_{1/2}$ 71 days; ß γ emitter). Labelled water is available in which one hydrogen atom of the normal molecule is replaced with tritium, the isotope hydrogen-3 ($T_{1/2}$ 12.3 years; ß emitter). This compound, *tritiated water*, is used, in vivo, to study electrolyte and water absorption problems. The relatively long half-life of tritium is tolerable because the beta ray emission energy is extremely small and the biological half-life of this compound is short, approximately 12 days. A tremendous variety of organic compounds labelled with hydrogen-3 (tritium) or carbon-14 ($T_{1/2}$ 5760 years; ß emitter) is available.

Capillary blockade

If radioactive particles in the size range 20 to 50 μm are injected into the vascular system they will partially occlude the first capillary bed they encounter (size of capillaries 8-10 μm). An intravenous injection of half a million ^{99m}Tc-labelled particles of macroaggregated albumin will block approximately 0.05% of the capillaries of a normal lung, thus permitting the visualisation of the vascular bed of the lungs. A protein such as albumin is chosen for production of the particles as it will be quickly broken down and removed from the lungs.

Exclusion

Pharmaceuticals may be selectively excluded from an organ except in the presence of disease. For example, because of the so-called blood–brain barrier normal brain tissue is relatively impermeable to substances such as [^{99m}Tc]sodium pertechnetate. Many mass lesions within the brain are more permeable than normal tissue and hence interfere with the blood–brain barrier. This allows the technetium to diffuse across the barrier, accumulate in the lesion and enable visualisation of the lesion.

Drug analogy

A pharmaceutical may be similar to a substance that is normally metabolised by an organ, and may be used as a substitute to investigate that organ.

1. To some extent the pertechnetate ion (TcO_4) behaves in the thyroid in a similar way to the iodine ion and the use of technetium-99m for the study of thyroid function is often an advantage since it gives a low absorbed dose to the gland.

2. The reticuloendothelial cells in the body have the capacity to ingest bacteria and small particles in the range 0.01–10 μm. This is known as phagocytosis. If a radiolabelled colloid is injected intravenously, the phagocytic action of the reticuloendothelial cells, in particular the Kupffer cells in the liver, will remove the colloid from the circulation, enabling the organ to be externally visualised. Areas of non-functioning liver tissue will not remove colloid material.

3. Thallium-201 is concentrated in muscle tissue in a similar manner to potassium. This can be used to image the heart muscle and detect areas of ischaemic and infarcted myocardium.

Excretion, secretion

Many drugs are excreted or secreted by body organs. These properties can be utilised to both visualise the organ and to quantify its level of physiological function.

1. The radiopharmaceutical [^{123}I]o-iodohippurate is taken up by the kidneys, passes through the tubules into the kidney pelvis, and is then excreted via the ureters into the bladder. The transit of the pharmaceutical through the kidney gives information about function.

2. [^{99m}Tc]Sodium pertechnetate is concentrated in the gastric mucosa and secreted into the lining of the gut. It can be used to visualise sites of ectopic gastric mucosas such as Meckel's diverticulum.

Compartmental localisation

The distribution of certain types of cells and molecules is restricted to particular body compartments. Radio-labelled forms of such cells can be used to visualise the compartment or to measure the volume of that compartment. ^{99m}Tc-labelled red cells, when re-injected into the patient from whom the cells have been withdrawn, will be retained almost exclusively within the vascular compartment. With the application of simple dilution analysis techniques the labelled cells can be used to measure the red cell volume of the compartment or by ECG gating the data collection they can be used to image the functioning heart.

Antibody–antigen reactions

Antigens are produced in low concentrations by normal tissue but are present in relatively high concentration on the surface of certain tumour cells. Monoclonal antibodies can be raised against specific antigens. If the antibodies are radiolabelled then the sites of antigen–antibody binding can be located.

Sterility and purity of radiopharmaceuticals

The radiopharmaceutical must not produce a pharmacological reaction within the patient. It must be chemically pure, non-toxic and contain only small quantities of chemical carrier and radionuclide.

The preparation of radiopharmaceuticals and the form in which they are made available for use in clinical departments is influenced by the method by which it is intended to introduce the product into the patient. For some tests oral administration is the preferred method and indeed sometimes the only suitable one. In this case clean, stable, palatable solutions are ideal. For many tests, however, intravenous injections must be used and for some cases intracavity or intrathecal (into spinal fluid) injection is necessary. In these cases great care must be taken to produce a radiopharmaceutical in a sterile solution of the correct pH value and free from pyrogens (foreign proteins arising from previous bacteriological activity).

The details of the necessary procedures are beyond the scope of this text but these requirements do influence the laboratory facilities necessary in hospital departments where radiopharmaceuticals are prepared. In addition to the radiation safety requirements discussed in Chapters 9 and 12, the needs of good pharmaceutical practice are also important.

The special laboratory facilities and equipment required are described in detail in other publications (see Bibliography). Many of the desirable design features necessary for the production of pharmaceuticals are also desirable for radiation safety. However there is one major area of conflict. For radiation safety, in order to contain any airborne contaminants, rooms where high activity levels are in use are often kept at a lower pressure than the surrounding environment. The requirements for a radiopharmacy are exactly the opposite. The preparation area must be bathed in a pure sterile air at a pressure higher than that of its surroundings so as to avoid leakage inward of non-sterile air and microorganisms.

RADIOPHARMACEUTICALS IN THE BODY

Consideration of the various processes through which the radiopharmaceutical may pass has shown that many of the compounds will at some stage be located in a particular organ or tissue, at least for a time. The localisation of iodine in the thyroid gland or of radioactive albumin particles of appropriate size in the lungs are good examples. This aspect of the behaviour of radioactive materials in the body is important in several ways: it capacitates the use of radionuclides in dilution analysis and metabolic function studies; it permits organ visualisation; it has an impact on radiation dose and the import of critical organs; and it allows for therapeutic applications.

Use for dilution analysis and metabolic function

Dilution analysis

The localisation of the radiopharmaceutical within a space or compartment enables an estimate to be made of the volume of that space within the patient. If a known amount of a radioactive material is introduced into a vessel containing an unknown volume of liquid and thoroughly mixed, it is easy to deduce the unknown volume by measuring the concentration of activity in a sample taken from the mixture.

An important example of the dilution technique is the measurement of the volume of the circulating red cells in the blood. For this purpose a sample of the patient's own red cells are used and the cells are labelled with either chromium-51 or technetium-99m. An accurately known volume of the labelled red cells is then re-injected into the patient and a smaller accurately known volume used to make up a standard. Twenty to thirty minutes after re-injection a venous blood sample is withdrawn from the patient. The radioactive assay consists of comparing the activity of equal volumes of the whole blood and of the standard solution. The red cell volume (RCV) is calculated from the formula:

$$RCV = \frac{A_s}{A_b} \cdot V \cdot D \cdot \frac{H}{100}$$

where A_s and A_b are the count rates from the standard and blood sample, V is the volume of labelled cells re-injected, D is the dilution factor used in preparing the standard and H is the percentage haematocrit of the venous blood sample.

Metabolic function

The investigation of a radioisotope's distribution about the body and the way in which this varies with time provides valuable information about the metabolism of the compound.

As we have mentioned previously a very common and important metabolic study is that of the element iodine which is involved in the function of the thyroid gland. Knowledge of iodine metabolism gives diagnostic information about thyroid disease (p. 357). The normal daily intake of iodine is about 100 µg. When the thyroid gland is functioning normally about half of this iodine is abstracted from the circulating blood by the thyroid gland and about half is abstracted by the kidney and excreted in the urine. The thyroid gland synthesises the thyroid hormones, of which the element iodine is one of the atomic constituents, and the hormones are transported throughout the body in the blood circulation to control the bodily functions influenced by these hormones. Between 150 and 200 kBq of iodine-131 in the form of a solution of sodium iodide is administered orally to the patient. An equal amount is stored in a small bottle for use as a comparison standard. The uptake of the radioiodine in the thyroid gland is observed by means of a collimated scintillation counter (see p. 167). Four measurements are required for an uptake measurement:

1. The activity in the thyroid gland in counts per minute, P.

2. By positioning a lead block between the patient's neck and the detector, a measure of the patient's non-thyroidal background activity, P_{bg}.

3. With the standard placed in a neck phantom underneath the detector, the activity of the standard, S.

4. With the phantom covered with the lead block a phantom background, S_{bg}.

It therefore follows that:

$$\% \text{ Thyroid uptake } = \frac{P - P_{bg}}{S - S_{bg}} \times 100$$

The curves of Figure 10.1 show the variation of uptake in the thyroid gland over 3 days following the administration of the tracer dose. The ordinates represent percentage of the administered dose taken up by the gland, and the three curves A, B, and C represent typical results: A in a patient with normal thyroid function; B in a case of hyperactivity, or thyrotoxicosis of the gland; and C in a case of hypoactivity of the gland leading to myxoedema. It should be noted that during the time of the test, sometimes up to 7 days, there will have been a physical decay of the iodine-131 and in the curves in Figure 10.1 the percentage of administered dose has in each case been corrected for this decay.

Use for organ visualisation

The localisation of a radiopharmaceutical within an organ makes possible the visualisation of that organ. Furthermore, if the distribution of the administered isotope in the organ concerned is abnormal, or changes with time, then deductions can be made about the function of the organ. Abnormal isotope distribution may appear as an increase in isotope concentration above the norm, revealing lesions as 'hot spots', or as reduced activity in the visualised pattern, revealing lesions as 'cold spots'.

The main purpose of organ imaging is to investigate the function of system pathology rather than anatomical definition. This may be achieved by the use of either static imaging, both planar and tomographic, or by dynamic imaging, the monitoring of changes in distribution with time. There follows a brief description of some of the more important clinical applications of radionuclide imaging. This is not meant to be a comprehensive list of every conceivable use, but more an introduction to the types of investigation possible.

Skeletal imaging

Bone is made up of collagen and minerals, mainly calcium, phosphates and hydroxides. The minerals form a crystalline lattice known as hydroxyapatite. Following intravenous injection, a bone seeking agent will be transported to the bone and become adsorbed on to the newly forming hydroxyapatite crystals, thus reflecting the bone forming activity at a given skeletal site. Hence areas where there is an abnormally high increase in bone turnover will show increased uptake and will appear as 'hot spots' on the image.

All current bone seeking radiopharmaceuticals are based on phosphate containing compounds which can be labelled with technetium-99m. A variety of these analogues are available but the most widely used is methylene diphosphonate (MDP). Typically, 400–600 MBq of [⁹⁹ᵐTc]MDP are administered intravenously and after a period of 2–4 hours 50–60% of the injected dose will be localised in the bone, the remainder being excreted via the kidneys. Multiple static views or a combination of a whole body image and selected static views are recorded. The appearances of the normal bone scan are shown in Figure 10.2, where it can be seen that each of the bones is well demonstrated.

Bone scan changes occur when there is increased osteoblastic activity, and increased or decreased blood flow to a lesion. The bone scan is a very sensitive technique for demonstrating bone lesions, but the findings are non-specific. An abnormal distribution of activity must be interpreted together with the relevant clinical history and appropriate X-rays.

Applications of skeletal imaging include those described below.

— The detection of metastases in bone, particularly from breast and prostate tumours. Figure 10.3 shows a patient with extensive metastatic involvement, from a

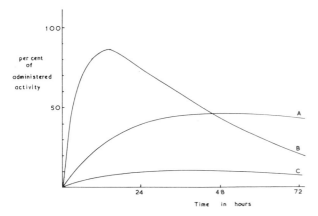

Fig. 10.1 Uptake of radioiodine in the thyroid gland. A, Normal thyroid function; B, hyperactive thyroid gland — thyrotoxicosis; C, hypoactive thyroid gland — myxoedema.

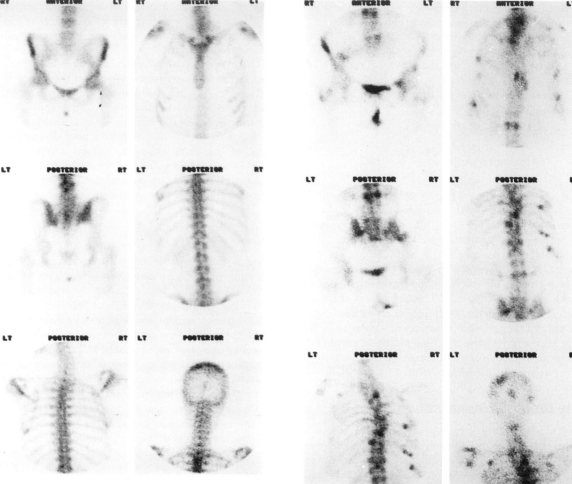

Fig. 10.2 Normal bone scan 4 hours post intravenous injection of [^{99m}Tc]MDP.

Fig. 10.3 Bone scan showing multiple metastatic deposits from carcinoma of the breast.

primary breast carcinoma, as demonstrated by the multiple areas of increased uptake. Figure 10.4 shows just three focal 'hot spots', one in the dorsal spine, one posteriorly in a left rib, and the third in the right side of the sacrum. This high activity pattern is typical of metastases from a prostate tumour. Radionuclide bone imaging provides earlier diagnosis of a lesion than X-ray techniques, since for a lesion to be apparent on an X-ray there needs to be about a 50% decrease in calcium content.

— The diagnosis of functional changes caused by metabolic bone disease. These techniques depend on the quantitative estimates of the uptake and clearance of a bone seeking radiopharmaceutical.

— Monitoring the progression and regression of known active disease or the response of a lesion to treatment.

— Detection of bone infarction or aseptic necrosis,

where the lesion will appear as an area of decreased activity, not as a 'hot spot'.

— The evaluation of stress fractures. Figure 10.5 shows the bone scan image of the tibia and fibula of an athlete in heavy training. Areas of increased uptake can be seen down the edges of both tibia demonstrating the clinical condition of 'shin splints'.

Brain

The brain is divided into the right and left hemisphere, the cerebellum and the brainstem. The falx cerebri separates the cerebral hemispheres, and the tentorium separates the hemispheres from the cerebellum. The brain is supplied with blood by branches of the carotid

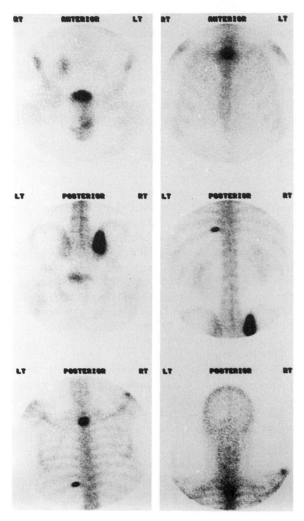

Fig. 10.4 Bone scan showing high activity focal 'hot spots' from prostatic metastases.

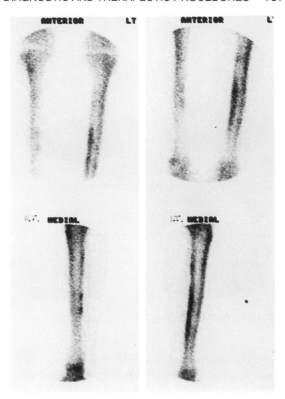

Fig. 10.5 Bone scan of stress fracture 'shin splints' in a top class athlete.

The incidence of brain scanning will vary from centre to centre depending on the availability of other facilities such as CT and MRI. These other modalities give superior image resolution for the detection of space occupying lesions. Nevertheless radionuclide imaging is a sensitive procedure and is still in use for the detection of neoplasms, abscess, subdural haematoma and the evaluation of vascular disease.

Three radiopharmaceuticals are in current use: [99mTc]pertechnetate; [99mTc]diethylene triamine pentaacetic acid (DTPA); and [99mTc]glucoheptonate. Pertechnetate is the least expensive, but the other two have at least two important advantages. They are not accumulated in the normal choroid plexus, salivary glands or thyroid, and hence do not require the predosing of the patient with potassium perchlorate. Image quality is usually better, with higher lesion to brain ratios being achieved in less time.

Typically 400–700 MBq of the radiopharmaceutical are administered intravenously. The imaging may then consist of two distinct phases: an immediate dynamic or vascular phase, and a static phase approximately 1 hour later. A normal pertechnetate scan is seen in Figure 10.6. This shows the blood within the skull and

and vertebral arteries; the blood eventually drains into the venous sinuses. The superior sagittal sinus lies in the upper margin of the falx cerebri and, as its name suggests, drains in the sagittal plane from the frontal region posteriorly to the occipital protuberance. The transverse sinuses run laterally in the margin of the tentorium and join with the sagittal and other sinuses at the occipital protuberance. These are all clear landmarks seen on a conventional brain scan.

The blood–brain barrier is a mechanism by which most substances are prevented from passing out of the blood into the brain tissue. This barrier appears to break down in the presence of tumours, abscesses, etc. This allows for the localisation of a suitable radiopharmaceutical, seen as a 'hot spot', in these lesions.

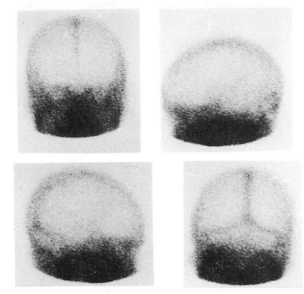

Fig. 10.6 Normal brain scan.

scalp, the sagittal and transverse sinuses, and the face. There is a lack of activity in the brain tissue and the area of the orbits. Figure 10.7 shows a tumour close to the centre of the brain. Increased uptake can be seen to a greater or lesser extent on all four views.

A second type of nuclear medicine brain scan involves the use of a radiopharmaceutical which is capable of crossing the normally intact blood–brain barrier and diffusing into the brain tissue. Such techniques demonstrate the regional cerebral blood flow and are being used to understand mental disorders such as Alzheimer's disease. Plate 6 shows a normal SPECT scan of local cerebral blood flow, following the injection of [^{99m}Tc]hexamethylene propylamine oxime (HM-PAO).

Thyroid

The normal function of the thyroid gland includes the concentration of iodine from the circulation, and the synthesis and storage of thyroid hormones. Iodine may also be trapped in the salivary glands and the gastric mucosa. Iodine-131 was once the radionuclide of choice for thyroid imaging, but because of the relatively high radiation dose to the patient it has now been superseded by iodine-123 and [^{99m}Tc]pertechnetate. The latter is the most readily available and is trapped in the thyroid gland by an active transport mechanism in the same way as iodine. However, it is not incorporated into the thyroid hormones.

An intravenous injection of 40–80 MBq of [^{99m}Tc]pertechnetate is administered and a static image of the thyroid gland acquired approximately 30 minutes later. Imaging may be performed, with a parallel hole collimator, on a small field of view mobile gamma camera, or on a conventional gamma camera using either a pin-hole or converging collimator.

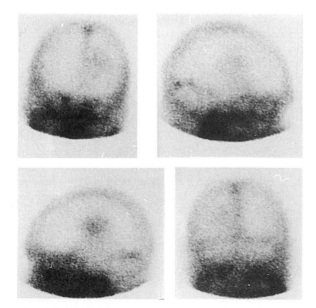

Fig. 10.7 Brain scan showing a large tumour in the parietal region.

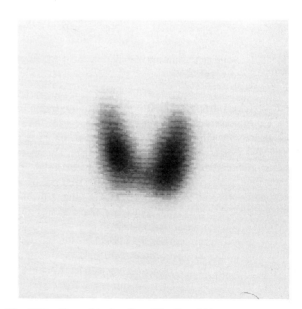

Fig. 10.8 Normal technetium-99m thyroid image.

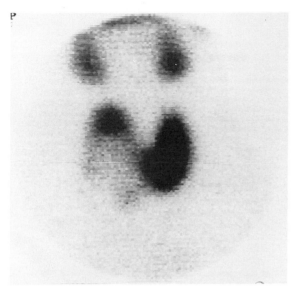

Fig. 10.9   Technetium-99m image of a 'cold' thyroid nodule corresponding to an area of swelling in the neck.

The commonest clinical conditions evaluated by this technique are: the differentiation between benign and malignant nodules; assessment of the size of the gland in hyperthyroidism; and the localisation of metastatic thyroid cancer. Figure 10.8 shows uniform uptake to a normal bilobed thyroid gland.

A non-functioning 'cold' nodule, corresponding to the visible mass in the patient's neck, is seen in the right lobe of the thyroid gland of Figure 10.9; also visible at the top of the image are the submandibular salivary glands. Thyroid malignancies do not concentrate radioisotopes and appear as cold nodules, but only 20% of the cold nodules detected are malignant.

Parathyroid

The four parathyroid glands, weighing only 35 mg each, are situated at the poles of the thyroid gland. The primary use of parathyroid imaging is the localisation of parathyroid adenomas.

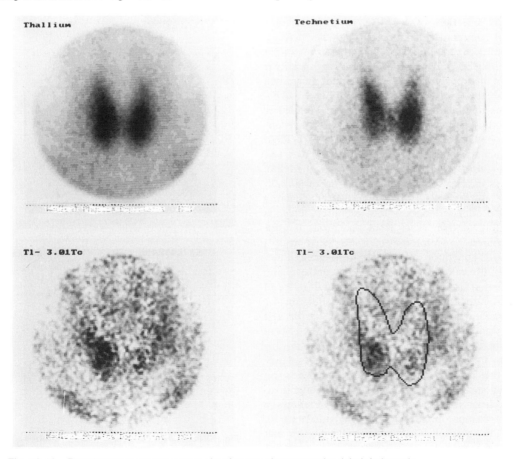

Fig. 10.10   Parathyroid subtraction scan showing an adenoma at the right inferior pole.

The technique involves the combined injection of 40 MBq of [^{99m}Tc]pertechnetate and 40 MBq of thallium-201 followed by subtraction imaging. Thallium-201 is localised in both the thyroid gland and in parathyroid adenomas. Technetium-99m is localised in the thyroid gland but not the parathyroid glands. Two images are taken and stored on computer, one using the technetium-99m window, the other using the thallium-201 window. The images are then normalised and the technetium-99m image is subtracted from the thallium-201 image. An example of such a procedure is given in Figure 10.10, where, following subtraction, a para-thyroid adenoma is seen at the inferior pole of the right lobe of the thyroid gland.

Lung

The function of the lungs is to exchange gases between the air and the blood. There are therefore two mechanisms to be investigated: the regional perfusion, and the regional ventilation.

Regional perfusion is studied by administering an intravenous injection of 80 MBq of [^{99m}Tc]macro-aggregated albumin. The albumin particles have a diameter of between 10 and 20 μm and after mixing in the heart will be trapped in the pulmonary arteriolar or capillary bed of the lungs. The resultant image will show the areas of lung which are perfused (Fig. 10.11B).

Lung ventilation is studied by the inhalation of either an inert radioactive gas such as xenon-133 or krypton-81m or a radioactive aerosol such as [^{99m}Tc]DTPA. All have their advantages and disadvantages. Xenon-133 is cheap, readily available and has a long shelf life. However, it emits a low energy gamma ray of 80 keV, making it less than ideal for gamma camera imaging because it produces images of low resolution, and it is only possible to take views from one projection for each examination. Krypton-81m is produced from a rubidium-81 generator. It has an ideal gamma ray energy of 190 keV, a half-life of 13 seconds, giving a low radiation dose to the patient, and a full range of views can be obtained. Unfortunately the rubidium-81 in the generator also has a short half-life, has limited availability and is very expensive. [^{99m}Tc]DTPA aerosol can be inhaled by the patient and has all the advantages of any [^{99m}Tc] radiopharmaceutical. The residency time of the activity within the lungs depends on the physiological state, but it is usually possible to obtain at least four views. Figure 10.11A shows a normal ventilation lung scan following inhalation of [^{99m}Tc]DTPA aerosol. The main disadvantage is that the same radionuclide, technetium-99m, is used for both the ventilation and perfusion phase of the study.

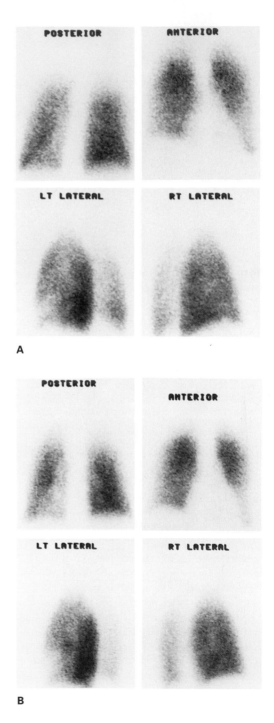

Fig. 10.11   A Normal lung ventilation images using [^{99m}Tc]DTPA aerosol; **B** normal lung perfusion images using [^{99m}Tc]MAA.

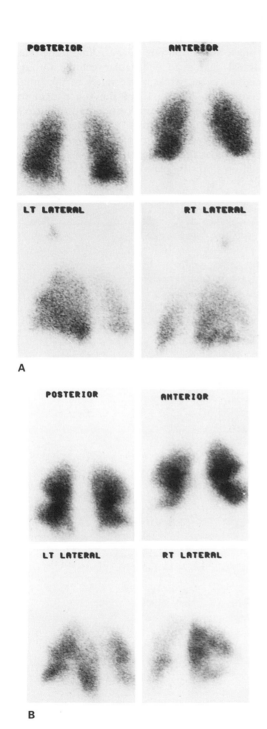

POSTERIOR   **ANTERIOR**

LT LATERAL   **RT LATERAL**

A

POSTERIOR   **ANTERIOR**

LT LATERAL   **RT LATERAL**

B

Fig. 10.12 A Normal lung ventilation; **B** lung perfusion images showing wedge-shaped filling defects. These are not matched on the ventilation images and are indicative of pulmonary embolism.

This means that the ventilation image must be acquired before the perfusion image and, depending on the physiological status, a time gap between the two stages of the investigation may be necessary.

The most common clinical application of lung scanning is the differential diagnosis of pulmonary embolism. Here the ventilation capacity of the lungs is normal, and hence the ventilation image is normal (Fig. 10.12A), while the perfusion pattern is abnormal in the regions occluded by the clot (Fig. 10.12B). These normally appear as wedge-shaped or segmental defects on the perfusion image.

Cardiac

The heart is a muscular organ divided internally by a muscular septum into right and left sides, each side having two chambers. The right and left atria collect the blood returning from the pulmonary and systemic circulations. The right and left ventricles are pumping chambers and are more muscular, particularly the left ventricle which pumps the blood to the systemic circulation. A single cardiac cycle or heart beat has three phases: contraction or systole; dilatation or diastole; and a period of rest. Many cardiac conditions can be investigated using nuclear cardiology but the two most important are studies of the adequacy of the myocardial perfusion and studies of the left ventricular action of the heart.

Thallium-201 is currently the most widely used perfusion agent, having physiological characteristics similar to those of potassium. Typically 80 MBq of thallium-201 chloride are administered intravenously at peak exercise and the exercise continued for a further 30 to 60 seconds. Multiprojection imaging is performed immediately (stress study) and again 3 hours later (rest study). The thallium is distributed throughout the myocardium according to the muscle mass and the regional blood flow. In fact only about 4% is taken up by the heart.

In normal subjects the myocardial blood flow increases during exercise in line with the increased oxygen demand of the muscle. In patients with coronary artery disease, although there is usually normal blood flow at rest, the blood vessel is unable to meet the increased demand placed upon it during exercise. This is known clinically as angina. In a normal heart a uniform distribution of thallium-201 is seen within the walls of the left ventricle on both the stress images and the rest images (Plate 7), while in a patient with diseased coronary arteries we will see areas of reduced perfusion on the stress study, with evidence of redistribution on the rest images (Plate 8).

The ventricular action of the heart is investigated by means of gated blood pool imaging—multigated acquisition (MUGA). Twenty to thirty minutes following a cold injection of pyrophosphate, or stannous fluoride, 400–800 MBq of technetium-99m is administered intravenously and in vivo labelling of the patient's red cells takes place. By using the patient's ECG to gate or control image acquisition, a series of images (16–24) is recorded and stored on computer during each cardiac cycle. Data collection continues for several minutes. High spatial resolution images are then obtained by summing images of identical time segments in consecutive cardiac cycles. The images can be processed to assess regional wall motion, and give ventricular ejection fractions. Functional images of stroke volume and paradoxical motion can be obtained together with phase and amplitude images. Amplitude refers to the actual change in ventricular volume throughout the cardiac cycle, while phase refers to the timing of the contraction. Figure 10.13 shows a patient with a normal ventricular ejection fraction and uniform heart muscle contractions. Figure 10.14 demonstrates an abnormal ejection fraction of 15% and a small area of dyskinesia at the apex of the left ventricle. This can be seen on both the paradoxical image and the phase image.

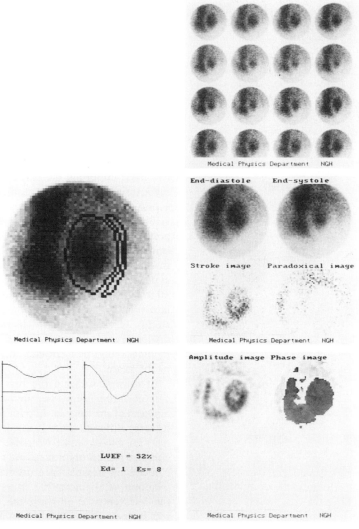

Fig. 10.13 Multigated acquisition study of a normally functioning heart—normal ventricular ejection fraction of >50%, normal contraction of the ventricle in systole, uniform amplitude and phase images.

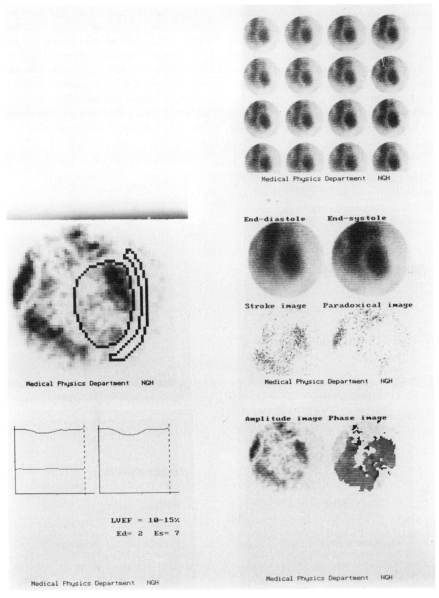

Fig. 10.14 Abnormal MUGA study with low ejection fraction and a small area of dyskinesia at the apex of the left ventricle.

Renal

The kidney produces urine and disposes of metabolic waste products. It is divided into an outer cortical and an inner medullary region. Urine drains from the medullary region via the renal pelvis into the ureter and thence into the bladder. Several radiopharmaceuticals are available for imaging the kidney and investigating renal function. The choice of pharmaceutical depends on the specific renal function measurements required and the clinical condition being studied. There follows just one example of a renal investigation.

The most widely used radiopharmaceutical is [^{99m}Tc]DTPA. It is suitable for the assessment of glomerular filtration, individual kidney function, and detection of drainage obstruction. With the kidneys, bladder, and if possible the heart, in the field of view of the gamma camera, up to 300 MBq of [^{99m}Tc]DTPA is injected intravenously. For the following 25–30 minutes a series of images (e.g. 90 20-second frames) are collected and stored on computer. Regions of interest can then be drawn around the kidneys, the bladder and the heart and, after suitable background correction, time–activity curves can be calculated for each region. This is known as a renogram.

Figure 10.15 shows the renogram data from a patient with one normally functioning kidney and one obstructed kidney. The top two pictures show the changes in the kidney images with the passage of time. The centre left image shows the regions of interest associated with each kidney. The bottom left image shows the net kidney curves. The renogram from the normal left kidney is seen to contain three phases: a vascular phase denoted by an initial sharp rise; a secretory phase denoted by a slower steadier rise peaking after about 4 minutes; and an excretory phase

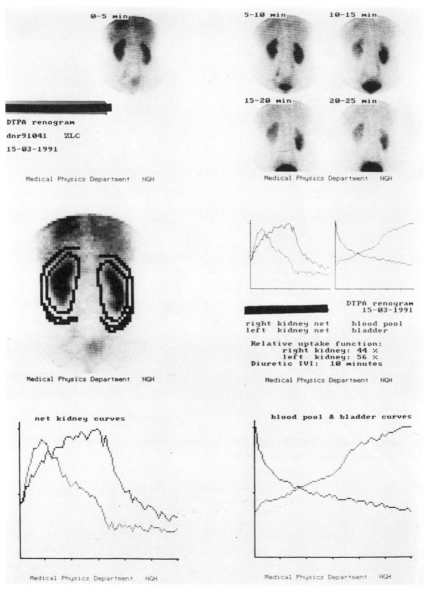

Fig. 10.15   [99mTc]DTPA renogram showing a normal left kidney and a right kidney with pelvic retention until the administration at 15 minutes of a diuretic.

denoted by the falling slope. An injection of a diuretic, which enhances renal excretion, was administered part way through the excretory phase and is seen as a rapid fall in the curve. The abnormal right kidney shows pelvic retention on the images and a continuously rising obstructive pattern on the renogram. There is a fall in the curve following administration of the diuretic. Other images show the accumulation of activity in the bladder and the clearance of tracer from the circulation. Values for relative kidney function have been calculated and these are displayed on the centre right picture.

Tumours

It is possible to produce monoclonal antibodies targeted against specific tumour types. The antibodies can be labelled with iodine-131, technetium-99m or indium-111. When injected into the patient the radiolabelled antibodies will seek out the tumour associated antigens. However the absolute uptake in the tumour is normally less than 1% and image quality is rather poor. Work in this field to refine the specificity of the antibodies continues.

Table 10.1 gives a list of some commonly used radiopharmaceuticals and includes notes on their more important uses, details of the maximum recommended activity, the absorbed dose to the critical organ and the effective dose equivalent.

Radiation dose and critical organs

The localisation of the isotope material even temporarily in some organ or tissue means that the absorbed dose of ionising radiation which a patient receives following the administration of a radioactive material is rarely uniform. In any isotope test it is always necessary to ensure that the whole body and each organ in the body receives an acceptably low dose. Some knowledge of the metabolic processes involved is essential in calculating the doses received by the patient in these procedures. It is possible that, because of retention of the isotope in one particular organ, that organ may receive a dose approaching the reasonable limit for that organ before the limit for the whole body is reached (p. 213). The organ which is most vulnerable in this sense is called the *critical organ* and calculations of absorbed dose involved must take account of the possible concentration of the isotope in the critical organ.

The definitions for absorbed dose, dose equivalent and effective dose equivalent are given in Chapter 12. Absorbed dose, measured in grays, is the quantity of energy imparted by ionising radiation to a unit mass of tissue. The dose equivalent, measured in sieverts, is

equal to the absorbed dose multiplied by a factor that takes into account the way in which different radiations deposit their energy in tissue. The effective dose equivalent, also measured in sieverts, is the sum of the products of the dose equivalent to various organs and a risk weighting factor for each organ. The effective dose equivalent is very important in nuclear medicine procedures as it allows for a variety of non-uniform distributions of dose equivalents in the body to be expressed as a single number representing the risk to health.

Dosimetry

The radiation dose to a patient resulting from the administration of a radiopharmaceutical depends on the amount of energy deposited by the radiation in the patient. When a radionuclide is absorbed in a local site in the body it disappears from that site roughly exponentially, with an effective half-life determined by the physical decay and the metabolic process which may remove it from the site. The energy of the beta particles which it emits is absorbed almost entirely in the immediate vicinity of the active material. However the gamma rays emitted by the active material will not be absorbed appreciably in the immediate vicinity. In general, depending upon the energy of the photons, a proportion will be absorbed elsewhere in the body, but most will escape altogether from the body. The photons that are absorbed will produce secondary electrons by the processes described in Chapter 4.

Calculation of the dose distribution of a radiopharmaceutical requires a knowledge of the *cumulative activity*, the *equilibrium dose constant*, and the *absorbed fraction*. Organs are divided into *source* organs, in which activity is accumulated and which therefore become a radiation source and irradiate other organs, and *target* organs which are the organs for which the dose is being calculated.

The cumulative activity, A_c, measured in kBq h, in each organ depends upon the percentage uptake in the organ, the effective half-life and the administered activity (i.e. the time integral activity). The equilibrium dose rate, Δ, measured in joules per becquerel per second or kg Gy kBq^{-1}h^{-1}, depends only on the radionuclide used and for gamma rays is analogous to the specific gamma ray constant. It represents the average amount of energy, either beta or gamma, emitted per disintegration. The absorbed fraction, ø, (no units), depends on the organs involved, their sizes and relative distances apart. The absorbed dose, D, is given by:

$$D = \frac{\Delta \times ø}{m} \times A_c \qquad 10.1$$

Table 10.1 Examples of some radiopharmaceuticals in common use

Radionuclide	Chemical form	Clinical use	Max activity (MBq)⁻¹	Half-life	Route	Critical organ	Absorbed dose (mGy MBq⁻¹)	Effective dose equivalent (mSv MBq⁻¹)
Chromium-51	Sodium chromate solution	Labelling red blood cells for RBC volume, survival and splenic sequestration	4.0	27.8 days	i.v.	Spleen	1.6	0.26
Cobalt-57	Cyanocobalamin capsules and solution	Diagnosis of pernicious anaemia and vitamin B_{12} malabsorption	0.04	270 days	p.o.	Liver	24	2.7
Cobalt-58				71 days			36	5.1
Gallium-67	Gallium citrate	Tumour imaging; localisation of inflammatory lesions	150	78.3 h	i.v.	Bone surfaces	0.59	0.12
Indium-111	Indium oxine labelled white cells	Infection, abscess imaging	40	2.8 days	i.v.	Spleen	5.5	0.59
Iodine-123	Sodium iodide capsules and solution	Diagnosis of thyroid function; thyroid imaging	20	13.2 h	p.o.	Thyroid	0.9	0.15
Iodine-125	Human serum albumin	Plasma volume determination	0.2	60 days	i.v.	Heart	0.69	0.34
Iodine-131	Sodium iodide capsule and solution	Diagnosis of thyroid function	0.2	8.1 days	p.o.	Thyroid	500 (35% uptake)	15
		Treatment of hyperthyroidism	600		p.o.	Thyroid	790 (55% uptake)	24
		Treatment of thyroid carcinoma and metastases	8000		p.o.			
Iron-59	Ferrous citrate	Ferrokinetic studies of iron metabolism	0.4	44.6 days	i.v.	Heart	32	13
Krypton-81m	Gas	Pulmonary ventilation	3600	13 s	Inhalation	Lungs	0.0002	0.00003
Phosphorus-32	Sodium phosphate	Treatment of polycythaemia vera	300	14.3 days	i.v.	Bone surfaces	11	2.2
Selenium-75	Selenomethyl	Adrenal imaging	8	119.8 days	i.v.	Adrenals	5.1	1.7
Technetium-99m	Sodium pertechnetate	Brain imaging	500	6 h	i.v.	GI tract	0.062	0.013
		Thyroid imaging	80		i.v.			
		Diagnosis of Meckel's diverticulum	400		i.v.			
Technetium-99m	Albumin aggregated (MAA) Albumin microspheres (HAM)	Lung perfusion imaging	100		i.v.	Lungs	0.067	0.012
Technetium-99m	Etefenin (EHIDA) injection	Hepatobiliary imaging	150		i.v.	Gall bladder	0.11	0.024
Technetium-99m	Exametazime HM-PAO	Region cerebral blood flow Leucocyte labelling	500 200		i.v. i.v.	Lacrimal Spleen	0.068 0.157	0.018 0.016
Technetium-99m	Glucoheptonate	Brain imaging Kidney imaging	500 300		i.v. i.v.	Bladder wall	0.056	0.009
Technetium-99m	Medronate (MDP) injection	Bone imaging	600		i.v.	Bone surfaces	0.063	0.008

Table 10.1 cont.

Radionuclide	Chemical form	Clinical use	Max activity (MBq)$^{-1}$	Half-life	Route	Critical organ	Absorbed dose (mGy MBq^{-1})	Effective dose equivalent (mSv MBq^{-1})
Technetium-99m	Pentetate (DTPA)	Brain imaging	500		i.v.	Bladder wall (4 h void)	0.08	0.063
		Kidney imaging, renograms	300		i.v.		0.047	0.007
		Lung ventilation imaging	80		Aerosol inhalation			
Technetium-99m	Stannous fluoride	Heart blood pool (Tc-RBC)	800		i.v.	Heart	0.023	0.0085
Technetium-99m	Succimer (DMSA)	Kidney imaging	80		i.v.	Kidneys	0.17	0.016
Thallium-201	Thallous chloride	Myocardial perfusion imaging	80	73.1h	i.v.	Kidneys	0.54	0.23
Xenon-133	Gas	Pulmonary ventilation imaging, cerebral blood flow	40	5.25 days	Inhalation	Lung	0.0011	0.0008

where m is the mass, in kg, of the organ whose absorbed dose is being measured. The contribution to the absorbed dose from the beta particles and the gamma rays must be calculated separately. If mathematical modelling is used, values for the masses and separating distances of the organs can be assumed and Δ and ϕ can be used to draw up a table of the dose from one organ to any other organ for unit deposited radioactivity, of a given radionuclide, in unit time. These are known as S values. Tables of Δ, ϕ, and S can be found in the publications of the Medical Internal Radiation Dose Committee (MIRD), the International Commission on Radiation Units and Measurements and the International Commission on Radiological Protection (Publication 53) (see Bibliography).

Let us consider the absorbed dose to the thyroid gland from an administered dose of 200 kBq of iodine-131, where the uptake is 35% and the mass of the gland is 20 g. The equilibrium dose rate for the beta particles is 0.110×10^{-6} kg Gy kBq^{-1} h^{-1} and for the penetrating radiations 0.217×10^{-6}. In this example the source and target organ are one and the same so the absorbed fraction for the beta particles will be 1; the absorbed fraction for the penetrating radiations is 0.03.

If we assume that none of the radioiodine leaves the thyroid gland then the effective half-life equals the physical half-life of 8.1 days (194.4 h) and the mean life (p. 20) will be 1.44×194.4 h. The cumulated activity, A_c, will therefore be:

$$200 \times 1.44 \times 194.4 \times 0.35$$
$$= 1.964 \times 10^4 \text{ kBq h}$$

From equation 10.1 the absorbed dose can be calculated as follows:

the absorbed dose from the beta particles will be

$$\frac{0.110 \times 10^{-6} \times 1}{0.02} \times 1.964 \times 10^4$$
$$= 0.108 \text{ Gy}$$

the absorbed dose from the gamma rays will be

$$\frac{0.217 \times 10^{-6} \times 0.03}{0.02} \times 1.964 \times 10^4$$
$$= 0.006 \text{ Gy}$$

and hence the total dose to the thyroid gland is 0.114 Gy.

The effective dose equivalent can also be calculated. Once the cumulated activity in the source organ is known then the dose to other target organs can be calculated by use of the S value tables. Each target organ dose can then be weighted according to the risk factor for that organ. The sum of the weighted doses in the target organs gives us the effective dose equivalent. For the 200 kBq of iodine-131 used in the example above the effective dose equivalent is 3 mSv.

Therapeutic applications

If a suitable radioactive compound is concentrated in one particular organ it seems feasible to give a very high radiation dose to the organ, which could be effective for therapeutic purposes. Unfortunately this possibility is only feasible if the ratio of the concentration of the material in the tumour to that of the body in general is very high. For example if the administration of a dose of 50 Gy to a particular organ is the aim while keeping the general whole body dose to say 0.05 or 0.1 Gy a *concentration ratio* of 500 or 1000 to 1 is required. This is hardly ever possible with available radiopharmaceuticals. The concentration ratios normally observed are at the most 10 or 100 to 1. These are suitable for diagnostic purposes since it is easy to detect and measure such concentration ratios, but they are impracticable for therapy. However, a limited number of radionuclides are suitable for therapeutic administration and these are discussed below.

Iodine-131

Iodine-131 is the most important and most extensively used unsealed therapeutic radionuclide. It decays by beta particle emission with a physical half life of 8.1 days and a principal gamma ray energy of 364 keV. The average energy of the beta particles is 246 keV and the maximum range in tissue is about 3 mm. As we saw earlier in this chapter, iodine is concentrated in the thyroid gland. This allows us to deliver a high radiation dose to the gland and a low dose to the rest of the body.

Two distinct disease states are treated by iodine-131 therapy. The first is the non-malignant condition of thyrotoxicosis, where the thyroid gland is overproducing thyroid hormones. The administered activity will depend upon the size of the gland and the degree of hyperactivity, but is usually in the range 150 to 500 MBq. With a normal sized gland and a percentage uptake of 55 the absorbed dose to the gland will be 790 mGy/MBq and the effective dose equivalent will be 24 mSv/MBq. About 90% of the absorbed dose will be due to the beta particles and 10% to the gamma rays. Radioiodine therapy for thyrotoxicosis is contraindicated in persons under the age of 40 and in pregnant or lactating women. The second condition which can be treated by radioiodine is in well-differentiated thyroid tumours and their metastases. The administered activity in this situation is much higher than for hyperthyroidism, being of the order of 2 to 8 GBq, as the aim of the treatment is to ablate all the thyroid-like tissue. The treatment may be repeated at 6-monthly intervals until no residual thyroid tissue remains.

Phosphorus-32

Phosphorus-32 comes close to being the ideal unsealed therapeutic radionuclide. It is a pure beta particle emitter with a physical half-life of 14.3 days. The average energy of the beta particles is 695 keV, resulting in a maximum range in tissue of about 8 mm. It is normally administered intravenously as sterile sodium phosphate, and is used in the treatment of polycythaemia vera and related blood disorders.

Treatment regimens vary and are a matter for clinical judgement but typical activities fall in the range 150 to 350 MBq. Following intravenous injection approximately 50% of the phosphorus-32 accumulates in the blood forming bone marrow. The absorbed dose to the bone surface and to the red marrow is 11 mGy/MBq and the effective dose equivalent is 2.2 mSv/MBq. In order to control the disease, treatment may be repeated at intervals of 6 to 12 months.

Yttrium-90

Yttrium-90 is also a pure beta particle emitter. It has a physical half-life of 64.2 hours, an average beta particle energy of 923 keV and a maximum range in tissue of about 11 mm. Although yttrium-90 is a pure

beta emitter the high energy of the beta particles can give rise to bremsstrahlung radiation.

An injection of a sterile suspension of colloidal yttrium silicate in aqueous solution is given for a variety of disease states. The activity administered will vary with the disease being treated. For example 120 to 240 MBq is injected into joints for the intra-articular treatment of arthritis, while 1 to 4 GBq is injected intrapleurally or intraperitoneally for the intracavity treatment of malignant effusions. The absorbed radiation dose to the patient will depend upon the nature of the disease state.

Strontium-89

Strontium-89 decays by beta particle emission with a physical half-life of 50.5 days. The average energy of the beta particles is 500 keV and the maximum range in tissue is about 7 mm. It is used for the palliation of pain from bone metastases secondary to prostatic and breast carcinoma. Administered activity is typically 150 MBq given intravenously as sterile strontium chloride. The absorbed dose will be dependent upon the degree of concentration of the strontium within the metastases, but can be expected to be of the order of 300 mGy/MBq. The effective dose equivalent is 2.9 mSv/MBq.

Special precautions must be observed in the care and management of patients undergoing unsealed radionuclide therapy and these have been discussed in Chapter 9.

11. Neutron and proton therapy

OXYGEN ENHANCEMENT RATIO (OER)

The results of radiobiology experiments and the experience of practical radiotherapy have demonstrated that cells starved of an oxygen supply (i.e. hypoxic cells) are very resistant to conventional forms of ionising radiations when compared with similar cells with a plentiful supply of oxygen. Some tumours and the centres of others, whose cells are starved of oxygen, therefore, are much more resistant than those containing well-oxygenated cells—they need a much larger dose of ionising radiation to produce a comparable biological effect and this larger dose might cause unacceptable normal tissue damage. To quantify this effect, an *oxygen enhancement ratio (OER)* is defined as:

$$\text{OER} = \frac{\text{Dose required in the absence of oxygen}}{\begin{array}{c}\text{Dose required in the presence of oxygen}\\ \text{to produce the same biological effect}\end{array}}$$

For ionising radiations such as X-rays and gamma rays, this ratio is large—between 2.5 and 3.0. In the ideal situation the ratio would be unity. One attempt to overcome this resistance was to use hyperbaric oxygen therapy, where the patient was treated using megavoltage X-rays in a sealed tank made of thick Perspex filled with oxygen at a pressure above the normal atmospheric pressure. In this atmosphere, the oxygen level in the blood and in the tissues was inevitably raised above normal. The technique has now been largely abandoned because the survival figures failed to show any significant improvement. The alternative is to use a radiation which does not differentiate between the hypoxic and well-oxygenated cells. It has been found that the OER decreases with the increasing linear energy transfer of the radiation.

LINEAR ENERGY TRANSFER (LET)

As a charged particle passes through an absorbing medium it loses its kinetic energy by producing ionisations and excitations in the atoms of the absorber. Insofar as the energy required to ionise any atom in the absorber is almost constant, the number of ionisations produced by a particle in motion will be proportional to its initial energy. Furthermore the distance travelled in the absorber will also be determined by its initial energy. The rate at which its energy is transferred to the absorber is known as the linear energy transfer (LET) and measured in keV per micrometre of track. Although average values can be quoted (e.g. the initial energy divided by the range), the actual LET increases as the particle energy falls and the distance travelled between ionisations decreases. This is portrayed in what is known as the Bragg curve. For an individual particle, the Bragg curve is pointed because the peak LET is reached as the particle comes to rest, whereas for a beam of particles it is more rounded (Fig. 11.1) with a definite tail due to the small spread of the energies present in the beam.

Electrons set in motion by the gamma radiation from cobalt-60 have a LET of approximately 0.25 keV μm^{-1}, or 250 eV μm^{-1}. If it is assumed 25 eV is required to produce one ionisation in tissue and less than half that

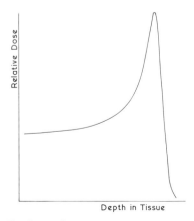

Fig. 11.1 The Bragg Gray curve.

to produce an excitation, then each electron will produce less than 10 ionisations per micron. Heavier charged particles (protons (hydrogen nuclei), alpha particles (helium nuclei) and the nuclei of other atoms) have LET values several hundred times greater. (The electrons released through the ionisation of atoms by particle radiations are known as *delta rays* and may be given sufficient energy in the process to produce further ionisations, perhaps remote from the track of the heavy charged particle. Where this may be significant the LET quoted may only refer to delta ray energies of less than, say, 100 eV, in which case a suffix will be given, i.e. LET_{100} and all the energy will be deposited close to the track. LET_{inf} is the total LET and is approximately double the LET_{100}.)

The biological damage is dependent on the energy deposited in each cell, which in general will be less than 1 μm in diameter. Thus low LET radiations will deposit less energy in each cell, minimising the chance of biological damage being caused. On the other hand, high LET radiations increase that chance, but there is a peak beyond which the biological damage no longer increases with LET—a state of 'overkill' takes place where more energy is being deposited in each cell than is necessary to kill the cell. The *relative biological effectiveness (RBE)* is the ratio of the X-ray dose to the high LET dose required to produce the same level of biological damage. The RBE peaks at a LET value of about 100 keV μm⁻¹.

Although a variety of high LET heavy particle radiations are generated, most require very high energy cyclotrons or synchrotrons operating at several hundred million electron volts. These will not be considered further.

PROPERTIES OF NEUTRONS

Neutrons have a mass slightly greater than the mass of a proton (1.67×10^{-27} kg) but no charge. They can therefore pass freely through the cloud of electrons orbiting the nucleus of an atom. The simplest interaction is the elastic collision of the neutron with a nucleus, which in turn is set in motion. This positively charged heavy ion (the nucleus) loses its energy by producing intense ionisation, while the neutron continues on its path with reduced energy. The lighter the nucleus, the greater the energy transferred from the neutron to the nucleus. Hydrogen being the lightest element is, therefore, the most efficient absorber of neutrons. Hydrogen compounds, especially paraffin wax, are invariably used as protective barriers against neutrons. Steel is also useful. The human body contains considerable quantities of hydrogen (10%) and

therefore readily absorbs neutrons—the elastic collision being the dominant process. Neutrons may be captured by the hydrogen nuclei and produce 2.2 MeV photons, the so-called (n, gamma) reaction.

Other light elements readily capture neutrons and produce alpha particles which in turn produce intense ionisation which is readily detectable and absorbed. For example, boron:

$$^{10}_{5}B + ^{1}_{0}n \longrightarrow ^{7}_{3}Li + ^{4}_{2}He$$

This emission of an alpha particle forms the basis of several neutron detectors, boron trifluoride gas-filled ionisation chambers, boric oxide/zinc sulphide scintillation crystals and boron/silver bromide emulsions for photographic plates. The ionisation chamber is generally used for dose and dose rate measurements in neutron therapy. Developments in the design of ionisation chambers now enable them to be made tissue equivalent in terms of the hydrogen content by the careful selection of wall material and enclosed gas, for example polyethylene and ethylene oxide respectively. (Note. Tissue equivalence takes into account the interaction processes of the radiation and therefore a tissue equivalent ionisation chamber for X-rays is not necessarily tissue equivalent for neutrons.)

It will be explained in Chapter 12 that the dose equivalent for neutrons is some 10 times greater than for X- and gamma rays, and therefore the permitted leakage radiation levels are smaller by a similar factor (p. 213).

Radioactive isotopes may be produced in any material which is irradiated with neutrons, but, fortunately, the quantities and the half-lives of the isotopes produced in the radiotherapy department are small. The half-life of the isotopes produced are in the range of 2 to 150 min. The additional dose given to the patient as a result of neutron activation within the patient is insignificant. On the other hand, and despite special care in the choice of materials in the manufacture of neutron therapy beam installations, the treatment couch and the treatment room walls, etc. may constitute a radiation hazard to staff unless strict controls are observed. For example, the use of the neutron beam will be restricted so as to limit the production of radionuclides, thereby keeping the background radiation down to a safe level. The protected walls may be of concrete, with a limestone base rather than sandstone, and lined with a hydrogenous material such as polyethylene, to absorb the thermal (low energy) neutrons. The use of aluminium and manganese (commonly found in steel) has to be avoided because they readily absorb thermal neutrons which give rise to high levels of radioactivity. On some older machines, the beam applicators become particularly active because of their proximity to the source and a means had to be provided whereby they could be changed by remote control and stored in a protected enclosure.

SOURCES OF NEUTRONS

The early experience of neutron therapy in California in the 1940s was discouraging but the development work done by the Medical Research Council in the 1960s at Hammersmith in London was more optimistic and other centres in the UK and abroad began investigating the technique. The most recent results from Clatterbridge, however, suggest that neutrons are only advantageous for a number of relatively rare tumours occurring mainly in the head and neck region. Initially the cyclotron was thought to be too large and the available dose rate too low to be clinically useful and the D-T generator was preferred. However the failure to solve many of the technical problems of the generator means the cyclotron is again the preferred source for neutron beam therapy. Interstitial and intracavitary therapy can be carried out with neutrons from the radioisotope californium-252.

Californium-252

Californium is a transuranic element which decays by both alpha emission and spontaneous fission, producing both gamma rays and neutrons, with an effective half-life of 2.65 years. The fission spectrum neutrons have an energy of about 2 MeV and the complex gamma spectrum falls between that of caesium-137 and that of cobalt-60. The active content of the sources is smaller than for radium at a few micrograms of the element, but otherwise the structure of the source is similar to those shown in Figures 8.2 and 8.15, only thinner.

The mixed radiation—neutrons and gamma rays—gives rise to problems in dosimetry and in general the measurement of dose is assessed separately. The actual ratio of neutron dose to gamma dose varies with the design of the source and the distance from the source. The oxygen enhancement ratio is about half of that for X-rays at low dose rates but increases with dose rate, making the use of high dose rate techniques of little value. Remote afterloading techniques are, however, recommended even at low dose rates. Bedshields to protect nursing staff exposed to sources in situ would have to be very massive as they would have to include both lead to attenuate the gamma rays and hydrogenous material to absorb the neutrons.

The RBE for californium-252 neutrons at low dose rate is approximately seven, suggesting that a dose of 9 Gy of californium-252 neutrons would produce the same biological effect as 60 Gy of radium gamma radiation over the same period of time, typically 7 days.

The size and cost of the necessary protective shield prohibits the use of californium-252 as a source of neutrons for teletherapy.

D-T generator

After the early work with cyclotrons, the D-T generator appeared to be the more practical source of neutrons for teletherapy. It is essentially a sealed tube—about the size of an orthovoltage X-ray tube insert—in which deuterons (deuterium nuclei) are accelerated to about 200 kV to bombard tritium nuclei. Hence the abbreviation D-T. Deuterium and tritium are isotopes of hydrogen, and the process occurring in the target is given by the equation,

$$_1^2H + _1^3H \longrightarrow _2^4He + _0^1n + 17.6\,MeV$$

the surplus energy being shared between the neutron (approximately 14 MeV) and the alpha particle. The generator has the advantage that it is relatively small and compact and can be readily mounted on an isocentric gantry in a conventional design of treatment room. The operating costs are less than for a cyclotron. However, one of the problems of the system is that the tritium target has only a limited life and so far efforts have not produced a clinically acceptable tube, i.e a tube

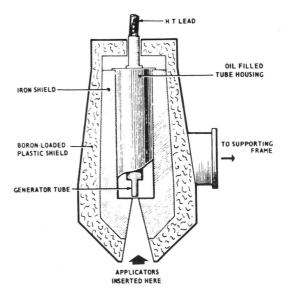

Fig. 11.2 The D-T generator. (Reproduced with permission from Meredith & Massey 1977.)

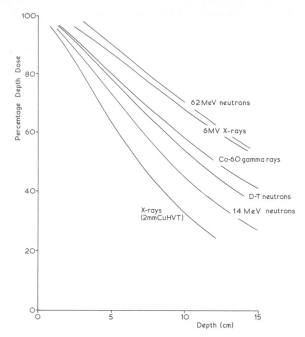

Fig. 11.3 Depth dose curves for neutrons compared with those for photons.

which will run for several hundred hours producing an acceptable dose rate (greater than 0.20 Gy per minute) with an emission of 10^{13} neutrons per second.

The tube has to be housed in a protective shield in which both the neutrons will be slowed down and the gamma rays will be attenuated (Fig. 11.2). The shield is essentially made of iron surrounded in boron-loaded polythene to absorb the low energy (thermal) neutrons which penetrate the iron. The collimating applicators are of similar construction, but using steel instead of iron. The collimators are some 50 cm long. The D-T tube produces neutrons of a higher energy than the cyclotron and their penetration is correspondingly deeper. The depth dose is still less than that for cobalt-60 gamma rays, however, even at 125 cm SSD (Fig. 11.3).

The technical problems of target life and dose rate have not been overcome and the D-T tube is now of historic interest only.

Cyclotron

The operation of the cyclotron has been discussed earlier (Ch. 2) and there is no need to repeat that outline here other than to stress that the cyclotron is capable of accelerating any type of charged particle. For any one cyclotron, the lighter the particle, the higher its final energy, but because of relativistic effects the theoretical maximum energy increases

with the mass of the particle. The proton (the hydrogen nucleus) can be accelerated to higher energies than electrons. Also almost any target material may be used, but it is found that low atomic number targets are more prolific in producing neutrons. Beryllium ($Z = 4$) is the most common. Bombarding a beryllium target with protons produces the reaction:

$$^1_1p + ^9_4Be \longrightarrow ^9_5B + ^1_0n - 1.85 \text{ MeV}$$

The dose rate available from this reaction is, however, small. The alternative is to accelerate the deuteron (the deuterium nucleus consisting of a proton and a neutron) which reacts with the beryllium target as follows:

$$^2_1d + ^9_4Be \longrightarrow ^{10}_5B + ^1_0n + 3.79 \text{ MeV}$$

as in Hammersmith (London) and Edinburgh. Although the neutron energy is lower, the dose rate from this deuteron-beryllium reaction is more satisfactory.

The larger cyclotrons, such as the 62 MeV proton cyclotron at Clatterbridge, Liverpool (Fig. 11.4), use the proton–beryllium reaction because, with the higher energy, both the beam penetration and the dose rate are improved. Operating at 150 cm source–axis distance the Clatterbridge cyclotron produces a neutron depth dose similar to 8 MV X-rays at 100 cm SSD (approx. 70% at 10 cm deep). At these higher energies, there is a low energy neutron component which has to be filtered out using a polythene filter several centimetres thick. The resulting dose rate is typically 0.5 Gy min⁻¹.

It is normal practice to have the cyclotron in one room with the treatment facility in an adjacent room, with a fixed horizontal beam in the early installations. With the development of *beam transport systems*, it has been possible to construct a neutron beam therapy

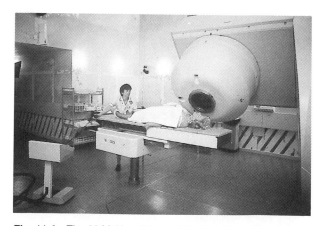

Fig. 11.4 The 62 MeV cyclotron at Clatterbridge. (Courtesy of the Medical Research Council Cyclotron Unit, Clatterbridge, UK.)

unit on an isocentric gantry. The large electromagnets required to bend the beam may mean these units are limited in practice to less than 60 MeV. Those that have been built have been limited to a gantry rotation of ± 120° unless a movable floor facility is included. As with the D-T generator, the beam sizes are selected by interchangeable applicators, often made of wood, benelex or water-based polymer. Variable collimators made of iron and boronated polythene are in use on the Clatterbridge unit, and multileaf collimators are being used in some centres.

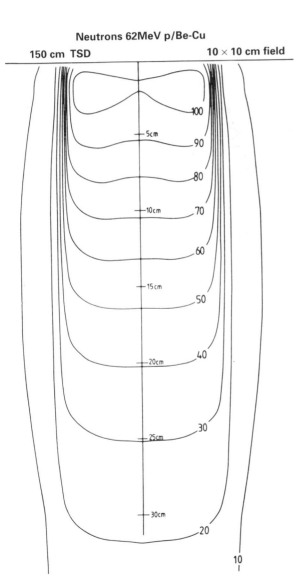

Fig. 11.5 A neutron beam isodose chart. (Courtesy of the Medical Research Council Cyclotron Unit, Clatterbridge, UK.)

NEUTRON TREATMENT PLANNING

The complexity of the collimator system means the range of field sizes available is limited: 5×5 to $30 \times 30\ cm^2$ being typical. The isodose curves for neutron beams are characterised by their rounded appearance due to the scatter generated within the beam and a relatively large penumbra (Fig. 11.5). This dependence on scatter means the use of wedges is handicapped by a decreasing wedge angle with increasing depth (a problem previously encountered when wedges were introduced at orthovoltage X-ray energies). The wedges may be made of polyethylene or of iron. The planning processes are therefore similar to those outlined in Chapter 6 for photons. Bolus may also be used providing it has the same scattering and attenuation properties as soft tissue. This requires some 10% hydrogen.

Within the tissues of the body, bone is low in hydrogen and absorbs less dose than soft tissue, whereas fat is high in hydrogen and absorbs more than the soft tissues —both processes having the opposite effect to those in a photon beam. Where the resulting skin dose is high, it is more often due to the superficial fat than to the lack of skin sparing properties in the beam.

Neutron radiography may be used to verify the therapeutic beam but the image quality is no better than one expects from megavoltage X-rays, the only visible contrast being between the tissues and air cavities. The large source size not only gives rise to the large penumbra on the therapy beam but also to poor image quality on the portal film. The gamma radiation generated within the patient by the neutrons further degrades the image quality.

The unique complicating factor is that with any neutron beam there is a significant gamma contamination from the bombardment of the hydrogen nuclei, and therefore any statement of dose needs to include either a separation of the two components or a statement of total dose with an indication of how the two components have been weighted in the summation. The statement is required to include the primary neutron spectrum, namely the type and energy of accelerated particle and the type of target. Phantom measurements suggest the gamma dose component increases with depth, reaching some 15% of the total (n + gamma) local dose at a depth of 20 cm, reflecting the importance of the (2.2 MeV) gamma rays produced within the tissues by the capture of thermal neutrons. Field size and collimator design are also important factors.

The numerical magnitude of the gamma component is, however, misleading in that it is biologically much smaller in comparison with the neutron component after the RBE has been taken into account. To this end some centres, particularly in Europe, calculate and quote an effective neutron dose using a formula such as:

$$D_{eff} = D_n + D_{gamma}/3$$

but this is not universally accepted and has to be used with caution.

PROPERTIES OF PROTONS

Protons are hydrogen nuclei and therefore are positively charged particles of a mass approximately equal to that of a neutron. Protons accelerated to high energy travel in straight lines—they are less easily scattered than neutrons—and have a precise range in tissue determined by their energy. Following the Bragg curve, the energetic proton loses its energy progressively along its track, with most of its energy deposited near to where the particle comes to rest. Protons have a LET in the range from 5 to 100 keV μm^{-1}, and therefore not very different from that for electrons (X-rays and gamma rays). The RBE is approximately 1.10.

The dosimetry of proton beams is simpler than the dosimetry of neutron beams in that there is less 'contamination' of the proton beam with gamma radiation. Calorimetry (p. 77) is the primary dose standard for proton beams. The absorbing block is mounted on insulators in an evacuated chamber, as it is for photons, but for proton dosimetry it is also operated in a magnetic field to deflect secondary electrons back into the absorber. The secondary standard may be an ionisation chamber used in isolation or in conjunction with a Faraday cup which measures the number of protons in the beam. The 'cup' is an absorber of sufficient thickness to stop all the protons and the secondary particles (electrons). Each proton carries a single positive charge. A measure of the total charge collected enables the total number of protons absorbed to be calculated, providing the loss of charge is minimised.

For practical dosimetry, ionisation chambers may be used—transmission chambers monitor the output dose rate from the proton beam generator and smaller parallel-plate chambers may be used to measure doses in a phantom. The composition of the chamber wall is less critical than for photons, but the choice of gas is more critical—oxygen-free nitrogen is often used. Thermoluminescence and photographic film may also be used with protons.

SOURCES OF PROTONS

Just as the high energy electron beam can be extracted from a linear accelerator by removing the X-ray target, so the proton beam can be extracted from a cyclotron but, rather than removing the beryllium target, the protons are extracted through a separate beam line and through an energy modulator. Because of the sharp Bragg peak, the energy of the proton beam needs to be modulated to spread the peak over the thickness of the target tissues. This may be done mechanically using an energy modulator—a fan with Perspex blades of varying thickness rotating about an axis parallel to the beam axis so that the protons pass through the blades or a Perspex wedge passing through the beam. A selection of fans (or wedges) enables the Bragg peak to be spread over the desired range. After passing through this energy modulator, the proton beam is scattered by passing it through a metal foil to produce a broad beam. The final collimation of the proton beam is a brass aperture tailored to the shape of the tumour, again analogous to the cut-outs used in electron beam collimators. The proton dose rate is typically 0.5 Gy min[1].

Unfortunately the proton energy required to treat tumours at depth is very large. The cyclotron at Clatterbridge in the UK can produce a neutron beam with a mean energy of 30 MeV capable of treating tissues anywhere in the body, but its 60 MeV protons will only penetrate to a depth of about 3 cm of soft tissue. The Clatterbridge team are therefore limiting themselves to treating eyes and ocular melanoma in particular. They are conducting the first formal clinical trial of proton therapy in the treatment of this disease.

Proton beam energies of about 250 MeV are required if treatments are to be effected anywhere in the body. Unfortunately most of the equipment capable of these high energies is based in physics research laboratories and not in hospitals. Nevertheless, patients have been treated effectively in places like Tsukuba in Japan, using a 250 MeV beam from a 500 MeV research machine, and in Uppsala, Sweden, although the patient numbers remain small. The collaboration between the Harvard Cyclotron Laboratory and the Massachusetts General Hospital has resulted in the largest number of patients being treated in this way—despite being limited to a horizontal beam. More recently a proton synchrotron has been built for the Loma Linda University Medical Center in California to produce proton beams up to 250 MeV. The synchrotron uses an eight magnet ring 6 metres in diameter to feed the proton beam to one of four radiation rooms—in three of these treatment rooms the gantries are 35 ft (10–11 m) in diameter and weigh 90 tons (91×10^3 kg).

TREATMENT PLANNING WITH PROTONS

Because of the Bragg peak, a single beam of protons can deliver a higher dose to the target at depth than to the intervening tissues with a negligible dose to the

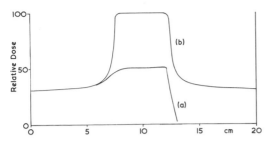

Fig. 11.6 (a) The spread out peak for a proton beam and (b) the dose profile resulting from the addition of an identical but parallel opposed beam.

tissues beyond (Figs 11.6 and 11.7). The penumbra edge (80% to 20%) may be as small as 2 mm, giving the beam a very sharply defined edge.

Higher energy protons justify the use of the parallel opposed or cross-fire techniques of conventional radiotherapy (Ch. 6). Figure 11.6B shows the distribution along the common axes of a parallel opposed pair, and should be compared with Figure 6.3.

The use of three and four field techniques enhances the target-healthy tissue dose ratio even further, thus eliminating many of the side-effects associated with the unnecessary irradiation of healthy tissue. The range of the energetic proton is primarily dependent on the electron density of the absorbing medium and therefore small changes in tissue density may not be important, whereas volumes of air in the beam will need compensation. Compensators made of Perspex may be used to correct for curvature of the incident surface, but more frequently they are used to modify the shape of the dose distribution to fit the shape of the target tissues more closely and/or to protect adjacent healthy tissues.

This dependence on electron density means the CT data may be used for the detailed three-dimensional treatment planning needed where the target tissues are in close proximity to sensitive healthy tissues—the narrow penumbra makes proton therapy the preferred option for these cases.

Strict immobilisation is essential prior to any CT scan to ensure the patient's position is maintained throughout the planning and treatment programme.

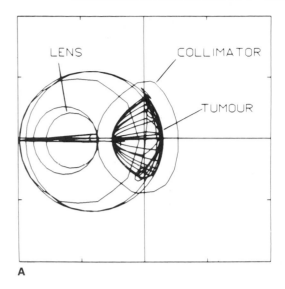

A

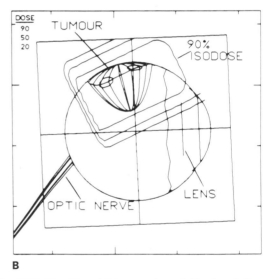

B

Fig. 11.7 The Clatterbridge eye dose distribution: **A** the beam's eye view of the target tissues and **B** the principal isodose curves. (Courtesy of the Medical Research Council Cyclotron Unit, Clatterbridge, UK.)

12. Radiation protection

INTRODUCTION

The biological effects of ionising radiation on a single component cell and a complete organism such as the human body are described briefly in this chapter; there is more detail in Part 2 of this book. Arising from the study of these effects, levels of radiation dose which can be accepted in a normal working environment and in the environment as a whole have been specified by authoritative international expert committees, principally the International Commission on Radiological Protection (ICRP). This chapter contains an account of the acceptable dose levels, and the steps which must be taken to keep within these dose levels in practice. However in order to appreciate the problems involved in establishing adequate control of the radiation hazard, and also to understand the apparently complicated specifications of a dose limit, it is necessary to summarise the available knowledge of the effects produced in human beings by low doses of ionising radiations. Radiation hazards are a matter of great concern to members of the general public. Radiographers are professionally in an important position to help ensure that the public, particularly patients in hospital, have an appreciation of the hazards, of the steps taken to control them, and of the relative dangers of using ionising radiation compared to other activities of normal living.

BIOLOGICAL EFFECTS OF RADIATION

It is well known that a variety of injuries can result from excessive doses of ionising radiation. The following list illustrates the need to consider a wide variety of possible working conditions and techniques when safety rules are drawn up:

1. Injuries to the skin arising from exposure of the epidermis to radiation of quite low penetrating power, such as beta rays or low energy photons.
2. Changes in the blood-forming organs and in the number and nature of the circulating blood cells. These changes will arise from exposure of the bone marrow to penetrating radiations received externally, or from radiations from internally distributed radioactive materials.
3. Cancer produced in both bones and other tissues by exposure to radiation arising from either external or internal sources.
4. Cataract formation due to irradiation of the eye lens by radiation of low penetrating power.
5. Genetic effects arising from the production of mutations by the irradiation of the reproductive system.

To specify levels of radiation exposure so as to avoid these injurious effects, detailed quantitative information is needed relating the incidence of the effects to the radiation doses which produce them. The information available is not complete but it is sufficient to enable dose limits to be incorporated in the various regulations and recommendations published in many countries.

EVIDENCE OF DAMAGE BY LOW DOSES

There are five main sources of information on the long-term effects of relatively low doses of ionising radiation or of the effects of higher doses of radiation which can be used to estimate the effects of low doses.

Early history of radiation damage

The radiation damage received by many early workers with X-rays and radium has been studied in detail. It was realised in the early days when the medical use of radiation was growing rapidly that there could be a long time interval, often of many years, between the radiation exposure and the observable damage. It was not realised that long periods of exposure at low dose rates could be as damaging as shorter periods at higher dose rates. The damage suffered by the early radiologists was predominantly of two types. First, damage to the tissues of the hands resulting from exposing them to the direct beam of X-rays (Plate 9), or handling radium sources with the fingers. (In these early days, radiologists practised both radiodiagnosis and radiotherapy.) This damage was often very serious, giving rise to malignant and sometimes fatal changes. Second, damage to the haemopoietic system, the site of blood cell formation in the bone marrow. This arose generally from exposure of the whole body to scattered radiation over long periods or the ingestion of radionuclides, again giving rise to fatal conditions. Though these two effects were eventually recognised, the magnitude of the dose to which the workers had been subjected years before could never be established accurately. In the nuclear industry today, some of those occupationally exposed may be receiving doses close to the recommended limits, and the doses may be assessed, but the numbers of workers are small and the exposures too recent, in comparison to the latent period, to correlate the effects accurately.

Evidence from radiation accidents

A great deal of evidence about radiation damage has been obtained from the study of accidental exposures to X-rays and to radionuclides in industrial and research processes and in medical practice. In spite of extreme care, accidental exposures do occur and detailed investigations into such events reveal valuable information of two kinds. First, a consideration of the circumstances which led to the accident may suggest improved techniques for the safe control of the radiation facility. These may become incorporated into the regulations and recommendations in an attempt to avoid any repetition. Second, if it is possible to observe the clinical damage produced and obtain a reasonable estimate of the dose involved, the information can be valuable in establishing further data on the dose–effect relationships. The Chernobyl disaster of April 1986 has precipitated a great deal of evaluation and investigation in this area of dose and effect.

Long-term effects of atomic weapons

The use of the atomic bombs on the Japanese cities of Hiroshima and Nagasaki at the end of World War II in August 1945 exposed large populations to a sudden acute radiation dose. The immediate effects of these explosions were due mainly to the intense heat and the explosive violence of the event and only in part to the high dose of radiation. However, large numbers of survivors in both cities have been studied continuously since 1945. The incidence of disease amongst these survivors, and the incidence of possible effects on those irradiated in utero, or the offspring of irradiated parents, have all been matched carefully against a similar population believed to be unirradiated. The radiation dose which the victims received at the time of the explosion has been estimated in a number of ways, including investigations of the position of the subject with respect to the explosion centre. The effects of this single dose of gamma rays and neutrons have been followed over a period of nearly 50 years, and the results have contributed valuable data on which safety levels can be based. A recent re-evaluation of the doses received by the survivors has suggested that early estimates were too high and the subsequent injuries were due to lower doses than previously thought. This study played a major part in the decision in the late 1980s to lower the 'safe' dose limits.

Results of animal experiments

Radiobiology has developed greatly over the last 40 years and much information has been obtained by experimental irradiation of various animals. In this case, both the irradiation effects and the administered dose can be very precisely observed. The fact that radiation damages chromosomes is well established, but a quantitative estimate of the magnitude of these effects could not be observed in human beings. Experimental data have to be obtained from species in which the generation life is short enough to enable adequate observation of effects. Most of the quantitative evidence comes from experimental work on the fruit fly and on mice.

The extrapolation of experimental animal data to humans accounts for the doubt, for example, of the exact radiation dose which would double the naturally occurring mutation rate in humans, though this is estimated to be about 0.5 Gy. There is also some uncertainty about the exact relationship between effect and dose for very low dose rates. Conservative extrapolations are invariably used when deducing appropriate safety standards so as to err on the safe side.

Evidence from radiotherapy

Finally, a great deal of careful observation and long experience in radiotherapy give a firm correlation of radiation effects against administered dose for a wide variety of conditions. However, this evidence always relates to dose levels between perhaps 1 Gy and (say) 50 Gy to selected tissues. Sadly, there have been a few accidental irradiations to higher levels of dose but again to small selected volumes of tissue. It is doubtful if these data can be used to estimate the effect of a few milligrays on the whole body.

RADIATION EFFECTS AT LOW DOSES

There are two facts about the possible effects of radiation at low dose levels which make precision very difficult. The first is that the predicted effects cannot be distinguished from the same conditions which occur spontaneously without the influence of additional ionising radiation. For example, there is a natural incidence of malignant disease, and the incidence rate varies with the type and site of the cancer, and with the environment to which the population is subjected. There are environmental causes of malignant disease other than radiation, though these causes are complex and only understood in a very incomplete way. The second fact that needs to be noted is that there is a natural radiation level in the environment to which all populations down the ages have been exposed and which it is impossible to avoid. It arises from a number of causes: cosmic radiation from extraterrestrial sources, the radioactivity in rocks and therefore in building materials, and in water sources and so on. There is natural radioactivity in the body, potassium-40 for example, which is a beta emitter of long half-life ($T_{\frac{1}{2}} = 1.3 \times 10^9$ years).

There is a possibility that some part of the natural incidence of malignant disease can be ascribed to natural sources of ionising radiation but the extent to which this occurs is not known. Radiation is certainly only one of many environmental factors which can lead to malignancies. The addition of man-made sources of ionising radiation to the environmental sources will give rise to an increase, albeit small, in both the incidence of malignant disease and of genetic abnormalities.

The effects of ionising radiation begin with the ionisation of an atom or molecule within a cell. On the basis that many million million ionisations are produced in the DNA alone every year by the naturally occurring radiations and only one in four deaths is attributable to cancer, then we must conclude that such cell damage is only rarely manifested in the formation of a cancer. The cell is not necessarily damaged. If it is damaged, the damage may be repaired by the body's defence mechanisms. If it is severely damaged, it may die or it may go on proliferating in a modified form and, after a latent period, produce a cancer. These effects are very much chance effects, starting from the ionisation of a single cell. There is therefore no threshold dose below which one can say it will not happen, but equally no dose above which it is certain to happen. The technical term

used to describe these chance effects is *stochastic* and where the effect is manifest in the person exposed the effect is said to be *somatic*. Somatic stochastic effects then are those which cannot be clearly ascribed to a particular dose of ionising radiation received by an individual. They can only be detected by observing an increased incidence of a known abnormality in a large group of individuals for whom an increase in radiation exposure has taken place.

Where the irradiated cells belong to the reproductive system (germ cells), the modified cells may be responsible for passing on incorrect hereditary information to the next generation. Such genetic defects may be trivial or may lead to serious disability or even death. However, these *hereditary* effects have only been suggested by experiments on plants and animals; they have not been detected in man.

In the event that the cell damage leads to a predictable loss of organ function, as revealed by some pathological condition, the effect is said to be *deterministic*. In contrast to the stochastic effect, the deterministic effect appears to require a threshold dose (or dose rate) below which the condition will not be observed—unless there are causes other than radiation contributing to its onset.

The effects of radiation on the developing embryo are very dependent on the time of exposure. At the early stages, there are few cells involved and exposure to radiation is likely to cause an undetectable death of the embryo rather than result in deterministic or stochastic effects in the live-born. After the third week, radiation may increase the probability of cancer or organ malfunction. Data from Hiroshima and Nagasaki on children exposed in utero suggest there may be a shift downwards in intelligence quotient (IQ), with the shift increasing with dose. The shift seems to be smaller where the exposure was after the 16th week of pregnancy. The probable mechanism is interruption of nerve cells migrating into the cerebral cortex. Mental retardation has been observed only in a few cases, where it amounted to about 30 IQ points per sievert of exposure.

NATURAL BACKGROUND RADIATION

To put these radiation effects into perspective, it is worth looking at the 'natural' radiations to which we are all exposed, and then at the 'artificial' radiations to which most of us are exposed at some time or other.

By natural radiations, we mean those radiations within the environment over which we have no control other than to protect ourselves by choosing a particular lifestyle. For example, cosmic radiations bombard the earth from outer space and their intensity will depend on the angle at which they strike the surface of the earth and the degree to which they are absorbed in the atmosphere. Our exposure to cosmic radiation will therefore depend on the altitude at which we live and the time we spend in high flying aircraft.

Perhaps the major source of 'natural' radiation is the gas radon, which permeates through the rocks into the atmosphere and through the foundations into our homes. The intensity of radon exposure varies considerably around the world and within the UK it is minimal in the fenlands of Lincolnshire, higher in parts of the Pennines and up to three times the average in Cornwall. Therefore the place we choose to live and the type of dwelling we choose to live in will determine our exposure to radon. The radon entering our homes will be determined by the design of the foundations and the choice of building materials. Where radon permeates into a well-insulated house, the concentration of the gas will be higher. A well-ventilated house with a special membrane incorporated into the foundations will have a lower concentration of the gas. Existing properties may be improved by increasing the under-floor ventilation, thereby diverting the radon before it enters the living areas. The exposure of miners to radon has been well-documented over the years, and pot-holers are becoming increasingly aware of the potential hazards of radon.

Small traces of potassium-40 can be found in the human body and are also present in many fertilisers, through which it enters the food chain. All these 'natural' sources contribute an average dose to the UK population of approximately 2.2 mSv per annum, of which about one-half is attributable to radon.

In addition, there is the smaller component from the 'artificial' or man-made sources of radiation, amounting on average in the UK to about 0.3 mSv per annum. Most of this comes from the diagnostic uses of X-rays. (Although the individual doses are small, large numbers of exposures are performed.) The total diagnostic medical exposure is so large that a major report published in 1990 has highlighted the need to reduce it by reducing the number of examinations (claiming that 20% contribute nothing to the diagnosis of the patient) and by optimising the exposure parameters and the equipment. Although the exposure to patients receiving radiotherapy is considerably greater than this, the relatively small numbers contribute little to the population average. The other 'artificial' sources of radiation often highlighted in the media contribute relatively insignificant levels to the overall background dose.

The UK average background dose is approximately 2.5 mSv per annum and breaks down as shown in the

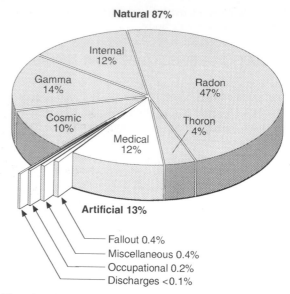

Fig. 12.1 The background radiation levels in the UK total an average of 2.5 mSv per year (by courtesy of the National Radiological Protection Board).

pie chart (Fig. 12.1); it should be remembered that regional variations are quite large.

DOSE LIMITATION

The deleterious effects of radiation have been recognised and the aim of radiation protection legislation and practice is to allow the benefits of radiation to be gained, both for the individual and for the population as a whole, without paying too high a price. To this end, the International Commission on Radiological Protection (ICRP) in 1990 elaborated on the three main features for dose limitation they laid down in 1977 (Publication 26) for any practice involving ionising radiation. (The extracts that follow together with Tables 12.1–12.3 are reprinted, with kind permission, from the Annals of the ICRP, Publication 60, H. Smith (ed), copyright 1991, International Commission on Radiological Protection.)

1. *Justification of a practice.* No practice involving exposures to radiation should be adopted unless it produces sufficient benefit to the exposed individuals or to society to offset the radiation detriment it causes.

2. *Optimisation of protection.* In relation to any particular source within a practice, the magnitude of individual doses, the number of people exposed, and the likelihood of incurring exposures where these are not certain to be received should be kept as low as reasonably achievable, economic and social factors being

taken into account. This procedure should be constrained by restrictions on the doses to individuals (dose constraints), or the risks to individuals in the case of potential exposures (risk constraints), so as to limit the inequity likely to result from the inherent economic and social judgements.

3. *Individual dose and risk limits.* The exposure of individuals resulting from the combination of all the relevant practices should be subject to dose limits, or to some control of risk in the case of potential exposures. These are aimed at ensuring that no individual is exposed to radiation risks that are judged to be unacceptable from these practices in any normal circumstances. Not all sources are susceptible to control by action at the source and it is necessary to specify sources to be included as relevant before selecting a dose limit.

The second of these statements has been widely known as the ALARA principle. Both (1) and (2) apply equally to those occupationally exposed as to those exposed as patients. There are no dose limits laid down for the exposure of patients, other than those deemed to be 'accepted practice'. Medical practitioners are legally responsible for ensuring their practice is within accepted guidelines. The exposure of patients should be the minimum consistent with the medical benefit to the patient.

Equivalent dose

Absorbed dose, D, has been defined (p. 72) as the energy absorbed per unit mass, and in the context of radiotherapy, the dose to water is an adequate measure, along with the statement of beam quality. It is, however, inadequate as a measure of the deleterious effects resulting from multiple sources of radiation. In radiotherapy, the dose is given under controlled conditions

whereas, in the context of radiation protection, the deleterious effect may result from an accumulation of exposures from different sources of radiation and maybe to different tissues of the body. The term *equivalent dose*, H_T, is the absorbed dose, D_{TR}, weighted by W_R, the radiation weighting factor (Table 12.1). The equivalent dose in sieverts ($J\ kg^{-1}$) is then given by:

$$H_T = \Sigma\ D_{TR} W_R$$

where the summation allows for the effects of a range of radiations to be taken into account. Equivalent dose cannot be used to assess the effects of radiotherapy or the early consequences of severe accidental exposures.

Effective dose

The probability of a stochastic effect is dependent not only on the equivalent dose but also on the organ or tissue receiving that dose. It is therefore necessary to

Table 12.1 Radiation weighting factors*

Type and energy range	Radiation weighting factor, W_R
Photons, all energies	1
Electrons and muons, all energies	1
Neutrons, energy < 10 keV	5
> 10–100 keV	10
> 100 keV – 2 MeV	20
> 2–20 MeV	10
> 20 MeV	5
Protons, other than recoil protons, energy > 2 MeV	5
Alpha particles, fission fragments, heavy nuclei	20

* All values relate to the radiation incident on the body or, for internal sources, emitted from the source.
(Reproduced with permission from ICRP 1991.)

Table 12.2 Tissue weighting factors*

Tissue or organ	Tissue weighting factor, W_T
Gonads	0.20
Bone marrow (red)	0.12
Colon	0.12
Lung	0.12
Stomach	0.12
Bladder	0.05
Breast	0.05
Liver	0.05
Oesophagus	0.05
Thyroid	0.05
Skin	0.01
Bone surface	0.01
Remainder	0.05†‡

* The values have been developed from a reference population of equal numbers of both sexes and a wide range of ages. In the definition of effective dose they apply to workers, to the whole population, and to either sex.
† For purposes of calculation, the remainder is composed of the following additional tissues and organs: adrenals, brain, upper large intestine, small intestine, kidney, muscle, pancreas, spleen, thymus and uterus. The list includes organs which are likely to be selectively irradiated. Some organs in the list are known to be susceptible to cancer induction. If other tissues and organs subsequently become identified as having a significant risk of induced cancer they will then be included either with a specific W_T or in this additional list constituting the remainder. The latter may also include other tissues or organs selectively irradiated.
‡ In those exceptional cases in which a single one of the remainder tissues or organs receives an equivalent dose in excess of the highest dose in any of the twelve organs for which a weighting factor is specified, a weighting factor of 0.025 should be applied to that tissue or organ and a weighting factor of 0.025 to the average dose in the rest of the remainder as defined above.
(Reproduced with permission from ICRP 1991.)

bring the tissue itself into the analysis of risk by applying a tissue weighting factor, W_T, to the equivalent dose, H_T. The summation of this product is called the *effective dose*, E, where

$$E = \Sigma \, H_T W_T$$

The recommended values of W_T are given in Table 12.2. In the event of the whole body being uniformly irradiated, the equivalent dose, H_T, is numerically equal to the effective dose, E, because $\Sigma W_T = 1$.

By implication, if only one tissue is irradiated, then the dose limit for that tissue would be the whole body dose equivalent limit divided by the appropriate weighting factor. Weighting factors are particularly important when isotopes may be taken into the body by inhalation or ingestion or through injuries or absorption through the skin. The radionuclide itself, or the label to which it is attached, will determine where the isotope is likely to be concentrated in the body and which organ or tissue will receive the majority of the dose. The length of the exposure will be determined by the effective half-life (p. 180) taking into account, as it does, the physical half-life of the isotope and its likely excretion rate or biological half-life.

Effective dose limits

The annual effective dose limits have largely remained unchanged over the last 35 years, but how they are applied in practice has changed. At one time, the permitted cumulative dose was limited to $50(n–18)$ mSv, where n was the age of the individual in years. This was abandoned in preference to a limit for the calendar year of 50 mSv, ignoring any previous lower levels of dose. The latest recommendation is that while the annual limit remains the same, the dose over any 5-year period should not exceed 20 mSv y^{-1} average for those occupationally exposed or 1 mSv y^{-1} average for those not occupationally exposed—implying an absolute maximum of 5 mSv in any one year. Occupational exposure is that exposure incurred at work to radiations considered to be the responsibility of management. Occupational exposure therefore generally excludes exposure to the natural background radiations, that is unless these levels are raised above average through the nature of the work, e.g. radon in mines, piloting high flying aircraft.

The effective dose limits (Table 12.3) apply to all those who are occupationally exposed and to all uses of radiation, but exclude the contributions from background radiation described above and personal exposures for medical purposes. They do not apply to patients undergoing medical exposures for diagnostic

Table 12.3 Recommended dose limits*

Application	Dose limit (mSv)	
	Occupational	Public
Effective dose	20 per year, averaged over defined periods of 5 years[†]	1 in a year[‡]
Annual equivalent dose in		
the lens of the eye	150	15
the skin[§]	500	50
the hands and feet	500	—

* The limits apply to the sum of the relevant doses from external exposure in the specified period and the 50 year committed dose (to age 70 years for children) from intakes in the same period.
[†] With the further provision that the effective dose should not exceed 50 mSv in any single year. Additional restrictions apply to the occupational exposure of pregnant women.
[‡] In special circumstances, a higher value of effective dose could be allowed in a single year, provided that the average over 5 years does not exceed 1 mSv per year.
[§] The limitation on the effective dose provides sufficient protection for the skin against stochastic effects. An additional limit is needed for localised exposures in order to prevent deterministic effects.
(Reproduced with permission from ICRP 1991.)

or therapeutic purposes. All those not occupationally exposed, i.e. other patients, visitors and contractors, etc., are subject to the lower 'public' dose limit.

Limits may also be derived from Table 12.3 for the accumulation of radioisotopes in the body by ingestion or inhalation. These dangers may arise from damage to sealed sources but, more frequently, from the use of unsealed sources in the form of solutions, aerosols, gases or powders. Using appropriate assumptions about the way in which the various isotopes are metabolised in the body, it is possible to deduce the concentration of isotopes in the air or in water which can be accepted in the working environment of a laboratory or in the environment of the general public. Similar figures can be derived for the total body content of the various isotopes which in time would lead to a given whole body dose, known as annual limits of intake (ALI).

Previously, women of reproductive capacity have been subjected to the same dose limits only on the understanding the exposure was crudely at a uniform rate. Under the new definitions, no distinction is made between men and women. Once a pregnancy has been confirmed, however, an effective dose limit to the surface of the woman's abdomen of 2 mSv is applied for the remainder of the pregnancy, together with the intake of radionuclides reduced to one-twentieth of the normal annual limit of intake. (These reduced dose limits cannot be applied retrospectively, and it is the woman's responsibility to formally notify her employer once the pregnancy is confirmed.) In hospital practice, the dose levels reported in recent years are so low that there is rarely any need for changes in duties resulting from the declaration of pregnancy *on the grounds of radiation dose*. The decisions must be based on local circumstances. However, the mutual concern for the welfare of the unborn child is such that staff are often only too willing to change their rosters to minimise the risk, however small it may be.

Basic principles

The following principles of dose limitation are discussed in isolation, but in practice it is often necessary to consider them together and to come to a compromise as to the most efficient means of minimising the radiation hazard.

Time

Total exposure is the product of exposure rate and time and therefore it is important to keep the exposure time as short as possible. In the case of diagnosis or treatment of a patient, the exposure has to be the minimum consistent with the desired result, and any further reduction may jeopardise the outcome and result in a repeat exposure. There is no such minimum exposure for a member of staff. Complex procedures should be practised using inactive sources until they can be performed efficiently and effectively. The time spent close to, or in the vicinity of, patients with brachytherapy sources in situ or unsealed sources in vivo should be restricted by only performing essential duties; other tests or procedures being arranged before the administration of the activity or postponed until after the source of radiation has been removed or decayed to a safe level. Where essential duties demand the presence of a member of staff, then the time may be shared with others to keep the individual doses to a minimum. Where patients need little more than a watchful eye, then relatives may be asked to cooperate.

Where fluoroscopy is practised, in diagnosis or on the simulator, then screening times should be kept short by the use of last frame hold facilities, for example.

Distance

Photons travel in straight lines and the intensity of radiation, and therefore the exposure rate, is reduced with increasing distance from the source, following the inverse square law. Long-handled forceps, long-handled lead pots and long-handled trolleys, etc. all increase the distance; pulling rather than pushing the trolleys further increases the distance between the source and the operator. Where patients have sources in situ, standing at 3 metres, distance is twice as effective as standing at 2 metres. In diagnostic radiology, increasing the focus–patient distance reduces the patient dose (although the exposure factors will have to be increased.)

Barriers

Wherever possible, an appropriate protective barrier should be used between the source of radiation and the patient or member of staff. It is important that the selected shielding is of a material appropriate to the radiation. The use of protected walls, benches, etc. is to be encouraged by careful design. A simple Perspex shield can be very effective against beta particles, whereas a lead rubber apron is totally ineffective against photons from caesium or iridium. Tungsten syringe shields combine attenuation with increased distance to reduce the finger dose by an order of magnitude. Lead glass spectacles may be usefully employed for screening procedures which require manipulation of the patient, but the hands must be kept well out of the beam, unless lead rubber gloves are worn. Lead rubber aprons must be worn, fastened at the sides, and the use of thyroid shields by staff is to be encouraged. Gonad shields, etc., are of course essential for the patient unless the shields will obscure the diagnostic information being sought.

Contamination

Where unsealed sources of radioactivity are used, a further factor has to be considered, namely the possibility of the operator becoming contaminated. This can occur by contact with, or by inhalation or ingestion of the isotope or by absorption of the isotope through the skin. Simple protective clothing—theatre clothes, for example—may be all that is necessary in most situations, with the addition of masks, plastic aprons, gloves and overshoes when appropriate. The laundering or disposal of theatre clothes is simpler than the operator's personal clothing.

Contamination of floors, benches, furnishings, etc. can be minimised by the use of lipped trays lined with absorbent tissues and the well-disciplined procedures detailed in the local rules (p. 217). Floors, benches and other surfaces should be finished with continuous impervious surfaces for ease of decontamination and to minimise the seepage of radioactive material into joints and cracks.

These simple precautions will help to reduce the exposure rather than eliminate it altogether. The practical measures taken to ensure that the exposures are kept within the agreed dose limits will now be discussed.

ADMINISTRATIVE STRUCTURE
Designation of areas

Some sources, including X-ray generators, or groups of sources of radiation are large enough to require strict controls to be implemented, both in the construction of the area in which they are to be housed and in their operation, if the dose limits are to be satisfied. The maximum permitted leakage of radiation from X- and gamma ray generators has been discussed in Chapter 3. Wherever possible, the sources should be housed in areas where sufficient protection is afforded to those outside, so that they need not be regarded as occupationally exposed. Where persons are required to work in or near radiation areas, then engineering controls and design considerations must be used wherever possible. For example, concrete protective barriers built into an installation are preferred to moveable lead screens which may or may not be used; an interlock is preferred to an instruction, which may or may not be obeyed. Current legislation in the UK lays down strict rules for determining whether or not a radiation area is to be designated as a *controlled area* or a *supervised area*. This is based on whether the potential exposure is likely to exceed three-tenths of any relevant dose limit or less than three-tenths but more than one-tenth, respectively. In general this requires areas where the potential exposure rate is likely to exceed 7.5 μSv h^{-1} or 60 μSv per 8 hour day to be designated controlled areas. Supervised areas are subject to one-third of these values. Similar criteria, based on the other dose limits, may require the area to be controlled.

The more recent ICRP recommendations have relaxed these definitions as being arbitrary and encourage local definitions of controlled and of supervised areas to be based on operational experience and judgement, taking into account the potential for accidents. The remainder of this chapter will assume radiation areas will be designated as controlled or supervised according to some locally agreed criteria, but where necessary the three-tenths criterion will be used.

Both controlled and supervised areas are required to be clearly defined, preferably by easily defined boundaries. For example, a permanent controlled area may be the treatment room and the maze corridor; a temporary controlled area may be the area within 2 metres of the patient on a ward. The radiation warning sign should be clearly displayed, together with words on a white or yellow background explaining the designation and the nature of the radiation: Controlled Area—Gamma Rays (Plate 4), X-rays, etc. The warning sign is a black trefoil on a yellow background within a black equilateral triangle, with its point uppermost. However the area is marked on site, the site must be fully described in the local rules. All staff working in the vicinity of radiation areas must be made aware of the meaning of the signs for their own safety and the safety of others. Only four groups of people are allowed to enter a controlled area:

— The patient undergoing medical diagnosis or treatment with radiation or persons participating in research (for whom there are very stringent controls, not considered here).
— Those who are authorised to inspect the areas for compliance with the regulations.
— Those who have been issued with a written system of work.
— Classified workers.

Occupationally exposed workers

Just as a controlled area is defined as where someone's accumulated dose might exceed three-tenths of any relevant dose limit, so a person who is occupationally exposed will be designated a *classified person* if his or her personal exposure might exceed three-tenths of any relevant dose limit. In hospitals, there are unlikely to be many staff classified in this way. Those practising manual techniques involving therapeutic activities of caesium-137, iodine-131, etc. may be classified. Some of those practising interventional radiology—cardiologists and orthopaedic surgeons—may need to be classified on the basis of their eye dose, assuming their whole body doses are kept low by the adequate use of lead rubber aprons, etc. Those operating radiotherapy beam equipment are unlikely to be classified.

A useful aid to maintaining the high standards of radiation safety is to establish a local guide to the expected radiation exposure of staff for different, but specific, procedures. These will, of course, be less than three-tenths of the effective dose limits. At the local level, an example may be where experience of a procedure has shown staff rarely exceed 7 mSv y^{-1}. The figure may be set at 6 mSv y^{-1} (or pro rata for each monitoring period). Using this locally agreed guide then justifies a local investigation into the circumstances surrounding any dose report suggesting it may be exceeded. These guide figures should be revised (downwards) from time to time as the practice improves.

At a national level, the UK has an agreed trigger level that any person on course for an accumulated dose of 75 mSv in 5 years will be subject to a thorough investigation.

Local rules

The majority of hospital staff required to enter controlled areas will therefore enter under a *written system of work*. The system of work is written into the local rules by the Radiation Protection Supervisor (RPS) for the Department and seeks to describe in detail how each procedure can be carried out in such a way that the exposure will not exceed three-tenths of any dose limit or the locally agreed action level. It may specify the techniques and/or the equipment to be used; it may limit the time spent in the area. It will include the precautions that need to be taken and the location and meaning of warning signs, alarms and emergency procedures to be followed should anything abnormal occur. The RPS is usually a member of the Department who is familiar with both the work of the Department and the requirements of the regulations governing their uses of radiation. It is, therefore, in his or her own interests to ensure the systems of work are practical and not prohibitive.

In anticipation of any foreseeable emergency, the local rules will contain a *contingency plan*, so that those responsible for radiation safety know exactly what to do and who to inform. Obvious contingency plans include the suspected loss of or damage to a sealed source (p. 159), the failure of the shutter mechanism on a gamma ray unit, the death of a patient following the administration of a therapeutic dose of iodine-131, etc. Other contingency plans will deal with problems such as the spillage of an unsealed radionuclide or the breakout of fire in the radiotherapy ward or department. Where unsealed sources are used or sealed sources are at risk of damage, then an emergency kit should be made available. Its contents and recommended procedures for use should be detailed in the local rules, so that any contamination can be dealt with promptly and efficiently.

The local rules will also contain a description of, and the extent of, each designated area, a list of the named officers responsible for radiation safety and the arrangements for personnel monitoring. The RPS is responsible for ensuring the regulations are implemented, that high standards of safety are maintained and the local rules are kept under review.

Operating procedures

Although not strictly a part of the administrative structure for radiation safety, the *operating procedures* play a vital part in ensuring the safety of staff and patients. The operating procedure is more than the operating instructions issued by the suppliers of the equipment, although they are a part. The operating procedure will specify the staffing levels and the responsibilities of each grade involved. They will include the operating parameters under which the equipment will be used and in particular the range of acceptable values, outside which the equipment should be taken out of clinical use. They will include those indicators which warn of malfunction. They will contain the programme of safety checks and their recommended frequency, the need for keeping an up-to-date log of the machine faults (p. 56), etc. and to whom those faults should be reported.

Radiation Protection Adviser

While the ultimate responsibility for ensuring the recommendations are put into practice lies with the employer, the employer will engage the services of an experienced radiation physicist as Radiation Protection Adviser (RPA) to determine the need to identify controlled areas and classified workers and to supervise the implementation of the radiation safety legislation. If classified workers are to be appointed then, an Employment Medical Adviser (EMA) should ensure their physical fitness is appropriate in the first instance and keep it and their annual accumulated dose under review. The EMA will also be responsible for counselling women who are, or may become, pregnant, those who are anxious about their personal exposure record and those who may volunteer themselves as subjects in radiation research.

The RPA is required to examine all proposals to instal new radiation equipment and subsequently to assess and report on the effectiveness of the equipment itself and its accommodation in the light of the recommendations. In return, the RPA needs to be kept informed of any changes of equipment or its use. The RPA will also be consulted on all matters relating to radiation safety, including the appointment of Radiation Protection Supervisors (RPS), the writing of the local rules, systems of work and contingency plans and the need for, and effectiveness of, radiation monitoring. The RPA will be involved in training and in the investigation of any abnormally high exposures.

In a large establishment, like a hospital, the employer will set up a radiation safety committee, where users, advisers and management can discuss matters relating to radiation safety, receive reports on the overall effectiveness of the measures adopted and on any incidents which may have occurred. While radiation is only one of many hazards covered by legislation in a hospital, its very technical nature suggests it should be discussed by a committee of specialists, who in turn report to a more open forum on health and safety matters.

BUILDING MATERIALS

Having described typical room layouts in Chapters 3 and 8, we now look at the materials available and their properties. The two materials in most common use are lead ($Z = 82$, $\rho = 11350\,kg\ m^{-3}$) and concrete ($\rho = 2350\,kg\ m^{-3}$) and a range of data is given in Table 12.4. Other materials are used in selected areas, but their use must be carefully monitored. For example, clay bricks ($\rho = 1600$–$2000\,kg\ m^{-3}$) may be adequate in a superficial therapy or diagnostic room, but they can vary both in their construction (density) and in their design (there may be weight-reducing cavities within each brick). The effectiveness of a brick wall will also be affected by the cement (mortar) used to bind the bricks together. There are many lightweight building blocks ($\rho = <1000\,kg\ m^{-3}$) in modern buildings, but they are totally unsuitable in themselves against radiation.

Where new rooms are planned, solid concrete is preferred for its cheapness and its contribution to the structure of the building, as well as its protection properties. For temporary accommodation or alterations to existing buildings, the use of lead bonded between plywood and secured to a supporting frame is probably the preferred material for diagnostic X-ray, superficial therapy rooms and nuclear medicine laboratories, but barytes plaster ($\rho \sim 2000\,kg\ m^{-3}$) on brick may be used. At megavoltage energies (including isotope therapy facilities), lead is too expensive. Large thicknesses of lead are best avoided; being a soft metal, it 'creeps' under its own weight and needs substantial support. Concrete is the preferred material. The addition of barytes to concrete, to increase its density (to approximately $3500\,kg\ m^{-3}$) is now prohibitively expensive for most applications. Lapped steel plate can be used in conjunction with concrete for a megavoltage installation where space needs to be conserved, but it is best avoided where neutron activation is likely (e.g. for installations generating photons of more than 10 MV).

The protective material used in or on walls must be continuous and without cracks or holes. For example, tie-bars are used to hold the shuttering in place whilst concrete is poured to form a wall; if these tie-bars are subsequently removed, the holes must be completely filled and not simply plastered over. Where lead panelling has been used effectively with overlapped joints it is easily ruined by drilling to fix wall accessories such as towel holders or pictures. (This hazard is even greater when the accessories are removed.)

Some perforations in the shielding have to be planned, for example, to admit electricity and water supplies, oxygen and vacuum lines, air conditioning, etc. These should be routed round the maze in a ceiling or floor void wherever possible, but, inevitably, some have to

Table 12.4 The properties of lead and concrete: approximate half and tenth value layers in lead and concrete for heavily filtered broad beams of X- and gamma rays

X-Ray energy/ isotope	HVL (mm Pb)	TVL (mm Pb)	HVL (mm Concrete)	TVL (mm Concrete)
50 kV	0.06	0.2	—	—
100 kV	0.30	0.95	—	—
150 kV	0.32	1.04	—	—
200 kV	0.43	1.42	—	—
300 kV	1.33	4.4	29	95
Iridium-192	5.5	20	45	140
Iodine-131	7.2	24	47	160
Caesium-137	6.5	22	50	165
Cobalt-60	11	40	65	205
4 MV	—	—	85	275
6 MV	—	—	105	340
10 MV	—	—	120	390
20 MV	—	—	140	460

Note. These values are for illustration purposes only, the filtration effect of any protective barrier changes the energy spectrum of the radiation and therefore the thickness of the HVL and TVL.

pass through an otherwise protective barrier. They must not be allowed through a primary barrier. Routes through secondary barriers can be accommodated providing they are designed to adequately trap the scattered photons, either by carefully angling the duct against the radiation or creating angles in the duct, e.g. by taking supplies through a wall below the level of the solid floor. Be wary of suspended floors and ceilings.

Lead equivalence

Table 12.4 gives some thicknesses of lead and concrete to attenuate radiations of different energies to one half (HVL) and to one tenth (TVL). For example, at 300 kV, 95 mm concrete provides the same attenuation as 4.4 mm Pb, whereas for cobalt-60, 205 mm of concrete has the same effect as 40 mm Pb. Putting these comparisons another way, we could say 'at 300 kV, 95 mm concrete has a lead equivalence of 4.4 mm Pb' and 'at cobalt-60 energies, 205 mm concrete has a lead equivalence of 40 mm Pb'. The effectiveness of any barrier, of whatever construction, can be stated in 'mm Pb equivalent', provided the photon energy is known. In practice, barriers are often specified in mm Pb equivalence before the material is decided. Protective barriers should be clearly labelled so that their effectiveness is not subsequently compromised.

ENVIRONMENTAL MONITORING

The aim of environmental monitoring is to check that the design of the protective shielding provides an adequately safe environment both for those working in the department and for the members of the general public and workers in other departments who may be exposed to radiation through their presence in or near the radiological department. It is particularly important to survey any new department and to repeat the survey whenever modifications have been made to the structure of the building, to the equipment or to the working practices. An environmental survey is also often necessary if personnel monitoring reveals excessive doses are being reported, as these may indicate the need for some further modification to the shielding or to the working practice. Environmental monitoring will include the measurement of radioactive contamination of surfaces and air concentrations of radioactivity in areas in which unsealed sources are being processed (p. 173).

Environmental monitoring equipment

Measurements of exposure rates around departments can be made by portable ionisation chamber monitors

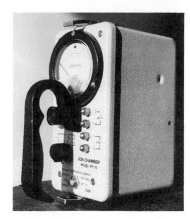

Fig. 12.2 A hand-held survey dose meter incorporating a 200 ml ionisation chamber.

(p. 74). The exposure rates likely to be encountered will be in the range from $0.01\ \mu Sv\ h^{-1}$ to $1\ mSv\ h^{-1}$ and therefore a large volume chamber will be required. Hand-held instruments with chamber volumes of up to 500 ml and battery driven amplifiers are available (Fig. 12.2), but have the disadvantage that they have a long time constant, i.e. they do not respond quickly to changes in the incident radiation intensity.

Instruments involving Geiger counters or scintillation detectors (Chapter 9) are more sensitive than ionisation chambers and use detectors of smaller size. They do, however, suffer from the disadvantage that for the measurement of X- and gamma radiation their sensitivity is more dependent on the radiation quality than ionisation chamber devices. It is therefore more difficult to rely on an accurate reading of the exposure rate. These instruments are more suited to checking for contamination in the isotope laboratory. Other portable instruments are available to which a number of different detector probes may be attached: scintillation probes with thin windows, being suitable for the detection of alpha and beta radiations and for the detection of contamination on benches, floors and clothing; and end-window GM tubes, which are more robust but not suited to alpha detection. Mains operated instruments (preferably with a battery back-up) may be permanently installed at strategic points to give audible and/or visual warning when a radiation level reaches a predetermined level. In laboratories, they can warn of an unsatisfactory increase in the radiation level, due to the accumulation of radioactive waste, for example, in an otherwise satisfactory working environment. Located at the exits from a radiotherapy ward and near sluices, they can monitor the passage of sealed sources and thereby help to prevent the inadvertent movement of sources in waste bins or in the clothing of patients or staff.

PERSONAL MONITORING

The personal monitoring of members of staff who are occupationally exposed to radiation is aimed at ensuring their individual exposures are within the limits laid down. This differs from the estimates made from environmental monitoring as it will be affected by the distribution of duties at different locations during the working day. It is carried out using small integrating dosimeters which can be worn on the clothing of the radiation workers. A number of different types of dosimeter are available including film badges, thermoluminescent badges, quartz fibre electrometers, solid state dosimeters and pocket-sized Geiger counters. These must be worn continuously during working hours, but kept away from radiation exposure out of working hours. The dosimeter should be worn on the front of the person between the waist and the shoulder to measure whole body dose, which in the main arises from scattered radiation and does not differ widely at different parts of the trunk. If protective clothing is being worn, the dosimeter should be worn underneath, since the whole body radiation to the trunk is the quantity being measured. Additional dosimeters may be worn to monitor the dose to particular sites, for example on the forehead to monitor the dose to the eyes. A thermoluminescent dosimeter can be small enough to attach to the finger to measure the extremity dose during brachytherapy or radiopharmaceutical procedures.

The quartz fibre electrometer, the pocket Geiger and solid state dosimeters permit immediate readings to be obtained. It is usual therefore for these to be worn during particular procedures attended by high exposure risk, such as the loading of new sources into gamma ray beam units. They may incorporate an alarm bleep to indicate the incident exposure rate. The film and thermoluminescent badges are more suited to measuring the accumulated dose over longer periods of time, of several weeks for example. Shorter periods are advised where the risks are higher. Personal monitoring is obligatory wherever classified workers are employed and their dosimeters must be processed by an approved laboratory or calibrated to a national standard. For other workers, personal monitoring provides reassurance that the protective measures in the environment and the working practices are satisfactory.

Personal monitoring for internal radiation hazards, aimed at estimating the radiation dose received by staff due to the accidental intake of unsealed radioactive substances, is more difficult than that for external radiation. The body content of gamma emitting isotopes can be measured using a whole body counter (p. 167) or simple counting equipment. Information can also be deduced, especially for beta or gamma emitting materials, by measuring the excretion of radioactive materials, particularly in the urine. A common example of biological monitoring is checking the accumulation of small quantities of iodine-131 in the thyroid gland of workers handling this isotope (p. 166).

Film badge

The use of photographic film for the measurement of radiation dose has been outlined in Chapter 5, and the properties and processing techniques have been described in Chapter 7. It is easy to obtain a rough estimate of dose by measuring the blackening produced by development under standard conditions. For a given radiation quality, the film density is roughly proportional to the exposure, if the exposure is small. Figure 7.7 shows the exposure–density relationship for a typical X-ray film exposed to gamma rays. The high atomic number of the silver halide in the film emulsion makes the film sensitive to radiation quality and much smaller exposures would be needed to produce the same film densities at say 100 keV. Curve A in Figure 12.3. shows that film is some 24 times more sensitive at 40 keV than it is at high energies. Add to this the fact that in radiation protection the radiation to be measured is mainly low energy scatter and the fact that the processing conditions can affect the characteristic curve, and it is easy to appreciate that film on its own will not give a very accurate estimate of the incident exposure. In spite of these disadvantages, the photographic film is extremely useful for personal monitoring. It is relatively cheap, easy to process and provides a permanent record of the exposure. In practice, the photographic films used for personal monitoring are used in a holder or cassette fitted with a variety of metal filters designed to improve the accuracy of the dose estimate. The absorption curve of the filter is designed to match the energy response of the film. At high energies, the filter has a negligible attenuation effect and the film is blackened in the normal way. The lower energy photons, to which the film is more sensitive, are attenuated in the filter, leaving fewer to penetrate the emulsion of the film. It is therefore conceivable that, if the degree of attenuation in the filter exactly balanced the increased sensitivity of the film over the whole range of photon energies, the energy sensitivity of the film–filter combination would be flat over a wide range of energies but in reality curve B in Figure 12.3 is as near as can be achieved.

A typical film badge is illustrated in Figure 12.4. The holder is a moulded polypropylene case into which is fitted a Kodak Radiation Monitoring film. The blackening under the different filters is a function of

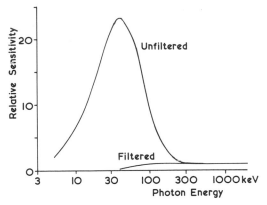

Fig. 12.3 The energy response of photographic film, (A) unfiltered and (B) filtered through the tin–lead filter.

the quality of the radiation to which the whole badge has been exposed. The badge has an open window (4) in the centre, through which the identification number stamped on the wrapping can be seen. The effect of the pressure applied in the stamping process enables the number on the film to be read after processing. The window also allows any radiation capable of penetrating the film wrapper to cause blackening on the film. There are two plastic filters, of 50 mg cm^{-2} (5) and of 300 mg cm^{-2} (6), corresponding to the critical depths of the skin and the lens of the eye respectively. The thin plastic filter attenuates beta rays and a comparison of the blackening under this filter compared with that under the open window enables beta and very soft X-ray doses to be estimated. The filter composed of 0.028″ tin plus 0.012″ lead (3) is chosen to give a response which is nearly independent of radiation

quality from 75 keV to 2 MeV. The filter (1) is an alloy of aluminium and copper 0.040″ thick, chosen to give an estimate of the dose for energies between 15 and 85 keV. Finally the 0.028″ cadmium plus 0.012″ lead filter (2) is used to estimate any dose from exposure to neutrons as neutrons interacting with cadmium produce gamma radiation which in turn causes blackening in the film. Where neutrons are unlikely to be encountered, badges may have the tin/lead filter extended to replace the cadmium. The 0.012″ lead edge shielding (7) extends round the edge of the tin/lead and the cadmium/lead filters to reduce errors due to the entry of low energy photons through the edge of the badge, producing blackening under those filters which could be misconstrued as a high energy photon exposure. Finally, 0.4 g of indium (8), may be added where appropriate to monitor accidental exposure in nuclear reactors.

The used films are developed with a set of suitable calibration films previously exposed to a range of known doses of gamma rays, together with unexposed films to estimate background and fog effects. A number of empirical methods are adopted by various laboratories to deduce the exposure from the densities measured under the various filters. For handling large numbers of films, an automated densitometer and computer programme are used to assess and record the estimated doses. In order to extend the range of exposure covered by the film, the Kodak RM film has a thick sensitive emulsion coated on one side of the cellulose-acetate base and a thin, less sensitive coating on the other. For normal use, the density through both layers is measured and the doses of a few per cent of the dose limit estimated. High doses make the sensitive emulsion too black for measurement, but it can then be stripped off and a measurement of the density of the thin emulsion alone can be made, leading to estimates of up to about 1 Sv.

Thermoluminescent dosimeters

The measurement of exposure by the thermoluminescent (TL) effect has already been outlined in Chapter 5. Lithium fluoride powder can be used in a variety of capsules or impregnated into plastic discs for use in cassettes. The advantages of this method of personal dose monitoring are: (1) freedom from dependence on photon energy because of the low atomic number of the phosphor, (2) the stability of the detector over long periods of time, (3) a very large dose range (0.1 mSv to 10 Sv) covered by a single dosimeter, (4) a reusable dosimeter and (5) ease of automatic processing. The TL badge usually consists of a metal plate, housing

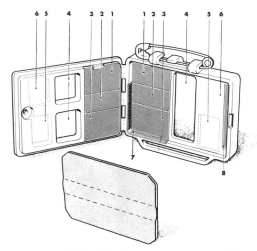

Fig. 12.4 The AERE/RPS film badge. (Courtesy of the Harwell Laboratory.)

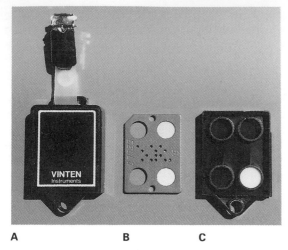

Fig. 12.5 A TL Badge. **A** The cassette, **B** the coded TL plate and **C** the cassette back.

two lithium fluoride loaded discs and carrying a binary coded identification number (Fig. 12.5). This assembly is loaded into a thin black plastic sheath and fitted into a plastic cassette of a similar size as the film badge. The plastic sheath is to keep the light from the phosphor and to avoid contamination of the plate; the sheath is monitored for radioactive contamination before the discs are read out. The TL cassette carries only two filters, one thicker than the other, to separate the low penetration radiations which only contribute to the skin dose from the more penetrating radiations which contribute to the whole body dose.

Solid state dosimeters

Integrated circuit technology using silicon diode

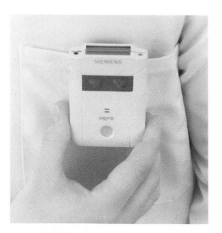

Fig. 12.6 The Siemens/NRPB electronic dose meter. (Courtesy of Siemens Plessey Controls, Ltd.)

radiation detectors is now available and offers a very robust and compact personal dosimeter, with instantaneous dose or dose rate display and preset dose rate alarm indication. The energy response is similar to the TL badge and film badge for both beta and gamma radiations and extends the integrated dose range from 1 µSv to 1 Sv. These instruments (Fig. 12.6) are currently undergoing trials, and once they are firmly established, they will compete with both the film badge and the TL badge in the whole body dosimetry field, being especially valuable where the risks are relatively unknown.

Quartz fibre electrometer

The pocket-type quartz fibre electrometer (QFE) is an instrument in which a direct and immediate reading of the dose can be obtained, and being the size of a pen torch, it is affectionately known as a 'pen monitor'. Its advantage therefore is that the worker can check his or her exposure at intervals during a particular procedure, instead of having to wait for laboratory processing of the dosimeter, which at best takes a day or two. In this instrument (Fig. 12.7), a metallised quartz fibre is mounted in a small ionisation chamber and illuminated by daylight shining through one end and viewed by a microscope built into the other end. The fibre system is charged to about 200 volts to bring the position of the fibre to the zero of the scale incorporated in the microscope—the fibre moves away

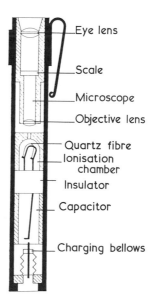

Fig. 12.7 The quartz fibre electrometer. (Courtesy of FAG Kugelfischer Georg Schafer KGaA, Germany.)

from a fixed fibre by electrostatic repulsion. On exposure to radiation, the ionised air causes the stored charge to fall and the fibre moves towards the fixed fibre, its shadow on the scale showing an increased exposure. A selection of sensitivities are available, with different instruments covering full scale deflections from 2 mSv up to 5000 mSv. The two disadvantages of the instrument are its energy dependence and the fact that doses over and above the full-scale reading are not recorded.

Pocket GM dosimeter/alarms

Microelectronics enable battery operated Geiger–Müller detectors to be made not much larger than the QFE and often with more facilities. They may have one of several specifications. The basic device will simply bleep slowly in normal background radiation at, say, one bleep every 20 to 30 minutes, the rate increasing with radiation level to a continuous tone above about $5 \mu Sv\,h^{-1}$. The second specification will mute the background bleeps below a preset threshold level. Neither of these instruments will have an on/off switch or any other operator controls and so continuously monitor their environment. Higher specifications may provide a digital read-out of the total accumulated exposure from the time the instrument was switched on, and an alarm signal, should the rate exceed one of several presettable levels.

DOSE MONITORING RECORDS

Reference has been made in a number of places to the necessity for keeping appropriate records in order that radiation protection procedures can be adequately controlled and to reduce the risk of accident through changes of working practice not known to the operators. Discipline in this matter is essential and good record keeping is important. The records required may be grouped as follows. First, there are those dealing with the safety of personnel, such as medical records, radiation dose records and records of any unusual exposure or contamination. A separate radiation record has to be kept for each individual classified worker and the recorded doses totalled for each calendar year and for the preceding 5-year period to ensure they are within the dose limits. These records must show a complete radiation history and are often kept at a central registry so that the record can be maintained even when the worker moves between jobs. If the central registry is not used, then the individual must be issued with a transfer certificate detailing his or her personal record of exposure on terminating one employment and moving to another. These dose records are of great assistance

to the EMA in the event of any worker receiving a dose in excess of accepted limits. The EMA must decide whether to carry out a special medical examination and to consider if any rearrangement of the duties of the exposed person is required. The reports of any investigation into a real or suspected overexposure of a member of staff or a patient must be kept for 50 years.

Second, there are records dealing with checks on the safety status of the department, such as the environmental monitoring and contamination monitoring of working areas. These records will include modifications to shields and barriers, to equipment, to controlled areas, warning signs and notices. Records of daily monitoring for radioactive contamination of personnel and the environment will need to be kept, in addition to those of annual inspections of the laboratory/ward areas. A number of records are required, dealing with the care and checking of tools and equipment whose malfunction could lead to a radiation hazard—these will be part of the quality assurance programme—and extend to the calibration of dosimeters. The movement, use, leak testing and disposal of radioactive sources must be recorded, along with the reports of investigations into any suspected loss of, or damage to, sealed sources. Full detailed records must be maintained of measurements of output dose rates and any modifications to therapy equipment which may affect the output beam dose rate or beam quality.

Properly organised record keeping is not an onerous, unnecessary chore but a disciplined activity contributing to a high level of radiation safety in the radiotherapy department. Gross radiation effects, such as that shown in Plate 9, should now be a thing of the past.

RELATED SAFETY MATTERS

The radiation hazard is not the only hazard with which the operators of radiation generators need to be familiar. They need to take precautions against the mechanical, electrical, fire and health hazards associated with their equipment. A variety of safety signs will be used around the department and about the equipment and these will need to be understood and observed by all members of staff and visitors. In the UK, the four groups of safety signs may be recognised by their shape and colour (Plate 10), as follows:

PROHIBITION signs give instructions about what you are not to do; the symbol is printed in black on a white background within a red circle with a red diagonal line through the symbol.

WARNING signs warn of risks or dangers; the symbol

is printed in black on a yellow background within a black equilateral triangle (point uppermost).

MANDATORY signs give instructions about what you must do; the symbol is printed in white on a blue circular background.

SAFE CONDITION signs give a white symbol or lettering on a solid green rectangular background.

These signs may be used singly or in conjunction with others appropriate to the situation and may be supplemented by explanatory wording in black lettering on a white background or in the colouring of the sign itself. They are required to be large enough to be clearly seen from the likely viewing distances.

In Chapter 3 it was stated that the acceptance tests on a new installation were to check the equipment's compliance with a previously agreed specification. That specification will detail the operating parameters and ranges for the equipment. In addition, the specification should also include statements requiring the installation to conform to the international and national recommendations on electrical and mechanical performance, on operating temperatures and on the inclusion of materials hazardous to health. Unless these recommendations are cited in the specification, the suppliers may not be legally bound to comply with them. As with radiation protection, internationally agreed recommendations are not necessarily legally adopted at national levels without modification.

Acceptance testing on a new piece of equipment does not guarantee its future performance and how it does perform will be largely determined by how it is handled and maintained.

Mechanical hazards

The one characteristic which is common to all radiological equipment is the weight. Radiation generators incorporate lead in large quantities, making them very heavy. Although the lead is usually supported on a substantial steel framework, the lead can be distorted under its own weight, particularly when its movement is stopped suddenly. The overall weight is further increased by the need for counterbalancing the movements. Where megavoltage equipment is concerned, merely rotating the gantry from one position to another involves the acceleration and retardation of several tonnes. This movement is generally controlled by an electric motor and gearbox. Rapid changes in speed or direction can put considerable strain on the gearbox, increasing the wear and tear, leading to early failure and the need for replacement. The movement of the gantry is easily appreciated, but the same consideration needs to be given to the movement of the collimators, couch, etc.

Superficial and orthovoltage therapy tube stands will incorporate either a counterbalance weight or a balance spring to counter the weight of the tube housing via a multistranded cable or chain. If these are not duplicated as a safeguard against the failure of one, then an automatic brake must be included in the design to arrest the free fall of the tube housing. Any apparent damage to, chafing of or broken strands in the cable or visual damage to the chain must be reported immediately and attended to as a matter of urgency.

Smaller weights, by comparison, which have to be handled regularly include the orthovoltage applicators and local shielding blocks, all of which are easily damaged if dropped.

All movements lead to wear and tear and the observant operator can report the early signs of damage before accidents occur or expensive repairs become necessary. Arresting movement is most easily achieved by reducing the speed first. The application of brakes should be regarded more as a means of stopping a stationary object from moving, than a means of bringing a moving object to rest. Brakes rely on the friction between two surfaces and abuse leads to the wearing away of those surfaces, reducing their effectiveness. The observant operator detects this reduction in effectiveness and may recognise the build-up of dust particles from the brake itself.

Plugs and sockets are mechanical devices for making electrical connections and rely on the mechanical pressure between metallic contacts. Inappropriate pulling and twisting of the plug or socket leads to a weakening of the contact pressure, which in turn leads to poor electrical continuity, sparking, oxidation and failure. Equally, they are not designed to support a lot of weight. Heavy cables should be supported independently, HT cables are particularly heavy and need that support.

New HT cables will flex fairly readily. Their inherent electrical resistance and the passage of electric current lead to internal heating of the heavy insulation, which in turn becomes hard and brittle. Unnecessary bending and strain will accelerate this hardening effect, leading to the eventual breakdown of the insulation—accompanied by large fluctuations in the displayed tube current and the smell of burning!

Electrical hazards

All electrical equipment is potentially dangerous—even low voltages can cause fatalities. Never operate electrical equipment with wet hands or wet shoes.

All major components of any installation should be visibly connected to 'earth', using either a continuous copper tape or a single core wire covered with a green or green and yellow sheath. These connections should all be brought together at a common earth reference terminal (ERT). The earthing of a metal frame or the screens of an HT cable are not regarded as alternatives. The resistance of each earth connection should be checked regularly. All potentially hazardous electrical and electronic circuitry will be housed in cabinets either behind fixed panels or locked doors. These doors must be kept locked and only opened by authorised personnel after isolating the supply. Furthermore, large capacitors are likely to hold their charge and special precautions need to be taken to discharge them before maintenance work is undertaken. Strict safety procedures must be followed. Maintenance staff must not work alone on electrical equipment.

The colour codes of indicator and control lamps and cables (Table 12.5) and the international markings and symbols should be understood.

Reporting of faults

Faults, however trivial they may seem, should be reported in a fault book and dealt with either immediately or as soon as possible in accordance with the locally agreed protocol. A separate fault book should be kept for each major piece of equipment. The faults recorded will include the failure of warning lights, the fraying or chafing of cables, the stiffness of movements, the ineffectiveness of brakes, the sticking of analogue meter movements, squeaks and rattles, nuts and bolts

Table 12.5 Some colour codes

Coloured indicator lights (e.g. on a control desk)	
RED	Warning of danger requiring urgent action to terminate an unintended state of operation
YELLOW	Requiring attention, caution (e.g. radiation on)
YELLOW (flashing)	Sources in transit (e.g. in remote afterloading equipment)
GREEN	Ready for action
WHITE	Equipment switched on but further operations required to bring it to the ready state

Coloured cables (single phase mains)	
BROWN	Live
BLUE	Neutral
GREEN/YELLOW	Earth

Coloured cables (three phase mains)	
BROWN/BLUE/YELLOW	Three live phases
GREEN/YELLOW	Earth

lost or found, etc., etc. All these are in addition to reporting any deviations from the normal parameters and conditions listed in the operating procedures (p. 217).

Fire hazards

Radiotherapy equipment uses a mixture of high current and high voltages with the consequent potential for fire. In the event of a fire, the mains electrical supply must be switched off immediately—an emergency 'off' control should be available in the treatment room and must be available at the control desk. A second isolator may have to be operated to completely isolate a linear accelerator's ion pump supply. Once isolated from the supply there is no radiation hazard from an X-ray generator. Isolating a gamma ray beam unit or remote afterloading unit from the supply should, by design, terminate the exposure and render the sources safe. This must be checked by using a pocket personal alarm or the independent gamma alarm in the treatment room—this is one reason for the instrument being powered independently from the treatment unit.

Water based fire extinguishers must not be used on electrical equipment of any sort. Carbon dioxide (CO_2) powder (black canister) may be used on electrical fires but halon (green canister) is preferred where computers are likely to be involved.

The radiological department will be designed to permit ready evacuation in the event of a fire. Therapy treatment rooms will rarely have an alternative escape route and the use of combustible materials in the construction or decoration should be minimised, particularly in the maze entrance. Early warning smoke detectors should be fitted either to the ceiling or in the extract air ducting and should be tested regularly, not only to check their operation but also to remind staff of the warning sound they emit, so that it is immediately recognised in the event of an emergency. Consideration and rehearsal of the evacuation of patients from the treatment rooms should include where access to the patient is difficult due to the height of the couch, the use of immobilisation devices or simply the rotation of the gantry, bearing in mind that the electrically controlled movements will not be available.

The evacuation of patients with brachytherapy sources in situ or following the administration of unsealed sources should be detailed in the local rules. The safety of the patient must take precedence, but the security of long-lived sealed sources must be ensured, whether the policy is to remove the sources before or after the evacuation. Where the source of radiation cannot be removed to a 'safe' position, then alternative safety precautions will need to be implemented. The procedures to be adopted should be agreed with the local emergency services in advance.

Ozone is generated wherever intense electron beams are used and, being both corrosive and hazardous to health, adequate air extraction facilities must be available to minimise the ozone concentration in the atmosphere.

PART 2

Radiotherapy and oncology

13. Cancer: epidemiology, prevention, early diagnosis and education

THE CANCER PROBLEM

In the UK and Europe cancer is a growing problem. It is a major cause of death in industrialised societies where life expectancy encompasses the maximum incidence of cancer in middle and old age. However it is less of a health care priority in countries where life expectancy is much shorter (e.g. in much of Africa) as a result of infectious disease and poor nutrition.

Cancer in Europe

With closer ties in the provision of health care within the European Community (EC) and with Eastern Europe, a European perspective is needed on the size of the cancer problem. The planning of the provision of cancer prevention and treatment within Europe will need to take account of the different current and future trends in cancer mortality. Within the combined population of 322 million in the EC, there are about three-quarters of a million deaths each year. The incidence of malignancy within the EC is rising and it is estimated that by the year 2000 two million people will have cancer and a million will die each year of the disease.

In Northern and Western Europe the commonest malignancies in males in rank order are lung, colorectal, prostate, bladder and oral and in females breast, colorectal, stomach, endometrium and cervix. These top five malignancies represent 60% of cancers for each sex.

Variations in cancer mortality in Europe

Within Europe there are striking differences in cancer mortality. For example the mortality from oesophageal cancer is much higher in Northern and Western France than across the border in Belgium. The reasons for this are not clear. Differences in the consumption of alcohol and tobacco are probably important. Less explicable is the higher incidence of oesophageal cancer in Irish and Scottish women or of stomach cancer in Bavaria compared with neighbouring parts of Germany.

Future trends in cancer mortality in Europe

When rise in population, increasing age and projected changes in risk are taken into account, increases in common cancers such as lung, large bowel, prostate and breast cancer are predicted in Northern Europe (including Great Britain). Stomach cancer is one of the few cancers likely to fall in incidence.

Cancer in the UK

In the UK 1 in 5 deaths is due to cancer and, after heart disease, it is the commonest cause of death. In England and Wales it accounts for 25% of all deaths. Between 1971 and 1983 the number of cancer registrations in the UK rose by 2.1% in men and 2.6% in women. If this rate of increase is maintained, the number of registrations by 1994 will have increased by 23.5% compared with 1983.

The incidence and mortality of common cancers in men and women in England and Wales are shown in Figure 13.1. Lung and skin cancer are the most common. However, whereas skin cancer carries very

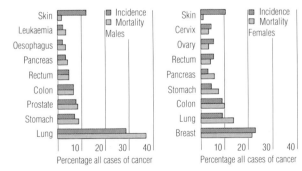

Fig. 13.1 Incidence and mortality of common cancers in England and Wales. (Reproduced with permission from Souhami R L & Moxham J 1990 Textbook of Medicine, Churchill Livingstone, Edinburgh.)

227

little mortality, the opposite is true of lung cancer, which accounts for nearly 40% of male deaths from cancer.

In the UK a consultant in radiotherapy and oncology will be referred on average 560 patients per year. That represents 12 new patients per week. Each consultant, if one includes patients on follow-up, will have about 2000 patients under his or her care at any one time. By 1994 it is estimated that 40% of all patients with cancer will require some form of radiotherapy. Approximately 110 000 new patients will need radiotherapy every year in England and Wales.

With the introduction of screening for breast cancer, increasing numbers of patients are being referred for radiotherapy as part of conservation therapy (p. 388). In Wessex, for example, a 20% increase in referral of early breast cancer has been noted between 1987 and 1991. Increasing numbers of cases of prostate, colorectal and AIDS related malignancy are likely to be referred to oncology departments.

EPIDEMIOLOGY OF CANCER

Terminology

Epidemiology is the study of the occurrence and distribution of disease. It can be divided into three main groups: descriptive, analytical and experimental.

Descriptive epidemiology is concerned with the retrospective analysis of the relationship between a disease and suspected aetiological factors.

Analytical epidemiology is the study of the relationship between different risk factors (e.g. age, sex, occupation) and the development of disease.

Experimental epidemiology involves observing the effects of controlling relevant suspected factors (e.g. stopping cigarette smoking).

The *incidence rate* of any disease is the total number of new cases occurring over a given period of time (usually a year) among a given number of people (usually 100 000 for cancer). This is different from the *prevalence rate* which is the number of cases of a particular disease existing at a given point in time.

The *mortality rate* is the incidence rate for the endpoint of death. The *crude death rate* is the number of deaths during a given period of time (normally a year) per thousand population. Crude death rates are of limited value since they do not take account of the differing proportions of people in particular age groups between populations. The crude death rate in a particular population may exceed that of another country simply because it contains a higher proportion of elderly people. The *age-specific death rate* takes account of the effect of age distribution on death rates. It is defined as:

$$\frac{\text{Number of deaths in a specific age group}}{\text{Mean population of that age group}} \times 1000$$

It provides a useful means of comparing mortality in different populations.

The *standardised mortality ratio* (SMR) is an overall measure of mortality which compares the observed number of deaths from a disease in a particular population with the expected number of deaths that would have been anticipated in a standard population if the age-specific death rates were the same.

$$\text{SMR} = \frac{\text{Observed numbers of deaths in given region}}{\text{Expected number of deaths in given region}} \times 100$$

SMRs are useful in comparing deaths from cancer in particular socioeconomic groups and occupations.

PROGNOSIS IN CANCER

We know what we mean by 'cure' of a simple fracture. We mean the uniting of the fracture and freedom from further trouble. But what do we mean by 'cure' of diabetes mellitus? We mean control of the underlying disease process but not its eradication. So in cancer we may talk of the 'cure' of, for example, a small basal cell carcinoma by surgery or radiotherapy where recurrence or persistent disease is uncommon. In other cancers such as breast cancer it is more appropriate to use the term 'control' since the tumour may recur locally or at distant sites after many years of freedom from the disease.

Indices of success

Survival rates

In measuring the success of treatment for cancer, a conventional yardstick is the proportion of patients who survive for a certain number of years—usually five. *Five-year survival* is sometimes interpreted as 'cure'. While this is true of many squamous carcinomas of the head and neck, it is not true of breast cancer, as seen above. For breast cancer, 10-, 20- or even 30-year survival figures (Fig. 23.13) are more appropriate end-points because of the long-term pattern of relapse and death from the disease.

Survival may be with or without evidence of cancer. For this reason the terms *disease-free survival* or *recurrence-free survival* are commonly used to define the outcome of treatment. These results require an elaborate system of clinic follow-up. Yet it is only from painstaking analysis of this kind that we can derive a sound knowledge both of the natural history of cancer and the effects of treatment. Survival data are commonly presented plotted graphically as curves (Fig. 23.13) which allow the comparison of different treatments for different stages of disease over time.

Crude survival. In studies of patients treated for cancer a variety of ways are used for analysing their survival. *Crude survival rate* refers to the number of patients alive a given number of years (*n*) after treatment. This is not valid unless all the patients included have been followed up for at least *n* years.

Actuarial survival. If a proportion of patients have been followed up for a shorter time than *n* years, the *actuarial method* (also known as log rank) is commonly used. The actuarial method assumes that all patients are subject to the same probability of dying from a particular cancer whether or not they have been withdrawn or lost from a study. It also assumes that for patients entering a study over a given period of time the probability of survival is constant. This method is used for calculating survival rates for deaths from cancer alone. Patients who die from causes other than cancer (i.e. from intercurrent disease) are considered to have been withdrawn from the study during the interval in which their death has occurred.

Age-corrected survival. Crude or actuarial survival rates do not take account of the mortality from natural causes of the patients studied. As a result the efficacy of treatment can be substantially underestimated. The crude survival rate can be corrected for age (*age-corrected survival rate*). The age-corrected *n* year survival rate is:

$$\frac{\text{Crude } n \text{ year survival rate}}{\text{Expected } n \text{ year survival rate in a normal population of the same sex and age composition.}}$$

The age-corrected survival rate enables direct comparisons between cohorts of patients of different ages and sex. It is the mortality specific to that particular disease. If a group treated for the same cancer has the same death rate from all causes as that of the normal population of the same sex and age, that group of patients can be considered cured. When the survival of the normal and treated groups are plotted semi-logarithmically, the point at which the two curves begin to run in parallel is the time at which the survivors can be considered cured. In breast cancer the mortality of the disease continues to exceed that of the normal

population even up to 30 years after treatment (Fig. 23.13). The curves never cross and patients can rarely be considered cured because of the long-term risk of relapse.

Outcome of palliative care

Survival figures are essential for estimating the success of treatment aimed at cure but are of limited value in assessing the effects of palliative treatment. The main aim of palliative treatment is the relief of distressing symptoms (p. 552). Palliative radiotherapy or chemotherapy may sometimes restrain tumour growth sufficiently to prolong the patient's life for a few months or sometimes years. However, as a goal, survival is subordinate to symptomatic relief.

EPIDEMIOLOGY AND THE PREVENTION OF CANCER

The principal role of epidemiological studies in oncology has been in the prevention of cancer. Such studies have played a major role in establishing occupational hazards in several industries (e.g. bladder cancer in aniline dye workers) and the link between lung cancer and smoking.

Epidemiology can assist in the prevention of cancer in a number of ways. First, it can show differences in the incidence of cancer in different populations and correlate them with differences in the prevalence of a potential causal factor. Secondly, it can test a hypothesis about the relationship between the occurrence of the disease to an aspect of the affected individual's constitution or exposure to some environmental factor. Thirdly, it can test the validity of a causal relationship by seeing whether the disease can be prevented or its incidence reduced by changing the prevalence of the suspected agent. A good example of the latter is the reduction in lung cancer observed among doctors since they gave up smoking cigarettes.

This analytical approach in the field of cancer has a long history. Percivall Pott in 1775 was the first to describe an occupational cancer. He established the relationship between cancer of the scrotum and exposure to soot in chimney-sweeps. Of wider significance has been the link established between cigarette smoking and lung cancer by Doll and Hill in 1964 in a survey of over 40 000 British doctors. Research of this type is important since it has opened the way to the prevention of certain malignant diseases by encouraging the population to avoid carcinogenic risk factors such as smoking and alcohol.

Latent period

One of the factors that makes the establishment of causal relationships between risk factors and particular cancers difficult is the long 'latent period' between exposure to the carcinogenic agent and the clinical appearance of the disease. For example, following the explosion of atomic bombs on Hiroshima and Nagasaki in 1945, solid tumours were not apparent until 15–20 years later in survivors. In most cases it is chronic rather than acute exposure to carcinogens that gives rise to cancer.

The latent period before cancer is clinically apparent will vary with the type of carcinogen, intensity and duration of exposure and age at the onset of exposure. Exposure to relatively small quantities of blue asbestos on a very limited number of occasions may induce pleural cancer several decades later. The risk of developing lung cancer is three times higher at the age of 60 for those who begin smoking cigarettes at about the age of 15 compared with those who start smoking 10 years later. It has been estimated that for lung cancer and skin cancer the risk of developing cancer roughly varies in proportion to the fourth power of the duration of exposure. For example, the carcinogenic effect after 40 years of exposure is 10–20 times that after 20 years of exposure. It may be that this biological principle holds true for many other tumours.

Sex, age and race in the distribution of cancer

Each tumour tends to have a typical sex distribution and age range. In some tumours these characteristics hold good anywhere in the world, e.g. for retinoblastoma. The sex distribution of retinoblastoma is roughly evenly balanced, with a peak incidence between 1 and 2 years of age.

In other tumours the age and sex distributions may vary. Bladder cancer in the UK is three times commoner in men than women and occurs in the sixth and seventh decades, with a peak incidence at the age of 65. However the disease may occur earlier in men in their forties and fifties if they have been occupationally exposed to aniline dyes in the rubber industry. There is wide racial variation in incidence: bladder cancer is twice as common in Caucasians as it is in Blacks. In other tumours the age range is more rigid, irrespective of country and race. Cancer is mainly a disease of the middle-aged and elderly. Skin, lung, colorectal and bladder cancer are typical examples. The rate of increase in incidence with age is non-linear and accelerates at and beyond middle age. Occasionally the disease may

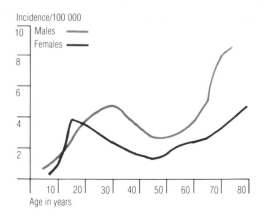

Fig. 13.2 Age-specific incidence of Hodgkin's disease (England, 1984). (Reproduced with permission from Souhami R L & Moxham J 1990 Textbook of Medicine, Churchill Livingstone, Edinburgh.)

have more than one peak. Hodgkin's disease has two age peaks. The first is at about 25 years and the second in the sixth decade (Fig. 13.2). These different age peaks suggest that different aetiological factors may be at work, with different latent periods between exposure and tumour development.

Changing incidence and mortality over time

Both the incidence and mortality of the disease may vary between males and females and change over time.

The male:female ratio for lung cancer increased from 2.0:1 after the First World War to 6.7:1 in 1959. By 1983 it had fallen to 2.8:1. Pipe smoking, virtually a male preserve, was a principal factor in the explanation of the increase in males from 1900 to 1925. In addition, lung cancer was commoner in non-smoking males. Recently there has been a small decrease in the male mortality from lung cancer but in females it continues to rise. The latter is thought to reflect the rise in the number of women who began smoking in the Second World War. The fall in male mortality has no obvious explanation since the number of cigarettes smoked over this period has remained relatively stable.

Sex ratios for some tumours may vary markedly between countries and also influence outcome of treatment. For example the male to female ratio of carcinoma of the oesophagus may vary from nearly 1:1 to 20:1. The prognosis is slightly more favourable in females.

Variation between populations

Differences in incidence of the same tumour between different countries certainly occur, although some may be explained by variation in case registration and medical practice. The incidence and death rates from breast cancer in the Far East are a tenth of those in the West.

Influence of migration

There is good evidence that the incidence of cancer among migrants often differs from the population that they left. Black migrants from Africa to the USA have rates of cancer more similar to white Americans than to the black population in Africa. Similarly, Japanese migrants to Hawaii have rates of colorectal cancer more comparable with those of caucasian Hawaiians than of the Japanese in Japan. This suggests that environmental factors in the country to which these groups have migrated play a part in the development of malignant disease.

Variation in incidence of cancer over time

While differences in incidence over time may reflect variation in standards of diagnosis, true changes have occurred. The incidence of cancer of the tongue has substantially declined in the UK. The reasons for this are unclear. It probably relates in part to improved oral hygiene. Gastric cancer has also declined in Western Europe in the last five decades (1930 to 1980).

Table 13.1 Proportion of cancer deaths attributable to different environmental factors (Reproduced with permission from Doll R, Peto R 1987 in Weatherall et al, Oxford Textbook of Medicine, 2nd edn, Oxford University Press)

Factor or class of factors	Best estimate of proportion (%)
Ionising radiation	
Background	1
Medical procedures	0.5
Industry	<0.1
Ultraviolet radiation	0.5
Occupation	4
Industrial products	<1
Pollution	
Atmospheric	1
Water	<1
Medical drugs	<1
Diet	30
Food additives	<1
Tobacco	30
Alcohol	3
Reproductive and sexual behaviour	7
Infection	(10)
Others and unknown	?

REDUCING THE RISKS OF DEVELOPING CANCER

Based largely on our current knowledge of the aetiology of cancer, it has been estimated that 80% of malignancies are preventable. To put the environmental causes of cancer in perspective their relative proportions have been summarised in Table 13.1. The striking feature is the high proportion due to dietary factors and to smoking (30% each). Smoking is discussed in more detail in Chapter 22. Changing dietary habits could potentially reduce the risk of cancer, possibly by a third. The main cancers involved are those of the stomach, colon and rectum and breast.

European code on the prevention of cancer

The EC has produced a 10-point code (Fig. 13.3) for the general public, summarising the ways in which certain common cancers can be prevented.

Reducing tobacco smoking

The UK Government has made health warnings mandatory on commercial tobacco products and on advertisements for tobacco. To achieve substantial reductions in tobacco consumption additional measures would be required. These could include banning advertising of tobacco, its consumption in public places and working environments, increasing taxation on tobacco, reducing tar content in cigarettes and setting up clinics for smokers to help them break the habit.

Alcohol

After smoking, alcohol is the second most important cause of cancer. It may be responsible in some countries for up to 10% of deaths from cancer. Cancers of the mouth, larynx, pharynx, oesophagus and liver are certainly caused in part by alcohol. It probably has a role in the aetiology of some breast and rectal cancers. For several tumours the risk rises with the quantity consumed to more than tenfold for lifelong non-drinkers.

Alcohol and tobacco smoking act as synergistic carcinogens (i.e. the combined effect is greater than that of either alone). This combination accounts for the very high incidence of these tumours in France, where they are often multifocal. Alcohol probably acts as a co-carcinogen rather than a carcinogen (i.e. it promotes rather than initiates carcinogenesis). Spirits may have a slightly stronger carcinogenic effect than other alcoholic beverages.

AVOIDING CANCER

A [10] POINT CODE...

THE EUROPEAN CODE

SMOKING IS THE GREATEST RISK FACTOR OF ALL...

Smokers, stop as quickly as possible. Cigarette smoking causes a third of all cancer deaths.

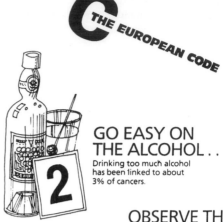

GO EASY ON THE ALCOHOL...

Drinking too much alcohol has been linked to about 3% of cancers.

AVOID BEING OVERWEIGHT...

Some cancers are associated with extreme overweight. Regular exercise and a sensible diet helps reduce weight.

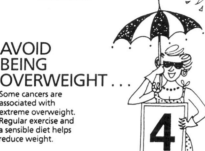

TAKE CARE IN THE SUN

Too much sun can cause skin cancer, so remember to protect your skin from sunburn.

OBSERVE THE HEALTH AND SAFETY REGULATIONS AT WORK

Some 40 or so chemicals and processes are known to cause cancer. If you are in any doubt, see your works doctor or health and safety representative.

CUT DOWN ON FATTY FOODS...

In countries where people eat a lot of meat, butter and other dairy products, there is a higher risk of breast and bowel cancer as well as coronary heart disease. Eat lean meat, try fish or chicken instead of red meat.

EAT PLENTY OF FRESH FRUIT AND VEGETABLES AND OTHER FOODS CONTAINING FIBRE

There is evidence that these foods may give some protection against cancer.

SEE YOUR DOCTOR IF THERE IS ANY UNEXPLAINED CHANGE IN YOUR NORMAL HEALTH WHICH LASTS FOR MORE THAN TWO WEEKS

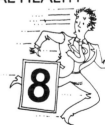

ESPECIALLY FOR WOMEN...

HAVE A REGULAR CERVICAL SMEAR TEST

The smear test can detect abnormal changes and very early cancer of the cervix when it can be successfully treated. Ask your doctor or family planning clinic for advice.

EXAMINE YOUR BREASTS MONTHLY

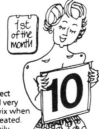

Women over the age of 50 should be screened by mammography at regular intervals. Self-examination should be done carefully. There are leaflets that tell you how. The NHS is setting up breast screening clinics and women aged 50-64 will be invited for screening every three years.

This leaflet was produced by the Cancer Education Co-ordinating Group of the United Kingdom and Republic of Ireland with support from the European Community and HEA, as part of the 'Europe against Cancer' campaign to reduce the number of deaths from cancer by 15%.

The Code has been approved by the European Community's Committee of Experts.

'EUROPE AGAINST CANCER' Campaign

Fig. 13.3 The European 10-point code against cancer.

Any policy on moderating the consumption of alcohol has to take account of a number of facts. First, many people find it pleasurable. Secondly, moderate amounts (2–3 units per day) protect against coronary thrombosis, though heavy drinking has other undesirable social consequences (e.g. violent behaviour and road accidents). Thirdly, its carcinogenic effects are largely in conjunction with smoking tobacco. Thus the risk of cancer induction by alcohol in non-smokers is relatively small.

Ultraviolet light

Exposure to ultraviolet light has been increasing with the reduction of the ozone layer caused by chemical pollution. An increase in the incidence of all forms of skin cancer can be expected. The principal culprits are the *chlorofluorohydrocarbons* (CFCs). These are components in, for example, aerosol sprays, refrigerants, and solvents for cleaning electronic equipment. However, to put the contribution of commercial sources of CFCs into context, one volcano in Antarctica emits 100 tons (100×10^3 kg) of chlorine every month, substantially more than the combined output of CFCs from deodorants over the same period. Nitrogen oxides from vehicle exhaust fumes also deplete the ozone layer. International agreements have been reached aimed at cutting the use of CFCs by 50% by 1998.

Occupational exposure

A wide variety of occupations are known to carry the risk of exposure to carcinogens. However they only represent a relatively small number of cases of cancer deaths (4% in the USA). In 1987, 246 agents were classified by the International Agency for Research on Cancer as definitely (50), probably (37) or possibly (159) carcinogenic to humans. These included industrial processes, industrial chemicals, pesticides, laboratory chemicals, drugs, food ingredients, tobacco smoking and related stimulants. Drugs and industrial chemicals represent the largest risks. There are many other occupations where an agent is thought to be carcinogenic to workers but a causal link has not been established. Some of the known occupational hazards are listed in Table 13.2. Of these, exposure to asbestos dust, aromatic amines and the products of burning fossil fuels are the commonest.

Measures to prevent occupational exposure include labelling of products as carcinogenic, and prohibiting the marketing and use of certain substances, e.g. the four aromatic amines (naphthylamine, 4-aminobiphenyl, 4-nitrodiphenyl and benzidine) and blue asbestos (crocidolite).

It is thought that preventive methods are likely to have little impact on the mortality from occupational cancers in the near future. The detection of tumours at an early stage by screening is likely to have a greater effect on mortality. Screening of urine by cytology among workers in the dyestuff and rubber industries has long been practised.

Diet

Diet influences carcinogenesis in a variety of ways: carcinogens may be eaten; food substances may be

Table 13.2 Occupational cancers

Occupation	Site of tumour	Agent
Dye manufacturers, rubber workers	Bladder	Aromatic amines
Copper and cobalt smelters: pesticide manufacture	Skin, lung	Arsenic
Manufacture of chromates from chrome ore	Lung	Chromium
Asbestos miners: asbestos textile manufacturers; insulation and shipyard workers	Lung, pleura, peritoneum, larynx	Asbestos
Workers with glues and varnishes	Marrow, e.g. erythroleukaemia	Benzene
Uranium and other miners; luminisers; radiologists; radiographers	Lung, bone, bone marrow	Ionising radiation
Nickel refiners	Nasal sinuses, lung	Nickel
Hardwood furniture manufacturers	Nasal sinuses	Agent unknown
Leather workers	Nasal sinuses	Agent unknown
Coal gas manufacturers; asphalters; roofers; aluminium refiners; workers exposed to tars and oils	Skin, scrotum, lung	Polycyclic hydrocarbons (soot, tar and oil)
Seamen, farmers	Skin	Ultraviolet light
PVC manufacturers	Liver (angiosarcoma)	Vinyl chloride

(Modified from Doll R, Peto R 1987 in Weatherall et al, Oxford Textbook of Medicine, 2nd edn, Oxford University Press.)

converted to carcinogens once ingested; and dietary components may modify the ways in which the body metabolises and responds to carcinogens.

The only component of food which has been found to be strongly linked to the development of cancer is *aflatoxin*. This is a product of the fungus *Aspergillus fumigatus* which often contaminates damp cereals in tropical countries. It causes primary liver cancer (see Ch. 22), although the data are unclear since there is a high incidence of hepatitis B, itself associated with liver tumours, in the same group of patients.

Bracken fern containing nitrates is suspected of causing oesophageal cancer, particularly among the Japanese. Salted fish is implicated in the aetiology of nasopharyngeal cancer (p. 327), possibly as a co-carcinogen with the Epstein–Barr virus.

Diet may be indirectly related to carcinogenesis. One example is fibre, which seems to have a protective effect against colorectal cancer (p. 368). A second is obesity, which is associated with an increased incidence of cancer of the endometrium and of the gallbladder in women. Consumption of saturated fat is implicated but not proven as a cause of breast cancer. A third is vitamin A (retinol) and its derivatives, retinoids, which may inhibit the full malignant transformation of cells and prevent tumour formation.

Dietary measures likely to reduce the risk of cancers are:

— High fibre diet
— Reducing saturated fats
— Plenty of fresh fruit and vegetables (due to the presence of antioxidants such as vitamin E).

Ionising radiation

The whole spectrum of sources of ionising radiations, both natural and man-made, has been calculated to contribute 1.5% of all fatal cancers. The sources of radiation exposure in the UK are shown in Fig. 13.4.

It is estimated that exposure to radon gas from domestic buildings may be responsible for 1% of lung cancer in Europe. Concentrations of radon gas in excess of 400 Bq/m^3 (about 1 in 1000 homes) will expose the occupants to 20 mSv per year. The lifetime risk of fatal cancer from this exposure is about 10%. The carcinogenic risks of ionising radiation have been revised upwards since 1988. Current estimates of risk are 2–5 times higher. However it is unclear whether these revised estimates apply to very low levels of exposure to natural background radioactivity.

The role of ionising radiation in the causation of cancer is mainly derived from occupational exposure. Early evidence came from the development of lung cancer amongst miners at Joachimstal in Czechoslovakia and Schneeberg in Germany. Lung disease had been known to occur amongst these workers since the 16th century. It was subsequently appreciated that the disease was lung cancer due to radioactive radon gas in the mines.

The main source of evidence of the effects of ionising radiation in man are the survivors of the atomic bombs dropped on Hiroshima and Nagasaki in 1945. The incidence of acute and chronic leukaemia was significantly raised within a radius of 1.5 km from the epicentre. The highest incidence occurred 6–8 years afterwards. For cancers other than leukaemia the

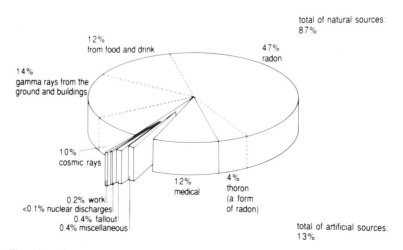

Fig. 13.4   Sources of radiation exposure in the UK population, 1988, based on data supplied by the National Radiological Protection Board. (Reproduced with permission from *Reducing the Risks of Cancers*, Open University, 1989.)

latent period was longer (15–20 years) among victims who received 1 Gy or more; indeed the incidence is still higher 40 years later.

It is assumed that there is no threshold below which cancers cannot be induced by ionising radiation. Indeed children who received only 0.01–0.02 Gy in utero when their mothers were irradiated had an additional 1 in 2000 risk of cancer. At low doses the risk of developing cancer is probably proportional to dose, although much uncertainty remains.

Reducing the levels of radon gas from domestic buildings requires a number of measures. First, systematic surveys are needed to identify buildings which pose a hazard. Levels of radon gas can be reduced by alterations to the floors and installation of extractor fans.

Pollution

Atmospheric. Atmospheric pollution has been suspected to be carcinogenic, ever since the incidence of lung cancer was found to be higher in cities than in the country. The combustion products of coal are known to contain carcinogenic hydrocarbons. However since the atmosphere is polluted by a wide variety of substances, often in small quantities, the assessment of carcinogenic risk is very difficult. The situation is further complicated by the contribution to atmospheric pollution of tobacco smoking. In the past pollution probably accounted for about 1% of cancers. Atmospheric pollution in the UK is now falling with stricter rules on the burning of fossil fuels. The evidence suggests that the current burning of fossil fuels, arsenic and asbestos will contribute to much less than 1% of future cancers.

Water. Ingestion of trihalomethanes from chlorinated drinking water may increase the risk of bladder cancer. Reduction of levels of these chemicals in drinking water is desirable.

EARLY DETECTION AND CANCER SCREENING

Early diagnosis of some cancers gives the best chance of cure. Sadly, symptoms of many tumours do not develop until the tumours are advanced and the prospect of cure limited (e.g. ovarian and small cell lung cancer). Some patients may conceal advanced tumours, typically of the breast, through fear of confirmation of the diagnosis or through ignorance. Here, however, we are concerned with presymptomatic diagnosis. Although we use the term 'early', it must be remembered that when a cancer is detectable, it is often 'late' in its natural

history and may already have seeded distant metastases (e.g. breast cancer). 'Early' is therefore a relative concept applied clinically. An early breast cancer that is only just palpable (or perhaps detected by mammography and not yet palpable) is a very different problem from an advanced tumour invading the chest wall.

Presymptomatic diagnosis

Presymptomatic diagnosis clearly involves a positive search for people who would not otherwise have consulted their doctors or feel the need to submit to any examination or test. *Screening* is the process by which particular tumours are detected at a stage in their development when treatment has a good prospect of cure. It involves submitting a large population (mass screening) to the same screening test, e.g. submitting all women between 50 and 64 years to mammography to detect breast cancer.

Criteria for screening

A number of criteria must be satisfied to carry out mass screening for a particular tumour:
— Treatment must have a good prospect of cure for disease detected at a early stage.
— The disease must be sufficiently common for a reasonable number of cases to be detected.
— The method of screening must have a high probability of detecting the disease when present (true positive) and a low probability of a positive result when the disease is absent (false positive).
— The screening method must be acceptable to patients, affordable, and practical to apply and interpret in trained hands.

Advantages of screening

1. Reduction in mortality. The main advantage of screening is that it can reduce the mortality from certain cancers (for example in women with breast cancer over the age of 50).

2. Reduced number of patients requiring radical treatment. The detection of premalignant changes and their eradication by simple measures (e.g. colposcopic laser therapy for severe cervical dysplasia, p. 402) reduces the need for radical radiotherapy or surgery.

3. Reassurance of patients whose screening test is negative.

Disadvantages of screening

1. Overdiagnosis of non-progressive lesions. Screening

may detect different degrees of cellular abnormality (e.g. in cervical smears). These may range from mild dysplasia to carcinoma-in-situ (p. 402). For some tumours there may be an orderly progression through these histological changes on the path to invasive malignancy. However more patients are detected with early changes than would be expected to progress to frank malignancy. Thus not all patients with dysplastic cervical smears will progress to malignancy. Screening is not therefore of benefit to all women with abnormal cervical smears.

2. Psychological and physical morbidity. Anxiety is commonly generated among patients about the technique of screening and its results. This is increased if the patient has to be recalled for further investigations, even if these eventually prove negative. Screening may be uncomfortable. Good mammography requires the breast to be compressed. Similarly laser therapy for a severely dysplastic cervix may be very painful without adequate analgesia.

3. False reassurance. If the screening test is negative, a tumour may still be present. The patient may feel reassured and perhaps ignore the symptoms of the tumour in the belief that she is free of disease. This may occur in early breast cancer where the mammogram is negative or in cervical cancer if the cervical smear has been incorrectly performed.

Measuring the effectiveness of screening

Before mass screening is introduced, a significant reduction in the mortality from the disease needs to be demonstrated on a large population of patients. This is by far the most important measure of the efficacy of screening. The best design is a randomised prospective trial in which a defined population is assigned randomly to screening or to an unscreened control group. All the deaths due to the particular tumour are recorded among each group over a period of years. Long-term follow-up of such patients is necessary since the transition from premalignant to malignant changes may be in excess of 10 years.

The shorter-term effects of screening can be measured in three ways.

1. The number of cancers detected. In general the number of cancers detected by screening should exceed the expected annual incidence. This is because screening has detected, and treatment prevented, some cases progressing to invasive cancer. For example the annual expected incidence of breast cancer in women between 50 and 64 years is 1.6 per 1000. The equivalent figure from the screened population is 5. On subsequent screening the incidence of tumours in the screened population should fall to about the same as the annual expected incidence.

2. Earlier stage of disease detected. If screening is effective the proportion of early tumours detected should exceed the expected proportion in an unscreened population. For example the proportion of early cases of colorectal cancer (Dukes' A) found by screening for faecal occult blood is 50%, compared with 10% in an unscreened population.

3. Comparison of survival of screening detected and unscreened cases—sources of bias. Better survival of patients whose tumours were detected by screening compared with those who were not does not necessarily confirm the benefit of screening. There are two reasons for this. First, the survival of screened cases is measured from the time of diagnosis. This point may be substantially earlier than the time at which symptomatic presentation would have occurred. The time of death may be exactly the same but the survival of the screened cases will be longer. This is known as 'lead-time bias'.

Secondly, the screened cases are likely to contain a higher proportion of slowly growing tumours. Faster growing tumours are more likely to have presented symptomatically before they are screened. Screened tumours are likely to be slower growing with longer survival.

An additional source of bias is the fact that participation in cancer screening is more likely among the better educated who are more conscious of their health. The difficulty is to obtain the attendance of those from lower socioeconomic groups who have a lesser appreciation of preventive medicine. Women who are prostitutes and at higher risk of cervical cancer frequently default from appointments for screening.

Methods of screening

In addition to simple self-examination, the available methods include:

— Periodic medical examination
— Cytological examination
— Radiological examination
— Highly specialised techniques—radioactive isotopes, biochemical and hormonal estimations, faecal occult blood, endoscopy.

Periodic medical examination

This form of screening has achieved limited popularity, applied either to selected groups such as business executives or offered commercially to those able to afford it. In addition to routine clinical examination, it includes a variety of laboratory blood and urine tests and a chest radiograph. Barium meal or sigmoidoscopy are occasionally carried out. It is unavoidably costly and unsuited to mass screening.

Cytological methods

Cytological methods differ from histological ones. The latter relate to cells organised in tissues, the former to cells isolated singly or in tiny clusters. Growing tumours shed (exfoliate) cells from their surface and these can be fixed and stained on a slide and examined microscopically. The expert can recognise abnormal features of cancer cells, for example of the appearance of the nucleus.

This technique of exfoliative cytology was developed by Papanicolaou in the USA. It is a simpler procedure than surgical biopsy.

Uterine cervix. Premalignant changes or early cancer can be detected by a cervical smear (p. 402). This is the most common application of cytological diagnosis.

Urinary tract (especially bladder). After centrifugation, cells deposited from the urine are examined for evidence of malignancy. This technique is useful for screening workers in dye and rubber industries who are at above average risk for bladder cancer. This method is more acceptable to the public than routine cystoscopy, though less accurate.

Lung. Malignant cells may be detected in the sputum. The need for bronchoscopy in some patients with obvious tumours on chest radiograph may thus be avoided.

Stomach. Gastric washings may yield cancer cells.

Radiological examination

— Mammography is able to screen for early breast cancer before it is large enough for either the patient or her doctor to feel.
— Chest radiographs have been used to screen for lung cancer.
— Barium meal examination using the double contrast technique, often in conjunction with endoscopy, has been employed to detect gastric cancer in Japan, which has a very high incidence of the disease.

Evaluation of screening programmes

In an ideal world, screening would only be introduced once the costs and benefits had been carefully assessed. Regrettably this is not always the case. Cervical screening, for example, was implemented in the UK before the evidence of benefit was certain. It was instituted because screening was felt by the public and medical profession to be worthwhile but it has never been submitted to a randomised controlled trial.

What can be learned from experience so far? Each cancer will be considered in turn.

Lung

Several mass surveys to detect lung cancer have been carried out by chest radiography and/or sputum cytology. Although there is an increased yield in the first screen, a shift towards the diagnosis of tumours at an earlier stage, and better survival of screen detected cases, no reduction in overall mortality has been demonstrated. The majority of screened cases were still inoperable.

There is no evidence at present that screening for lung cancer is worthwhile. A much greater impact could be made by reducing the smoking of cigarettes.

Cervix

Screening for cervical cancer has been shown from a variety of retrospective studies to reduce the incidence and mortality from invasive cervical cancer. Mass screening was introduced in Europe in the early 1960s in the absence of evidence of effectiveness.

Uncertainty about its benefits was reinforced by the fact that the mortality from the disease was declining in the UK and USA. There was no obvious acceleration in this decline with the introduction of cervical screening. Wide variations in the natural incidence of the disease in Britain, the earlier implementation of effective treatment of symptomatic disease and increasing rates of hysterectomy make the contribution of cervical screening difficult to assess. However in countries where screening has been quickly and comprehensively introduced the rise in incidence up to the age of 50 is interrupted, showing a fall corresponding to the time when screening was introduced.

The cervical smear is taken using a specially shaped spatula (Fig. 13.5), and the material transferred to a slide. In the UK cervical screening is repeated every 3–5 years in women of 35 years or older.

Although exfoliative cytology remains the cornerstone of current cervical screening, there is a need for more reliable methods since false-negative rates range from 20 to 40%.

There is an increasing trend towards an increased incidence of the disease in young women. This may be

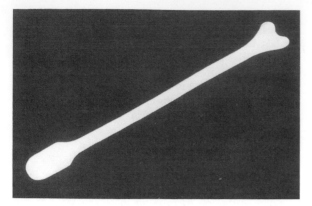

Fig. 13.5 Spatula for taking a cervical smear.

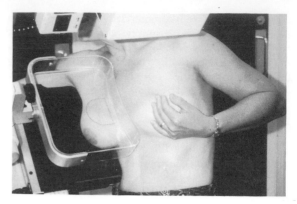

Fig. 13.6 Patient undergoing mammography. (Courtesy of the Rotherham Breast Screening Service.)

related to sexually transmitted viral infection. Some gynaecologists are recommending changing the criteria for describing a smear as positive to include more women with minimal cellular abnormalities. Such women are being recommended to have colposcopic treatment of even these minimal cellular changes. An assessment of cervical screening using new criteria for reporting cervical smears has yet to be made.

Carcinoma-in-situ has been replaced by the term *cervical intraepithelial neoplasia* (CIN). CIN is divided into three grades, of which CIN III is the most abnormal. All grades of CIN are precancerous. Initially it was thought that CIN I or mild dysplasia was benign. This is now considered to be premalignant and up to 25% of CIN I will progress to CIN III over a 2-year period. Transformation to malignancy has been reported in 18% of CIN III at 10 years and 36% at 20 years.

Patients with CIN should be submitted to colposcopy (illuminated magnification of the cervix). Colposcopic examination allows abnormal areas of the cervix to be biopsied. In many units all patients with CIN are treated. Where the whole abnormal area on the cervix can be seen at colposcopy, it is treated by laser evaporation. If the abnormal area is only partially defined, a cone biopsy (Fig. 24.4) or cylinder excision of the endo- and ectocervix is performed.

Breast cancer

This is an even more important cancer numerically, with over 13 000 deaths per year in the UK. One in every 12 women will be affected by the disease at some time in her life.

The value of screening for breast cancer has been more intensively studied than at any other tumour site. There is an increased yield of tumours at the first screen, a shift to earlier stage distribution and better survival in the screened population.

Two large randomised studies have shown a 30% reduction in mortality from breast cancer in women aged 50 or over. The reduction persists for up to 18 years, although it falls at that time to 23%. No benefit has been demonstrated in women below the age of 50.

Regular self-examination is the simplest and most obvious means of early detection of a lump in the breast. However it is not now recommended as a method of screening since it has brought about no reduction in breast cancer mortality. (However it remains true that at present, self-detection of a lump is the commonest way a breast cancer is detected.) The minimum size that can be detected by this technique is about 1.5 cm.

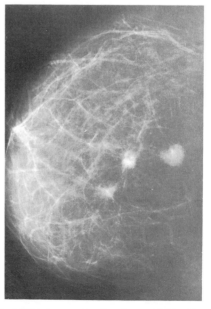

Fig. 13.7 Mammogram showing three spiculated tumours in the breast. (Courtesy of Dr R Peck, Sheffield.)

Mammography is the screening method of choice. A single oblique view of the breast (Fig. 13.6) delivers a dose of less than 0.01 Gy to the breast. It is of little value in the small fibrous breast, but very helpful, particularly in the large breast. It can detect tumours less than 1 cm in diameter.

The classic mammographic features of malignant lesions are: (1) a lesion with a dense centre and an irregular spiculated border (Fig. 13.7); and (2) stippled or punctate calcification (microcalcification), like grains of salt (Fig. 13.8). The presence of microcalcification is virtually pathognomonic of a carcinoma and occurs in about 30% of cases.

A national programme of mammographic screening was instituted in the UK in 1988 for women between 50 and 64 years. A single oblique view is used. Screening is repeated 3-yearly. Patients with abnormal or equivocal mammograms are recalled for clinical examination of the breast and, if necessary, additional mammographic views or ultrasound of the breast. Palpable abnormalities are subjected to fine needle aspiration. Impalpable lesions seen on mammography are localised and needled for cytology under radiological control.

Colorectal cancer

The mortality from colorectal cancer has remained unchanged. It would be of great value if screening could increase the detection of presymptomatic Dukes' A cancers. There is strong circumstantial evidence that many tumours develop from dysplastic adenomatous polyps. The value of screening for colorectal cancer is as yet unproven. A variety of methods have been used, including clinical examination, proctosigmoidoscopy and, if necessary, barium enema. The survival of cases detected by annual proctosigmoidoscopy (64–85%) among over 21 000 men and women was over twice that of symptomatic cases. However a reduction in overall mortality has yet to be demonstrated in a randomised controlled trial.

The most widely used test is that for the presence of faecal occult blood (*haemoccult test*). Disadvantages include the number of false positives, the sensitivity necessary to detect most cancers and polyps and limited acceptability of the technique to the public. It is the most useful test, if positive, for determining the need for proctosigmoidoscopy.

Reliance must still be placed on the immediate investigation of suspicious bowel disturbance or episodes of rectal bleeding, especially at and beyond middle age.

Stomach

No prospective evaluation of screening for stomach cancer has been undertaken. It is not clear what relative contributions the declining incidence and screening have made to the fall in the mortality from the disease. The situation is different in Japan where the incidence is much higher and many early cancers are detected.

Bladder cancer

Screening for bladder cancer by urinary cytology has been used for high risk groups. While an increased yield at first screening, detection of earlier stage disease and improved survival in screened cases have been demonstrated, no reduction in mortality from bladder cancer has been proved.

CANCER EDUCATION

Understanding about the nature and outcome of cancer treatments tends to vary with educational attainment. The better educated tend to take a greater interest in and are better informed about cancer. They may appreciate that cancer is not a single disease conferring a uniformly poor prognosis. This misconception is sadly still common. For a large proportion of the population, the ugly reputation of cancer persists. They are unaware that about 30% of cancers can be

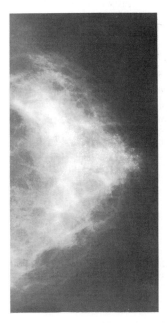

Fig. 13.8 Mammogram showing malignant calcification within the breast. (Courtesy of Dr R Peck, Sheffield.)

cured or controlled long enough to give patients an expectation of life not far from that of the normal population and that good palliation of symptoms can be achieved in most cases.

Concepts of radical and palliative treatment are not widely understood by the general public or by some members of the medical profession who have little contact with the management of malignant disease.

The need for a coordinated policy

The responsibility for cancer education should be shared between international organisations, national and local governments and the health service professions. A coordinated policy promoting the prevention and detection of early disease is required to have the maximum impact on the mortality of common diseases such as lung, breast and colorectal cancer.

International organisations

Since cancer is a global problem, there is a need for internationally agreed policies. The International Union Against Cancer (UICC) has provided a forum for formulating such policies. It has adopted a number of objectives in relation to tobacco smoking. These include:

— Achieving lower rates of smoking in all age groups.
— Encouraging non-smokers, especially young ones, to remain so.
— Stopping all forms of tobacco promotion.
— Encouraging smokers to reduce, as far as possible, their exposure to harmful components of tobacco smoke.
— Maintaining liaison with other health organisations and authorities to ensure maximum effectiveness and avoid conflicts of interest.

Educating the young about cancer

The behaviour patterns that predispose to some cancers, particularly smoking and cervical cancer, are often established in childhood or adolescence. Peer pressure is often a powerful factor in starting smoking. This pressure is often reinforced by tobacco advertising associating smoking with relaxation, confidence and being adult. Similarly, children whose parents smoke are more likely to do so themselves. However if their parents smoke but disapprove of their children doing so, children are less likely to become smokers. School policy, teacher and parental example may all contribute to a child's decision whether or not to smoke. Regular

smoking is not uncommon among 12- and 13-year-old children. Although smoking rates among boys have fallen, the rates among girls have declined more slowly.

Cervical cancer is known to be associated with starting sexual intercourse in the teens. There is evidence that the age at which the young are starting to have intercourse is declining. Often they have multiple partners. Both boys and girls need to be educated about cervical cancer. Schooling is the only period of a girl's life when her attendance at classes on cancer education is likely. On leaving school, the chances of reaching her with any message on cancer prevention declines sharply.

To prevent lung and cervical cancer it is therefore important to establish programmes of cancer education among children, to encourage behaviour which will avoid cancer and present a realistic picture of the disease in order to avoid unnecessary fear. The latter may reduce the likelihood of attendance for screening.

A child's perspective

A child's perspective of cancer differs from that of an adult. The idea of preventing cancer is difficult for them to comprehend. Children tend not to distinguish cancer from any other illness. The child may regard cancer simply as another type of infectious disease that he or she is likely to catch. Furthermore, talking about a disease which may affect a child several decades later is beyond the comprehension of most children. It seems too far-off to have any impact.

Cancer education for children: a different approach

The approach to cancer education among children has to be adapted to take account of the child's different perspective on disease. Teaching about health risks is likely to be non-productive. As one commentator says:

To children the facts are boring, the distant future is not relevant and some children like to take risks anyway... Imagine how many children hold most or even all of the following beliefs: it is part of life to smoke; all my family do; so do my friends and teachers; cigarettes are sold in ordinary shops, so they cannot be that bad; it is attractive to be as thin as possible, if not even thinner; fat people are ugly and laughable; it is good to be calm, cool, confident and sophisticated—cigarettes do this for you, films and advertising tell you so; it is old-fashioned not to have at least one boyfriend or girlfriend and quite unmentionable not to have sexual relations with them; it is beautiful to be tanned; not to eat meat every day is a sign of poverty; it is friendly and sociable to drink alcohol.

From the above statement it is clear that cancer education may conflict with a young person's firmly held beliefs. It is therefore necessary for the health educator to instil healthy behaviour into the lifestyle that the child has chosen.

Cancer education in schools

Successful cancer education within schools is dependent upon teachers having the necessary experience and teaching material. Teachers may have a number of reservations about teaching cancer education. They may feel (1) deficient in their own knowledge about, and fearful of, cancer; (2) that the children are too young to be taught about it; (3) that there is insufficient time within the curriculum.

However, rather than teaching cancer prevention as one subject or focusing a week of teaching on cancer education, teachers may be more amenable to incorporating it into part of their own subject area. For example dietary aspects of cancer prevention could be included in classes on home economics. The carcinogenic properties of certain industrial chemicals could be taught as part of chemistry. Children are more likely to take note of the messages of cancer prevention in this format.

Care needs to be taken that neither child nor adult is given to believe that they are wholly responsible for whether or not they develop cancer. This may induce feelings of guilt and disillusionment if they do contract the disease. It needs to be emphasised that following particular guidelines of behaviour does not always prevent cancer.

Good cancer education packages have been produced for use in schools, e.g. The Cancer Research Campaign Education and Child Studies Research Group package: 'Cells, Cancer and Communities'.

Cancer education within the local community

Each district health authority needs a coherent policy to communicate important information about prevention and early diagnosis of cancer and of services available for the care of patients with cancer and of their families. Such a policy requires coordination of a wide variety of groups, including health professionals, community representatives, school teachers and voluntary agencies.

The overall responsibility should lie with the District General Manager. There should be a District Health Promotion Unit which coordinates the publication and dissemination of educational material and organisation of meetings and provides advice to interested parties.

The Director of Education should be involved in developing a programme of cancer education in schools, providing training for teaching staff, encouraging the provision of healthy school meals and adopting non-smoking policies within schools.

The Director of Nursing may incorporate cancer education into basic and post-basic courses. He or she should support non-smoking policies in hospitals.

The role of the general practitioner

Members of the general public have most medical contact with their general practitioner. He or she is in a good position to offer simple advice on the prevention of cancer. Advice on stopping smoking is the most important. Patients may be referred to voluntary classes to help them stop smoking or to use non-carcinogenic nicotine substitutes (e.g. chewing Nicorette gum). The general practitioner can provide screening for cervical cancer and encourage women to accept invitations for breast screening. Young men can be given leaflets on self-examination for testicular cancer. The waiting areas of health centres offer a good site for displaying leaflets on the prevention and early diagnosis of cancer (e.g. the European 10-point code (Fig. 13.3).

Cancer education in the work place

Cancer education in the workplace can be channelled through environmental health officers, occupational medical and nursing staff, health and safety officers, management and trade unions.

Effective cancer education requires more than simply disseminating information about the causes. More important is the process of persuading people to change their lifestyle to reduce the risk of cancer. Exhorting people to stop smoking is easy. Persuading them sufficiently to stop doing so is much more difficult. One of the most effective methods of educational interventions is directed at small community groups. This may be based on locality, work or social network. Specially trained and influential members of target groups can be very effective in disseminating health education.

Cancer education in the workplace can be very effective if the following criteria are met. It must be part of a general health programme. It needs to be developed in consultation with management and unions. It should use existing networks within the workplace. It should be consonant with workers' own perceived health needs, i.e. what concerns them most. The programme should be popular, e.g. fitness or losing weight, and suited to the company's style.

The essential messages that need to be conveyed are:

1. Many cancers are preventable by changes in behaviour.
2. Some cancers are curable and prognosis for many is improving.
3. The quality of life of many patients with cancer is good.
4. Particular symptoms commonly associated with cancer should be reported promptly to a general practitioner.

14. Biological and pathological introduction

Radiotherapy is used almost exclusively for the treatment of cancer and related conditions. It is thus very important to have a reasonable understanding of this disease. This chapter contains an outline of the basic characteristics of cancerous cells, and the conditions that can cause cancer. There is consideration of the natural history of untreated cancer, and of the ways different types of cancer are named and classified.

GROWTH: PROLIFERATION AND DIFFERENTIATION

Growth is the process of increase in size and maturity of tissues from fertilisation through to the adult. When normally controlled, the different parts of the body take on their correct size and specialist functions, and relationship to one another. Furthermore, throughout life these attributes continue despite the need for replacement and repair. This is all a reflection of accurate control of the timing and extent of cellular proliferation, cell-to-cell orientation and organisation, and *differentiation*. Differentiation is the process of a cell taking on a specialised function; this is usually associated with a change in its microscopic appearance. It is also usually a one-way commitment, with relative or complete loss of the ability to continue proliferating.

Growth disorders

Hypertrophy is an increase in the size of an organ due to an increase in the size of its constituent cells. The left ventricle of the heart becomes hypertrophic if it has to work harder due to hypertension.

Hyperplasia is an increase in size because of an increase in the number of cells. The adrenal cortex will become hyperplastic if there is excessive adrenocorticotrophic hormone to stimulate it. However it will return to normal if the stimulus is reduced again.

Metaplasia is a change from one type of tissue to another. Smoking induces a change of the bronchial lining from the usual respiratory mucosa to a squamous epithelium, with resultant loss of mucus-producing and ciliated cells. It is also potentially reversible.

Neoplasia (literally a new growth), in contrast, is an irreversible process once initiated: it is the main subject of this chapter. It is also called cancer, or a tumour, though the latter is sometimes used to denote any swelling.

NEOPLASIA

A neoplasm, can be defined as 'a lesion resulting from the autonomous or relatively autonomous abnormal growth of cells which persists after the initiating stimulus has been removed; i.e. cell growth has escaped from normal regulatory mechanisms'. The abnormality affects all aspects of cell growth to varying degrees. Proliferation continues unabated, irrespective of the requirements of the organ in which the neoplasm is situated. This, combined with loss of control of the normal relationships between cells, often results in the new tumour cells replacing and insinuating themselves between the adjacent normal tissues, a process called *invasion*. Loss of differentiation accompanies, and often correlates with, failure of proliferation control and invasiveness.

Benign and malignant neoplasms

Neoplasia is not a single disease, but rather a common pathological process with a multitude of different varieties and clinical outcomes. One fundamental division is between *benign* and *malignant* tumours. Benign tumours will remain localised, with generally relatively little effect on the patient. In contrast, other tumours are locally destructive, may spread to involve other parts of the body, and ultimately result in the death of the patient. Figure 14.1 and Table 14.1 show some of the differences between benign and malignant

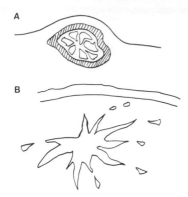

Fig. 14.1 Showing the difference between a benign tumour (A) contained by a definitive capsule and a malignant tumour (B) actively invading the tumour bed.

Table 14.1 Characteristics of neoplasms

Feature	Benign	Malignant
Growth rate	Slow	Variable, may be rapid
Margin	Encapsulated	Invasive
Local effect	Little	Destructive
Differentiation	Good	Variable, may be poor
Metastases	No	Frequently
Usual outcome	Good	Fatal

neoplasms. Further aspects of the classification of tumours are discussed later in this chapter.

The term *cancer* (Latin for 'crab') is very ancient, and there are several explanations for its usage. Some say it reflects the tenacious grip the disease has on its victim, some that it describes the radiating prominent veins that may surround an advanced superficial tumour. Others contend that it describes the irregular infiltrative profile of some tumours, e.g. of breast. Suffice it to say that cancer is a common colloquial term that is generally applied to any malignant neoplasm.

Though the behaviour of tumours, particularly malignant ones, may seem very odd it can generally be explained by the excessive or inappropriate expression of genes that are present in all cells. The tumour continues to be dependent upon an adequate blood supply (though many acquire the capacity to induce new vessels). Also, many of those which arise from hormone dependent tissues (e.g. breast, prostate) continue to show a degree of dependence on those hormones. This can be exploited to therapeutic advantage by giving antihormone treatment (Ch. 32).

CARCINOGENESIS

The causes of cancer are numerous, and mechanisms

of its production are complex, but some of the principles will be presented. There are two avenues of thought to follow: one at the molecular and genetic levels, the other concerned with causative associations. It is not always easy to relate these to each other. Underlying the mechanistic approach is the assumption that cell behaviour is controlled by the genes expressed (which ones, and how strongly), bearing in mind that these can be influenced by chemical messages relayed from outside the cell. Every cell contains the entire genetic code, but only expresses those genes appropriate to its own situation. In cancer this has gone wrong, particularly with respect to proliferation and differentiation. We can generalise to say that multiple abnormalities need to have occurred between normality and cancer, and that this reflects a *multistep* process. Only those cells capable of division are at risk of transforming into a neoplasm. This excludes terminally differentiated cells such as circulating red cells, the uppermost keratinised cells of the skin, and adult voluntary muscle and nerve cells.

Initiation

This describes the first step towards neoplasia. It reflects a change at the molecular level of how a cell can function, escaping in some small way from a control mechanism. Nothing can be seen microscopically at this stage. Substances that can initiate neoplasia are called *carcinogens*.

Promotion

No more will come of the initiated cell unless it continues to divide. Further abnormalities of cell function (i.e. gene expression) arise over a period of time. Substances that enhance this process are called *promoters*.

Progression

Neoplasms are *clonal*, i.e. are derived from a single cell. For this to happen, a cell and its progeny must acquire and sustain a growth advantage over other cells throughout succeeding cell divisions. This eventually results in visible alterations at the microscopic level. Not all the daughter cells will be identical, giving rise to differences between individual cells or subclones; this is called *pleomorphism*.

Clinical cancer

Finally, the neoplasm becomes manifest as a clinically

significant tumour. Unless removed, it will continue to progress with a general tendency towards further loss of growth restraint, and acquisition of the capacity to spread to other parts of the body (metastasise).

Oncogenes and tumour suppressor genes

Over the past few years, a large number of the genes have been identified as potentially involved in the above steps. *Oncogenes* (i.e. tumour genes) came to light in experimental systems where they caused 'tumours' to form in tissue culture. Many of the genes were found to be closely related to genes found in viruses capable of causing tumours in other species: this is reflected in their nomenclature. As a generalisation, many of these genes are normally concerned with various aspects of cell proliferation. Some tumours are found to have a mutation in an oncogene (e.g. *ras* gene in bladder cancer), which modifies its function in the direction of poorer control.

In contrast, *tumour suppressor genes* are those which, when totally absent or non-functioning in a cell, permit the emergence of neoplasia, i.e. their presence prevents neoplasia. Given that all normal cells will have two copies of each gene (one on each chromosome pair), the development of neoplasia by this means requires loss or mutation of both copies.

It must be stressed that clinical cancer does not reflect a solitary abnormality of one of these genes, but rather the final result of a combination of several errors of function. It may be that the ability to invade and metastasise depends on further classes of genes that do not fit this framework.

Heredity and cancer

The great majority of common tumours do not seem to have any relationship to hereditary factors. However some rare tumours do, and have led to an understanding of tumour suppressor genes. The pioneering work of Knudson on families of patients with multiple retinoblastomas (a tumour of the eye) indicated first that there must be two genetic events. In due course it became clear that one defective gene was inherited by the patient, while its corresponding gene on the opposite chromosome became defective, or was lost, in some cells during the growth of the eye. With both retinoblastoma (Rb) genes now defective the cells proceeded to neoplasia.

It is now apparent that a minority of common tumours, for example some breast and some colon cancers, run in families due to the same sort of mechanism. This is a rapidly developing field, with many new chromosomal abnormalities reported.

Physical agents

Ionising radiation

There is no doubt that ionising radiation can cause cancer. Direct damage to DNA (i.e. the chemical basis of genetic information), and damage mediated via ionisation of water can result in mutation of genes. The damage is randomly scattered throughout the genetic code, but can include sites critical to the development of cancer by the usual sequence of initiation, promotion and so on. This typically results in an interval of many years between exposure and clinical cancer. The source of radiation does not matter from the point of view of causing cancer, though it will affect the sites at risk.

Industrial exposure. Early workers with X-rays unknowingly induced tumours, and other radiation damage, in their hands. Today, diagnostic and therapeutic radiation also carry this risk to patients and staff alike, necessitating stringent safety regulations. Some mineworkers are exposed to high levels of radon, which is inhaled and may cause lung cancer (a risk increased by cigarette smoking). Another industrial association was with the painters of luminous watch dials. These ladies pointed their brush with their lips, thereby taking in minute quantities of radium. Some of the material remained near the jaw, while some was absorbed and passed to bone marrow, where the alpha emissions resulted in bone necrosis, tumours and marrow failure. In all cases there was the usual long time delay between exposure and clinical cancer.

Atomic bomb survivors have been followed up very carefully. There has been an excessive number of cases of leukaemia, mainly 7 to 12 years after exposure, and also a larger number of other cancers from about 20 years later onwards.

Ultraviolet light

The shorter wavelengths of solar ultraviolet light, UV B, are capable of damaging the DNA of various skin cells, resulting in mutations and eventually cancers. The common tumours, basal cell and squamous cell carcinomas, seem to result from chronic overexposure; malignant melanoma correlates better with acute and intense exposure.

DNA repair enzymes. The rare condition *xeroderma pigmentosum* (see p. 293) gives a useful insight into cellular function. Patients with this condition develop skin tumours after trivial exposure to the sun. They have been found to have an inborn defect resulting in failure of the normal enzymes that repair DNA damage inflicted by UV light. Presumably skin tumours in normal subjects represent overwhelming of these repair systems. Melanin pigment protects against UV penetration to the deeper layers of cells.

Chemicals

Coal tars, oils and cigarette smoke

Percival Pott, in 1775, described carcinoma of the scrotal skin in chimney-sweeps, and attributed it to the soot. Similarly, mule-spinners in mills developed tumours due to the oil that soaked their clothing, and even today motor mechanics are at risk from lubricating oils. However the greatest problem at present from this group of chemicals is cigarette smoke. This contains many known *carcinogenic* substances, including benzo[a]pyrene, a potent carcinogen also present in coal tars. Not only do smokers have a very greatly increased incidence of lung cancer, they also have a higher risk of cancer at several other sites, such as the bladder. Chemicals that are able to cause tumours are called *direct carcinogens*.

Aniline dyes and the rubber industry

Workers in the chemical industry, particularly those involved in making dyes, were found to develop bladder cancer. A similar risk was noted in the rubber processing industry. Unlike coal tars, the chemical implicated, β-naphthylamine, needs to be metabolised first before releasing the active ingredient into the urine. This is called a *procarcinogen*.

Asbestos

Many particulate minerals are now recognised as carcinogenic, including asbestos. The blue asbestos (crocidolite) particles used for insulation are easily inhaled when very small but are then retained within the lung. Over a period of decades they may then cause tumours of the pleura (malignant mesothelioma); they also correlate with bronchial cancer, particularly if associated with smoking.

Hormones

Are endogenous chemicals such as hormones carcinogenic? There is no doubt that hormone levels are important in hormonally responsive organs and their cancers. Whether the hormone is actually carcinogenic, or simply contributes to the process of carcinogenesis by promoting cell proliferation is debatable; the latter is more probable. The relationship between oestrogens and endometrial cancer is discussed in Chapter 24. Breast and prostate cancers are also likely to relate to hormonal influences. As mentioned earlier, hormonal manipulation is an important therapeutic tool in cancer treatment.

Viruses and cancer

As viruses contain genetic material, and gain access to the inside of cells, they have long been suspected of having a role in carcinogenesis. This speculation has been fuelled by finding close similarity between some viral genes and oncogenes. Viruses are clearly responsible for a variety of tumours in several species, such as leukaemias in mice and cats and sarcomas in chickens. In humans, common skin warts are a self-limiting benign tumour caused by a virus. Over recent years, these human papilloma (wart) viruses (HPV) have been found to be a large family of related organisms, some of which correlate closely with cancer of the uterine cervix and similar tumours. A direct causal link between virus and cancer is unproven, but the presence of these viruses in the cells seems to be an adverse factor. Similarly, Epstein–Barr virus, which is very widespread and causes infectious mononucleosis, is closely associated with tumours such as Hodgkin's disease, Burkitt's lymphoma (a high grade non-Hodgkin lymphoma), and nasopharyngeal carcinoma.

Infectivity and cancer. Some patients, or their relatives, worry that cancer may be infectious. It is possible to allay these fears and assure them that this is not the case. The association with viruses mentioned above is a rare sequel to agents widely present in the community; the cancer cannot be passed on.

Immunity and cancer

The immune system exists to detect and eliminate foreign substances, from isolated molecules to whole organisms. This is effected by antibodies and cells, principally lymphocytes. In the development of a tumour, it is quite possible for new or inappropriate substances to be produced. From this one would predict that tumours would sometimes be antigenic, i.e. provoke an immune response. This does seem to be the case. There are several examples of rare and common tumours with evidence of an immune response, generally the presence of numerous lymphocytes within and around the tumour. Tumours of rectum and breast, and seminoma of the testis all vary in the density of tumour-infiltrating lymphocytes. Studies of patients have correlated the density of lymphocytes with survival, often showing an advantage to those with an immune response. However the effect is not large, and is easily obscured by better treatment to all patients.

With malignant melanoma of skin, there is slightly more evidence to suggest a significant favourable immune response in some patients. Microscopic examination sometimes shows areas of apparent regression within the primary growth. There are also some patients with advanced melanoma who respond to stimulation of their immune system against the tumour (immunotherapy).

Despite these few encouraging observations, it is obvious that the majority of clinical cancer is beyond the capability of the patient's immune system. In some cases there is evidence that tumour cells may simply evade it.

Immune surveillance

The normal immune system actively seeks foreign material, apparently screening everything against its memory bank to distinguish self from non-self. This may allow the detection and elimination of some cancers before they are clinically established. For example, renal transplant patients require drugs to suppress their immune response in order for the new kidney to survive. These patients have many more skin tumours than would otherwise be expected, possibly as a result of loss of immune surveillance. Patients with AIDS suffer from a wide range of tumours, but this does not necessarily imply that loss of immune surveillance is the key event. Many patients with defects of the immune system (either as a result of disease or treatment), have an increase in tumours of lymphocytes, but this is probably a different phenomenon.

Injury and cancer

To be acceptable as a cause of cancer, an injury would need to be severe enough to have caused tissue damage, there must be evidence that the site was previously normal, and that the tumour arose at the site of injury. Finally, the time interval must be long enough to be plausible, generally several years. The mechanism is presumably via a non-specific induction of cell division as part of the repair process, rather than anything actually carcinogenic. There are a few instances that fulfil these criteria, but the usual circumstance is simply that the injury draws attention to a pre-existing tumour.

PRECANCEROUS LESIONS

There are a number of conditions in which there is an increased risk of the subsequent development of cancer. Some are disorders that are not of themselves neoplastic, but carry a risk of cancer. Others are more like a half-way house in which the process of development towards cancer is recognisable as neither normal nor cancer. Some are benign tumours that may change to be malignant. In none is the development of cancer inevitable, though the risk and time scale vary greatly. Some examples are given below.

— *Undescended testis* is an abnormality of development: it carries a high risk of neoplasia (p. 434).
— *Paget's disease of bone*, a condition of middle to late adult life, has a risk of osteosarcoma, a tumour otherwise seen in adolescence (p. 505).
— *Solar keratosis*, a warty skin lesion due to sun-exposure; it may progress to cancer.
— *Leucoplakia*, a whitish patch in the mouth (p. 311) or vulva (p. 420), is a descriptive term including several conditions. Some run the risk of cancer later.
— *Dysplasia* may be detected at several sites (e.g. stomach), and indicates a microscopic abnormality of cells with some, but not all, the features of cancer.
— *Carcinoma-in-situ*, may be seen on a surface (e.g. cervix, p. 402) or within the lumen of a duct (intraduct carcinoma of the breast, p. 384). This has all the microscopic features of cancer, but the cells are still confined to their normal anatomical limits, i.e. have not invaded.
— *Adenomatous polyp* of the large intestine is a benign tumour. However it may develop into a malignant tumour. In the condition familial adenomatous polyposis there are so many polyps (thousands) that malignancy becomes inevitable.

An important consideration is that the detection of some of these conditions allows surgical intervention before cancer becomes established.

Field change

Although an individual tumour arises from a single cell, within the vicinity of that cell there are often other cells part-way through carcinogenesis. Removal of the tumour, or its precursor lesion, may be followed by the local development of further lesions. This is regarded as a field change across the whole area. An example would be the appearance of cancer on the tongue following removal of one from the cheek.

NATURAL HISTORY AND SPREAD OF CANCER

As stated earlier, *benign* tumours remain localised,

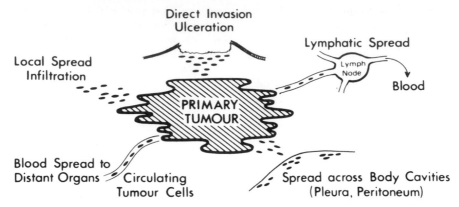

Fig. 14.2   Metastasis or secondary spread. Tumours can spread by a variety of routes including local spread, spread through the lymphatics, via the blood and across cavities. (Reproduced with permission from Calman, Smyth and Tattersall, Basic Principles of Cancer Chemotherapy, Macmillan, 1980.)

often separated from surrounding tissue by a capsule. This has relatively little effect on the adjacent structures, unless it arises in a particularly critical site, and surgical removal is curative. In contrast, *malignant* tumours show a capacity to invade, frequently recur after surgery, spread to other sites and result in the death of the patient. The initial or *primary* site of tumour growth thus gives rise to separate secondary tumours, or *metastases*. Some tumours, such as *basal cell carcinoma* of skin have an intermediate behaviour; they invade locally but do not give rise to metastases.

In summary, spread may occur in several ways (Fig. 14.2):

— By local invasion
— By lymphatic vessels
— By blood vessels
— Across cavities.

Local invasion

As the tumour invades, adjacent tissues are displaced and destroyed to be replaced by tumour. The tumour margin is ill-defined and irregular. Surgical removal therefore needs to include a generous extent of normal tissue. Failure to do so results in some tumour being left behind, which proliferates and gives rise to *local recurrence*. Radiotherapy is frequently used after surgery in order to prevent this situation. The invasion often follows anatomical tissue planes; it may be temporarily halted by some dense structure such as bone, until these are also eroded.

Functional effects

The effects a tumour produces will depend upon the site involved; a knowledge of anatomy and physiology allows prediction of many symptoms. Thus a tumour in the head of the pancreas will soon obstruct the bile duct, so that the patient becomes jaundiced. A tumour of the left lung may obstruct its bronchus, with resulting pneumonia from infection of retained secretions. Further local invasion of this mass will compress the recurrent laryngeal nerve; the patient's voice is altered. Further growth may obstruct the superior vena cava passing through the mediastinum, causing swelling of the face and arms.

A tumour just beneath the skin can so stretch it and impair its nutrition that it breaks down to form an ulcer. This is then liable to infection or bleeding. Pain and weakness will occur when peripheral nerves are affected, e.g. Pancoast tumour (p. 375) at the apex of the lung invading upwards to compress nerves to the arm and hand.

The extent of local invasion dictates the extent of surgery necessary to remove it, and indeed may render the tumour inoperable if critical structures are involved. However the usual reason why a tumour is 'inoperable' is because of metastatic disease. Sometimes it is worth debulking the tumour, but surgery alone is insufficient to cure the patient.

Metastasis

By lymphatic vessels

Invasive tumours readily penetrate the thin wall of lymphatics. Then fragments of tumour are carried downstream to lodge in one or more local lymph nodes. If the tumour cells survive this journey and proliferate in the node they form a *metastasis*, or secondary tumour. Further dissemination may proceed to other lymph nodes along the chain, e.g. from pelvic to para-aortic to supraclavicular nodes. Some primary tumours remain tiny, yet have massive nodal deposits. If the node capsule is breached by tumour, the whole mass becomes fixed to surrounding structures.

By blood vessels

Thin-walled blood vessels are similarly at risk of tumour invasion, and again fragments of tumour float passively downstream. (Single tumour cells are generally destroyed by non-specific defence mechanisms in the blood.) These then lodge in the next capillary bed, where they may develop into metastases. Though this can happen in any tissue, the liver, lungs and bone are by far the most frequent sites for secondaries.

Across cavities (transcoelomic)

Access to the *pleura* enables tumour cells to seed themselves around the pleural cavity, forming numerous further deposits or seedlings. These may be associated with secretion of fluid into the cavity, with resultant impairment of respiration. An identical process may occur in the peritoneum; the fluid accumulation is called *ascites*. Malignant cells may settle on the ovaries, or all over the omentum. Related to this, some intracranial tumours, such as medulloblastoma (p. 473) of the cerebellum, may disseminate by the cerebrospinal fluid, seeding over the surface of the brain and down the spinal canal.

Implantation

Occasionally cells may be implanted in the scar by the surgeon's knife while removing a tumour, or through a pleural or paracentesis drainage site.

Functioning tumours

Many tumour cells continue certain cell functions related to their tissue of origin, but in some this has a profound effect on the patient. Tumours of endocrine glands typically produce an excess of their hormone. The problem is that the tumour is no longer responsive to the usual control of secretion. Thus an adrenal cortex tumour will produce steroids despite switching off its pituitary drive, and Cushing's syndrome will result.

In other circumstances the hormone production is quite inappropriate for the tumour site. Many lung tumours produce parathyroid hormone, antidiuretic hormone, or adrenocorticotrophic hormone (p. 575).

Again it is not subject to the normal control of secretion, and the clinical consequences may be severe. Some of the other effects that tumours may have, such as profound weight loss, could be due to secretions as yet unidentified.

Cause of death from cancer

As the word 'malignant' implies, death is the natural consequence of untreated cancer. Sometimes the tumour will have grown locally and spread in an orderly manner. In other cases the primary site remains undetected despite widespread metastatic deposits. Some tumours show relentless progression, and run their course in a few months; others take many years, with long intervals of apparent dormancy.

Many patients with locally advanced or metastatic cancer become bedridden and die from bronchopneumonia, inanition and/or metabolic disturbance. Sometimes there may be liver failure due to numerous liver secondaries. Often the actual cause of death is unclear. It is important to consider carrying out a post-mortem examination if there is reasonable doubt about the cause of death. Patients with cancer are still at risk of non-neoplastic conditions such as coronary artery disease. This is particularly likely in patients who smoke. Indeed, smoking may have given rise both to the primary tumour (e.g. in the lung, oral cavity or pharynx) and to ischaemic heart disease.

It is important to make a judgement as to whether the patient died from cancer or from an unrelated condition, since this influences cancer mortality statistics. Where a patient has remained disease free from cancer for more than 5 years, and the cause of death is said to be cancer, this conclusion should be questioned. However, late relapses can occur after 5 years, in breast cancer for example. Alternatively, a new primary may develop, especially in head and neck cancer.

STAGING OF CANCERS

It is of the greatest practical importance in many cases to estimate the extent of the spread of a tumour. This process is called *staging*. Staging often influences the choice of treatment, and can provide valuable information on prognosis. Staging may include clinical, pathological, radiological, and biochemical information. This enables similar groups of patients to be compared between different oncology centres nationally and internationally. A number of staging classifications are in use. The simplest and oldest classification is as follows:

Stage 1:   Tumour confined to the organ of origin
Stage 2:   Local lymph nodes invaded
Stage 3:   Distant nodes invaded, or local spread beyond the organ of origin
Stage 4:   Blood-borne metastasis present

This is still used for carcinoma of the breast and cervix, with slight modification to bring in subcategories. The UICC (International Union Against Cancer) has worked towards international agreement on the staging of many tumours, coding them on the TNM system.

TNM classification

This includes a description of the primary tumour (T), nodal spread (N), and distant metastases (M). It provides a succinct summary of the extent of malignancy in the patient.

T1–3:   Generally based on the size and/or extent of the primary
T4:   The most advanced local disease, often with invasion of adjacent structures

N0:   No nodes palpable
N1:   Mobile nodes on the same side as the primary
N1a: Nodes not considered to contain tumour
N1b: Nodes considered to contain tumour
N2:   Mobile nodes on the opposite side (N2a and N2b as above)
N3:   Fixed, involved nodes

M0:   No evidence of distant metastasis
M1:   Distant metastasis present

Thus a very early cancer would be categorised as T1N0M0, and a very advanced one as T4N3M1. The TNM classification for breast cancer is shown in Table 23.3.

The clinical staging may differ from the pathological staging. For example, a tumour in the breast may be measured clinically as 2 cm in diameter and thus be staged as T1. However, when actually measured directly in the mastectomy specimen it might be 3 cm in maximum diameter, and thus be pathologically T2 (abbreviated as pT2). Most staging classifications are based on the clinical extent of spread.

Radiological information may influence staging. For example in carcinoma of the cervix the presence of an obstructed kidney on ultrasound or other investigation (in the absence of a non-neoplastic cause), automatically indicates stage 3b.

The staging of testicular cancer is an example where biochemical information (the presence of serum tumour markers alpha-fetoprotein and human chorionic gonadotrophin) is included. If the tumour is clinically confined to the testis but tumour markers are rising, it is classified as stage 1, marker positive (Mk+).

HISTOLOGICAL GRADING: DIFFERENTIATION

In an effort to predict the future course of a tumour, an estimate is made of how malignant it is for a particular site and type of tumour. Generally speaking, the closer a tumour cell resembles its normal counterpart, i.e. the better it is differentiated, the more orderly and slower its growth. Thus histological examination allows tumour *grading* on the basis of the extent of differentiation. Attention is given to the nucleus (how abnormal it is and how often mitosis is observed), and the cytoplasm (the extent to which normal structures are seen).

For most of the common tumours, the pathologist divides them into descriptive categories: well differentiated, moderately differentiated and poorly differentiated. Undifferentiated tumours lack sufficient features to allow more than a broad classification, as do anaplastic tumours (see below under Classification of Neoplasms).

Limitations of grading

Some tumours show a tight correlation between histological grading and behaviour, such that treatment is guided by this information. Cancer of the bladder is one of these. However the tumour stage is of overriding importance. Some tumours (e.g. pancreatic islet) have a very variable rate of clinical progression, but uniform histology: grading in this circumstance is misleading if attempted. Other tumours vary considerably from one microscopic field to another: in general the outlook will depend upon the worst areas, but these could be missed without adequate sampling. Finally, the organ of origin is important: a well differentiated cancer of the skin carries an excellent prognosis, whereas in the lung it does not.

GROWTH RATE OF CANCERS

As indicated in the section on carcinogenesis, there is usually a considerable time between initiation of a tumour and its clinical detection. Part of this time is taken by the process of becoming a cancer cell, and part by growing to sufficient size to be found. The latter can be measured as the time taken for it to double in diameter, its *doubling time*. A mass 1 mm diameter would represent about one million cells: this could result from one cell, and each of its subsequent daughter cells, dividing 20 times. A word of caution is needed before theorising further. Once a tumour exceeds about 2 mm it is essential for it to have its own blood supply: this, together with other supporting structures, is the tumour *stroma*. In some tumours the stroma is very scanty, while in others it constitutes the majority of the mass. (The character of the stroma also influences what the tumour feels like on palpation; most breast cancers are hard because of abundant, dense stroma.) Thus calculations about how many cancer cells there are in a tumour of a certain size will be incorrect if they ignore the stroma.

Another consideration is that the clinical growth of a tumour will be the result of the balance between cell proliferation and loss. It will be influenced too by the growth fraction or proportion of cancer cells actually proliferating. Many cancer cells in a tumour cease to proliferate as they differentiate, or produce nonviable daughter cells. Furthermore, if the vascularity of the stroma is inadequate there will be necrosis.

Though a cancer produces an expanding mass, this is a reflection of loss of control of growth. The actual rate at which individual cancer cells divide is *slower* than comparable normal tissues. If there is a very sudden increase in the size of a tumour, it will probably reflect internal haemorrhage or fluid accumulation. (On the other hand, a slow-growing mass which begins to grow faster may have changed from benign to malignant.)

Observation of established clinical cancers has shown that doubling times vary widely, but average about 2 months. Leaving aside the question of whether this is true for the first 20 doublings to reach 1 mm size, it would require about a further 10 doublings (i.e. 20 months) to reach 1 cm diameter, at which point it might be detectable. Many tumours are 2 cm or more in diameter before they produce symptoms, so a considerable time has elapsed between the first emergence of a clone of cancer cells and the clinical disease. In comparison with that, the remainder of its course, if unchecked, is liable to be over after five or so more doublings. Metastatic deposits may be disseminated during the preclinical period, only to appear after removal of the primary. If the doubling time is considerably more than 2 months the whole process takes on a much longer time scale.

Bearing these matters in mind, there is no fixed length of disease-free interval that equates with a cure. However, for practical purposes 5 years disease free is tantamount to cure for many of the common tumours, with breast cancer as a notable exception. The earlier detection of a cancer at a minute size increases the possibility of removal before metastases develop. However the tumour has been around for a long time. Prolonged postoperative survival in these patients may simply reflect 'earlier diagnosis' rather than 'longer survival', a phenomenon called *lead-time bias*.

Spontaneous regression of cancer

Occasionally a tumour may regress and disappear without treatment, though the original diagnosis could have been erroneous. Most of the reported cases are renal cell carcinoma, malignant melanoma and gestational choriocarcinoma. In all these instances, immunological mechanisms are thought to be responsible. Some cases of lymphoid tumours fluctuate in size, and may temporarily disappear, only to return later. In some cases of neuroblastoma, a primitive tumour of nerve cells, there is subsequent differentiation and growth ceases.

CLASSIFICATION OF NEOPLASMS

Table 14.2 lists examples of tumour nomenclature. In general, the names are built up from one part to describe the tissue type, and another to indicate its behaviour. All end in 'oma' to denote a lump, a suffix almost restricted to neoplasms, though a few other terms are in use, such as haematoma for an accumulation of blood. Most malignant tumours fall into the following broad categories:

— Carcinoma
— Sarcoma
— Lymphoma.

The majority of tumours arise from epithelium (surface lining cells). Benign ones are called *papilloma* or *adenoma*; malignant ones *carcinoma*, often with a prefix to give the cell type. Carcinoma is Greek for 'crab' but is used in a more restricted sense than cancer and applied only to epithelial malignancy, which makes up 75% of cancer.

Squamous epithelium lines the skin, where it is called epidermis, the upper aerodigestive tract (mouth, pharynx, larynx, oesophagus), anus, vagina and cervix. It is present in the bronchi if there is metaplasia. *Transitional cell epithelium* lines the renal pelvis, ureters and bladder.

Glandular (secretory) epithelium lines the gut from stomach to rectum, and forms the related secretory glands (salivary, pancreas, biliary tract and liver), endocrine glands (pituitary, thyroid, parathyroids, adrenals), kidneys, ovarian surface, endometrium and breast.

Sometimes the tumour name is combined with a description of shape or function. If a *cyst* is formed it may

Table 14.2 Types of neoplasms

Type	Benign	Malignant
Epithelial		*Carcinoma*
Squamous	Papilloma	Squamous carcinoma
Transitional	Papilloma	Transitional cell carcinoma
Basal cell	Papilloma	Basal cell carcinoma
Glandular	Adenoma	Adenocarcinoma
Mesenchymal		*Sarcoma*
Smooth muscle	Leiomyoma	Leiomyosarcoma
Striated muscle	Rhabdomyoma	Rhabdomyosarcoma
Fat	Lipoma	Liposarcoma
Blood vessels	Angioma	Angiosarcoma
Bone	Osteoma	Osteosarcoma
Cartilage	Chondroma	Chondrosarcoma
Lymphoid tissue		*Lymphoma*
		Hodgkin's disease
		Non-Hodgkin lymphoma
Plasma cell		Multiple myeloma
White blood cells		Leukaemia
Intracranial and neural		
Supporting cells		Glioma
Meninges	Meningioma	
Cerebellum		Medulloblastoma
Retina		Retinoblastoma
Sympathetic nerve	Ganglioneuroma	Neuroblastoma
Pigment cells		
Skin or eye	Mole or naevus	Malignant melanoma
Gonad		
Germ cells	Dermoid cyst	Malignant teratoma Seminoma
Placenta		
	Hydatidiform mole	Choriocarcinoma

be cystadenoma or cystadenocarcinoma, both of which are common in the ovary. Mucin-secreting variants would be mucinous cystadenoma.

Sarcoma denotes any tumour of mesenchymal origin (supporting structures). They are much less frequent than carcinoma. Metastasis from sarcomas is generally blood-borne, and few give rise to lymph node secondaries.

Lymphomas are malignant tumours of lymphoid cells; many are classified as Hodgkin's disease, leaving the remainder as non-Hodgkin lymphoma. Some are closely related to leukaemias (tumours of white blood cells).

There are many tumours that do not easily fit the guidelines mentioned: some are in Table 14.2 and others are referred to elsewhere in this book under the relevant organ.

Undifferentiated tumours

Some tumours lack obvious features to allow their identification or classification. An undifferentiated carcinoma, or sarcoma cannot be ascribed to any subcategory. An anaplastic tumour could be carcinoma, lymphoma or sarcoma. As these different categories have major therapeutic consequences, it is important to attempt a more detailed diagnosis. Simple microscopy can now be supplemented by special staining procedures, many of which involve detecting cell components with antibodies. Electron microscopy sometimes helps, and there are other approaches such as cytogenetics.

Most oncology centres arrange for many of their patients' tumours to be reviewed before treatment. Diagnosis and classification of rare or undifferentiated tumours form a considerable part of such work.

15. Principles of radiobiology

Radiobiology is the term applied to the scientific study of the effects of ionising radiation on cells and tissues, both normal and malignant. This chapter covers some of the main concepts in radiobiology and their application to clinical radiotherapy.

The science is a relatively young one, which rapidly expanded in the 1950s with the development of techniques for cell culture and the description in 1953 of the 'oxygen effect' by Gray (p. 260). Historically, dose and fractionation schedules in radiotherapy were developed empirically before their radiobiological basis was understood. Many of the concepts and models in modern radiobiology have been developed from the study of normal and malignant cells in experimental animals and in tissue culture. Disappointingly the clinical application of the important theoretical benefits of the oxygen effect derived from radiobiological research (hyperbaric oxygen, fast neutrons and hypoxic cell sensitisers) has not improved cure rates in common cancers. At present there are no in vitro or in vivo radiobiological tests which will predict the response of an individual patient's tumour to radiation. An understanding of the fundamental mechanisms of tumour radiosensitivity and resistance may help to select patients who would benefit from treatments (discussed later in this chapter) which are designed to overcome tumour hypoxia.

EFFECTS OF IRRADIATION ON CELLS

The biological targets of radiation are the cells which make up the body's various tissues. It is the interaction of X-rays with the cell which precipitates a chain of molecular events that results in the inhibition of cell division. Radiation is particularly lethal to cells during cell division (mitosis). In addition it delays the onset of mitosis. The end result is cell death or the loss of reproductive capacity. The exact mechanism by which the cell loses this capability is unknown.

The specific target of radiation damage is the de-

oxyribonucleic acid (DNA) molecule which lies within the chromosomes of the cell's nucleus and constitutes the genetic blueprint for future reproduction. The

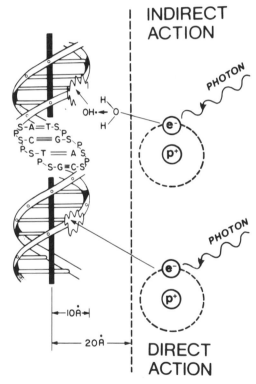

Fig. 15.1A Illustrating the direct and indirect actions of radiation. The structure of DNA is shown schematically; the letters S, P, A, T, G and C represent sugar, phosphorus, adenine, thymine, guanine and cytosine respectively. Direct action: a secondary electron resulting from absorption of an X-ray photon interacts with the DNA to produce an effect. Indirect action: the secondary electron interacts with, for example, a water molecule to produce an OH˙ radical, which in turn produces the damage to the DNA. The indirect action is dominant for sparsely ionising radiations such as X-ray. (Reproduced with permission from Hall, Radiobiology for the Radiobiologist, 3rd edn, Harper & Row, 1988.)

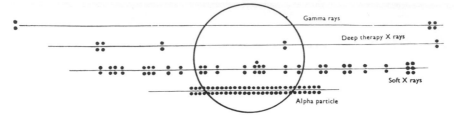

Fig. 15.1B   Diagram showing comparative ionisation densities along the tracks of various qualities of radiation. (The diameter of the circle is 27 millionths of 1 mm.) (Gray, British Medical Bulletin.)

two spiral threads of DNA twist around each other to form the 'double helix' (Fig. 15.1A). DNA is composed of purine and pyrimidine compounds, known as bases, and of phosphate and sugar molecules. The paired purine bases are *adenine* and *guanine* and the pyrimidine bases *cytosine* and *thymine*. DNA is composed of two complementary strands.

Effects of ionising radiation on DNA

Radiation may produce single or double strand breaks within DNA. The former are less important since they are more amenable to cellular repair. However double strand breaks are more difficult to repair and can irreversibly damage the cell. Cells may go through a few divisions before dying.

Radiation damage may result in changes (mutations) in the structure of DNA. The direct or indirect effects of irradiation may also result in breaks appearing in the chromosomes. Broken ends of different chromosomes may rejoin. This is known as *chromosomal rearrangement*. In chromosomal rearrangements it is double strand breaks in DNA due to the effect of ionising radiation or failure to repair them satisfactorily that are thought to be critical. The incidence of chromosomal abnormalities increases with the dose of ionising radiation.

The quality of radiation is also important to chromosomal damage. As ionising radiation passes through tissue it gives up energy along its track by setting electrons in motion. The amount given up per micron of tissue (1 million microns = 1 mm) is called the Linear Energy Transfer (LET). For radiation with a high LET, e.g. alpha particles, fast neutrons and soft X-rays, the high density of ionisation (Fig. 15.1B) increases the probability of damaging chromosomes along the track of the particle. For low LET irradiation, e.g. gamma rays, the density of ionisation per unit of distance along the track is lower and correspondingly the probability of chromosomal damage is reduced.

Radiation and the cell cycle

The growth of both normal and malignant tumours is influenced by the different proportions of cells in the cell cycle (Fig. 15.2). The cell cycle for proliferating cells is composed of four phases, S (DNA synthesis), M (mitosis) and the gaps before and after S phase, G_1 and G_2 respectively. Proliferating cells in this cycle constitute what is known as the *growth fraction*. It represents the proliferating portion of the total cell population. The proportion of tumour cells in the growth fraction may vary very widely from under 1% to nearly 100%. In general there is a correlation between the differentiation of the tumour and the size of the growth fraction. The more anaplastic the tumour the higher the growth fraction. Accordingly the less differentiated the tumour, the more cell killing a given dose of radiation is likely to achieve.

Cells that are not proliferating, i.e. they are resting, may be in a phase known as G_0 or be incapable of division (a sterile phase). Cells from the proliferating phase or the sterile phase may undergo cell death. The rate of cell death is known as the *cell loss factor*. The cell loss factor also varies widely among different histological types. It seems to be highest in tumours where the growth fraction is large.

There is a dynamic interplay between proliferating and resting cells. Cells may move from the resting phase into the cycle of proliferating cells and vice versa. However once cells have entered the sterile phase, they are unable to revert to the resting or proliferating phases.

Radiosensitivity in the cell cycle

The proportions of a cell population in proliferating, resting or sterile phases can affect the radiosensitivity of a cell population. In animal experiments it has been shown that there may be a fivefold variation in cell survival between the most sensitive phase of the cycle (M phase) and the most resistant (late S phase).

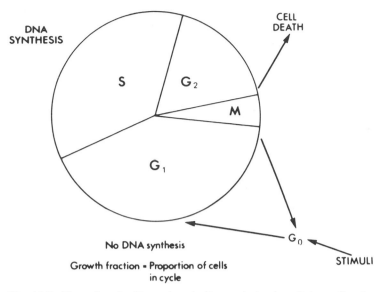

Fig. 15.2   The cell cycle. (Reproduced with permission from Calman, Smyth & Tattersall, Basic Principles of Cancer Chemotherapy, Macmillan, 1980.)

The duration of the cell cycle varies widely between different tumours and even between histologically uniform cells of the same tumour. Unfortunately there is no consistent difference in the duration of the cell cycle in normal and malignant cells that can be exploited therapeutically. Nor is there much difference in the average length of different phases of the cell cycle between different tumours in man.

Mitosis and cell division are among the cell's most sensitive processes. These processes are shared by both malignant and normal tissues. However in the malignant cell the normal control of cell division has been lost, resulting in inappropriate cellular proliferation. Cell division in both normal and malignant tissue is inhibited. *It should be emphasised that there is no intrinsic difference in the radiosensitivity of normal and malignant cells. However small differences in cell survival for a given dose are amplified by fractionation.*

Direct and indirect damage by ionising radiation

X-rays damage the reproductive capacity of the cell by the process of *ionisation*. Ionisation is the removal of an electron from one of the outer shells of an atom. It is the interaction of an incident X-ray (photon) with the atomic nucleus which results in the ejection of an electron. Ionisation is unique to X-rays and is due to their extremely short wavelength. Ionisation does not occur with electromagnetic radiation of longer wavelength (e.g. radio waves).

Radiation has both *direct* and *indirect* effects at a molecular level (Fig. 15.1). The direct action is the ionisation of atoms in the cell nucleus. Much more important in radiotherapy is the indirect action on the cell nucleus of radiation induced free radicals. When X-rays interact with water, free radical ions are produced (H_2O^+ and a free electron e^-). The H_2O^+ is chemically unstable and quickly forms a hydrogen ion (H^+) and a hydroxyl ion ($OH^\bullet$). The dot signifies an unpaired electron. These free radicals are highly reactive and result in breaks in the chromosomes. Much of this damage is repaired, possibly by repair or rejoining of the broken chromosomes. The lethal damage caused to the cell may be due to the delivery of a large amount of energy to particularly sensitive molecules within the nucleus.

These molecular events will affect the cell's metabolism and produce observable effects. Immediate cell death may result after massive radiation doses (e.g. 1000 Gy from an atomic bomb). At lower dose levels, as used in clinical radiotherapy, the chromosomal damage does not reveal itself until the cell attempts to go into mitosis.

BIOLOGICAL FACTORS INFLUENCING RADIOSENSITIVITY

1. Intrinsic radiosensitivity

While tumour cells are, in most cases, as radiosensitive as normal tissue, they do vary in their intrinsic radiosensitivity. These differences are expressed in the α/β ratio for early responding tissues. A relatively high α/β ratio occurs in very sensitive acutely responding tissues such as skin (p. 259) and low values in relatively radioresistant tissues such as connective tissue.

In conventional radical radiotherapy daily doses of the order of 2 Gy are delivered. After each dose the same proportion of 'sensitive' cells in particular phases of the cell cycle are killed. Each dose of 2 Gy roughly reduces the surviving tumour population by 50%. Fractionation exploits the different responses of rapidly dividing tumours and late responding normal tissues to ionising radiations. These differences may be explained by the following biological phenomena:

— Repair of cellular damage
— Repopulation by tumour cells
— Reoxygenation during the course of irradiation
— Redistribution of cells in the cell cycle.

2. Repair of cellular damage

Damage to DNA following irradiation is generally repaired over a period of a few hours. However the degree of repair will vary from tissue to tissue. Slowly responding tissues (e.g. connective tissue and spinal cord) have a greater capacity for repair than tumours, as long as the gap between treatment fractions is at least 6 hours, as it is with conventional once daily fractions.

Since cell killing is logarithmic rather than linear, the difference in survival between normal and tumour cells is increased exponentially. Thus if 65% of a late responding tissue's cells survive a given dose, compared with 50% of tumour cells, the relative survival of the late responding 'target cells' is $(65/50)^{30} = 2620$.

Sublethal and potentially lethal damage

A distinction is made between *sublethal* and *potentially lethal* damage. Sublethal damage (SLD) refers to irradiated proliferating cells where the damage caused is insufficient to kill the cell. Metabolic processes are thought to be important in the recovery of SLD. Recovery occurs fairly promptly after irradiation, usually within an hour. The amount of recovery from SLD varies with the amount of oxygenation within normal and tumour cells during and after irradiation. The lower the degree of oxygenation, the smaller the degree of recovery from SLD.

Potentially lethal damage (PLD) differs from SLD in at least two respects. First, it may occur in non-proliferating cell populations. Secondly, recovery from PLD is dose-dependent. Recovery increases with dose. The time to recovery from PLD is thought to be

similar to SLD. The damage is 'potentially lethal' because the degree of recovery can be modified by changing the environment of the cells following irradiation. For example lowering the temperature of growing tumour cells in tissue culture from 37°C to 20°C increases the amount of recovery.

Over the range of fraction sizes used in clinical radiotherapy, PLD, because of its dose dependence, is considered to play less of a role than SLD.

3. Repopulation by tumour cells

Following irradiation of normal and malignant tissue, dead cells are replaced by recruitment of resting cells (in G_0 phase) into the cell cycle. This process may be rapid in highly proliferative normal tissues and malignant tumours. The occurrence of repopulation in response to cellular injury is a major reason for fractionating radiotherapy rather than giving limited numbers of fractions. It enables acutely responding tissues, e.g. the mucosa, to tolerate much larger doses than would be the case with an equivalent dose in a single fraction. The rate of repopulation varies widely between tumours. However overall repopulation is greater in acutely responding normal tissues than in tumours. No similar therapeutic differential occurs between tumour and late responding tissues.

In tumours with a high growth fraction, repopulation of tumour cells between daily fractions may outstrip the tumoricidal effects of irradiation and lead to persistent disease after a course of radiotherapy is completed. There is evidence that in some tumours treatment may actually accelerate tumour growth. Previously it had been thought that tumour growth was autonomous. It may be that the activity of tumour growth factors is facilitated by a better vascular supply as the tumour shrinks.

Ideally it is preferable to deliver a radiation dose over as short a time as possible within the limits of acute radiation tolerance. Giving radiotherapy in several small doses at regular intervals during the day (multiple daily fractions, p. 565–6) may help to overcome tumour repopulation. Conversely excessive prolongation of radical external beam irradiation (Fig. 17.2A) over 7–8 weeks may allow significant tumour repopulation.

4. Reoxygenation during the course of irradiation

As tumours grow, their increased demand for nutrients often cannot be met by their vascular supply (p. 261). Poorly vascularised tumours are therefore prone to hypoxia and necrosis. Hypoxic tumours are known to be 2–3 times more radioresistant than well-oxygenated cells. About 15–20% of tumours are thought to contain hypoxic cells. Even a small population of hypoxic cells may prevent a tumour being cured. Tumour cells which are hypoxic improve their oxygenation and radiosensitivity during treatment as they are closer to a vascular supply once the radiosensitive population has been eliminated by the previous dose. Reoxygenation is a counterbalance to hypoxia. The amount of reoxygenation that occurs during fractionated radiotherapy varies widely between tumours. It may be influenced by the interval between fractions. One of the reasons for using multiple daily fractions (p. 565–6) is that it may enable the radiosensitive population to be removed several times a day. After each dose the hypoxic cell population has the opportunity of reoxygenation and being removed by the next dose of radiation.

5. Redistribution of cells in the cell cycle

The radiation sensitivity of cells varies markedly according to which phase of the cell cycle they are in at the time of radiation exposure. The most sensitive phase of the cell cycle to radiation is the mitotic (M) phase. Once the radiosensitive cell population has been killed and removed, the residual cell population is virtually synchronous in radioresistant phases of the cell cycle. The normal 24-hour period before the next dose of radiation allows cells to progress towards a more radiosensitive phase. Since the rate of cell division varies markedly in most tumours, synchrony in the cell cycle is soon lost after the last dose. None the less the radiosensitivity of the asynchronous tumour population still exceeds that of the cell population remaining just after the radiosensitive component has been removed.

Redistribution in the cell cycle applies to both acutely responding normal tissues and to tumours. Redistribution is not, however, a major factor in the response of late responding tissues. Thus for late responding tissues redistribution has a neutral rather than favourable effect.

Cell survival following irradiation

The survival of a single cell, whether normal or malignant, which has been irradiated is measured by assessing its ability to form a colony of daughter cells in tissue culture. The number of colonies formed is a measure of the capacity of surviving cells to proliferate. The percentage of cells which develop into colonies is called the *plating efficiency* (PE).

If the number of colonies of a given size is counted it can be plotted graphically against radiation dose. The cell survival curve represents the relationship

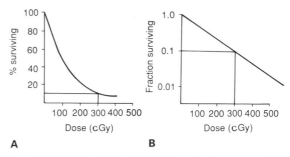

Fig. 15.3 To show the basis of cell survival curves, survival is plotted against dose. Dose is plotted in linear fashion in both graphs, i.e. double the distance represents double the dose. Survival is plotted linearly in **A** but logarithmically in **B**, i.e. double the distance represents double the percentage survival in **A** but ten-fold in **B**. A plot such as **B** is called 'semilogarithmic', and the effect is to convert the exponential curve of **A** into the straight line of **B** which is simpler to use. The dotted lines show an example such as might be found in an experiment: a dose of 300 cGy yields a survival of 10% (0.1).

between the number of cells surviving following irradiation and the dose of radiation delivered (Fig. 15.3A). A logarithmic scale (Fig. 15.3B) is used to express the surviving fraction of cells.

$$\text{Surviving fraction of cells} = \frac{\text{Number of colonies counted}}{\text{Cells seeded} \times \text{PE}/100}$$

The higher the dose, the smaller is the proportion of surviving cells. The greater the fractional kill, the steeper is the slope of the curve (i.e. the greater the radiosensitivity). A given dose will kill a certain percentage of cells. The remaining cells, after temporary inhibition of mitosis, will recover. If the same dose is applied again, the same percentage of cells will again be killed. We can thus determine experimentally the effects of variations of dose and fractionation.

If the simple percentage of surviving cells is plotted against dose, the relationship is an exponential curve (Fig. 15.3A). This is known as a *cell survival curve*. This exponential relationship is typical of mammalian normal and malignant cells.

After moderate doses of radiation, there is a temporary 'shoulder' (Fig. 15.5B) before the curve becomes a straight line (exponential). The shoulder region reflects the repair of sublethal damage. If the scale of the surviving fraction is logarithmic, the exponential curve of Figure 15.3A is converted into a straight line (Fig. 15.3B). Such a plot is semilogarithmic.

D_o and D_q

The shapes of cell survival curves following different single doses of irradiation can be compared using the parameters D_o and D_q (Fig. 15.5B). D_o represents the slope of the exponential part of the curve that follows the initial shoulder. D_o is defined as the dose (c Gy) needed to reduce the surviving fraction to $1/e$. e is the exponential function and $1/e = 0.37$. D_o is the mean lethal dose. In Figure 15.5B D_o is measured from the vertical axis as the added dose to induce a fall from 10^{-2} cells to 3.7×10^{-3}. D_o expresses the intrinsic radiosensitivity of the cell population.

The 'shoulder' of the curve is expressed by extrapolating the exponential part of the curve upwards and backwards to the vertical axis. It meets that axis at a point referred to as the *extrapolation number* (n). The point at which the extrapolated line crosses the horizontal axis (Fig. 15.5B) at 100% survival is known as D_q or the *quasithreshold dose*. D_q approximates to the amount of radiation energy 'lost' following exposure to a high single dose due to sublethal damage (p. 256).

Alpha and beta

In the linear quadratic model of cell survival (described later in this chapter) the initial shallow slope (α) of the cell survival curve is followed by a steeper final slope (β).

Effect of dose rate on cell survival

Most mammalian survival curves are based on single exposures of radiation at standard dose rates of 0.1 Gy/minute. However when irradiation is given continuously, for example by an iridium implant, over a long period (Ch. 19), the cell survival curve is less steep. The explanation for this difference is that continuously irradiated cells have the capacity to repair sublethal damage at a constant rate.

Influence of linear energy transfer and relative biological effectiveness on cell survival

The higher the *linear energy transfer* (LET), the higher is the efficiency of cell killing for a given level of dose. Thus for high LET radiation the size of the shoulder on the cell survival curve is smaller and the slope of the curve is steeper. Figure 15.4 illustrates this for high LET radiations (neutrons and alpha particles) and for low LET gamma rays.

The biological efficiency of irradiation is expressed as its *relative biological effectiveness* (RBE).

RBE is defined as the ratio of the dose of a standard low LET radiation (normally X-rays or gamma rays) to the dose of the test radiation which results in the same biological effect. There is no unique figure for

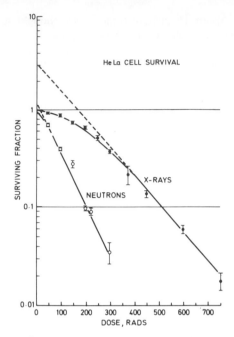

Fig. 15.4   Survival curves for HeLa cells irradiated with 300 kv X-rays or 14.7 MeV neutrons in air. (Reproduced with permission from Duncan W & Nias A H W 1977 Clinical Radiobiology, Churchill Livingstone, Edinburgh.)

RBE. It will vary not only with the quality of the radiation but with fraction size and the tissue in which it is measured.

RBE and fast neutrons. Because of the small shoulder of the survival curve for fast neutrons (Fig. 15.4) compared with X-rays, RBE varies markedly over the range of doses used in conventional radiotherapy. The smaller the dose per fraction for neutrons, the higher is the RBE (Table 15.1).

The RBE for a given dose or dose per fraction of fast neutrons is highest for intestinal epithelium and

Table 15.1   Variation of RBE with survival level

Survival (%)	Neutron dose (rads)	X-ray dose (rads)	RBE
90	15	65	4.3
80	30	115	3.8
70	45	160	3.6
60	60	200	3.3
50	80	240	3.0
40	100	280	2.8
30	125	335	2.7
20	160	400	2.4
10	210	515	2.4
3	305	695	2.3

(Reproduced with permission from Duncan W & Nias A H W 1977 Clinical Radiobiology, Churchill Livingstone, Edinburgh.)

lowest for lung. The RBE for skin is intermediate between the two. The RBE tends to be higher in normal tissue than in malignant tissue. This difference is thought to be due to the higher proportion of well-oxygenated and therefore more radiosensitive cells in normal tissue.

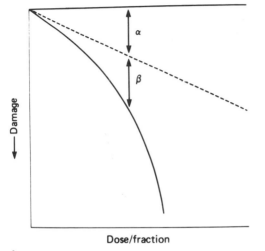

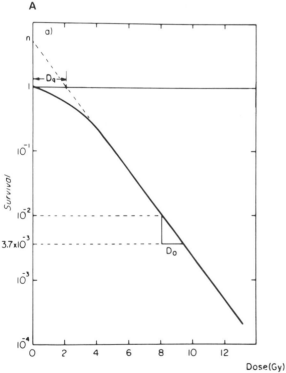

Fig. 15.5A The derivation of the α/β ratio, a dose which describes the curviness of the dose effect relationship. (Reproduced with permission from Hope-Stone 1986.) **B** D_o and D_q (reproduced with permission of McGraw-Hill from Tannock & Hill, The Basic Science of Oncology, Pergamon, 1977).

MODELS OF CELL SURVIVAL

There are several mathematical models that may be used to describe mammalian cell survival curves. However the linear-quadratic model seems best to fit observed mammalian survival curves and be consistent with clinical experience.

Linear quadratic model

In the linear quadratic (L-Q) model it is assumed that for cell killing to occur an interaction must occur between two lesions. Both lesions might arise from a single ionising track. In this circumstance cell killing would be directly determined by the level of dose. Alternatively, the interaction might occur between lesions arising from two or more separate tracks of ionisation.

The shape of the cell survival curve defined according to the L-Q model (Fig. 15.5A) on a semilogarithmic plot is concave downwards. At no point is it linear (exponential).

α is the parameter used to refer to the probability that the interacting lesions originate from a single track. α is responsible for the linear component of the cell survival curve (single hit, irreparable damage). β refers to the probability of interacting lesions arising from two independent tracks. β is responsible for the increasing 'curviness' of the shoulder (multi-hit, reparable damage).

The α/β ratio describes the dose (Gy) at which the cellular damage attributable to α and β are equal (Fig. 15.5A) This ratio varies from tissue to tissue. The range of values for α/β ratios is three to four times greater for acutely responding compared with for late responding tissues. For example the α/β ratio for skin desquamation is about 10 Gy, for the colon 8 Gy and for the testis 14 Gy. For late reacting tissue, α/β is about 0.2–0.4 Gy for the lung, 0.40–4.0 Gy for the kidney and about 2.5–5 Gy for the spinal cord. This means that the cell survival curve (Fig. 15.6) for early responding tissues (e.g. skin) and possibly some tumours is much less 'curvy' than for late responding tissues (e.g. connective tissue).

For tumours the values of α/β tend to be higher than late responding tissues and occasionally higher than early responding tissues. α/β for most tumours is rarely less than 0.5 Gy.

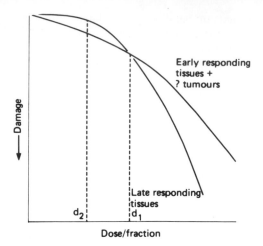

Fig. 15.6 Most late responding tissues have less 'curvy' dose response relationships than do most early responding tissues, possibly including tumours. (Reproduced with permission from Hope-Stone 1986.)

THE OXYGEN EFFECT

Oxygen has an important effect in modifying the biological response to irradiation. The presence of oxygen enhances the physicochemical reactions in tissue following exposure to ionising radiation. Oxygen reacts with free radicals ($R^{\bullet}$) in the following reaction:

$$R^{\bullet} + O_2 \longrightarrow RO_2^{\bullet}$$

The product $RO_2^{\bullet}$ is an organic peroxy radical, an unrepairable form of the target molecule. Thus the presence of oxygen 'fixes' radiation damage.

The oxygen concentration in most normal tissues is about that of the ordinary atmosphere (21%). The sensitivity of tissues irradiated in air is approximately three times that of the same tissues irradiated in an atmosphere with a substantially reduced oxygen concentration (hypoxic conditions). The absence of oxygen seems to interfere with the intracellular biochemical events that follow irradiation.

The radiosensitivity of cells increases rapidly as the oxygen concentration in their immediate neighbourhood during radiation treatment increases, up to a critical level. Above this level (21% oxygen concentration) sensitivity does not increase appreciably (Fig. 15.7). The oxygen effect is so potent that it is clearly desirable to increase the oxygen concentration in tumours during treatment. Many tumours tend to outstrip the available blood supply because of the accumulation of cells and consequent compression of surrounding blood vessels, leading to slowing of the local circulation and partial necrosis with oxygen deficiency. Thus the outermost parts of a tumour may be

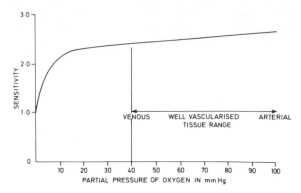

Fig. 15.7 Relationship of radiosensitivity to oxygen concentration. (Redrawn from Deschner and Gray, 1959, courtesy of Duncan W & Nias A H W 1977 Clinical Radiobiology, Churchill Livingstone, Edinburgh.)

well supplied with blood vessels and oxygen while the centre is liable to be much poorer in both, i.e. relatively hypoxic. Such hypoxic areas will be less radiosensitive than the rest of the tumour. The larger the tumour the more likely is the centre to be anoxic and the greater the bulk of anoxic cells. This helps to explain why large tumour masses are more radioresistant and require higher doses for eradication than small masses. Even a small proportion of anoxic cells may substantially reduce the prospect of cure.

Oxygen enhancement ratio

The degree of sensitisation to oxygen is described by the *oxygen enhancement ratio* (OER). It is defined as: 'the ratio of the doses necessary to achieve the same biological effect in the presence or absence of oxygen.' If a dose D is required to cause a certain amount of damage in fully oxygenated (aerobic) conditions, then a larger dose xD is required to cause the same damage in anoxic conditions. The ratio of xD to D is the OER.

The OER for most tissues irradiated in vitro or in vivo with X-rays or gamma rays varies from 2.5 to 3.3. Cell survival curves are the best means of comparing OERs in different tissues.

The oxygen concentration of most normal tissues is equivalent to a partial pressure of 40 mmHg. As a result they are wholly sensitive to irradiation. By contrast the majority of tumours contain a significant proportion of hypoxic cells. The proportion of hypoxic cells in experimental animal tumours is commonly 10–20%. Unfortunately the proportion of hypoxic cells in human tumours is not known since there is no means of measuring their numbers. A figure of 10% hypoxic cells would probably fit the cell survival curve for some tumours in clinical radiotherapy. However the range of the proportion of hypoxic cells is likely to be wide over the whole spectrum of human malignancy. There is, however, some indirect evidence to suggest that significant populations of hypoxic cells do occur in some human tumours.

It has been shown that these hypoxic cells tend to lie in areas at a fairly constant distance from the capillaries carrying oxygenated blood. This turned out to be the same distance that oxygen would be expected to travel by simple diffusion from the blood supply. Beyond a certain distance from the capillaries the oxygen concentration is inadequate to meet the demands of the tumour. Tumour necrosis and hypoxia are the result. An alternative explanation to the presence of hypoxic cells is the possibility that the flow through blood vessels within the tumour fluctuates. When the flow falls, some areas of the tumour become hypoxic until the normal blood flow is restored. Hypoxia is therefore transient and will depend upon which blood vessels have reduced flow at any particular time. There is some evidence that both models may apply in tumours. The influence of each model may vary from one tumour to another.

METHODS OF OVERCOMING TUMOUR HYPOXIA

Correction of anaemia

Anaemia from any cause will have a similar effect. It is important therefore that patients should maintain a normal haemoglobin concentration during a course of radiation. A blood transfusion may be required before or during treatment. In support of this is the fact that patients with cervical cancer undergoing radical pelvic irradiation have a poorer prospect of survival if their pretreatment haemoglobin level is below 12 g/dl compared with patients with a haemoglobin greater than 12 g/dl.

Hyperbaric oxygen

Since tumour hypoxia is an important factor in radiation resistance, it is logical to try to increase the oxygen supply to a tumour during irradiation. The oxygen concentration breathed by the patient can be raised by placing the patient in a hyperbaric oxygen (HBO) tank and gradually increasing the pressure to three times atmospheric pressure. This is maintained during treatment and then gradually lowered back to normal. The oxygenation of the whole body is increased including, it is hoped, that of the tumour. The radiosensitivity of normal tissues will be little affected, since it is normally at its maximum. However any increase in tumour oxygenation will be valuable.

Clinical trials comparing patients with advanced head and neck and cervical cancer irradiated in air or HBO have been conducted. A significant improvement in local control (65% versus 47% at 2 years) and in survival (71% versus 50% at 2 years) in advanced head and neck cancer was demonstrated in a randomised study of patients undergoing radiation in HBO compared with radiation in air. HBO conferred some but a lesser improvement in cervical cancer over treatment in air. Local control was increased in stages IIIb, IIIa and IVa from 20% to 24% 2–5 years after irradiation. The benefit was greatest for patients with stage III tumours.

Hyperbaric oxygen has not been widely adopted, largely for two reasons. First, the benefits in local control were considered only modest and, secondly, the technique poses considerable difficulties for both patients and staff. Patients are sometimes unable to tolerate treatment because of claustrophobia. The treatment set-up is also complex and time consuming.

Despite these shortcomings the application of HBO did demonstrate that the 'oxygen effect' does have an effect in conventionally fractionated radiotherapy.

Hypoxic cell sensitisers

An alternative to increasing the oxygen concentration delivered to the tumour is to enhance the sensitivity of tumour cells to the killing effects of ionising radiation. Chemical compounds which do this are called *radiosensitisers*. The most potent radiosensitiser is oxygen itself (Oxygen effect, p. 260). However a number of chemical compounds can mimic the radiation sensitising effect of oxygen. These are known as hypoxic cell sensitisers. These substances, like oxygen, are *electron-affinic*. It is this property that is thought to account for the radiosensitising effect. Overall clinical benefit over conventional irradiation alone in common tumours has been disappointing. In future their use, as with fast neutrons, may be best directed at tumours where reoxygenation can be identified to be relatively inefficient.

Nitroimidazoles

The nitroimidazole chemical group has been most extensively investigated. Of this group, *misonidazole* has undergone the most intensive laboratory and clinical assessment. In tissue culture, the sensitising effect of misonidazole is dose dependent. It has the additional advantage of not sensitising well-oxygenated cells. This would otherwise increase the acute and late effects of radiation on normal tissue and offset the gain in killing hypoxic tumour cells (i.e. there would be no therapeutic gain). Misonidazole is administered intravenously before irradiation. Unfortunately the highest oxygen enhancement ratio that can be achieved clinically is 1.8. This compares poorly with the enhancement ratio of oxygen at 3.0. Treatment with misonidazole and fractionated radiotherapy at a variety of tumour sites (head and neck, cervix, brain) has shown no useful gain in local control against radiotherapy alone. One important reason may be that during fractionated radiotherapy some hypoxic tumour cells become reoxygenated, so negating the selective radiosensitising of these cells by misonidazole. Escalating the dose of misonidazole in an attempt to increase radiosensitisation is limited by neurotoxicity. The latter is cumulative.

More recently developed nitroimidazoles which lack the neurotoxicity are under laboratory and clinical evaluation. At present, however, none of the nitroimidazoles can be recommended for routine clinical use.

Halogenated pyrimidines

Another group of compounds, the halogenated pyrimidines, can also sensitise cells to irradiation. However they are not specific to hypoxic cells and do sensitise normally oxygenated cells. They are incorporated into DNA instead of the base, thymidine, where they enhance damage to DNA. Their clinical application has been limited by their acute toxicity on normal tissues.

Fast neutrons

Fast neutrons (see also p. 201) have an OER of 1.6, much lower than that of X-rays and gamma rays, as well as a higher RBE and LET. The oxygen effect is therefore of much less importance for neutrons. This means that for the same amount of damage to normal (well-oxygenated) tissue, neutrons cause greater damage to anoxic tissue than X-rays or gamma rays. This potential therapeutic advantage in killing tumour cells resistant to conventional X-rays has unfortunately not proved to be as useful in practice as had been hoped. The application of neutron therapy in treating tumours thought to contain significant proportions of hypoxia cells (head and neck, brain, bladder, rectal and cervical cancer) has on the whole proved disappointing. The reasons for this are not clearly understood. It may be that the doses of neutrons used have been able to reduce but not eradicate the population of hypoxic cells

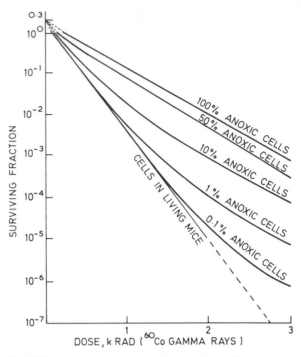

Fig. 15.8 Survival curves for cell populations with various proportions of anoxic cells. The lowest curve applies to well-oxygenated cells, in which a dose of 2000 rad (2 Gy) can be seen to give a survival of only 10^{-5} (i.e. 1 in 100 000). In the presence of 1% anoxic cells, survival is 10^{-1} (1 in 10 000) and with 10% anoxic cells it rises to 10^{-3} (1 in 1000). (Reproduced with permission from Hewitt and Wilson. Courtesy of Duncan W & Nias A H W 1977 Clinical Radiobiology, Churchill Livingstone, Edinburgh.)

within the tumour. As has been shown in experimental animals (Fig. 15.8), only a 0.1% proportion of hypoxic cells significantly increases resistance to X-rays.

THERAPEUTIC RATIO AND THERAPEUTIC GAIN

Therapeutic ratio

The aim of curative radiotherapy is to eradicate a tumour with minimal damage to normal tissue included in the treated volume. Steering a course between the Scylla of failure of local control and the Charybdis of late normal tissue injury is a difficult task. This is particularly true of tumours such as head and neck cancer where a high dose is usually needed for cure and critical structures such as the spinal cord lie within or close to the high dose volume. This delicate balance is expressed in the form of the *therapeutic ratio*. It is defined as: 'the ratio of the probability of eradicating tumour within the irradiated volume to the probability

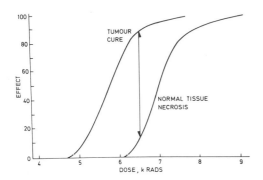

Fig. 15.9 Dose response curves for tumour cure and normal tissue necrosis. (Reproduced with permission from Duncan W & Nias A H W 1977 Clinical Radiobiology, Churchill Livingstone, Edinburgh.)

of causing severe late damage to normal tissue.' Increasing the therapeutic ratio may be achieved by increasing the cure rate for the same level of normal tissue injury of conventional treatment.

The relationship between dose and normal tissue injury and tumour cure is shown in Figure 15.9. Below a certain threshold dose no cures are obtained. With higher doses the cure rate rises steeply. The curve for normal tissue injury is similar to that of tumour cure, except that for reasons of fractionation and other physical and biological factors it is shifted to the right. It can be seen from Figure 15.9 that a total dose of 65 Gy can achieve a 90% cure rate at the expense of a normal necrosis rate of 15%. However, the steepness

of the slope for normal tissue necrosis is such that very small increments in dose beyond 65 Gy achieve little increase in cure rate but a substantial rise in normal tissue necrosis.

The therapeutic ratio is essential to the safe and effective practice of radiotherapy and is the main criterion by which any new application of therapeutic radiation to malignant disease should be judged. For example most of the trials of fast neutron therapy (p. 261) have shown a reduction in the therapeutic ratio. The reason for this is that, in comparison with conventional photon therapy, severe late morbidity is increased in head and neck, bladder and rectal cancer without any significant improvement in tumour cure.

By contrast, early experience of hyperfractionated radiotherapy (p. 565–6) in advanced head and neck cancer suggests a possible increase in the therapeutic ratio. Local cure rates are higher than with conventionally fractionated radiotherapy, without any significant increase in late morbidity. These findings await confirmation from randomised trials comparing hyperfractionated and conventional radiotherapy (p. 566).

Therapeutic gain factor

The *therapeutic gain factor* is used to describe the ratio of the radiobiological effectiveness (RBE) of any form of radiation on a tumour to the RBE for normal tissues. An improvement in the therapeutic gain factor can only be achieved by increasing the RBE to the tumour relative to normal tissue, or vice versa.

16. Effects of radiation on normal tissues

The radiobiological events described in Chapter 15, when ionising radiation passes through tissue, result in damage to DNA, mainly through the effects of free radicals. The pathological effects of ionising radiation on cells are due to chemical changes which, although involving only a small part of the DNA molecule, cause major or irreparable damage.

While we understand much about the molecular events following irradiation, it is uncertain how they are converted to changes at a tissue level. Damage to DNA may result in immediate cell death or, at the next mitosis, be fully repaired or result in a permanent change in genotype which is transmitted to future generations of cells. Which of these outcomes is effected will depend on the dose delivered and the radio-sensitivity of the cell. Low dose irradiation is most likely to cause a change in the genotype since it may be below the threshold for cell death. The abnormal genotype may therefore survive in subsequent cell divisions.

The dose given will influence this outcome, as will the radiosensitivity of the cell. Tissue and organ changes will reflect the overall reactions in the component parts.

Acute cellular effects

The most marked acute effects of radiation on normal cells will be on those with the highest mitotic activity (e.g. gut and bone marrow). The renewal of the cell population from a pool of less differentiated cells is stopped either permanently or temporarily, while the process of cell loss continues. There is also damage to the vascular lining (endothelium), which results in protein and fluid leakage.

Chronic cellular effects

The pathogenesis of the chronic cellular changes of irradiation are less well understood than the acute ones. The relative importance of different factors is contested.

The lining of collagen is exposed when the vascular endothelium is damaged. Exposed collagen may act as a focus for platelets to gather and thrombosis to be initiated. Vascular endothelial cell loss will result in exposure of the underlying collagen. This will prompt platelet adherence and the formation of thrombus, which is then incorporated into the vessel wall. The intimal lining of vessel wall proliferates. This process is known as *endarteritis obliterans*. Chronic vascular insufficiency may lead to atrophy and fibrosis of the tissues supplied.

Recovery from radiation damage

Recovery from the cellular effects of radical therapeutic irradiation is very limited. The doses given are often close to the tissue tolerance of the particular organ. For this reason radical irradiation is not generally repeated for fear of precipitating tissue breakdown (radionecrosis). It may be possible to repeat palliative courses of radiotherapy (e.g. 30 Gy in 10 daily fractions) as long as the combined dosage remains within tissue tolerance.

Tumour induction

Ionising radiation causes tumours, probably due to mutation in DNA. This is well documented for relatively high doses, but at low dose there is more uncertainty. The risk of malignant transformation and dose is nearly linear. However, as the dose increases, the proportion of cells lethally irradiated also rises. The surviving fraction able to be transformed to malignant cells accordingly decreases. It is tempting but not necessarily justified to extrapolate from the data on tumour induction at high dose to that at low dose. Unfortunately the numbers of tumours induced at low dose are too small to establish a threshold below which neoplastic transformation is unlikely to occur. The role of ionising radiation in carcinogenesis is discussed in Chapter 14.

RADIATION TOLERANCE OF NORMAL TISSUES

The purpose of radiotherapy planning is to confine the X-rays to the tumour and minimise the dose to normal tissues. This is clearly easier for superficial than deep seated tumours. Inevitably some normal tissue is included in the target volume to cover microscopic spread beyond the visible limits of the tumour (Ch. 6). There are definite limits to the amount of radiation that normal tissues will tolerate. This maximum dose of radiation that a tissue will tolerate is referred to as the *tolerance dose*. Exceeding this dose may result in major, and sometimes fatal complications. The tolerance dose will vary with the type and amount of tissue irradiated, the quality of radiation and its fractionation (Ch. 15).

Radiosensitivity

The term 'radiosensitivity' means the relative vulnerability of cells to damage by ionising radiation. Radiosensitivity is measurable in cell survival curves (p. 257–8), using the capacity to reproduce as the endpoint. Both normal and malignant tissues have different sensitivities, mainly determined by their different growth rates. This is the basis of the Law of Bergonié and Tribondeau (1904): 'The biological action of Roentgen rays is greater, the higher the reproductive activity of the cell, the longer the period of its mitosis and the less the degree of differentiation.' They studied the testis of the rat and found the radiosensitivity of the rapidly dividing germ cells to be high. It is no surprise that the cells of a malignant tumour of the germ cells of the testis (seminoma) are also very radiosensitive. By contrast a slow-growing soft tissue sarcoma shares the low sensitivity of its parent tissue. Radiosensitivity is discussed further on page 283.

The various tissues and organs have a wide spectrum of radiosensitivity. The highly sensitive are readily damaged by fairly low doses. The most radioresistant can withstand much higher doses without obvious ill-effects.

High sensitivity
— The epithelium of the skin (epidermis)
— The epithelial lining (inner surface) of the alimentary tract
— The cells in the bone marrow which produce the blood cells, i.e. the haemopoietic tissue
— The reproductive cells of the ovary and testis.

Intermediate sensitivity
— Liver, kidney, lung and many glands (e.g. thyroid).

Low sensitivity
— Muscle, bone, connective and nervous tissue.

RADIATION EFFECTS ON INDIVIDUAL TISSUES

The skin

This is a subject of prime importance since we are bound to irradiate the skin in most treatments, even if it is not the site of the tumour. Before the development of megavoltage irradiation with its skin sparing property, the tolerance of the skin to orthovoltage irradiation was often a limiting factor in delivering radical radiotherapy to deep seated tumours. Skin reactions are still of fundamental importance. Inappropriately marked skin reactions should alert the clinician to the possibility of an error in the calculation of the dose to be delivered or in the calibration of the output of the treatment machine.

Microscopic alterations

The changes in the skin reflect its composition from epithelium, connective tissue and blood vessels. Epidermis will suffer the consequence of cessation of mitosis, with desquamation and hair loss. Provided enough stem cells survive, hair will regrow, and any defects in epidermal coverage can be re-epithelialised. The regenerated epidermis will lack rete ridges and adnexa. Damage to keratinocytes and melanocytes results in melanin deposition in the dermis where it is picked up by phagocytic cells; these tend to remain in the skin and result in local hyperpigmentation. Some fibroblasts in the dermis will be killed, while others are at risk of an inability to divide, or to function correctly. As a consequence, the dermis is thinned, and histology shows bizarre, enlarged fibroblast nuclei.

The vessels show various changes depending on their size. Endothelial cell loss or damage is the probable underlying factor; they show vacuolation. Small and thin-walled vessels will leak fluid and protein, and mimic the inflammatory response; in the long term, they can be permanently dilated and tortuous (telangiectatic). Larger vessels develop proliferation of the intima and may permanently impair blood flow.

In summary, the skin is at first reddened with desquamation, and subsequently shows pigmentation. Later it is thinned with telangiectasia; if damage is too severe, it will break down and ulcerate (radionecrosis).

Acute skin reaction

The characteristic acute reaction on skin is erythema (Greek for 'redness'). Before the roentgen and the rad were defined, the 'erythema dose' was actually used as the measure of radiation dosage. In the orthovoltage era, skin reactions were a very useful guide in actual treatment and could give warning signals to the therapist. In a conventionally fractionated course of radical radiotherapy (e.g. over 4 weeks), there is an interval of time (latent period) before erythema appears. This is because the reaction is an inflammatory one following the breakdown of cells in the basal layer, the most actively dividing cells in the epidermis.

Radiodermatitis

Radiodermatitis may be acute or chronic.

Acute. This occurs typically in patients undergoing a radical course of radiotherapy (e.g. postoperative chest wall irradiation for breast cancer).

Chronic. This includes late effects seen in: (1) patients—months or years after treatment; (2) workers exposed to radiation (usually in industry) or patients accumulating small doses over many years without passing through the acute reaction.

Stages of the acute reaction. The acute reaction to conventionally fractionated radiotherapy follows a fairly predictable series of stages. The time at which each occurs will depend on the energy, dose and fractionation. Typically, during a 4 week course of chest wall irradiation following mastectomy for breast cancer, no skin changes are observed during the first fortnight, apart from faint erythema.

At about 14 days, hair loss (epilation) occurs. During the third week the main erythema develops. Initially this is punctate but then coalesces. The skin is warm, red and oedematous. Dusky pigmentation is common. Itching and discomfort are reported by the patient. During the fourth and fifth weeks of irradiation, dry desquamation occurs, sometimes progressing to moist desquamation. In moist desquamation the skin surface is shed, with inflammatory and serous discharge. Regeneration of new skin from the periphery of the irradiated fields or from small areas within the irradiated fields starts about a week after the end of irradiation. Recovery is normally complete by the third week after treatment. Sweat gland function is normally resumed within 2 weeks of the end of treatment. However the secretion of sebaceous glands usually does not recover, even if moist desquamation has not occurred. Hair begins to regrow by about 2 months after treatment. Its colour may be darker in patients with fair or white hair.

The skin reaction increases with both dose and the area irradiated. In practice high skin doses for curative purposes are normally confined to skin cancers where the field diameter is small (2–4 cm). For the cure of skin tumours, the skin is treated to its tolerance. If this is done, radiation induced skin necrosis will occur in about 5% of cases. It is more likely to occur in treated skin that has been previously damaged and its blood supply compromised, and with increasing field size.

Different parts of the body vary in their skin sensitivity to radiation. The more sensitive areas include those subject to moisture and friction (axilla, groin, vulva, anus) and those with a poor blood supply (back of the hand, back and sole of the foot, midline of back) and areas overlying cartilage (e.g. pinna) and bone (e.g. shin).

Chronic radiation dermatitis. After treatment to high dose, the skin will show some radiation effect for a long time, usually permanently, especially after superficial or orthovoltage irradiation.

All the following changes are now seen far less frequently since the introduction of megavoltage with its skin sparing effects.

Ischaemia. Many of the late effects of therapeutic doses in the skin or any other organ are due to the destruction and narrowing of local blood vessels with consequent ischaemia, often associated with fibrosis. We shall have occasion to refer to this when discussing particular treatment, e.g. complications of intracavitary caesium therapy in cervical cancer (p. 412) and effects on other tissues, e.g. brain, bone and bowel (see below).

Pigmentation. This may vary from light to very dark brown and will show the size of the irradiated field. It may be distributed in a patchy manner, especially at the edges of a treated area, and may be mingled with whitish patches of depigmented atrophic skin.

Thickening. The skin may heal with considerable fibrosis of the dermis, giving a typical leathery feel with loss of elasticity.

Telangiectasia. Telangiectasia refers to dilatation of thin-walled blood vessels. Destruction or narrowing of the small arteries of the skin may lead to compensatory dilatation of capillaries, which can be very disfiguring.

Late ulceration. An atrophic area is always vulnerable to injuries that would normally be of negligible importance. A scratch or burn, even years later, may lead to a persistent breakdown. This is late necrosis. It is very slow to heal and may require excision and grafting.

Secondary malignancy. This is a complication of chronic radiation exposure. In pioneer X-ray and radium workers, before the dangers were appreciated, skin changes appeared, especially on the fingers. The skin became dry, lost its elasticity and erythema formed around the nails, which became fissured and irregular and might be shed. Later, warts and fissures appeared on the skin and eventually, after some years, malignant change.

Similar changes also happened in some patients subjected to repeated courses of irradiation, especially for non-malignant conditions such as psoriasis and pruritus.

Management of skin reactions

Explanation to patients. Patients should always be given a simple explanation of the probable effects of treatment on the skin and any other organs likely to be affected such as bowel and bladder. It is useful to have a leaflet to hand out at the start, informing them of the likely reactions and of the precautions to take to minimise them. If moist desquamation is expected, they should be warned of the probable breakdown and discharge, crusting and eventual healing after 2 weeks or more. They should be assured that these are normal reactions, not 'burns'.

In milder reactions, little or no special treatment may be necessary, e.g. in dry desquamation, unless the part is exposed to friction, when a simple covering may be useful until the skin has healed. For small areas of moist desquamation (e.g. small basal cell cancer on the face), it is often quite satisfactory to leave it alone, allow it to crust over and leave healing to proceed until the crust drops off the new epidermis. If infection is suspected, it may be removed with forceps. If infection is present or threatens during the course of treatment, an antiseptic cream such as chlorhexidine (Hibitane) or cetrimide can be used.

In the first- and second-degree reactions, the chief complaint is usually of simple irritation or itching. An ordinary dusting of talcum powder may be used but, as many of these contain a heavy metal (zinc or bismuth), they should not be put on before treatment has finished, because the metal gives rise to secondary radiation which increases the skin dose and therefore the severity of the reaction. A simple baby powder should be used instead. For the same reason zinc oxide strapping should be avoided and Sellotape or micropore used instead. In areas of friction, lanolin or tulle gras may be applied. When the full course of radiation is over, creams or ointments containing metals may be used freely, e.g. zinc and castor oil. Cold air from a fan also has a soothing effect.

The patient should be cautioned against all forms of irritation to the treated area. The patient was often advised in the past against washing the treated area until the acute reaction had settled. This is usually 2–3 weeks after the end of treatment. Lack of local hygiene over so long a period is unpleasant and inconvenient for the patient. As long as the patient does not rub the treated area vigorously, washing after chest wall irradiation does not significantly worsen the radiation reactions. This is almost certainly true at other sites.

If skin marks have been outlined on the patient for the radiographer's guidance, they must not be washed off. They tend to come off as a result of sweating and friction, especially in hot weather, and then need to be re-marked.

Oropharyngeal mucosa

The mouth and pharynx are lined by mucous membrane covered by non-stratified squamous epithelium. The major and minor salivary glands produce secretions which keep the mucous membranes moist. Below the mucosa lies the lamina propria, containing blood vessels, nerves and minor salivary glands. Since mucous membranes proliferate rapidly, the effects of radiation are expressed at an early stage.

The acute mucosal reaction to conventionally fractionated irradiation is the killing of the stem cells in the basal layer of the epithelium. This has no immediate clinical effects. However the supply of new cells to replace those lost from the mucosa by wear and tear is cut off. There is therefore a lag phase before the mucosa is denuded. Residual stem cells that have survived irradiation proliferate to try to repopulate the mucosa.

Following the start of irradiation, cells which are dividing in the basal layer degenerate and undergo necrosis. Oedema with neutrophil infiltration develops in the lamina propria and submucosa. This is associated with dilation of capillaries and swelling of their endothelial lining, accounting for erythema which is observed clinically. When a radical dose (55 Gy) is given in daily fractions over 4–4.5 weeks, a confluent mucosal reaction occurs in which the mucosa is denuded. This starts at the end of the second week. Histologically there is a pseudomembrane consisting of cell debris, fibrin and leucocytes. The mucosal reaction is maximal in the middle of the third week. It has normally settled by the 5th–8th week. If the same dose is given over 5–6.5 weeks, the intensity of the mucosal reaction is reduced.

Where radical irradiation has been given in multiple daily fractions (p. 565–6) (e.g. 48 Gy over 2 weeks at three fractions of 1.6 Gy 3–4 hours per day, followed by a 3–4 week gap and then further irradiation on the same fractionation schedule to 70 Gy over 6–7 weeks), severe confluent erythema has occurred by day 13 but healed by day 22. Regeneration of mucosal stem cells is thought to be greater during the rest period between a 'split-course' of radiation such as this than between conventional single daily fractions of radical irradiation.

Within a month of a 6–7 week course of radiation, the epithelium has regenerated. Later changes occur as a result of the process of repair, with fibrosis in the lamina propria and the submucosa. Telangiectatic capillaries and thickening of the walls of arterioles are seen. As a result of scarring, the mucosa is subsequently more than normally susceptible to ulceration following minimal trauma.

Salivary glands

Some portions of the major salivary glands (parotid, submandibular and sublingual) are almost invariably included during irradiation of tumours in a variety of sites in the head and neck, especially of the oral cavity. Most of the unpleasant side-effects of head and neck radiation relate directly or indirectly to irradiation of the major salivary glands. Together these glands secrete 60–70% of saliva at rest and following stimulation. The parotid gland is the main source of saliva. Most of the resting saliva is secreted by the submandibular gland.

The minor salivary glands are widely spread in the mucosa of the tongue, cheeks, lips, tonsils and palate. They mainly secrete mucus.

Following irradiation an acute inflammatory reaction occurs in the major salivary glands. There is rapid loss of secretory acini corresponding to the development of xerostomia (dry mouth). The dose at which xerostomia is permanent varies widely, from 4.5 to 40.5 Gy. This wide range is probably explained by individual variation in pretreatment salivary flow rates. Permanent inhibition of salivary secretion is probable in 80% of patients after 40–60 Gy, conventionally fractionated. At or beyond 60 Gy total xerostomia occurs in all individuals. If the sublingual and submandibular glands are irradiated and the parotid largely excluded, late sequelae are rare. Patients with the greatest pretreatment taste discrimination tend to experience the quickest loss of taste after irradiation. The relative contribution of direct damage to taste buds by irradiation or as an indirect effect of reduced salivary flow is uncertain. However saliva is considered important in maintaining the sense of taste.

Intestine

The surface epithelium of the small intestine is renewed every 24–48 hours. A significant dose of irradiation will therefore result in loss of protective and absorptive functions over a similar time scale; diarrhoea and the risk of infection then follow. If a high dose is given to a localised region, the mucosa will regrow, although often with a less specialised cell type, and with the probability of mutations in the remaining cells. The muscle coat will also have been damaged, and there is the risk of granulation tissue causing the formation of a stricture later.

The tolerance dose to limited volumes of the small bowel, as in conventionally fractionated pelvic irradiation for cervical or endometrial cancer, is 45 Gy over 4 weeks.

Clinical effects

In the mouth the membranous reaction is initially white and may be mistaken for thrush. It then becomes yellowish and gradually decreases in size as healing proceeds, as decribed above.

In the mouth and pharynx these reactions may cause unpleasant dryness, loss of taste, sore throat and dysphagia. In the oesophagus, which is bound to be involved in the treatment of the lung and mediastinum, there may be soreness, painful spasm and dysphagia. Recovery of taste usually occurs 2–4 months after treatment. Xerostomia is permanent if substantial amounts of the parotid glands have been irradiated.

Treatment of mucosal reactions

As a prophylactic measure, dental treatment should be carried out where necessary in cases of head and neck cancer (Ch. 20).

When the mouth and throat are involved, the diet should be light. Drinks of high calorific value (e.g. Build-up or Complan) are helpful. Mouthwashes with aspirin mucilage or a local anaesthetic such as Mucaine before meals are recommended. Hot or spiced food (vinegar or pickles) should not be given. Smoking and alcohol should be discouraged.

Bowel reactions are common and important in the treatment of abdominal and pelvic lesions. Drugs may be required to control vomiting (metoclopramide), spasm (propantheline) or diarrhoea (codeine phosphate or diphenoxylate hydrochloride (Lomotil). If bowel reactions are marked, treatment may have to be interrupted for a few days or, in extreme cases, stopped entirely.

In the bowel, when abdomen or pelvis is treated, there may be spasm and diarrhoea which can lead to dehydration and also to bleeding. When cancer of the cervix is treated, the rectum (immediately behind the vagina) receives a considerable dose and some degree of proctitis is usual, with irritation, tenesmus, passage of mucus and possibly blood. In the bladder, reactions may cause dysuria with pain and frequency.

Late effects on mucosal surfaces may appear after weeks, months or years. In the mouth, reduction in salivary flow gives rise to dental caries. The fall in pH and in the secretion of antibodies encourages the growth of bacteria responsible for dental decay. These bacteria produce acids from breaking down foodstuffs. The acid in turn dissolves tooth enamel and dentine. There may be malabsorption, adhesions, fibrosis and stenosis, leading to obstruction, fistulae and bleeding. Surgical intervention may be needed for any of these.

Effects on blood-forming tissues

Haemopoietic tissue—mainly bone marrow and lymphoid tissue—is highly radiosensitive. The most marked effects are on the parent (stem) cells of the leucocytes, lymphocytes and platelets. Red cells are much less radiosensitive, as their life cycle is much longer, about 4 months, compared with a day or less for most white cells.

In patients the effect on the blood count is very variable. It depends on a number of factors, particularly the area of bone marrow irradiated and the dose. There is a fall in total white cells (leucopenia) and in platelets (thrombocytopenia) but red cells may hardly be affected at all. If only a very small part of the body is under treatment, the effect on the blood will be negligible, and in superficial therapy, e.g. for skin cancer, there is no need to monitor the blood count. High dose irradiation of small volumes of the bone marrow will not alter the blood count, but it will result in local loss of haemopoiesis and fibrosis of the marrow cavity. But the larger the field and the more penetrating the radiation, the greater will be the effect on haemopoietic tissue. Whole body irradiation exposure (see below) may result in bone marrow failure. In the absence of a bone marrow transplant this is often fatal.

During most courses of wide field radical therapy covering substantial amounts of the bone marrow (e.g mantle or inverted Y for Hodgkin's disease), the blood should be measured twice weekly. More frequent measurements, e.g. daily, are necessary if the blood count is falling rapidly or is close to the threshold for suspending treatment.

There is a risk of inducing leukaemia, as happened in patients who underwent low dose spinal irradiation for ankylosing spondylitis (p. 524).

Effects on reproductive organs

The gonads (ovary and testis) contain two separate types of tissue:

— Reproductive, for the formation of germ cells (ova and sperm). They are among the most radiosensitive.
— Endocrine, for the production of sex hormones (oestrogens and androgens).

Males

The germ cells of the seminiferous tubules of the testis provide a self-renewing supply of sperm. The Leydig cells of the supporting tissues produce testosterone, the male sex hormone. The germ cells are much more radiosensitive than the Leydig cells. However there is variation in radiosensitivity between different stages of development into mature sperm. With single doses as low as 2–3 Gy the maturation of spermatocytes is stopped. For spermatids 4–6 Gy causes damage. Doses as low as 0.78 Gy have been reported to cause azoospermia. Due to this variation in radiosensitivity, depletion of sperm following irradiation is gradual. This may take as long as 22 weeks. Recovery is also dose dependent. The lower the dose the more rapid the recovery. For doses less than 0.1 Gy this occurs in 9–18 months. For doses of 4–6 Gy recovery may take over 5 years. Over 6 Gy no recovery of sperm production occurs. Some dose to the testis is almost invariable from abdominal irradiation (e.g. inverted Y to para-aortic and pelvic nodes for lymphomas or 'dog-leg' irradiation to the paraaortic and ipsilateral pelvic nodes for testicular seminoma). Azoospermia and permanent sterility usually develop after inverted Y irradiation. However recovery usually occurs 20–40 weeks following 'dog-leg' fractionated irradiation where the dose is less than 0.6 Gy, and 50–90 weeks after doses over 0.6 Gy. In excess of 2 Gy permanent azoospermia is likely.

Total doses of fractionated radiotherapy to the testis should be less than 1 Gy. Sperm storage should be offered to patients with an adequate sperm count prior to treatment. The dose to the testis from scattered irradiation from 'dog-leg' irradiation can be reduced by lead shielding.

At low doses (<1 Gy), testosterone production from the Leydig cells is maintained, although the levels of the gonadotrophins FSH and LH may rise. Hormone replacement therapy is unlikely to be necessary in the range of doses received by the testis in normal clinical practice.

Females

Sterility can similarly be induced by radiation but depends on physiological age. However the effects of different doses on the ovary are difficult to assess because it is not possible to measure the absorbed dose to the ovary directly. Hormonal effects are more obvious and of greater clinical significance in the female than in the male. Production of oestrogens can be reduced or abolished with temporary or permanent cessation of menstruation. This effect is used in the induction of an artificial menopause (p. 521). It is not known what the minimum dose is to induce ovarian failure. Amenorrhoea will follow single doses of 6 Gy in prepubertal girls. The dose needed to induce a menopause is probably less with increasing age. This might be due to the reduced number of oocytes in the ovary. Permanent amenorrhoea occurs in only 30% of women aged between 30 and 35 years after 5 Gy but in 80% aged between 35 and 40 years. The dose required to induce the menopause is between 10 and 20 Gy. A dose of 12 Gy in four daily fractions is recommended to induce a radiation menopause for breast cancer.

Genetic effects of radiation

It is well established that ionising radiation does cause gene mutations, i.e. changes in the structure of the genetic material. In man, however, there is little information on which to judge the risks of exposure to particular doses. There was no evidence of an increase in genetic abnormalities among children born to survivors of the atomic bombs dropped on Nagasaki and Hiroshima in 1945 where one or both parents had been exposed to radiation.

The term 'doubling dose' is used to describe the dose of irradiation which doubles the spontaneous mutation rate. The doubling dose in man is estimated to be approximately 1 Gy.

Mutations may occur both in somatic and germ cells. Mutations in somatic cells may be carcinogenic, particularly after exposure to low dosage. Mutations in the germ cells are important since they may have an impact on subsequent generations.

The genetic defects which may be induced are chromosomal abnormalities, changes in autosomal or sex-linked characters, spontaneous abortions and genetic deaths. Genetic death is the term given to the termination of a cell line either due to fetal death early

in pregnancy or to reduced fertility. It is thought that most germ cell mutations do not result in offspring that survive. For this reason abnormal children are very rarely fathered by men whose testes have received low dose scattered irradiation (e.g. from abdominal node irradiation after orchidectomy for testicular seminoma). When it is realised that a single dose of 0.4 Gy to the testis will result in the death of 90% of germ cells, it is understandable that germ cell mutations rarely have the opportunity to be expressed in offspring.

Radiation in pregnancy

Radiation should be avoided in pregnancy. Damage may be done either to the mother's ovaries or to the fetus. Potentially, genetic mutations may occur in the ovaries of mother and fetus, resulting in abnormal later children or future generations. The fetus is particularly vulnerable in view of the relatively enormous growth rate and the extreme immaturity of all its tissues. The first 3 months (first trimester) is the most dangerous period. Even low dose irradiation (e.g. from diagnostic X-rays) can produce birth defects such as hare lip and cleft palate. More importantly, evidence from women irradiated by the atomic bomb in Japan in 1945 shows that the developing brain may be impaired, causing mental deficiency at low doses (0.04 Gy) and microcephaly at higher doses between 8 and 25 weeks of pregnancy. Larger doses will kill the fetus and lead to abortion.

Fetal irradiation probably increases the risk of childhood leukaemia, although the relationship is not definitely proven. For this reason, diagnostic X-ray departments, before taking films of the pelvis, enquire routinely about the date of the last menstrual period, to avoid exposure in women of reproductive age if there is a possibility of pregnancy.

Kidney

The kidney is an organ of intermediate radiosensitivity. It is mainly a late responding tissue, although functional and histological changes may be observed within a few weeks of irradiation. The low tolerance of the kidney to irradiation was first appreciated from the study of patients who underwent irradiation for abdominal metastases from testicular cancer. Five clinical syndromes were described:

— *Acute radiation nephritis*, associated with hypertension and proteinuria, occurring 6–13 months after treatment.
— *Chronic radiation nephritis*, associated with urinary protein and casts, nocturia, loss of ability to

concentrate the urine, occurring 1.5–4 years after treatment.

— *Benign hypertension*, associated with proteinuria, occurring 1.5–5 years after treatment.

— *Proteinuria*, lasting 5–19 years, as the only evidence of renal damage.

— *Late malignant hypertension*, occurring 1.5–11 years after treatment.

In adults the limit of tolerance if both kidneys are irradiated is 28 Gy in 5 weeks. The risk is less if only part of or the whole of one kidney is irradiated, since the kidney on the opposite side may hypertrophy and compensate for the loss of renal function.

The pathogenesis of renal damage is controversial. It may be due to damage to the endothelial cells lining the glomeruli (parenchymal damage) or to the larger blood vessels (vascular damage). The critical target cell population has not been firmly identified.

Damage to the renal tubules precedes glomerular damage and sclerosis. Radiation nephropathy is slowly progressive and irreversible, in spite of tubular regeneration and epithelial proliferation.

Care should be taken to determine the position of the kidneys when the pelvis, abdomen and spine are treated. The soft tissue shadow of the kidney can often be seen on a plain abdominal film. If there is any uncertainty about their position, an intravenous urogram should be carried out. It should be remembered that pelvic or horseshoe kidneys occur. A pelvic field, which would normally exclude the kidneys in their normal position, may unwittingly include the kidneys in such anomalous positions.

In general most of one kidney should be excluded from the radiation field or shielded by lead blocks if the other kidney has to be irradiated.

Where part of both kidneys has to be included, for example in abdominal node irradiation for lymphoma (p. 448) and seminoma of the testis (p. 437), the area irradiated should not exceed a third of each kidney.

It is generally safe to irradiate the whole kidney to 20 Gy. Beyond this dose the kidneys should be shielded by lead blocks (e.g. in whole abdominal irradiation for ovarian cancer, p. 418).

Nervous system and eye

The radiation pathology and tolerance of the central nervous system and the eye are described in Chapter 27.

Bone and cartilage

In growing bone, as in children, irradiation of an epiphysis is likely to retard growth. The tolerance dose for 5% damage at 5 years after irradiation for growing cartilage is 10 Gy. For children under the age of 3 years, the equivalent tolerance dose is lower (8 Gy). The effects on growth are much more marked when the long bones are irradiated than when the vertebral column is irradiated. Both limb shortening and scoliosis may occur in children.

For mature bone, the tolerance dose for 5% damage within 5 years of irradiation is 60 Gy. Both direct damage to osteocytes and indirect damage due to radiation-induced vascular injury may play a part in the pathogenesis of osteoradionecrosis (p. 321). Radionecrosis of the mandible may occur following radical radiotherapy for oral cancer (p. 321 and Fig. 20.12).

The threshold level for osteoradionecrosis may be lowered in patients who have received both radiotherapy and steroid-containing chemotherapy for lymphoma. Radionecrosis of the femoral head is the most important example of this (p. 449).

Cartilage necrosis can occur in the outer ear (pinna and external auditory meatus), nose (ala nasi) and larynx. All these changes are aggravated or precipitated by trauma and infection. Dental caries is an example discussed on page 314.

Lungs

The inflammatory reactions in lung tissue (radiation pneumonitis) may cause serious scarring (fibrosis) which prevents the lung expanding properly. Vital capacity is thus reduced. Care is taken to minimise the amount of lung irradiated in treating the chest wall for breast cancer (Fig. 23.6). Radiation pneumonitis is described in more detail on page 379.

RADIATION SICKNESS

This is a general reaction which is liable to occur during a course of treatment. Its severity depends on the part of the body and the volume of tissue which is irradiated. If a small skin tumour is treated, there will be no general reaction at all. However if the upper abdomen is irradiated for a deep seated tumour (e.g. for gastric lymphoma), there may be marked general upset. By contrast similarly large volumes of a lower limb can be irradiated with minimal systemic upset.

The clinical features of radiation sickness are nausea (sometimes with vomiting), headache, tiredness and weakness. In very sensitive or debilitated patients there may be prostration.

The cause of radiation sickness is unknown. It may be that the products of the breakdown of tissue, particularly rapidly dividing cells of the gastrointestinal tract, contribute largely to the stimulation of the vomiting centre in the brainstem. There is much individual variation between patients in response to the same dose of irradiation to a similar volume. Anxiety about treatment may exacerbate symptoms and can often be relieved by a clear explanation of what is to be expected.

Treatment with sedatives (e.g. Motival) and antiemetics (prochlorperazine or metoclopramide) may help. More recently the 5-hydroxytryptamine ($5HT_3$) receptor antagonists (ondansetron and granisetron) have proved to be very effective in preventing radiation sickness. An adequate daily fluid intake of 4–5 pints (2–2.5 litres) should be maintained.

WHOLE BODY IRRADIATION

As a therapeutic procedure this is now rarely used except before bone marrow transplantation (e.g. for acute leukaemia). However chronic exposure is natural and unavoidable (Ch. 13). We are subject to radiation from natural sources and man-made appliances. The current exposure of the population in the UK to these sources is shown in Figure 12.2.

Acute radiation syndrome

The acute radiation syndrome describes the clinical effects of whole body exposure to single doses in excess of 0.5 Gy. The best documented evidence of the effects of such doses is derived from the explosion of atomic bombs at Hiroshima and Nagasaki in Japan in 1945. The radiation doses have been estimated and the survivors followed up and observed. Other episodes have been the unintentional exposure in the Marshall Islands in the Pacific in 1954 in the course of bomb testing, affecting nearly 300 people, and the explosion of the nuclear reactor at Chernobyl in 1986. All these, in addition to observations of experimental animal work, give us a detailed picture of the effects of acute radiation damage.

The time of onset, extent and duration of symptoms are all dose dependent. Three main clinical syndromes are described, reflecting the most radiosensitive organ systems. Their principal features are summarised in Table 16.1.

— The haematological syndrome
— The gastrointestinal syndrome
— The central nervous (CNS) syndrome.

These are preceded by a prodromal syndrome.

Prodromal radiation syndrome

After exposure to whole body doses of 0.5 Gy, radiation sickness begins within 1–2 hours. This is accompanied by headache, lassitude and sometimes vertigo. At much higher doses of 1 Gy the onset is within minutes.

Haematological syndrome

The threshold total body dose for the development of the haematological syndrome is 1 Gy. At a dose of 2 Gy the syndrome is almost invariably fatal. It comprises two successive phases.

In the first phase the direct target is the bone marrow, where parent cells of the peripheral blood cells are killed or their differentiation inhibited. The immediate result is leucopenia and thrombocytopenia. Of the white cells, the lymphocytes are affected earliest and most profoundly, followed by other white cells and megakaryocytes. The red cell precursors are also sensitive, but since the red cell has a life span of about

Table 16.1 Acute radiation syndromes following whole body irradiation

Features	Syndromes		
	CNS	Gastrointestinal	Haematopoietic
Main organ affected	Brain	Small bowel	Bone marrow
Major pathology	Vasculitis, encephalitis, oedema (CNS)	Depletion of intestinal epithelium, infection	Bone marrow atrophy, pancytopenia, haemorrhage, infection
Threshold dose for onset (Gy)	20	5	1
Threshold dose for death (Gy)	50	10	2
Onset following exposure	0.25–3 hours	3–5 days	2–3 weeks
Typical clinical features	Lethargy, tremor, seizures, ataxia	Malaise, anorexia, nausea, vomiting, diarrhoea, fever, electrolyte imbalance, circulatory collapse	Malaise, fatigue, exertional dyspnoea, leukopenia, thrombocytopenia, purpura
Time of death	Within 2 days	3–14 days	3–8 weeks

(Adapted from Rubin P & Casarett G W 1968 Clinical Radiation Pathology, W B Saunders, Philadelphia.)

4 months, anaemia develops later than leucopenia and thrombocytopenia.

In the second phase a haemorrhagic anaemia develops; this may be a consequence of widespread damage to the vasculature of the viscera and mucous membranes.

The following clinical sequence is seen:

Within hours: Anorexia, nausea, vomiting, diarrhoea.
24–36 hours: Symptoms subside; patient feels well.
3 weeks: Malaise, fever, anorexia, fatigue, exertional dyspnoea, alopecia, pharyngitis, swelling and ulceration of tonsils, swelling and bleeding of gums, petechiae and bruising, diarrhoea.
5–6 weeks: Agranulocytosis, anaemia, bacterial infection.
8 weeks: If patient recovers, resolution of symptoms and signs.

Prognosis. The absolute lymphocyte count at 48 hours (without blood transfusion) is a useful guide to outcome:

1200+   Unlikely to be fatal
300–1200 Lethal range
<300   Almost certainly fatal.

Gastrointestinal syndrome

In the gastrointestinal syndrome the main organ affected is the small bowel. The threshold dose is 5 Gy. The time of onset of nausea and vomiting followed by diarrhoea varies from within half an hour of exposure to several hours. These symptoms may persist from the start or subside after 2–3 days, recurring on the fifth day when the gastrointestinal epithelium has been denuded. Diarrhoea becomes bloody. Fluid and electrolyte imbalance develops, eventually leading to circulatory collapse, coma and death.

CNS syndrome

The onset of the CNS syndrome is prompt, with death rapidly supervening. The pathological processes are vasculitis and encephalitis leading to cerebral oedema. Apathy and drowsiness develop, increase in severity and progress to prostration. Seizures ranging from muscle tremor to grand mal type are followed by ataxia if the dose is in excess of 50 Gy.

Effect on unborn children

In those who survived the atomic bomb, a special hazard involved pregnant women. Abortions and stillbirths were brought about. If the child survived in utero, its brain development was liable to be retarded and it might be born with a small head (microcephaly) and mental deficiency.

Late effects of atomic bomb explosions

There are special dangers of radioactive 'fall-out'. This is the radioactive dust containing fission products (p. 27) carried to great heights in the atmosphere with the vaporised material from the bomb. The fine particles are carried in air currents, settling down gradually to earth. These dust clouds can travel great distances, even encircling the earth many times. A bomb exploded in Nevada in the USA produces fall-out detectable in England 5 days later.

A particular hazard of fall-out concerns radioactive strontium, a fission product. This is soluble and is absorbed by plants and grazing animals (e.g. cattle and sheep) and reaches humans in the diet and water. Biochemically it behaves like calcium and is deposited in bone tissue after absorption. It is therefore potentially capable of producing late effects comparable to those in luminous dial painters (p. 245).

17. Principles of management and dosage

Once a diagnosis of malignancy has been reached, some important management decisions must be made:

1. To select necessary investigations
2. To undertake curative (radical) or palliative therapy
3. To choose appropriate palliative or radical treatment
4. To choose appropriate support services (e.g nursing and social services) for patient and family.

This chapter concentrates on items (2), (3) and (4). The appropriate staging investigations are covered by tumour site in Chapters 18–29.

Radical or palliative treatment?

This is perhaps the most important decision that the clinical oncologist has to make. The decision will depend on the history, clinical examination and investigations. The oncologist has to weigh the factors outlined below in coming to a decision.

Radical treatment means the attempt to kill or remove all the malignant cells present. Cure or local control is the aim. Some morbidity, and occasionally mortality from treatment has often to be accepted if cure is to be achieved.

Palliative treatment is aimed at relieving the symptoms of cancer (for example pain, dysphagia, dyspnoea) or restraining temporarily the growth of the tumour. Any side-effects should be minor. Palliative and continuing care is considered in detail in Chapter 33.

ASSESSMENT BEFORE TREATMENT

Multidisciplinary management

The increasing complexity of curative cancer management for many tumours, with different combinations of surgery, radiotherapy and chemotherapy for different stages of disease, requires a coordinated multi-

Table 17.1 Surgery alone—the treatment of choice

Lower oesophagus, stomach, colon, pancreas, kidney
Thyroid
Melanoma
Hepatocellular carcinoma
Keratoacanthoma

Table 17.2 Radiotherapy—the treatment of choice

Oral cavity, lip, tongue, cheek
Nasopharynx
Oropharynx
Hypopharynx
Nasal cavity
Larynx
Skin cancer (except melanoma)
Cervix
Bladder (except T1)
Testis—seminoma
Hodgkin's disease (early)
Non-Hodgkin lymphoma (early)
Medulloblastoma (following surgical debulking)
Astrocytomas (grades 3 and 4)
Retinoblastoma

Table 17.3 Cytotoxic therapy—the treatment of choice

Acute and chronic leukaemias
Hodgkin's disease (advanced)
Non-Hodgkin lymphoma (advanced)
Testicular teratoma
Choriocarcinoma
Small cell lung cancer
Rhabdomyosarcoma
Neuroblastoma

disciplinary approach. The correct initial choice gives the best prospect for cure or good palliation. Tables 17.1–17.3 summarise the tumours for which surgery, radiotherapy and chemotherapy, respectively, are the treatments of choice. For many early tumours, e.g. of the oral cavity, surgery and radiotherapy give equally good results. The choice between them may depend on local expertise.

In patients with potentially curable disease, inappropriate initial treatment may compromise both the quantity and quality of survival. In curative treatment, it may also increase the risk of complications when surgery or radiotherapy for residual disease has to be added after incorrect primary therapy has failed. Occasionally, for example, a Wertheim's hysterectomy for early cancer of the cervix (p. 404) is not completed because the extent of disease preoperatively has been underestimated. The risks of pelvic morbidity from radical pelvic irradiation following pelvic surgery are much higher than if primary radical radiotherapy had been given alone.

Patients with malignant disease may present before, during or after treatment as a medical or surgical emergency—e.g. with respiratory failure (from large volume lung metastases from testicular teratoma), with acute upper airway obstruction requiring tracheostomy (laryngeal and thyroid cancer), with spinal cord compression (breast and lung cancer, myeloma) or with pathological fracture (breast cancer)—requiring the attention of the ear, nose and throat, orthopaedic or neurosurgeon.

Joint clinics

Where the choice is between surgery, radiotherapy or a combination of both, assessment by an oncologist at a joint clinic with a specialist surgeon, dermatologist, gynaecologist or haematologist is often helpful.

The success of such clinics depends on a collaborative spirit and on each specialist knowing the strengths and limitations of each modality of treatment. In some situations equally good results can be achieved by different treatments, e.g. by surgery and radiotherapy for early cancer of the cervix. The choice may be determined by the relative morbidity of each treatment or by the experience of the specialist or the treatment facilities. For instance, the best results of radical surgery for ovarian cancer are obtained in the hands of a gynaecologist undertaking this form of surgery on a regular basis.

The lines of communication between specialists need to be clear so that the timing of surgery, radiotherapy and chemotherapy are properly synchronised. Each specialist, referring doctor and the patient's general practitioner should be kept informed of the patient's progress. The patient should know which member of the multidisciplinary team to contact for advice.

Advantages. There are a number of potential advantages. Delay incurred by referral to more than one clinic is avoided. The patient may feel reassured that all treatment options have been considered before embarking on the chosen course of treatment. Joint clinics provide a good basis for the audit of treatment and for clinical trials to assess new therapies.

Disadvantages. If the number of medical staff attending the clinic is large, the patient may find attendance intimidating. This can be minimised if, once all the relevant specialists have examined the patient and withdrawn to discuss management, the specialist undertaking the primary management returns alone to explain the planned treatment to the patient and to answer questions.

Information required for a decision on treatment

In every case all the relevant information must be gathered about the patient in general and the tumour and its extent of spread in particular.

Age and general medical condition. The latter includes coincident disease (e.g. diabetes mellitus, chronic respiratory disease, peptic ulceration).

Tumour spread—local, regional nodes, distant metastases. Staging is the term applied to determine the extent of the disease. Staging may include clinical, radiological or laboratory findings. Local, regional or distant spread is assessed by:

1. Clinical examination—especially for accessible cancers, e.g. skin, oral cavity, larynx, cervix and breast. This includes palpation of the regional nodes, e.g. the cervical nodes for the oral cavity, larynx and pharynx, and the axilla and supraclavicular fossae for breast tumours.

2. Instrumental endoscopy—e.g. bronchoscopy for lung, cystoscopy for bladder, sigmoidoscopy for colon and rectum.

3. Radiology—radiographs of the chest for secondary deposits in the lungs, skeletal survey for deposits of myeloma, intravenous urography (IVU) for identification of tumours of the bladder, ureters and kidneys, CT scanning for pelvic, para-aortic and mediastinal nodes.

4. Isotope scans—radioactive tracer studies may detect primary or secondary deposits in thyroid, bone, brain and liver.

Histology. Histological confirmation of the tumour should be obtained, if at all possible. If there is no clinical doubt about the diagnosis (e.g. of a basal cell carcinoma on the face) and the patient's condition is very frail, biopsy may be omitted. Similarly in superior mediastinal obstruction a clinical diagnosis of lung cancer is also often made without pathological confirmation. This is because bronchial biopsy may precipitate serious haemorrhage in the presence of raised venous pressure. Biopsy of brainstem gliomas is often avoided because of the risk of causing a major neurological deficit. Occasionally biopsy of an obvious bronchial tumour is negative. This may happen if the biopsy is taken unwittingly from adjacent inflammatory tissue.

Where the pathological type is likely to influence management, i.e. the patient would be fit for chemotherapy if the histological diagnosis was small cell lung cancer, the biopsy should be repeated. If the patient would only be fit for palliative radiotherapy whatever the histology, further biopsy is often avoided.

Review of histology by specialist tumour pathologist. The histological classification of some tumours, particularly the lymphomas and sarcomas, requires a great deal of experience. In these circumstances, or where the pathologist is uncertain of the diagnosis, the pathological specimens should be reviewed by a specialist histopathologist. The distinction in a neck node between a poorly differentiated carcinoma and a high grade lymphoma is essential since the management of each tumour is different. Unless emergency treatment is required (e.g. for stridor from thyroid cancer), a firm pathological diagnosis should be made before starting treatment.

CHOICE OF RADICAL OR PALLIATIVE TREATMENT

When the relevant investigations on these lines have been completed, consideration has to be given as to whether treatment is to be radical or palliative.

The choice between radical and palliative treatment may be straightforward or difficult. A fit young woman with a stage II carcinoma of the cervix should be treated by radical radiotherapy with curative intent. An elderly but otherwise fit patient with localised bone pain from metastatic cancer should be offered a short course or single fraction of palliative radiotherapy. However, often the general condition of the patient is too poor, even if the disease is localised, to sustain the stress of anticancer treatment. Where the decision is borderline, reassessment after correction of anaemia and electrolyte and fluid imbalance is often helpful before a final decision is taken.

The following factors relating to the tumour, the patient and available resources can influence the decision. The importance of each factor will vary from patient to patient.

1. The tumour
   a. Site
   b. Size
   c. Spread (locoregional/metastatic spread)
   d. Operability
   e. Radiosensitivity/chemosensitivity
   f. Histology (including differentiation)
   g. Clearance of surgical resection margins.
2. The patient
   a. Age and general condition (physical and mental)
   b. Morbidity and mortality
   c. Function and cosmesis
   d Reliability of follow-up after treatment
   e. Preference of patient.
3. Resources: technical expertise, experience and equipment.

1. Features of the tumour

Site. Some tumours are unsuited for primary radiotherapy because of (a) the poor tolerance of the tissues to radical radiation doses, e.g. the skin over the shin, or (b) the proximity of dose limiting structures (e.g. the spinal cord in head and neck cancer). Other tumours (e.g. nasopharangeal carcinoma) are unsuitable for surgery because their deep position and proximity to critical structures would require hazardous and mutilating surgery.

Size. In general the larger the tumour, the lower is its radiocurability. This is related to the size of the clonogenic tumour cell population and the increased proportion of radioresistant hypoxic cells. For example, the local control rate of virtually all squamous cancers of the head and neck declines with increasing tumour bulk.

Spread. The pattern of spread of tumour will strongly influence the choice of treatment and will vary with site and histology. Early tumours confined to the primary site, with or without regional nodes, may be suitable for radical surgery or radiotherapy. This applies, for example, to early squamous cell carcinomas of the floor of the mouth. However carcinomas of the oral cavity which have invaded the mandible are unlikely to be controlled by radical radiotherapy. Radical surgery with reconstruction of the mandible gives a better prospect of cure. Similarly locoregional spread of Hodgkin's disease to the cervical, axillary and mediastinal nodes can be encompassed by wide field 'mantle' irradiation (p. 446). Chemotherapy also has a role in treating a limited number of chemosensitive tumours with locoregional spread (e.g. pelvic and para-aortic nodes in testicular teratoma).

For metastatic disease, local treatments (with the

exception of, for example, the surgical removal of isolated lung metastases in osteosarcoma) are generally inappropriate. For chemosensitive tumours systemic cytotoxic or hormonal chemotherapy is the main form of treatment. Radical radiotherapy does have a role in the lymphomas in treating residual locoregional disease following clearance of bulky local and metastatic disease by chemotherapy. Palliative radiotherapy may be necessary to relieve local symptoms of metastases (e.g. in bone).

Operability. This depends on two factors.

Fitness for surgery. Patients with a variety of general medical illnesses (e.g. chronic obstructive airways disease or ischaemic heart disease) affecting cardiorespiratory function may represent an unacceptable risk for general anaesthesia. This may, for example, exclude from curative surgery some patients with localised lung cancer. Similarly some patients with endometrial cancer may be too obese for hysterectomy.

Complete removal of the tumour. For radical surgery to be successful the surgeon must be able to remove all the macroscopic disease with a margin of normal tissue. Residual disease at the resection margins is likely to give rise to local recurrence. Early carcinomas of the breast are operable, whereas a more locally advanced breast tumour invading the chest wall is inoperable.

Fixity to adjacent structures usually contraindicates radical surgery. This applies, for example, to neck nodes in squamous cancer of the head and neck (p. 320) and to cervical cancer extending to the pelvic side wall.

In the brain, complete tumour removal of high grade gliomas is impractical because of widespread microscopic dissemination well beyond the macroscopic tumour margins and the need to avoid damage to surrounding normal brain.

Radiosensitivity/chemosensitivity. The sensitivity of tumours to radiotherapy and chemotherapy varies widely (Tables 17.4 and 17.5). Cure may be anticipated in a high proportion of cases of Hodgkin's disease which is highly sensitive to both chemotherapy and radiotherapy. In contrast melanoma is relatively resistant to both chemotherapy and radiotherapy, and even palliation is difficult to achieve.

Histology. The degree of differentiation is relevant to management. In general, undifferentiated (anaplastic) tumours are liable to behave more aggressively than well-differentiated tumours. For example, a well-differentiated carcinoma of the thyroid may be curable

Table 17.4   Radiosensitivity of different tumours

Highly sensitive
Lymphoma
Seminoma
Myeloma
Ewing's sarcoma
Wilms' tumour

Moderately sensitive
Small cell lung cancer
Breast cancer
Basal cell carcinoma
Medulloblastoma
Teratoma
Ovarian cancer

Relatively resistant
Squamous cell carcinoma of lung
Hypernephroma
Rectal carcinoma
Bladder carcinoma
Soft tissue sarcoma
Cervical cancer

Highly resistant
Melanoma
Osteosarcoma
Pancreatic carcinoma

(Reproduced with permission from Souhami R L & Moxham J 1990 Textbook of Medicine, Churchill Livingstone, Edinburgh.)

Table 17.5   Chemosensitivity of different tumours

Highly sensitive (which may be cured by chemotherapy)
Teratoma of testis
Hodgkin's disease
High grade non-Hodgkin lymphoma
Wilms' tumour
Embryonal rhabdomyosarcoma
Choriocarcinoma
Acute lymphoblastic leukaemia in children
Ewing's sarcoma

Moderately sensitive (in which chemotherapy may sometimes contribute to cure and often palliates)
Small cell carcinoma of lung
Breast carcinoma
Low grade non-Hodgkin lymphoma
Acute myeloid leukaemia
Ovarian cancer
Myeloma

Relatively insensitive (in which chemotherapy may sometimes produce palliation)
Gastric carcinoma
Bladder carcinoma
Squamous carcinoma of head and neck
Soft tissue sarcoma
Cervical carcinoma

Resistant tumours
Melanoma
Squamous carcinoma of lung
Large bowel cancer

(Reproduced with permission from Souhami R L & Moxham J 1990 Textbook of Medicine, Churchill Livingstone, Edinburgh.)

by subtotal thyroidectomy and radioiodine, whereas anaplastic thyroid cancer is usually unresponsive to any form of local therapy and does not take up radioiodine.

Clearance of resection margins. Curative surgery aims to remove the tumour in its entirety with a margin of normal tissue. If the resection margins are clear of tumour further therapy is often not required. If there is gross or microscopic disease at the resection margins (e.g. an inadequately excised basal carcinoma of the skin) postoperative radiotherapy is needed to prevent recurrence. Sometimes the pathologist finds that the margin of normal tissue around the resected tumour is very slender, perhaps a few millimetres only. In this circumstance clearance of the tumour may be considered inadequate and postoperative radiotherapy advised or further resection carried out to clear the margins more definitively (e.g. following initial lumpectomy for early breast cancer).

2. The patient

Age and general condition. It is important to assess the patient's fitness for any major procedure, whether it be surgery, radiotherapy or chemotherapy.

Age. Tolerance to both radical radiotherapy and chemotherapy diminishes with age. For example, an elderly person over the age of 70 with inoperable oesophageal cancer may appear medically fit for radical radiotherapy. Such patients often tolerate treatment poorly. Radiotherapy may have to be suspended permanently or the total dose reduced, with consequent compromise of tumour control.

The anticipated rise in the population of elderly in the UK will make this difficult decision a more frequent one. Aggressive treatment of the elderly is likely to result in greater treatment related morbidity and mortality without increasing cure rates.

Coincident diseases. A similar argument applies to coincident diseases which compromise fitness to treat. For example a patient with chronic obstructive airways disease and severely impaired pulmonary function (forced expiratory volume in 1 second (FEV_1) of less than 1 litre) is likely to made more breathless by radical radiotherapy for a lung tumour. Impaired respiratory function may also contraindicate a pneumonectomy. Patients with arteriosclerosis are subject to poorer tissue perfusion. This compromises the ability of normal tissue to recover from radiation injury.

Performance status. An objective assessment of the performance status of the patient (Ch. 34) is a useful guide to fitness to treat. It has been shown, for example, in small cell lung cancer that performance status is a very important prognostic factor in the response to chemotherapy. Poor performance status at presentation tends to be associated with shorter life expectancy. Anaemia and dehydration often accompany malignant disease and impair performance status. They should be corrected before a decision on eligibility for radical treatment is taken, since the patient's general medical state may sometimes be improved sufficiently to undergo radical treatment.

Morbidity and mortality. Surgery may involve unacceptable risks of morbidity and mortality. Examples are:

— *Brainstem tumours*, where cranial nerve nuclei and sensory or motor tracts may be damaged, resulting in serious and permanent neurological deficit.
— *Oesophageal cancer*. Surgery of carcinomas of the middle third of the oesophagus carries an operative mortality as high as 30%.
— *Paediatric cancer*, where the role of radiotherapy has declined with the appreciation of its long-term adverse effects on growth and development. At many sites higher cure rates have been achieved with chemotherapy alone, with fewer long-term complications.
— *Cervical cancer*. In young women with cervical cancer Wertheim's hysterectomy (p. 404) should enable a functional vagina to be preserved. Radical pelvic irradiation, however, results in progressive narrowing of the vagina due to fibrosis, limiting sexual intercourse.

Function and cosmesis. Radical surgery, particularly in the head and neck region, can be mutilating, although advances in plastic reconstruction of tissue defects with skin flaps and bone grafts from other sites have improved cosmetic and functional results. Radical surgery of carcinoma of the maxillary antrum involves a maxillectomy. A facial prosthesis is required to fill the tissue defect. Radical radiotherapy of tumours at this site which have not extended into the pterygoid fossa are therefore often treated with radical radiotherapy (p. 330) to avoid facial disfigurement.

Before the advent of cytotoxic chemotherapy, amputation well above the site of the tumour was standard treatment for osteogenic sarcoma of a limb bone. Preoperative and postoperative adjuvant cytotoxic therapy has allowed limb-conserving surgery (Fig. 28.4) to be carried out, with much improved functional results.

In early breast cancer lumpectomy and postoperative radiotherapy can avoid mastectomy in most women with operable tumours 4 cm or less in size (p. 388).

For carcinomas of the lower rectum and anal margin

and canal, radical radiotherapy may allow the anal sphincter to be preserved and a colostomy avoided.

Reliability of follow-up. Some patients are less likely to attend follow-up appointments on a regular basis. This may be due to factors such as concurrent physical or mental illness, shift working, unstable home circumstances, lack of transport, distance from the clinic, fear of hospitals or lack of appreciation of the seriousness of their condition or the need for early detection of persistent or recurrent cancer. Early detection of recurrent disease suitable for salvage surgery may thus be compromised. For unreliable attenders, e.g. alcoholics with head and neck cancer, prophylactic neck irradiation carried out at the same time as treatment of a primary tumour may be preferable to treating the neck only when nodes become palpable. Similarly in early breast cancer a mastectomy, with or without postoperative radiotherapy may be preferable to lumpectomy and postoperative radiotherapy (breast conservation) where regular clinical and mammographic follow-up of the treated breast for local recurrence is impractical.

The preference of the patient. Some patients prefer surgery or radiotherapy for a variety of reasons. Older patients with operable breast cancer often prefer to have a mastectomy rather than a local excision and radiotherapy because they feel more confident that all the disease has been removed. Young women often prefer a conservation approach because it can preserve breast symmetry and a normal cleavage.

3. Resources

Staff and equipment. Sometimes specialised expertise and treatment may not be available in a patient's district general hospital (e.g. a gynaecologist experienced in carrying out Wertheim's hysterectomy for stage I carcinoma of the cervix in young women). In these circumstances radical radiotherapy by intracavitary, with or without external beam, treatment is preferable. In most cases patients can be referred to hospitals which can provide the necessary technical expertise. In the UK the practice of referring patients with very rare curable tumours, e.g. for retinoblastoma (p. 497) and choriocarcinoma (p. 421), to national treatment facilities is well established. However in parts of the world where cancer services have a lower health priority, availability of resources may have a greater impact on the choice of anticancer treatment.

Clinical experience. This is one of the most important criteria in choosing treatment. Long personal experience of assessing and treating patients for tumours of different sites and stages is one of the best guides to the probability of cure or effective palliation.

Deciding not to offer anticancer treatment

Occasionally, an oncologist may decide not to recommend anticancer treatment but supportive care only. It is even more difficult to persuade the patient and family that this is the right decision if they anticipate that anticancer treatment will be offered. Some patients have such advanced disease and their general medical condition is so poor that they are unfit for any form of anticancer therapy. Much pressure may be put on the oncologist by the patient, the family or the referring physician or surgeon to offer some form of active anticancer therapy. This must be resisted if the oncologist believes that little benefit will accrue. An open discussion with the patient, the family and referring doctor, emphasising the upset that anticancer therapy would cause, for little benefit, and the positive aspects of symptom control by other means, may persuade all concerned to accept the oncologist's advice.

Clinical assessment in radiotherapy

The radiotherapist and oncologist is both a physician and a technical specialist. Decisions on the management of individual patients depend on balancing clinical and technical factors. If the tumour is a small basal cell carcinoma on the cheek, radiotherapy is a comparatively simple matter. A few brief outpatient attendances suffice. The treatment reaction is predictable and the probability of cure very high. More complex is the choice of target volume, beam directed technique, dose, fractionation and respect for the tolerance of normal tissue and critical organs in the treatment of head and neck cancer.

Inpatient or outpatient treatment?

The majority of patients undergoing radiotherapy can manage to attend as outpatients if they are well enough or within reasonable daily travelling distance of the cancer centre. Relatives may be able to transport them. Failing this, an ambulance can be arranged. Elderly patients often tolerate long journeys poorly and are best admitted. The same applies to patients who are very anxious about their treatment. Hospital admission gives greater opportunity for nursing and medical staff to offer explanation and reassurance about treatment. Many cancer centres have a hostel for patients who are admitted for geographical reasons and who have minimal nursing requirements. Other patients with heavier nursing requirements (e.g. malignant spinal cord compression), undergoing more intensive therapy (e.g. complex chemotherapy regimes) or interstitial or intracavitary therapy (for purposes of radiation protection) will need to be admitted to the main wards.

General medical care

Good medical condition is important in achieving cure, whatever the modality of treatment. Dehydration and poor nutrition are common in advanced malignant disease. Intravenous fluids to correct fluid and electrolyte balance, blood transfusion for anaemia, antibiotics for infection, and calorie and vitamin supplements for malnutrition are often needed.

Review during treatment

A course of radiotherapy, especially to a radical dose, is usually a strenuous undertaking for many patients. One or more of the radiation effects described in Chapter 16 are likely to cause some discomfort and may last for several weeks before healing. Regular weekly review of treatment is necessary to monitor the patient's clinical state and response to treatment. Sometimes the severity of the treatment reaction will require treatment to be suspended, and occasionally stopped definitively. Frequent explanation and reassurance is needed since anxiety often hinders patients' recall of what they have been told initially about diagnosis and treatment.

Palliative radiotherapy

Palliative radiotherapy is aimed at relieving local symptoms of advanced disease. The following criteria should be applied to achieve good palliation:

1. Prompt relief of symptoms
2. Minimal upset from treatment
3. Simple treatment technique
4. Limited number of fractions.

Assessment

Patients with advanced disease may have a life expectancy ranging from a few days to many months. A judgement has to be made as to whether the patient is likely to benefit within his or her expected life span. In most cases benefit from palliative radiotherapy is seen during or within a few days of treatment. Where life expectancy is only a few days, every effort should be made to control the patient's symptoms at home by medical means without recourse to radiotherapy.

Palliative radiotherapy should relieve symptoms with minimal side-effects. The amount of upset varies with site, dose and fractionation.

Site. Sites which tolerate palliative radiotherapy poorly are the upper abdomen (sensitivity of the stomach and duodenum), oral cavity (soreness and dysphagia) and perineum (painful skin and vaginal reaction).

Single fractions of 8 Gy to the lower thoracic and upper lumbar spine are likely to cause vomiting since some of the duodenum will be incorporated in the field. Fractionated treatment is better tolerated.

Palliative radiotherapy is of value at a wide range of tumour sites. Here are a few examples.

— Relief of haemoptysis, cough, dyspnoea and mediastinal obstruction in lung cancer.
— Control of bleeding in advanced bladder, rectal and cervical cancer.
— Relief of pain from bone metastases.
— Relief of symptoms of raised intracranial pressure due to brain metastases.
— Healing of ulcerating breast tumours.

Dose and fractionation

Relative low doses are adequate to relieve most symptoms. Single fractions of 8 Gy using orthovoltage, cobalt-60 or megavoltage are suitable for ribs, upper thoracic spine, and long bones. Fractionated doses, e.g. 20 Gy in four daily fractions or 30 Gy in 10 fractions are suggested for bony metastases in the cervical, lower thoracic and upper lumbar spine and for malignant spinal cord compression.

Technique

The treatment set-up should be as simple as possible, with single or parallel opposed fields to limit the duration of each treatment.

Palliative surgery

This may be required for:

1. Obstruction, e.g. transurethral resection in prostate cancer, colostomy in bowel cancer, laser therapy of bronchial and oesophageal cancer.
2. Pain, e.g. pinning of a pathological fracture.
3. Paraplegia—laminectomy for relief of spinal cord compression.
4. Hydrocephalus—ventriculoperitoneal shunting for relief of obstruction of CSF pathways by tumour.
5. Fungation—toilet mastectomy for fungating breast cancer.

6. Ascites—insertion of a LeVeen shunt from the peritoneal cavity into the superior vena cava for recurrent ascites.

Palliative chemotherapy

Palliative cytotoxic chemotherapy is less widely used than radiotherapy because unpleasant side-effects are more common and difficult to justify according to the criteria for good palliation (see above). Palliative hormonal chemotherapy (Ch. 32) is more widely used because of limited toxicity. The use of palliative chemotherapy is considered by site in other chapters.

In general, palliative cytotoxic chemotherapy is best avoided in frail and elderly patients, who are more prone to toxicity. Similarly, poor performance status is associated with poor outcome of treatment. However poor performance status may be related to the effects of the tumour (e.g. the patient bed-bound due to severe dyspnoea from lung metastases). If symptoms are potentially reversible by chemotherapy, poor performance status is not per se a contraindication to treatment.

1. Hormonal therapy
   a. Antioestrogens, progestogens, steroid inhibitors, androgens in advanced breast cancer
   b. Progestogens in advanced and metastatic endometrial cancer.
2. Cytotoxic chemotherapy
   a. Advanced breast cancer
   b. Lung cancer (except possibly limited stage small cell lung cancer)
   c. Alimentary tract (including liver and pancreas)
   d. Cervix and ovarian cancer
   e. Bladder cancer
   d. Melanoma
   e. Soft tissue sarcomas
   f. Low grade non-Hodgkin lymphoma.

Technical factors in radiotherapy

In any radiation treatment the clinician has to define the following parameters:

1. Tumour volume
2. Target volume
3. Treatment volume
4. Radiation energy and quality
5. Number of fields
6. Arrangement of fields
7. Use of wedges, tissue compensators or bolus
8. Dose
9. Total number and frequency of fractions
10. Overall treatment time.

(1)–(7) have been covered in Chapter 6. Dose, fractionation and treatment time are considered here.

Dose, fractionation and overall treatment time

It is essential to specify dose, energy, number of fractions and overall treatment time together since each has an effect on the biological response. Stating a dose without specifying its energy, fractionation and overall treatment time is meaningless.

Dose in radical and palliative radiotherapy

Radical. In radical radiotherapy the choice of dose and fractionation regime will depend on the radiosensitivity of the tumour, the size of the treatment volume, the proximity of dose limiting critical structures and the quality of radiation used.

Relatively radiosensitive tumours such as testicular seminoma can be controlled by total doses of 30 Gy at megavoltage fractionated over 4 weeks. Higher doses of the order of 50–55 Gy are needed to control most squamous carcinomas of the head and neck.

The maximum tolerated dose of radical radiotherapy to different volumes of tissue varies in different parts of the body. For example field sizes in excess of 60 cm^2 for head and neck cancer rarely tolerate more than 50 Gy in 20 daily fractions over 4 weeks. Similarly, the tolerance of the small bowel limits the dose to the whole pelvis in cervical/endometrial cancer to 45 Gy fractionated over the same period.

The presence of critical structures such as the brainstem and spinal cord may limit the dose that can be delivered to tumours, for example of the head and neck, lung and oesophagus. This problem can be obviated in treating nodal areas overlying the cord in the head and neck by the use of electrons of limited penetration. The appropriate energy can be chosen to ensure that the cord is not overdosed (Figs 20.17 and 20.18).

The relative biological effectiveness (RBE) of the quality of irradiation chosen will influence the choice of dose. Fast neutrons have a higher RBE than photons. The RBE of neutrons varies in different tissues and increases as the dose per fraction falls (p. 258). The radical doses of neutrons equivalent to photons are therefore much lower.

Homogeneity of dose distribution across the target volume is important to achieve maximum tumour kill. Areas of underdosage may give rise to local recurrence and overdosage to morbidity. For this reason the variation in dose across the target volume should not vary by more than ±5% of the intended dose.

Palliative. Homogeneity of dose distribution is much

less important than in radical radiotherapy. Thus simple treatment techniques by single or parallel opposed fields will suffice for most purposes. Since dose homogeneity is not essential, computerised planning and the use of wedges to improve the dose distribution are not needed. Treatment volumes should be more generous than for radical radiotherapy since the doses delivered should be well below normal tissue tolerance.

Fractionation. Fractionation refers to the division of the total dose into a number of separate fractions, conventionally given on a daily basis, usually 5 days a week (Monday to Friday).

In assessing the value of any fractionation regime, whether for cure or palliation, the effects on both the tumour and the normal tissues have to be considered together (see Therapeutic ratio, p. 262). Normal tissue tolerance is dose limiting at many sites in radical radiotherapy (e.g. the spinal cord in head and neck irradiation). As shown in Figure 15.9, at high dose a small increase in cure may be at the expense of substantially greater morbidity. Similarly, high dose per fraction is poorly tolerated with even palliative doses at sensitive sites, as discussed earlier in this chapter.

Hyperfractionation, multiple daily fractions. The terms *hyperfractionated* or *multiple daily fractions* refer to the delivery of more than one fraction per day. It is now appreciated that significant repopulation of some rapidly dividing tumours may occur over the weekend period when traditionally there has been a break in radiotherapy. Tumour repopulation reduces the chance of cure by radical radiotherapy. For this reason hyperfractionated radical radiotherapy schedules in which the patient is treated every day are under evaluation (continuous hyperfractionated accelerated radiotherapy (CHART)). Early experience suggests improved cure rates in non-small cell lung cancer and head and neck cancer (p. 566). The rationale for hyperfractionation is described later in this chapter.

Historical aspects of fractionation. The development of dose and fractionation in the early part of the 20th century was largely empirical. Initially most treatments were given as single large fractions for a wide variety of conditions, both benign and malignant. The energy of the early treatment machines was low and the measurement of their radiation output was clinical and crude (Ch. 5). Skin reactions were the most frequently used, the so-called *erythema dose*. Later, scientific (as opposed to clinical) methods were introduced to gain a deeper insight into the mode of action of radiation and to find a rational basis for dose, fractionation and overall treatment time, i.e. what factors gave the best probability of tumour cure with acceptable normal tissue morbidity. This is the modern science of *radio-*

biology. In Vienna in 1914 a radiologist named Schwarz noted that a mediastinal tumour which had failed to respond to a single large fraction of radiation had regressed several months later when exposed to small fractionated doses. There was still no consensus on the merits of fractionated radiotherapy until, in 1919, Coutard achieved the first cures of tumours of the larynx and tonsil giving one or two small fractions daily over a period of weeks. Coutard's dosage and fractionation were designed to achieve a severe but recoverable acute mucosal reaction. He assumed that the population of cancer cells had the same sensitivity as the normal regenerating epithelial cells. Further confirmation of the therapeutic gain of fractionation was derived from fractionation experiments on the rabbit testis. It was shown that fractionating the same total dose in four fractions caused more damage to the seminiferous epithelium of the testis and less skin reaction than did a single fraction.

In the early 1930s Coutard observed that the acute tolerance of normal tissues treated at high dose per fraction deteriorated with increasing field size. He therefore treated larger volumes with lower daily doses over longer overall times.

In the 1930s Paterson at the Christie Hospital in Manchester combined the low dose rate Paris system of intracavitary radium therapy with the extended treatment times of the Stockholm technique to treat cancer of the cervix. Initially each 48 hour radium insertion was repeated four times over a 4 week period. Subsequently the overall treatment time for intracavitary radium alone was shortened to 2–3 weeks.

In 1935 radical external beam irradiation to small volumes for tumours in the head and neck was initiated in Manchester. Practice at the Christie Hospital was widely adopted in the UK. Daily fractions were given from Monday to Friday over 5–6 weeks to total doses of 5500–6000 R. Reduction in overall treatment time at the Christie Hospital, e.g. 52.5–55 Gy in 15–16 fractions, was brought about because of the pressure on treatment facilities and beds of large numbers of patients. Radical treatments over 3 weeks result in 'hotter' acute reactions. Longer overall treatment times (e.g. 6 weeks) with milder acute reactions have been adopted, particularly in the south of England. Many centres have adopted a middle way (i.e. treating radically over 4 weeks). The cure rates achieved by radical treatments over 3–6 weeks are very similar.

Radiosensitivity. There is a wide spectrum of radiosensitivity among tumours, as illustrated in Table 17.4. Some comment has already been made on radiosensitivity (p. 255).

We know that the sensitivity of a cell, normal or

malignant, depends in part on its position in the cell cycle. Those cells in mitosis (M phase) or between G_1 and S are more sensitive to killing by radiation than those in S phase. This variation in radiosensitivity during different phases of the cell cycle is less marked with neutrons than with photons and with low dose rate brachytherapy (p. 305).

According to the Law of Bergonié and Tribondeau (1904), radiosensitivity increases with the amount of proliferative activity within tissues at the time of radiation. This is now thought not to be the case. The proliferative state of cells at the time of radiation exposure is not critical. However for radiation to have an acute effect, cells need to be in a proliferative state at or within a short time of exposure. Anaplastic (or poorly differentiated) tumours have a higher proportion of their cell population in mitosis at any given time than do well-differentiated tumours. It follows that anaplastic growths are more likely to be more radiosensitive. This is borne out in clinical practice.

A single dose of 20 Gy may suffice to cure a small basal cell carcinoma of the skin, but if given in five daily fractions (5 × 4 Gy) it would be insufficient. To achieve a comparable result would require 5 × 6 Gy (30 Gy). If we took 2 weeks (10 treatment sessions), the dose would be 10 × 4.5 Gy (45 Gy). As a general rule, the longer the overall treatment time, the higher the total dose required.

Protracted fractionation takes advantage of the better tolerance of the normal tissues and the difference in recuperative ability (see below) between normal and malignant cells. The sequence of events is illustrated in Figure 17.1. Tumour cells suffer progressive damage

as the course proceeds and the gap between them and normal cells widens. Eventually, if cure is obtained, all the tumour cells are irreversibly damaged, while normal cells can still recover. If the overall treatment time is too long (Fig. 17.2A), cure may not be obtained because tumour repopulation occurs. If the regime is too short (Fig. 17.2B), the tumour population may remain at a level capable of giving rise to local recurrrence.

Fractionation is clearly of great importance in any scheme of therapy, whether radical or palliative. Many patterns of fractionation have been tried, often empirically and without appropriate scientific evaluation of randomised trials.

Influence of time and dose. Both experimental evidence and clinical experience show that variation in the parameters of fractionation influences acute and late normal tissue reactions. The tolerance of normal tissue is affected by the total dose, the dose per fraction, the separation between fractions and the overall duration of treatment.

The severity of the *acute reaction* will depend on the rate of accumulation of dose and the balance between cell killing and regeneration within the irradiated tisssues. With shorter overall treatment time (e.g. 3 weeks) acute reactions will be more severe than those given over 6–8 weeks. Healing of the acute reaction requires a minimum number of normal stem cells to survive to allow repopulation of the damaged area. If the rate of accumulation of dose or the total dose is too high, the stem cell population will be eradicated and radionecrosis will occur.

Late reactions typically occur in tissues with a

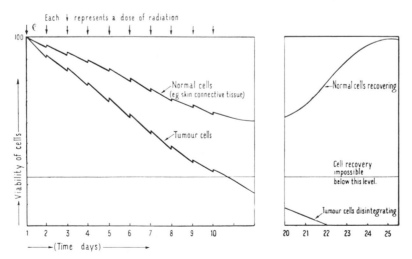

Fig. 17.1 Diagrammatic representation of a successful course of radiation treatment. For explanation see text.

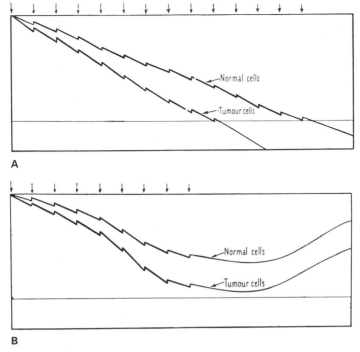

Fig. 17.2 Diagrammatic representation of unsuccessful courses of radiation treatment. **A** Course too long, resultant permanent injury to normal tissues and inability to heal. **B** Course too short, some tumour cells remain active to seed later recurrence.

slower cell turnover (e.g. connective tissue). They do not manifest the effects of cell death until after a course of radical radiotherapy has been completed. For this reason the overall treatment time and the rate of accumulation of dose have little influence on late reactions. However the total dose, size of dose per fraction and the interval between fractions do have a major effect on the severity of late reactions. The rate at which cellular damage is repaired is slower in slow reacting tissues. For this reason short intervals between fractions may allow inadequate time for repair and result in more severe late reactions. An interval of at least 6 hours is required between fractions for adequate repair in man.

Number of fractions per day

1. *Conventional fractionation.* Daily treatments from Monday to Friday with a gap at weekends remain standard for most radical treatments. However there is wide variation in the overall treatment time. This varies from 15–16 fractions in 3 weeks in Manchester, with a fraction size of 3.3–3.6 Gy, to 35–40 fractions over 7–8 weeks in the USA, with fraction sizes of 1.8–2.0 Gy.

2. *Hyperfractionation (accelerated fractionation).* Instead of treating once a day, the number of daily fractions

can be increased, in practice rarely to more than three. This approach has been explored in tumours where conventionally fractionated radiotherapy has often failed to cure tumours (e.g. cerebral gliomas and advanced lung and head and neck cancer). The rationale for giving more than one fraction per day is based on the four Rs of Radiobiology (p. 256).

a. Dose per fraction. There is experimental evidence that as the dose per fraction decreases, so too does the oxygen enhancement ratio (p. 260). Theoretically, with multiple small daily fractions the importance of hypoxia as a cause of radioresistance in tumours should be less marked compared with normal tissues.

b. Morbidity. In general, accelerated or hyperfractionated treatments are associated with more severe acute reactions. As stated above, acute reactions are determined by the rate of accumulation of dose. Unless small field sizes are used, the mucous membranes of the head and neck will not tolerate fraction sizes of 2 Gy or more given three times a day or more than 55 Gy in 2 weeks.

Late reactions are influenced by fraction size and the interval between fractions. Late reactions are generally worse when the interval between fractions is less than 4.5 hours.

3. *Hypofractionation.* Hypofractionation refers to the practice of giving less than the conventional five daily fractions per week. This approach is illogical for treating most tumour sites since long gaps between fractions may allow tumour repopulation. In a trial comparing three fractions (hypofractionated) versus five fractions (conventional fractionation) per week in laryngeal cancer, there was a tendency for a higher local recurrence rate in the patients treated with three fractions a week.

Hypofractionation is more logical in treating tumours with a higher capacity for repair, e.g. melanomas and soft tissue sarcomas, and in palliative radiotherapy. A limited number of large fractions may take advantage of the higher fractionation sensitivity of such tumours compared with normal tissues.

In palliative radiotherapy single fractions of 4–15 Gy for bone metastases are in general as effective as multiple fractions to total doses of 20–40 Gy. As good and prompt pain relief can be achieved by a single fraction of 8 Gy as by 30 Gy in 10 daily fractions. Two fractions of 8.5 Gy given a week apart are as effective in relieving the symptoms of non-small cell lung cancer as 30 Gy in 10 daily fractions.

Split course therapy. In split course treatments, a gap is planned between the first and second halves of the treatment. The duration of the gap may typically be up to a month. The purpose of the gap may be to allow patients, especially the elderly, to recover from the acute reaction of their treatment and to exclude from further morbidity those who have tolerated the first half poorly or whose disease has progressed despite treatment. Split course therapy is sometimes applied to elderly patients undergoing radical radiotherapy for bladder or prostate cancer. It is commonly used in the radical treatment of lung cancer, since the development of clinically overt metastatic disease during continuous radical radiotherapy over 4–6 weeks is not uncommon. Patients who develop metastases during the month's gap can be spared further toxicity.

Split course therapy has the disadvantages of the possibility of tumour repopulation during the rest period in rapidly growing tumours and the difficulty of designing split course regimes biologically equivalent to conventionally fractionated treatments. Furthermore, if both parts of the split course are given, there is no reduction in late morbidity.

Isoeffect formulae. Mathematical formulae (e.g. nominal standard dose (p. 287) and cumulative radiation effect (p. 287), have been developed to predict the different dose and fractionation regimes which will achieve the same effect on the tumour (isoeffect). Though helpful, the limitations of these formulae should be appreciated. Observations of the effects of different fractionation regimes in experimental animals, both on tumour cure and morbidity, cannot necessarily be extrapolated to man.

1. Strandquist isoeffect curves. One of the earliest and most influential pieces of work was that of Strandquist. He constructed a series of isoeffect curves to relate total dose to overall treatment time. These included curves for skin necrosis, the cure of squamous skin carcinoma and skin erythema (Fig. 17.3). Each line represents the total dose required to achieve these end-points over a given treatment time. Doses above the middle line resulted in late radiation damage and below the line in tumour persistence or recurrence. In the absence of previous guidelines, Strandquist's isoeffect curves were enthusiastically adopted. However it was subsequently appreciated that his observations were not applicable to normal clinical practice. It is now accepted that differences in the sensitivity of the skin and squamous skin carcinoma cannot be determined by this method for a variety of reasons. First, the time scale of a third of a day for a single fraction is out of step with normal clinical practice. Secondly, most of his patients had basal and not squamous

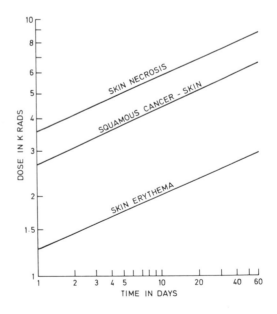

Fig. 17.3 Isoeffect curves relating total dose and overall treatment to skin necrosis, cure of squamous cell carcinoma and erythema. (After Strandquist, 1944. Courtesy of Duncan and Nias, Clinical Radiobiology, Churchill Livingstone, 1977.)

carcinomas and, thirdly, the number of patients on which his curves were based was small.

2. More recent isoeffect formulae. These include nominal standard dose (NSD), cumulative radiation effect (CRE), time, dose and fractionation (TDF) and, most recently the α/β ratio. The α/β ratio is discussed on page 259.

It should be emphasised that none of these formulae should be relied upon clinically to predict the effects of different fractionation regimes. All of the predictive formulae have limitations in their applicability to a greater or lesser degree.

Ellis introduced in 1967 an isoeffect formula, the *nominal standard dose.* This proposed that the tolerance of normal tissues (*D*) could be related to the overall treatment time (*T*), and the number of fractions (*N*) by the following formula:

$$D_N = (NSD) \, T^{0.11} . N^{0.24}$$

The formula was widely adopted, particularly since it enabled less than five fractions a week to be given. This was attractive to centres treating larger numbers of patients. Radical treatments were sometimes reduced to two fractions a week.

Other formulae such as CRE and TDF were derivatives of the Ellis NSD concept.

Cumulative radiation effect (*R*) was developed to predict the effects of doses below tolerance on normal tissues.

$$R = D_N \cdot T^{-0.11} . N^{-0.24}$$

The concept of NSD is only applicable to full normal tissue tolerance doses. It cannot be calculated for two parts of a fractionated course of treatment. The concept of *partial tolerance* is useful for the calculation of the modified treatment regime which has to be given if a continuous course of fractionated radiotherapy is interrupted unintentionally (e.g. by illness or machine breakdown) or intentionally in split course therapy. The sum of the partial tolerances of the two halves of treatment can be added. Thus if *N* fractions are needed for a full NSD value of *Y* rets, then the partial tolerance (PT) from fewer fractions, *n*, is as follows:

$$PT = (n/N) \times Y$$

Tables of TDF factors equivalent to the partial tolerance doses have been constructed for fractionation regimes of one, two, three, four or five fractions a week.

Complexity of factors determining biological effects of fractionation. In any fractionated course of radiotherapy, there is a wide range of interacting physical and biological variables operating which determine the biological effect. In addition to the four Rs, treatment energy, dose rate, distribution of cells in different phases of the cell cycle, rate of cell loss and of 'scavenging' of dead cells by phagocytosis all play a part. In so complex a situation it is difficult to assess the contribution of any one factor. In the laboratory, where spontaneously occurring animal tumours or human tumours transplanted into animals can be irradiated, the effects of different treatment parameters can be studied. For example the effect can be observed on normal tissue and tumour of different numbers of fractions of the same total dose while keeping the energy, tissue, field size, dose rate and overall treatment time constant. None the less, great caution should be taken in extrapolating from radiobiological laboratory experiments on animals to man.

Normal tissue tolerance. The tolerance of normal tissue is of great practical importance to the radiotherapist. Exceeding it may result in major morbidity and, sometimes, mortality. Since radical doses often need to be at or close to normal tissue tolerance to achieve cure, some degree of morbidity almost always has to be accepted. For example, a major morbidity rate of up to 5%, mainly due to bowel and bladder damage, has generally to be accepted in treating cervical cancer by radical radiotherapy. The degree of risk accepted will depend on the seriousness of the morbidity. The more serious the complication, the lower the probability of its occurrence is the clinician likely to accept. For example less than a 1% risk of spinal cord damage would be accepted for 'mantle' radiotherapy (p. 449) for Hodgkin's disease.

Probability of complications. Tolerance doses of ionising radiation are commonly expressed in terms of the doses which give a certain probability of a particular complication. Typically the probabilities cited are 5% ($TD_{5/5}$) and 50% ($TD_{50/5}$). Examples of $TD_{5/5}$ and $TD_{50/5}$ for different tissues are shown in Table 17.6.

There is wide variation (up to 20-fold) in the sensitivity of normal tissues from the most radiosensitive to the most radioresistant. The sensitivity of tumours derived from normal tissues tends to be similar. The testes, ovaries, lymphoid tissue and bone marrow are among the most radiosensitive, as are seminomas of the testis, dysgerminomas of the ovary and lymphomas. Bone, cartilage, nervous tissue and kidney, and correspondingly the tumours derived from them (gliomas, osteosarcomas and renal cancers), are relatively radioresistant.

It is now clear that normal tissue and organ tolerance is relative rather than absolute and can be altered by a variety of factors. These include treatment factors (e.g. dose, volume, fractionation, chemotherapy, radiosensitisers, radioprotectors, biological response modifiers) and patient factors (age, concurrent disease,

Table 17.6 Tolerance doses of normal tissues to conventionally fractionated irradiation

Tissue/organ	$TD_{5/5}-TD_{50/5}$ (Gy)
Testes	1–2
Ovary	6–10
Eye (lens)	6–12
Lung	20–30
Kidney	20–30
Liver	35–40
Skin	30–40
Thyroid	30–40
Heart	40–50
Lymphoid tissue	40–50
Bone marrow	40–50
Gastrointestinal	40–50
Vasculoconnective tissue	50–60
Peripheral nerve	65–77
Mucosa	65–77
Brain	60–70
Bone and cartilage	>70
Muscle	>70

(Courtesy of Vaeth & Meyer 1989.)

trauma, direct and indirect effects of tumours). The injury inflicted on normal tissue depends upon the capacity of the stem cell population to supply new cells and the timing of its expression on the cell cycle time for renewal.

Between 20 and 50 different cell types are represented in normal tissue, although the number of different stem cells is more restricted. This cellular heterogeneity is similar to that observed in tumours. It is therefore hardly surprising that since a fixed dose does not kill all tumour cells, the effect on normal tissues is non-uniform. It also explains why isoeffect formulae (see above) oversimplify normal tissue tolerance and do not reliably predict tolerance in vivo. Each subpopulation of normal cells may vary in its response to different doses, fraction sizes and timing of exposure. The overall response of a given tissue to different dose and fractionation regimes is extremely complex.

Factors influencing radiosensitivity of normal tissues

1. Treatment factors

a. Quality of radiation and RBE. The quality of radiation and its RBE strongly influence normal tissue tolerance. Megavoltage irradiation with its skin sparing effects and reduced absorption in bone causes much less skin reaction and risk of bony injury than orthovoltage irradiation. High LET irradiation, such as fast neutrons, with its high absorption in fat can cause substantial damage to tissue with a high fat content (e.g. the bowel). Fast neutrons have a higher RBE (approximately 5.2) for the central nervous system compared with photons, with increased risk of inducing radionecrosis.

b. Dose. The dose that irrevocably damages normal tissue is not absolute but depends on fractionation.

c. Fractionation. The fraction size and the interval between fractions largely influence the severity of acute and late effects. Hyperfractionation and hypofractionation will modify normal tissue tolerance.

d. Volume. Normal tissue tolerance is influenced by the volume of the organ that is irradiated. The tolerance of the whole lung to conventionally fractionated photon irradiation is 20 Gy in 20 daily fractions over 4 weeks. However, limited volumes of lung (e.g. $8 \times 8 \times 8$ cm) will normally tolerate 50 Gy similarly fractionated. The same principle applies to the kidney. If no more than a third of the kidney is treated on each side during prophylactic abdominal node irradiation for seminoma, 30 Gy in 20 daily fractions over 4 weeks are tolerated without serious renal damage. This is because there is adequate functional unirradiated kidney tissue to compensate. The tolerance dose for conventionally fractionated irradiation of the whole kidney irradiation is lower (20 Gy).

e. Time. The time interval between exposure of normal tissue to irradiation and the expression of damage is determined by the kinetics of different cell subpopulations.

f. Chemotherapy. Chemotherapy can influence the tolerance of normal tissue. An example is the reduced lung tolerance to radiation following treatment with bleomycin.

g. Other agents. Radiosensitisers such as the hypoxic cell sensitisers (e.g. misonidazole, p. 261) can increase the radiation reaction in some normal tissues (e.g. the skin) and possibly in the CNS, liver and other organs. This may be due to the presence of small numbers of hypoxic cells within normal tissues.

2. Patient factors

a. Age. In utero, in infancy and at puberty, when growth is rapid, normal tissues are particularly sensitive to radiation damage. For example extended field irradiation before the age of 13 of mediastinal or para-aortic nodes overlying the spine in Hodgkin's disease may impair sitting and standing height by about 5%. Over the age of 13, there is little effect on growth even if it has not been completed.

b. Concurrent disease. A variety of conditions such as anaemia, diabetes mellitus and arteriosclerosis can reduce the supply of oxygen to tissues. This in turn may impair the cellular repair of normal tissue injury and increase both acute and late reactions.

c. Trauma. Irradiated tissue is particularly vulnerable to traumatic damage. For example if the skin of the nose is irradiated for a basal cell carcinoma, subsequent exposure to very cold temperatures may precipitate skin necrosis (p. 295). Similarly, radionecrosis of the mandible following radical irradiation for cancer of the floor of the mouth may be precipitated by minor accidental trauma or tooth extraction (p. 321).

3. Tumour factors

a. Local invasion. The presence of tumour may directly or indirectly affect normal tissue tolerance. Direct invasion of normal structures, e.g. the bowel in extranodal non-Hodgkin lymphoma, may result in perforation of the bowel after abdominal irradiation or chemotherapy. Indirect damage may be caused by mechanical effects, such as ureteric obstruction resulting in hydronephrosis and renal failure.

b. Radiosensitivity. This is another factor of obvious fundamental importance. Tumours, like normal tissues, vary in their vulnerability to radiation and this depends chiefly on their rate of growth.

Table 17.4 lists some of the most important tumours in order of their relative radiosensitivity. It is a useful approximation. There are exceptions: some lymphomas may prove radioresistant, even at high dosage.

The highest proportion of successes is achieved in the epithelial cancers (especially squamous) of moderate sensitivity, such as the skin, mouth and cervix.

The most important factor is the biological nature and behaviour of the particular cell type of an individual tumour. At present there is no reliable method of predicting in advance the responsiveness of an individual patient's tumour to radiation.

FOLLOW-UP

Once patients have completed anticancer treatment, it is customary to assess them on a regular basis as outpatients. In general the longer patients remain well, the less frequently they need to be seen.

Aims

The reasons for following up patients are:

— Confirmation of response to treatment and of resolution of its side-effects
— Detection of persistent or recurrent disease at a stage when curative 'salvage' treatment is possible
— Detection of late complications of treatment
— Reassuring the patient that he or she is free of tumour

— Management of patients with persistent or progressive disease or complications of treatment
— Evaluation of new and existing treatments.

Frequency

The frequency of hospital follow-up will depend on a number of factors. These include:

— The period during which the risk of recurrence is highest
— The development of complications of treatment
— Persistent or progressive disease
— Age and performance status
— Geographical, e.g. distance from the patient's home to the outpatient clinic
— Availability of transport to and from the clinic.

Practice varies widely. For an activity that occupies so large a part of an oncologist's professional time, there is a surprising lack of information on the optimal frequency of follow-up of patients with tumours of different stage and site.

Risk of recurrence

Head and neck cancer. In most cases of head and neck cancer treated with curative intent, recurrence, if it occurs, is most likely to do so within the first 2 years. Thus monthly appointments in the first year after treatment, 2-monthly appointments in the second year and less frequently in subsequent years are generally sufficiently frequent to detect most relapses at a stage when curative salvage treatment can be attempted. A similar intensity of follow-up is applicable to cervical cancer, which has a similar time-scale of relapse.

In general, local relapses after 5 years are uncommon in squamous carcinomas. If they do occur they are often due to new primary tumours close to the original site.

Often the distinction between a new primary and relapse of the original tumour is impossible to make. For these reasons such patients probably need at least 10 years of follow-up.

Lymphomas. Relapse more than 5 years after treatment is not uncommon in the non-Hodgkin lymphomas. It is less common in Hodgkin's disease. Lifelong follow-up is recommended.

Breast cancer. The follow-up of patients with breast cancer illustrates a number of principles applicable to other tumours.

Most local relapses tend to occur within 5 years of mastectomy. Surveillance for at least 5 years is therefore desirable.

Although metastatic relapse may occur at any time

after treatment, there is no evidence that detection at scheduled as opposed to 'interval' appointments (i.e. arranged between routine appointments) improves survival. Most metastatic relapses are symptomatic. Patients usually present to their general practitioner with symptoms, for example, of dyspnoea from lung metastases or pleural effusion or with pain from bony metastases. The offer of an appointment at the next oncology clinic can avoid unnecessary appointments when the patient is symptom free.

Many clinicians still undertake lifelong follow-up of patients with breast cancer in view of the risk of death persisting for at least 30 years (Fig. 23.13). However, since the tumour is very common, such a policy, particularly in oncology centres serving large populations, can result in very large numbers of women attending the oncology clinic. This pressure can be reduced by surgeon and oncologist seeing patients alternately at an agreed frequency.

SUPPORT SERVICES

Treatment includes not simply the delivery of specific therapy such as surgery or radiotherapy but physical, psychological and social support.

There is a wide range of support services available to meet these needs. Some are specific to patients with particular tumours (e.g. mastectomy or stoma care nurses). Others such as medical social workers have a wide role in assisting patients and their families with their social and financial concerns.

Mastectomy/breast care nurse

Experienced nurses provide counselling to patients who have undergone mastectomy. They are familiar with dealing with the psychological distress of a patient following mastectomy. They can also, in conjunction with the surgeon, offer advice on breast conserving surgery, the range of prostheses available to compensate for the loss of the breast and the surgical reconstructions of the breast that are possible.

Stoma care nurse

Stoma care nurses provide practical advice on the management of bowel (colostomy, ileostomy) and urinary (urostomy) stomas.

MacMillan nurses

MacMillan nurses are based both in hospitals and in the community. Their role is to provide, in conjunction with the patient's general practitioner, advice on symptom control at home and psychological support for both the patient and the family.

District nurse liaison

District nurses may have a specific responsibility for liaising between the hospital and the community in the care of patients with malignant disease. They may identify nursing needs at home and bring these to the attention of hospital staff. This assists the appropriate provision of support services when the patient is discharged home.

Prosthetic services

The prompt provision of prostheses (to replace, for example an eye, nose or breast) or wigs (following chemotherapy or cranial irradiation causing hair loss) can be extremely important in maintaining a patient's appearance and morale.

Department of Social Security (DSS) advisory service

Each patient has access to an advisory service within the DSS on sources of financial help. In some areas an adviser may visit a hospital on a regular basis. Financial assistance is of considerable practical importance to patients who are unable to work temporarily or permanently because of disability.

Day care unit

A day care unit can provide patients with support during the period of acute reaction after radiotherapy. The first unit for this purpose was established in Sheffield.

Dietician

Adequate nutrition is important in both radical and palliative therapy of malignant disease. Anorexia and weight loss commonly accompany malignancy and its treatment by chemotherapy and radiotherapy. Maintaining an adequate protein and calorie intake is vital to recovery from radical surgery, radiotherapy and chemotherapy. In incurable disease, dysphagia, vomiting, anorexia and constipation all influence dietary intake.

A hospital dietician should be available to advise inpatients and outpatients with dietary problems related to their malignancy or its treatment. Close liaison is necessary with the hospital catering department and pharmacy to provide for the special dietary needs of patients. This may include selection of foods that are appetising to the patient, oral food supplements (e.g. Complan or Build-up drinks) and nasogastric feeds. Patients being treated with curative intent may sometimes require intravenous feeding (total parenteral nutrition (TPN)). Many hospitals have a team of surgeons, specialist nurses and dieticians who provide such a service.

Medical social work department

Medical social workers are familiar with the social and financial problems faced by patients and their families. They can provide practical advice on grants available, such as mobility and attendance allowances and travel expenses. They liaise with medical and nursing staff and with social services in the community. They may apply on the patient's behalf and with medical support for financial assistance from charitable bodies.

Support and self-help groups

Newly diagnosed patients and their relatives may benefit from attending a support or self-help group. Awareness of how other patients have coped with the emotional and physical side-effects of treatment may enable a patient to cope better with cancer and its treatment.

Bereavement counselling

Some form of bereavement counselling service can help relatives come to terms with the loss of a member of the family.

Spiritual care

Spiritual support of the patient and family can be provided by the church and other religious organisations.

CONFIDENTIALITY

It is important to clarify with the patient, if well enough, what medical information he or she is willing to have disclosed, so that confidentiality is not breached. Often well-intentioned relatives ask to speak to the doctor without the knowledge of the patient. To do so without the patient's permission is a breach of confidentiality. Where the patient is too unwell to grant permission, immediate relatives or, in their absence, close friends may be informed.

18. Skin and lip

SKIN CANCER

Pathology

Epidemiology

Skin tumours are the commonest of all neoplasms in the UK, as in many other countries with a predominantly white population. Non-melanomatous skin cancer represents 10% of all cancers but only 0.3% of cancer deaths. They are rare in dark-skinned races. They are most common in the seventh and eighth decades of life. There is a male predominance (sex ratio 1.5:1). Secondary deposits also occur in the skin.

There are three main varieties: basal cell carcinoma, squamous cell carcinoma and melanoma. Non-melanomatous skin cancer is of considerable importance to the radiotherapist since it is the most accessible of cancers, tends to present early with localised disease and is eminently radiocurable.

Aetiology

1. Sunlight. Ultraviolet light is the most important aetiological factor for skin cancer. Basal and squamous carcinomas arise most frequently on exposed skin, though they can arise elsewhere. For melanoma it is thought that intense exposure to the sun is more important than the total life-time exposure.

2. Ionising radiation. Basal and squamous cell carcinomas may occur many years after exposure to therapeutic irradiation for benign conditions in childhood (e.g. for ringworm of the scalp—a practice long abandoned).

3. Chemical carcinogens. Prolonged exposure to many oil and tar products may cause squamous carcinomas. Arsenic salts, which used to be prescribed in low dosage for prolonged periods for a variety of common diseases, gave rise to keratoses, typically on the palms of the hands. Some of these underwent malignant change.

4. Chronic ulcers and granulomas. Occasionally a longstanding ulcer may develop carcinoma from its margin.

5. Scar tissue. Especially after wounds or burns soft tissue may rarely undergo malignant change.

6. Immunosuppression. Squamous cell carcinomas of the skin are commoner following drug-induced immunosuppression (e.g. with steroids) after kidney transplantation.

7. Genetic factors. (a) Basal cell naevus syndrome (Gorlin's syndrome) is an autosomal dominant disorder giving rise to multiple basal cell carcinomas developing from childhood onwards. (b) Xeroderma pigmentosum is a rare autosomal recessive disorder in which there is a defect in the capacity to repair DNA (p. 245). It predisposes to the development of squamous skin cancer after normal light exposure. This seems to illustrate the important normal function of DNA repair enzymes.

Premalignant conditions

There are a number of conditions to consider: some may undergo malignant change.

1. *Hyperkeratosis.* Small warty nodules, may be due to sunlight, actinic or solar keratosis, tar, or X-rays.
2. *Papilloma.* These are generally viral warts.
3. *Bowen's disease.* This is a form of carcinoma-in-situ, and may progress to invasive malignancy.

BASAL CELL CARCINOMA

Pathology and clinical features

This tumour accounts for 80% of skin tumours. It arises from the basal aspect of the epidermis and grows as nests of darkly staining cells, often palisaded peripherally. There are a number of clinical varieties.

1. Noduloulcerative. This is the commonest variety (Plate 11). It appears as a pearly papule. The epidermis is thinned and abnormal blood vessels (telangiectasia)

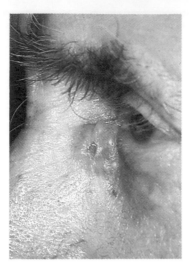

Fig. 18.1   Basal cell carcinoma at the inner canthus.

can be seen over the surface. As it grows the central part ulcerates.

2. Superficial spreading. This variety is a reddish macule with a thin pearly border and atrophy of the epidermis. The tumour can sometimes be discontinuous or multicentric, so surgical excision sometimes leaves some tumour behind.

3. Morphoeic. This rarer variety appears as a plaque of scar-like tissue with an ill-defined border making diagnosis difficult and often late. It occurs virtually exclusively on the face. Microscopically, there is a dense stroma with thin strands of basal cells. At the periphery the tumour blends with the surrounding dermis, so there is a great risk of leaving some behind at operation.

4. Cystic. In this form the tumour is typically raised with a smooth surface and underlying cystic degeneration.

The commonest sites are on the face: nose, cheek, temple, eyelid and scalp. Growth is slow, often over several years, with only a gradual increase in size, but superficial ulceration and slight bleeding are common. Infection of the ulcer is common. However their capacity to grow and destroy tissues locally gives them the common name of 'rodent ulcer'. Typically they are up to 3 cm in diameter at the time of diagnosis. Occasionally, in patients who are mentally impaired or who have neglected themselves or deferred presentation for fear of the diagnosis, the tumour may measure several centimetres in diameter. It may have caused extensive damage by its 'rodent' activity, invading the eye or the skull vault. Death may eventually occur from haemorrhage (erosion of a large blood vessel) or meningitis (erosion of the skull). They do not metastasise.

SQUAMOUS CELL CARCINOMA

Pathology

Squamous carcinoma forms about 15% of skin cancer. It tends to grow more rapidly than basal cell carcinomas and may spread to the regional nodes. Microscopically the typical appearance is of a well-differentiated keratinising tumour extending downwards from the epidermis into the dermis. The majority are due to sunlight and are of low grade malignancy. A small proportion behave fairly aggressively.

Clinical features

Squamous carcinomas may occur anywhere on the body surface but are usually, by reason of occupational exposure, seen on the head and neck, hands, forearms and scrotum. There are two main clinical varieties. The commonest is an ulcer with a raised rolled edge and slough at the base (Plate 12). Less common is a slow growing variety, presenting as a nodular mass. The more advanced form of the latter can be a keratinised horn, for example on the pinna of the ear. Lymph node metastases are commoner with the ulcerated form.

OTHER FORMS OF SKIN CANCER

1. *Basi-squamous carcinoma* is a mixture of basal and squamous carcinoma with the metastatic potential of the latter.
2. *Malignant melanoma* represents about 5% of skin cancer and is considered later in this chapter.
3. *Miscellaneous.* Sweat gland tumours are uncommon. A variety of cysts and benign tumours also occur.
    a. *Keratoacanthoma* (Fig. 18.2) resembles squamous carcinoma but is distinguished by its

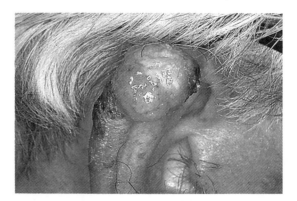

Fig. 18.2   Keratoacanthoma.(Courtesy of Dr D Gawkrodger, Sheffield)

well-defined edge and central plug of keratin. It typically develops rapidly over a few weeks. It is a benign lesion and often heals without treatment or after curettage. Biopsy may not distinguish it from a squamous cell carcinoma. If there is any doubt about the histology it should be treated as a squamous cell carcinoma with radical radiotherapy.

b. *Skin glands*. Sebaceous and sweat glands rarely give rise to benign tumours (adenomas) or malignant (adenocarcinomas). Tumours of the sebaceous glands occur more frequently on the head and neck. Lymph node spread is rare. Tumours of the sweat glands arise most often in the axilla, scrotum and vulva. Surgery is preferable in these areas since they tolerate irradiation poorly.

c. *Lymphoma*. Skin lesions (lymphoma cutis) may be an early manifestation of lymphoma. The most serious is mycosis fungoides (p. 458).

d. *Secondary carcinoma* often appears as nodules just below the epidermis, especially from a lung or breast primary (of which it may be the first clinical evidence). The diagnosis may be confirmed on fine needle cytology or excision. Local radiotherapy is helpful in relieving pain.

Treatment

Basal and squamous cell carcinomas can be cured in over 90% of cases by a variety of techniques, including curettage and cautery, cryosurgery, local excision and radiotherapy. Practice will vary with local expertise and facilities.

Close liaison should be established between dermatologist, radiotherapist and plastic surgeon in determining the best form of treatment.

Factors which influence the choice of treatment are the aetiology, site, size, local extent and number of lesions, the cosmetic and functional effect, the age, occupation, general condition and convenience of the patient.

Surgery

Surgery is generally recommended for the following categories:

— Radiation induced tumours
— Persistent or recurrent disease following radiotherapy
— Scarred or unhealthy skin (e.g. dermatitis or chronic infection)
— Patients under the age of 50 (better cosmesis)
— Sites tolerating radiotherapy poorly (dorsum of the hand, abdominal wall, perineum, shin and sole of the foot)
— Sites adjacent to structures likely to be damaged by radiation (e.g. lateral third of upper eyelid overlying lacrimal gland)
— Very large lesions, e.g. >5 cm
— Tumours involving cartilage or bone
— Multiple lesions (e.g. Gorlin's syndrome)
— Occupational exposure to extremes of heat and cold.

In general, surgical excision is preferred to radiotherapy in the younger patient because the scar is often less noticeable than the coin-shaped area of pale skin with overlying telangiectasia which characterises the late effects of radiotherapy. However, where loss of tissue is likely to cause cosmetic or functional impairment, e.g. lower eyelid, lip, nose, inner canthus and ear, radiotherapy is generally preferred.

Sites which tolerate radiotherapy poorly (and are more prone to radionecrosis) are the back of the hand, abdominal wall, perineum, shin and the sole of the foot. Surgical excision is preferable at these sites. Similarly, tumours of the upper eyelid are best excised because of the proximity of the lacrimal gland behind the lateral third. Inhibition of the production of tears from the lacrimal gland will result in a dry eye and the risk of corneal ulceration.

Very large lesions, e.g. over 4–5 cm, are less likely to be controlled by radiotherapy. Surgical excision with skin grafting should be considered.

Tumours invading cartilage or bone, e.g. on the ear or nose, are best treated surgically since radiotherapy may precipitate necrosis of cartilage or bone. Pain is a common symptom of cartilage or bony invasion. This is less of a problem where electrons of suitable energy are available in view of their limited absorption in cartilage or bone.

Multiple lesions, e.g. in basal cell naevus syndrome (Gorlin's syndrome), are best treated by local excision since otherwise many weeks will be occupied by multiple courses of radiotherapy. There may also be difficulty in avoiding overlap with previously irradiated areas.

Elderly patients and those in poor medical condition may not be fit for surgery. However excision may be possible under local anaesthetic and may be preferable to several visits to hospital for radiotherapy. For the very frail, single fractions of radiotherapy are an alternative.

Patients whose occupations expose them to extremes of heat or cold are best treated by surgery. Such exposure increases the risk of radionecrosis, even many years after treatment.

Small lesions are excised with a margin of normal tissue. This tends to be narrower on the face to achieve a good cosmetic result. Inadequate excision is more likely to occur on the face than in other sites where a more generous margin of normal tissue can be afforded.

Radiotherapy

Target volume

For most basal cell carcinomas the target volume is the tumour with a 0.5 cm margin of surrounding normal skin. Particular care is needed in determining the ill-defined edge of morphoeic lesions. This can often be better appreciated by stretching the lesion between both thumbs. For morphoeic basal cell carcinoma and all squamous cell carcinomas this margin should be larger, i.e. 1 cm.

Technique

Single fields are appropriate for the vast majority of basal and squamous cell carcinomas. Where the contours of the skin may result in considerable fall-off in dose, e.g. over the tip of the nose, a wax block attached to the nose and treatment by opposed lateral fields at orthovoltage makes the dose distribution more even across the target volume. The concavity or convexity of the skin can often be overcome by flattening the tumour and surrounding skin with the treatment applicator.

At some sites (e.g. the inner canthus) it is not possible to bring the applicator to the level of the lesion because the applicator is obstructed by the adjacent nose and cheek or because the lesion is below the surface of the skin (positive 'stand off') (Fig. 18.3A). In these circumstances, the tumour is treated at a slightly longer SSD (e.g. 20.5 cm instead of the normal 20 cm). Conversely, lesions protruding above the surface of the skin (negative 'stand off') are treated at a shorter SSD (Fig. 18.3B). The distance from the end of the applicator to the surface of the lesion is measured by passing a thin wooden stick through the middle of the applicator so that it touches the surface of the tumour. The applicator is removed with the stick held in the same position. The distance that the stick protrudes from the end of the applicator is then measured with a ruler.

To avoid a sharply punched out border, which is unsightly, the inner edge of the lead cut-out can be bevelled. This results in a more gradual fall-off in dose at the periphery. The late radiation induced skin changes are less noticeable since they blend with the surrounding normal skin. Without bevelling, the irradiated area is more clearly demarcated.

Surface radium moulds had a long vogue but are now rarely used as they involve expensive preparation, hospitalisation and unavoidable radiation exposure to hospital staff.

Tumours around the eye. The cornea and the lens of the eye are particularly sensitive to radiation. Every effort should be made to protect the eyes from irradiation where possible.

Eyelid. Lesions on the eyelids are common, usually basal cell carcinomas, e.g. at the medial ends near the bridge of the nose (inner canthus, Fig. 18.1). Tumours of the upper eyelids are generally best treated by surgical excision because a radiation field covering the tumour and 0.5 cm safety margin will almost invariably include the lacrimal gland, which lies behind the lateral third of the eyelid.

Tumours of the lower eyelids can usually be treated by superficial radiation. An internal eye shield is

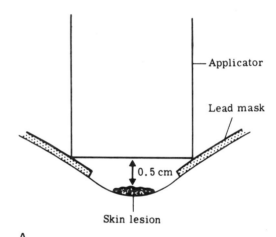

A

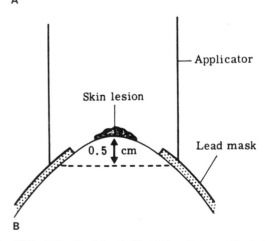

B

Fig. 18.3   A Positive 'stand-off' of 0.5 cm between the lesion and applicator. **B** Negative 'stand-off' of 0.5 cm. (Reproduced with permission from Dobbs J & Barrett A 1985 Practical Radiotherapy Planning, 1st edn, Edward Arnold, London.)

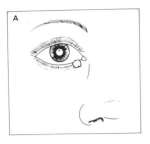
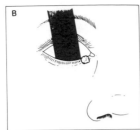
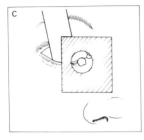
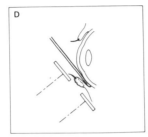

A

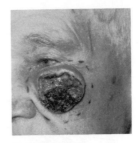
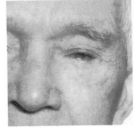

B (i)   (ii)

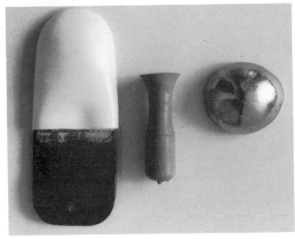

C

necessary. This is in form of a contact lens, but made of lead (1 mm thick). It has a smooth surface to avoid scratching the cornea or conjunctiva. Eye shields may be kept in an antiseptic solution (chlorhexidine gluconate) and rinsed before use in sterile water. They should be regularly inspected for damage and cracks. Local anaesthetic (1% amethocaine hydrochloride) is instilled into the eye, followed by 1–2 drops of sterile paraffin. The patient should be advised that the local anaesthetic will sting briefly before its anaesthetic action takes effect. If the eye shield (Fig. 18.4C) is to be inserted under both lids, the patient is asked to look down and the eye shield is inserted under the upper lid first. The patient then looks up and the shield is placed behind the lower eyelid. For tumours of the lower eyelid, a spatula-like lead shield can be inserted behind the lid margin and taped temporarily to the forehead (Fig. 18.4A).

Tumours of the ala nasi. If the ala nasi is treated, some protection to the inside of the nose can be given by a narrow strip of lead (covered with wax to absorb the secondary electrons from the lead) inserted into the nostril during treatment.

Dose and energy

Choice of energy, dose and fractionation will depend on the site, diameter and thickness of the lesion and the age and general condition of the patient. For superficial and orthovoltage the energy is chosen which delivers 50% of the surface dose to the base of the tumour (the half-value layer). For example, for 100 kV at 15 cm SSD the half-value layer is 1.5 mm of

Fig. 18.4 A Treatment of skin cancer on lower eyelid (reproduced with permission from Souhami RL & Tobias JS 1986 Cancer and its Management, Blackwell Scientific, Oxford). **B** Squamous carcinoma of the cheek (i) before and (ii) after treatment with 6 MeV electrons (courtesy of Dr A.Champion, Sheffield). **C** Protection of the eye during radiotherapy: (left to right) (1) lead shield inserted below lower eyelid, (2) rubber applicator for (3) gold full internal eye shield.

aluminium. The depth doses of different energies are shown in Figure 18.5. Basal cell carcinomas at certain sites, e.g. in the retroauricular sulcus (behind the ear), inner canthus and nasolabial fold, are prone to deep extension. This should be suspected if lesions at these sites appear fixed. For deeply penetrating lesions, excision and skin grafting are indicated.

For most basal carcinomas up to 0.5 cm thick, superficial X-rays (90–120 kV) are adequate. For thicker lesions, orthovoltage (250–300 kV), or electrons (6–8 MeV) are required (Fig. 18.4B). Open-ended circular applicators are used (2–4 cm diameter, e.g. on a Pantak machine at 20 cm FSD). A series of lead cut-outs (0.5 mm thick for 90 kV and 2 mm for 140 kV), both circles and ovals, should be available in all standard sizes.

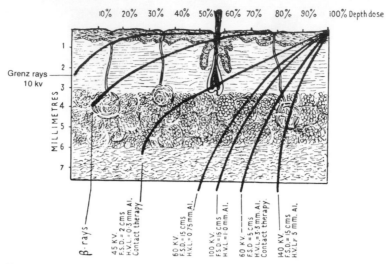

Fig. 18.5 Depth dose absorption curves of various qualities of radiation, superimposed on a cross-section of the skin.

For widespread superficial skin infiltration from mycosis fungoides whole body low energy (3 MeV) electrons or beta irradiation from a strontium-90 source are advised (p. 458).

For lesions up to 3 cm diameter and up to 0.5 cm thick:

45 Gy applied dose in 10 daily fractions over 2 weeks (90–120 kV)

For lesions over 3 cm diameter or >0.5 cm thick:

50 Gy in 15 daily fractions over 3 weeks (250–300 kV)
or

55 Gy in 20 daily fractions over 4 weeks (megavoltage or 6–8 MeV electrons with bolus to bring the maximum dose to the surface)

Protracted fractionation is particularly important on the cartilaginous areas of the ears and the nose, to minimise the risk of late necrosis.

It is possible to cure small lesions of less than 2.5 cm in diameter with single fractions of 22.5 Gy, and from 2.5 to 4 cm with 18–20 Gy. This is particularly useful for the elderly and frail where a single attendance for treatment is desirable.

Radiation reactions

Acute. When 45 Gy is given in 10 daily fractions, erythema develops in the last few days of the course. The colour deepens for a week and then fades, or goes on to moist desquamation. After moist peeling, a scab usually forms. Healing proceeds underneath the scab. The scab falls off when healing is complete, usually in 4–5 weeks after the end of treatment. Pigmentation may follow, especially in dark-skinned individuals, but usually fades in a few weeks or months.

The acute reaction is more marked in those with fair complexions.

Late reactions. Late skin changes are hypo- or hyper-pigmentation, atrophy, alopecia and telangiectasia. These changes become more obvious as the field size increases. Irradiated skin remains at long-term risk of damage. Patients should be advised to avoid excessive exposure of the treated area to sun, cold wind and trauma. The nose and the ear are particularly vulnerable. Cartilage and bone necrosis are now rare with the wider availability of electrons (see above).

Treatment of reactions. If possible, the area should be kept dry and undisturbed, uncovered by any dressing or application. However, for treated lesions which are discharging, some coverage at night to avoid soiling bedlinen is desirable. A simple non-adherent dressing, e.g. tulle gras covered by gauze, suffices in most cases. Thick or infected crusts are best removed to enable the lesion to be cleaned and healing to progress. Greasy applications should be avoided since they prevent natural discharges and encourage infection. Topical antibiotics based on culture and sensitivities of a swab of an infected lesion may occasionally be needed.

Cosmetic creams may help conceal the stigmata of late radiation skin changes.

Patients should be encouraged to apply a high factor sun blocking cream (e.g. 15) to block UVA and UVB radiation if exposed to the sun.

Follow-up

Patients with basal cell carcinomas should be followed at least until the lesion has healed. This is normally 4–5 weeks after the end of treatment. Longer term follow-up may be needed if there are other areas of hyperkeratosis or the patient is at particular risk of further skin malignancy (e.g. basal cell naevus (Gorlin's) syndrome, xeroderma pigmentosum) for which lifelong surveillance is warranted.

Closer surveillance is required for squamous carcinomas because of the additional risk of lymph node spread. Three-monthly follow-up in the first 2 years, 4-monthly in the third year and 6-monthly in the fourth and fifth years are suggested. Follow-up can usually be discontinued at 5 years since relapse thereafter is rare. Patients should be encouraged to report back if they notice nodularity or ulceration in an irradiated area which had previously healed.

Recurrences following radiotherapy

Recurrences may occur, especially at the edges, due to a 'geographic miss'. This is more likely in the morphoeic variety of basal carcinoma where the margins are poorly defined. Recurrences are best treated surgically.

Results of treatment

The overall cure rates of surgery and radiotherapy for small basal cell carcinomas of the skin are excellent at about 90–95%. Cosmetic results of surgery are generally better than those of radiotherapy. Cure rates are slightly less good for squamous cell carcinomas due to their tendency to metastasise.

MALIGNANT MELANOMA

Melanoma is a malignant tumour arising from cells (melanocytes) that produce the black pigment, melanin, and lie in the basal layer of the epidermis. Melanoma of the eye is described in Chapter 27.

Pathology

Benign melanocytic naevi are almost universal. Most people have 10–20 congenital brownish spots or moles. These naevi lie just in the deepest part of the epidermis. The surface may be smooth, warty or hairy. Malignant change is higher in congenital (about 12% for lesions over 2 cm) than acquired melanocytic naevi. The majority of acquired melanocytic naevi do not undergo malignant change.

Malignant change may occur in dysplastic naevi sporadically or as part of a familial syndrome. In the familial variety (inherited as an autosomal dominant) the incidence of malignant melanoma is substantial.

Epidemiology

The incidence of melanoma continues to rise. It represents 0.8% of all cancers and 0.6% of cancer deaths. The highest incidence is in Australia and New Zealand (40 per 100 000 population in Queensland). It is lowest in Japan and Hong Kong (0.2 per 100 000). In the UK the disease is commoner in females (sex ratio 2:1). In white races the lower limb and the head are the commonest sites in females, and on the trunk and the head in males. However melanoma can arise from any part of the skin. Rare sites are the nose, vulva, vagina, anus and penis.

Pattern of growth

Situated at the dermal–epidermal junction, proliferating melanocytes may grow either radially (horizontally) or vertically. Most varieties have an initial radial growth phase, with vertical invasive growth later. Nodular melanoma only shows vertical growth. In general the prognosis depends on the thickness of the tumour.

Growth rate is very variable. The clinical course may be very long (10–15 years) or rapidly fatal over a few months. Lymph node and metastatic spread is often rapid. Lymph nodes are often palpable in the absence of satellite nodules around the primary. Spread is then to the regional nodes (to the inguinal nodes from the lower limb, and to the axilla or inguinal nodes from the trunk). Blood-borne metastases are common, particularly to the lungs but also to the brain and liver.

There are four principal clinicopathological varieties:

1. Lentigo maligna
2. Superficial spreading
3. Nodular
4. Acrolentiginous.

Lentigo maligna (Plate 13) occurs in an older age group (6th–7th decades) and develops mainly on the face. The superficial spreading variety, which accounts for about 70% of all melanomas, occurs in a younger age group (4th–5th decades), mainly on the legs in women and on the trunk in men. The nodular form (Fig. 18.6) develops in an intermediate age group (5th–6th decades), mainly on the trunk, head and neck in men and on the legs in women. The acrolentiginous form develops on the palms of the hands and on the soles of the feet.

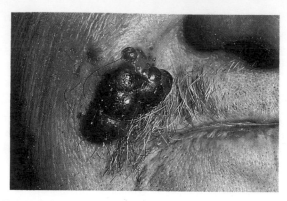

Fig. 18.6   Skin melanoma (nodular variety). (Courtesy of Dr M Kesseler, Rotherham.)

Diagnosis and staging

Early diagnosis is essential for curative treatment. Health professions and the general public need to be alert to the symptoms and signs of malignant change in any pigmented lesion. These are:

1. Change in pigmentation
2. Persistent or intermittent itching
3. Change in size or shape
4. Erythema or bleeding
5. Ulceration.

The regional nodes are palpated. The clinical diagnosis is confirmed by excisional biopsy and enables the pathologist to assess the depth of invasion. Staging investigations should include chest X-ray and a liver ultrasound for evidence of metastases. These are not essential for thin melanomas. A commonly used staging system for melanoma is shown in Table 18.1. The prognosis of melanoma is principally influenced by the thickness of the primary tumour at the time of diagnosis.

Treatment

Surgery

For stage I disease, less than 1 mm in thickness, excision with a 1 cm margin of normal tissue can be curative (Clark levels I and II). A skin graft may be

Table 18.1   Staging system for malignant melanoma

Stage	Clinical findings
I	Primary tumour only
II	Regional lymph node spread
III	Distant metastases including internal organs

necessary. For thicker lesions a wider resection margin of 3 cm is required.

If the regional lymph nodes are not palpable, their removal is probably unnecessary since survival is not altered. Lymph nodes in excess of 1 cm in diameter should be removed by block dissection.

Radiotherapy

Malignant melanoma is a relatively radioresistant tumour. Radiotherapy (with the exception of ocular melanoma, p. 496), has no primary role in the treatment of the disease, if the patient is fit for surgery. Occasionally radical radiotherapy may be attempted in those unfit for or refusing surgery. The main but limited role for radiotherapy is in palliation of advanced disease. The indications are:

1. Primary or nodes
   a. Painful infiltration
   b. Bleeding
   c. Ulceration
2. Metastases
   a. Bone
   b. Brain.

Technique

For the primary a single field usually suffices, and for the regional nodes (axilla, groin or neck) a parallel opposed pair. Bone metastases are treated using single fields or a parallel opposed pair. A parallel opposed pair of fields is used for brain metastases (Fig. 27.5A).

Dose and energy

For small solitary nodules (<1 cm) single fractions of 30 Gy using superficial X-rays (90 kV), or 6–8 Gy weekly for larger fields, is recommended. For bone metastases 20 Gy in four daily fractions at orthovoltage or megavoltage is suggested, and for brain metastases 30 Gy in 10 daily fractions over 2 weeks.

Chemotherapy can be given on a regional basis (isolated limb) or systemically. Systemic therapy may be given as an adjuvant to deal with micrometastatic disease or for overt metastases. In none of these situations has a curative role been established.

Regional chemotherapy (isolated limb perfusion)

This involves isolating the limb using a tourniquet under general anaesthesia and injecting cytotoxic agents into the isolated arterial supply. Its use should be restricted to specialist centres with surgical oncologists familiar with the technique. The chemotherapeutic agent of choice is DTIC. The main indication is local recurrence not amenable to surgery. Good palliation can be achieved. Local toxicity is minimal. Bone marrow toxicity is dose dependent. In advanced disease it may delay or avoid amputation for pain and ulceration uncontrolled by other means.

Adjuvant cytotoxic therapy

There is no good evidence that adjuvant cytotoxic therapy given postoperatively following the removal of the primary improves disease-free or overall survival.

Chemotherapy for palliation

Modest palliation is achievable with chemotherapy for advanced disease. Single agent therapy is as good as and less toxic than combination therapy. Vindesine and DTIC are the preferred agents, with response rates of 20–30%. Suggested doses are shown in Table 18.2. DTIC causes severe nausea and vomiting in most patients and myelosuppression in 15%. For vindesine bone marrow toxicity is normally the limiting factor. Alopecia occurs in 80–90% of patients. Neurotoxicity is common and cumulative (as with other vinca alkaloids).

Immunotherapy

Immunotherapy may have a role to play in the treatment of melanoma if the body's own immune response is important in influencing the growth of melanoma. Great care must be taken in interpreting the results of immunotherapy since spontaneous remissions are known to occur.

BCG (Bacille Calmette-Guérin) can be injected into small areas of local recurrence and skin deposits. Responses can be obtained in over 75% of patients. These indications are very limited since recurrence is usually extensive and skin deposits multiple.

Human interferon shows about a 10% response rate in metastatic melanoma. Its role in adjuvant therapy is being evaluated in prospective studies but cannot be recommended for routine use.

Biological response modifiers such as interleukin 2 (IL2), which stimulate the production of T lympho-cytes and may help control the immune response to melanoma, are also under evaluation as an adjuvant and for palliation of advanced disease.

Table 18.2. Palliative chemotherapy for melanoma

Agent	Regime
Vindesine	3 mg/m^2 i.v. weekly
DTIC	250 mg/m^2 i.v. for 5 days. Repeated every 21 days

Prognosis

When the tumour is confined to the epidermis, 5-year survival is 95–100%. It falls to 90% when the dermis is infiltrated and to 65% when tumour extends to the papillary–reticular junction. If there is deeper spread to the subcutaneous tissues or reticular dermis, 5-year survival is about 50%.

Skin metastases

Secondary carcinoma often appears as nodules just below the epidermis, especially in lung and breast cancer. It may be the first evidence of disease. Skin metastases may be symptomless, painful or ulcerate. They often respond well to palliative, superficial or orthovoltage radiotherapy (5 Gy in single fraction or 20 Gy in 4 daily fractions).

LIP

Cancer of the lip is the commonest oral cancer, representing 25% of the total cases. It accounts for 0.2% of cancers and 0.04% of cancer deaths. It arises from the vermilion border of the lip. Strictly speaking, tumour arising from the inner aspect of the lip and the commissures are tumours of the buccal mucosa. The lower lip is involved far more frequently than the upper lip (ratio 10:1) and in males more than females (sex ratio 10:1).

Pathology

Exposure to the sun and pipe-smoking are the main risk factors. Virtually all are squamous carcinomas. Basal carcinomas on the adjacent skin may impinge on to the lip. Tumours of the lower lip tend to be well differentiated and those of the upper lip less so. The central portion of the lower lip drains to the submental nodes and the lateral portions to the submandibular nodes. The upper lip drains to the upper deep cervical nodes.

Clinical features

Presentation is usually with a superficial ulcer or chronic cheilitis with an overlying scab. Minimal trauma may cause bleeding. Less frequently there is a nodule, indurated plaque, fissure or exophytic growth. There may be associated leucoplakia. Local spread may involve the whole of the lip, the skin below or the oral mucosa, and eventually the mandible.

Tumours at the angle of the mouth are particularly

Table 18.3   TNM staging of lip cancer

T stage	Clinical findings
T1	Tumour confined to the lip, 2 cm or less in greatest dimension
T2	Tumour confined to the lip, more than 2 cm but not larger than 4 cm in greatest dimension
T3	Tumour confined to the lip, more than 4 cm in greatest dimension
T4	Tumour extending beyond the lip to neighbouring structures, e.g. bone, tongue, skin of neck

likely to invade the buccal mucosa. This makes radiation treatment more difficult because of the changing tissue contours.

Nodal spread is uncommon at presentation in well-differentiated tumours (10%) but increases with tumours sited at the angle of the mouth, large size and anaplasia. Nodal metastases are present in 40% of poorly differentiated tumours.

Diagnosis and staging

The diagnosis is confirmed by biopsy. Staging is according to the TNM system (Table 18.3).

Treatment

The main treatments are radiotherapy and surgery. T1 and T2 tumours can be treated by surgery or radiotherapy. Radiotherapy is preferable in T2 tumours since excisional surgery may leave a substantial tissue defect which is cosmetically and functionally unsatisfactory.

Surgery

For very superficial tumours, a 'lip shave' and advancement of the vermilion can be carried out. Excision with primary closure is possible for small tumours, with good cosmetic and functional results. Surgery is the treatment of choice for lip tumours with adjacent leucoplakia. T3 and T4 tumours are best treated by surgery since the control rates from radiotherapy are only moderate and overt bone invasion increases the risks of radionecrosis.

There is no advantage in prophylactic block dissection of the cervical nodes. If nodes are >2 cm in diameter and operable, a radical neck dissection is carried out on the affected side.

Radiotherapy

The choice of technique and energy will depend upon the site and size of the tumour. Electron beam and interstitial implantation with iridium-192 (Fig. 19.5B) are now the preferred methods. Interstitial implantation is discussed in Chapter 19. Previously, superficial and orthovoltage therapy were commonly used before the wider availability of electrons. They have the advantages of the energy being chosen to suit the thickness of the lesion and the sharp fall-off in dose beyond the depth of the target volume.

The cosmetic results of superficial and orthovoltage are less satisfactory due to greater late radiation fibrosis and contracture of the lip. However they can still be used if electrons are not available.

A double 'sandwich mould technique' was also used in some centres but has been largely abandoned because of the complex planning and the radiation exposure to staff.

Tumours 1 cm or less in thickness. Such tumours can be treated by interstitial implant alone (Fig. 19.5B) using the plastic tube technique (Fig. 19.4A). Three parallel lines in a triangular configuration are often adequate (Fig. 19.5A). More sources may be needed for tumours extending on to the lip.

Tumours more than 1 cm in thickness

Technique and target volume
Electron beam is preferred. A single field with a lead applicator of suitable size is chosen. The target volume should include the tumour and 1 cm margin of adjacent normal tissue. The treatment volume should be 1 cm wider than the target volume to take account of the penumbra of the electrons. To protect the buccal mucosa, tongue, teeth and mandible, a shaped lead strip is positioned behind the lip. It is lined with wax to absorb the secondary electrons generated by interaction beween the incident beam and the lead.

Dose
50 Gy in 20 daily fractions over 4 weeks

Results of treatment

For tumours less than 3 cm in diameter without palpable nodes, the 5-year local control rate is about 90%. Where nodes are palpable or the tumour exceeds 3 cm in diameter, the local control rate falls to 60%.

19. Interstitial implantation

Interstitial implantation refers to the temporary or permanent insertion within the body's tissues of sealed radioactive sources. Interstitial implantation together with intracavitary therapy (Ch. 24) make up the two forms of brachytherapy (literally treatment at short distances (from the sources)). Implants are normally employed either alone or in conjunction with external beam therapy in the cure of localised tumours. Occasionally they are used for palliation (e.g. of metastatic neck nodes).

Implants may be temporary with caesium-137 needles or iridium-192 wire or permanent with gold-198 or iodine-125 seeds. Permanent implantation with gold seeds is limited by the unevenness of dose distribution resulting from the difficulty of implanting small individual seeds with good geometry. Implantation with iodine seeds is largely limited by the high cost of each seed. Temporary implants are most commonly practised in the UK, with iridium-192 progressively replacing caesium-137 for reasons discussed below.

This chapter concentrates on the clinical aspects of temporary removable implants. The principles of the two main systems of dosimetry used in the UK (Paris and Manchester) are described in Chapter 8. Implantation of the anterior two-thirds of the tongue using iridium hairpins and caesium needles, and of the breast and anus with plastic tubes and hollow rigid needles, illustrate both systems. The specific indications for implants at these and other sites are considered in the other clinical chapters.

Implantation is predominantly carried out in tumours which are readily accessible to the radiotherapist, e.g. floor of mouth, tongue, lip, skin, pinna, nose, breast, vagina and penis. However even more deeply seated structures, e.g. the nasopharynx, can be implanted, as can selected prostate, bladder and soft tissue tumours. The latter two require the assistance of the surgeon to provide access but the prostate can be approached percutaneously. More recently endobronchial (Fig. 19.1) and endo-oesophageal (Fig. 19.2) brachytherapy using

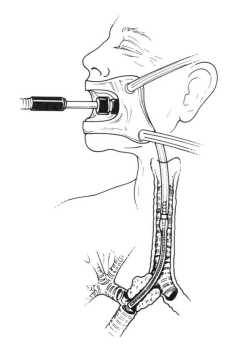

Fig. 19.1 High dose rate (HDR) iridium-192 for endobronchial brachytherapy for palliation of non-small cell lung cancer of right main bronchus using *microSelectron-HDR*. (Courtesy of Nucletron.)

high and low dose rate afterloading has been applied in the palliation of selected lung and oesophageal tumours.

While the value of implantation has been demonstrated in many personal series of cases by skilled brachytherapists, randomised trials comparing it with other forms of therapy (e.g. surgery or external beam) have rarely been attempted.

HISTORICAL ASPECTS

It was in the 1920s in Paris that the first attempts were made to seal radium salts as a source for brachytherapy.

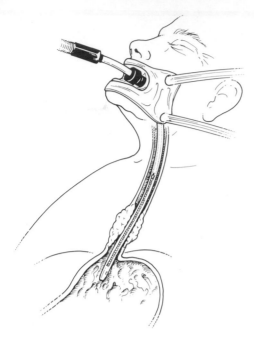

Fig. 19.2 Low dose rate (LDR) remote afterloading iridium-192 oesophageal brachytherapy for palliation of lower third carcinoma using *Selectron LDR*. (Courtesy of Nucletron.)

Dosimetry for the early radium tubes and needles was crude. Doses which could eradicate tumours while not exceeding normal tissue tolerance were derived empirically. The Paterson–Parker system (also known as the Manchester system) of radium dosage was described in 1934. This system enjoyed, and in some departments still enjoys, wide usage throughout the world. However the rigidity of the radium needles (and caesium that replaced radium) meant that the implant was not always best suited to the configuration of the tumour and surrounding normal structures. In addition, radiation exposure to the operator implanting the needles could be substantial.

In the early 1950s the flexible 'afterloaded' plastic tubes containing gold seeds were developed in the USA at the Memorial Hospital in New York. The advantages of afterloading are described on page 152. Afterloaded interstitial iridium-192 has substantially reduced radiation exposure to the operator.

In France in the mid 1950s the techniques of modern afterloading techniques were elaborated. The Paris system of dosimetry for implantation, based on afterloaded iridium-192, was published in 1966. The Paris system of dosimetry and its rules of implantation are described in Chapter 8. In the last 15 years the Paris system has been adopted by increasing numbers of radiotherapy departments in the UK and has largely

replaced the Manchester system. However some departments in other parts of the world where supplies of iridium wire are less reliable have retained stocks of caesium-137 needles because of its long half-life (p. 141). Iridium-192 wire with a much shorter half-life (p. 148) is more difficult to re-use unless a department undertakes implantation very frequently.

ADVANTAGES OF INTERSTITIAL IMPLANTATION

Interstitial implantation has the following physical and biological advantages over external beam irradiation.

1. High dose to tumour with reduced dosage to adjacent normal tissues

Due to the inverse square law (p. 60) the dose is inversely proportional to the square of the distance from the source. The dose therefore drops markedly with increasing distance from the source. The implant is normally confined to the tumour-bearing area. This limits the dose, and consequent morbidity, to adjacent normal tissues. By contrast external beam irradiation, e.g. of the head and neck, often includes substantial volumes of normal salivary tissue, resulting in a dry mouth.

The doses around the sources can be very much higher than can be achieved by external beam while still remaining within normal tissue tolerance.

2. Flexible conformation to tumour and normal structures

The flexible nature of iridium-192 wire enables it to follow the changing contours of tumour and adjacent normal structures. For example it can be threaded along the arch of the soft palate. It can be looped around the posterior part of the inner aspect of the cheek where the insertion of rigid needles is hindered by the posterior intermaxillary commissure. Using a mould to keep it in place, it can be inserted into the nasopharynx. The adaptability of iridium wire to local anatomy has permitted the role of interstitial implantation to be greatly extended.

3. Continuous low dose rate

There are a number of radiobiological advantages of low dose rate brachytherapy.

a. Repair of sublethal damage. Repair of sublethal damage increases in importance as the dose rate falls. At low dose rate accumulated sublethal damage contributes less to cell killing. At very low dose rates (i.e. <1 Gy/hour), it is direct radiation damage that accounts for most cell death. At low dose rate the tissues with a large 'shoulder' (or low α/β ratio, p. 259), for example late responding vascular endothelium and connective tissue, are better protected against damage than tissues with a small shoulder (or high ratio), such as basal epidermal cells of the skin. Late responding tissues thus have a greater capacity to absorb and repair sublethal damage. It also explains why interstitial therapy at lower than conventional dose rates (e.g. 10 Gy per week as opposed to 10 Gy per day) may be tolerated by tissues which have previously received tolerance doses of radical external beam therapy. At higher dose rates (i.e. >1 Gy/hour) the duration of irradiation is insufficient for sublethal damage to be repaired.

It is uncertain whether any correction to the total dose needs to be made to take account of differences in dose rate. It is thought that at conventional rates of 40–50 cGy/hour (5–6¼ days for a radical dose of 60 Gy) no correction is necessary. For high dose rate some correction would seem appropriate but has yet to be established.

b. Distribution in the cell cycle. It is known that cells in the G_1 phase of the cell cycle (Fig. 15.2) are more radiosensitive than in late S phase. It seems probable that during an implant over 6 days, tumour cells in the more sensitive phase of the cycle have longer periods of radiation exposure than during daily fractionated external beam therapy.

c. Tumour hypoxia. At low dose rates hypoxic tumour cells have a reduced capacity to repair radiation damage compared with normal tissues. This is because repair is an oxygen dependent process. Better oxygenated normal tissues are preferentially repaired compared with hypoxic tumour cells.

d. Reduced tumour proliferation during irradiation. The short overall treatment times of curative implants, commonly 6–7 days, do not allow increased tumour proliferation to occur during treatment. This is in contrast to external beam irradiation where tumour proliferation may occur in the conventional 24 hour gap between fractions.

CHOICE OF IMPLANTATION TECHNIQUE

In the Manchester system caesium needles are the only sealed sources used, whether it be for the tongue, vagina or anus. In the Paris system, both hairpins (Fig. 19.3), afterloaded plastic tubes (Fig. 19.4) and hollow needles (Figs 19.5, 19.9 and 19.11) are used. Plastic tubes can be used for implanting soft tissue

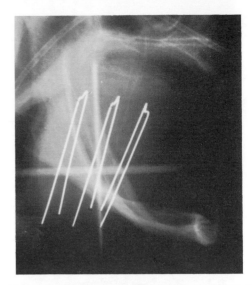

Fig. 19.3 Lateral radiograph showing iridium-192 hairpin implant of squamous carcinoma of the lateral border of the anterior two-thirds of the tongue.

sarcomas where longer target volumes need to be treated than can be encompassed by hairpins. Some radiotherapists also use plastic tubes for breast implants, while others prefer hollow needles. Hollow needles are used with templates to obtain more rigid geometry in the lip (Fig. 19.5A & B), breast (Fig. 19.9), penis (Fig. 19.6) and anus (Figs 19.10 and 19.11).

Anterior two-thirds of tongue

See page 317 for indications.

Iridium

Implantation with iridium hairpins can be carried out under either local or general anaesthesia. Local anaesthesia is less hazardous and has the advantage that the normal tone of the musculature is retained, allowing a similar distribution of the sources during and after the implant. Under general anaesthesia, where muscle relaxants are given, the distal end of the sources tend to bunch together as the normal tone of the tongue's musculature returns postoperatively. None the less, for the comfort of the patient most radiotherapists in the UK prefer to carry out the implant under general anaesthesia.

A double plane hairpin implant is best suited to most early carcinomas of the anterior two-thirds of the tongue. If the tumour is wider than 12 mm, the standard width of iridium hairpins, additional hairpins or single

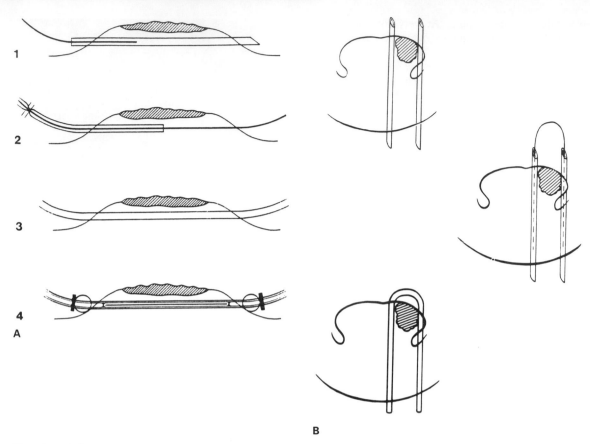

Fig. 19.4   A Steps in performing afterloaded plastic tube implant. (1) Stainless-steel guide needle inserted and nylon cord passed down needle. (2) Guide needle removed and outer plastic tubing passed over nylon cord and clamped. (3) Plastic tube in position ready for afterloading. (4) Plastic tube afterloaded with iridium-192 wire encapsulated within inner tubing. Nylon ball and lead discs placed to fix implant in position. (Redrawn from Hope-Stone 1986.) **B** The loop technique for iridium wire implantation. (Reproduced with permission from Dobbs et al 1992.)

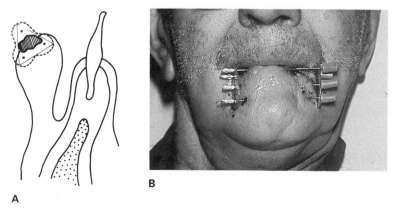

Fig. 19.5   A Cross-sectional diagram of a typical triangular implant pattern for a small exophytic lip cancer. Reference isodose is indicated by the dotted line. (Reproduced with permission from Pierquin et al 1987.) **B** Iridium implant of the lip using a template. (Courtesy of Dr D Ash, Leeds.)

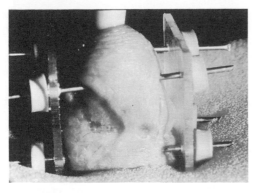

Fig. 19.6 Iridium-192 implant of the penis using hollow needles and template. (Courtesy of Dr D Ash, Leeds.)

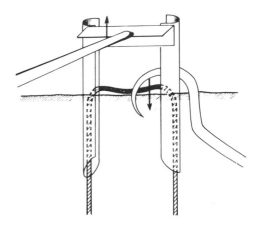

Fig. 19.7 Method of substituting hairpin for guide gutter. The pin is held against the tissue being implanted with a surgical hook while the guide gutter is removed with a needle-holder. (Reproduced with permission from Pierquin et al 1987.)

pins may be required. Alternatively, where the width of the tumour exceeds that of the hairpins, the plastic loop technique may be used which permits greater widths (up to 20 mm) to be implanted.

A dental impression is made of the floor of the mouth, including that of the tumour. Lead protection is incorporated in the periphery of the mould adjacent to the implant to reduce the dose to the mandible. A similar mould not containing lead (and therefore radiolucent) is used so as not to obscure the position of the pins on the verification radiographs.

For a hairpin implant, the tumour is inspected and palpated to confirm its boundaries. Local anaesthetic is infiltrated around the margins of the tumour.

The most posterior guide gutter is introduced first, with its bridge lying transversely and its limbs at the margin of the target volume. Additional hairpins are implanted anteriorly, keeping an anteroposterior separation of 12–15 mm between each hairpin. The length of the hairpins is chosen according to the depth of extension of the tumour. Ideally, the position of the guide gutters should be verified using a screening facility in theatre. If this is not available, peroperative orthogonal radiographs (Fig. 19.3) are an alternative. Adjustments are made if necessary to the position of the guide gutters to ensure that they are equidistant and parallel. When the geometry is satisfactory, a silk suture is passed under the bridge of the most posterior hairpin and through the substance of the tongue. This is repeated for the hairpins lying anteriorly. The free ends of the threads are clipped to the surgical drapes to the side of the mouth. Each hairpin is gently grasped by one limb and each limb introduced into the guide gutter, starting with the most posterior hairpin. Care should be taken not to bend the hairpins by applying undue pressure when inserting them into the guide gutter. While applying firm but gentle pressure to the centre of the bridge of the hairpin with a specially

designed hook, the guide gutter is removed (Fig. 19.7) by forceps held in the other hand. Each hairpin is then sutured to the tongue at the midpoint of its bridge.

For lesions close to the mandible, the dose to the mandible can be reduced by shortening the limbs of the most anterior hairpin by 0.5–1 cm. Rarely are more than three hairpins required. Exceeding this number substantially increases the risk of radionecrosis if the limbs of the hairpin lie close to the mandible.

Dosimetry. This is based on the plane perpendicular to the midpoint of the sources (p. 149). The position of the sources in this plane can be determined from tomograms taken through the central plane or reconstructed from orthogonal radiographs using a computerised dose planning system (p. 94). Ideally both manual and computerised dosimetry should be carried out independently, since errors in one may be exposed by the other.

Caesium needles

Implantation with caesium needles is carried out under general anaesthesia in the operating theatre. The therapist can make a preliminary calculation, based on the size of the lesion. In the example shown (Fig. 19.8) a single plane of needles will be adequate, covering a rectangular area. Needles of 1 and 2 mg of caesium are generally of most use in this type of case. Precise details of a typical case using the Paterson and Parker rules are given on page 144. In this case the dose will be worked out at 0.5 cm from the plane of the needles, i.e. it will suffice to dose adequately a 1 cm thickness of tissue, which should include all the malignancy.

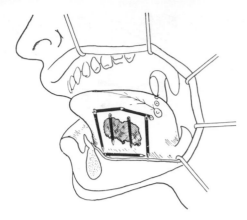

Fig. 19.8 Diagram of radium needles for single plane implant of the lateral border of the anterior two-thirds of the tongue. The layout is applicable to caesium needles. (Reproduced with permission from Paterson, Treatment of Malignant Disease by Radiotherapy, 2nd edn, Edward Arnold, 1963.)

Based on these calculations, the operator will have ordered the requisite types and number of needles. It is helpful to pass a suture through the tip of the tongue at the beginning of the procedure. Grasping the threads enables the position of the tongue to be manipulated for the purposes of implantation. The needles are inserted, starting at the posterior margin of the tumour. Needles should be inserted in a posterior oblique direction since they tend to move towards the front of the mouth as the tongue recovers its normal tone after anaesthesia. The distances and separations are carefully measured with a ruler to ensure the correct layout as calculated. A safety margin of 1 cm of normal tissue is included within the area implanted. The needles are held in special grooved long-handled forceps and pushed home with special 'pushers'.

Gold grain implants

Gold grains can be used as a permanent implant, especially in elderly people as they allow free tongue movement and so lessen the risk of postoperative pneumonia. Gold grains are only suitable for small single plane implants.

Postoperative care (iridium and caesium implants)

The patient is nursed in a protected room. An implant is a painful procedure once the anaesthetic has worn off and adequate analgesia (usually 4-hourly diamorphine) is essential. The position of each hairpin should be checked at least once a day to confirm that the sutures are securely fastened and the position of the hairpin is as intended. A soft diet and fluids are necessary to minimise movement of the tongue.

Iridium hairpins can normally be removed without anaesthetic. A general anaesthetic is usually necessary for the removal of the caesium needles. A soft diet should be continued for a further 3 weeks, by which time the acute reaction has normally settled.

Breast

Interstitial implantation as a boost to the tumour site can be carried out as a peroperative procedure following local excision or, more often, postoperatively following external beam irradiation of the breast. If carried out peroperatively, the radiotherapist has the advantage of knowing the exact site of the tumour. Alternatively, the surgeon can be asked to place radiopaque clips at the poles of the tumour or to draw on the skin, following closure of the wound, the area corresponding to the underlying tumour. If the surgeon makes the incision over the centre of the tumour, the radiotherapist can use the scar as the site to be boosted. In most cases a two plane implant (Fig. 19.9) is required, where the depth of breast tissue allows. The plastic tubes are loaded with dummy inactive iridium wire. The patient is transferred to the simulator after recovering from the general anaesthetic and anterior and lateral radiographs are obtained for planning. The Paris system of dosimetry is recommended (Ch. 8). To ensure adequate coverage of the tumour bearing area, the active wire will extend beyond the margins of the target to allow for colder areas occurring between the ends of the wires. Implantation is best done with rigid needles and a template to maintain good geometry.

Anal cancer

Implantation is carried out under general anaesthesia or, for those less fit, under spinal anaesthesia. The patient is placed in the lithotomy position. The circumferential extent, depth and proximal limits are assessed by inspection and palpation. A silver grain is embedded at the proximal and distal limits of the tumour to assist the positioning of the afterloaded sources. To maintain the parallelism of the sources, a crescentic Perspex template, predrilled with holes at regular intervals around its circumference (Fig. 19.10), is sutured against the perineum. Not more than two-thirds of the circumference of the anus is implanted to reduce late anal stenosis. Hollow steel needles of appropriate length are inserted through the holes in the template, through the perineal skin and then under

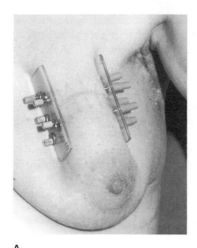

A

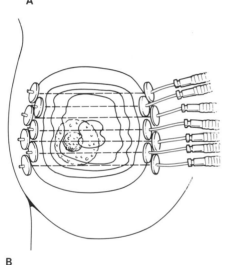

B

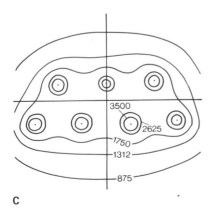

C

Fig. 19.9   A Iridium-192 breast implant with hollow needles and template. (Courtesy of Dr D Ash, Leeds). Dosimetry of breast implant **B** in plane of sources and **C** in cross-section.

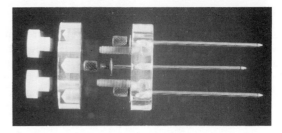

Fig. 19.10   Perineal applicator. (Courtesy of Dr D Ash, Leeds.)

the submucosa of the anus and rectum. Care should be taken not to pierce the rectal lumen. This is difficult to avoid in women in whom it is necessary to place the needles anteriorly in the rectovaginal septum without penetrating either the vagina or the rectum. To verify this it may be helpful to insert the first needle through the rectovaginal septum since, if done later in the implant, the field of vision may be limited. Between five and seven needles are commonly required. The average length is 5–7 cm. Inactive wire is inserted into each steel needle and drawn back under screening until it is correctly positioned in relation to the silver seeds. The appropriate length of iridium wire to be afterloaded can be calculated. Verification lateral and anteroposterior radiographs are taken to confirm the position of the needles and of the inactive wire (Fig. 19.11). It should also be checked that the position of the needles is not significantly altered by extending the patient's legs. The proximal ends of the needles are crimped at their entry points into the template to ensure that the needles are immobilised. Computerised dosimetry is carried out. Sources are afterloaded manually or using an afterloading machine (*micro-Selectron*).

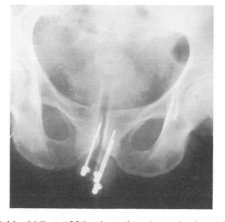

Fig. 19.11   Iridium-192 implant of anal canal using rigid hollow needles and template. (Courtesy of Dr D Ash, Leeds.)

Care during the implant

One or two enemas to clear the bowel are recommended before implantation. The patient should be nursed prone or on the side in a protected room. Regular 4-hourly opiates are given orally to control the discomfort and to keep the patient constipated during the implant. At the end of the implant, the template and attached needles are removed under a further general anaesthetic.

FUTURE DEVELOPMENTS

It is likely that better definition of the target volume will be made possible from computerised tomography, magnetic resonance imaging and ultrasound. Integrating this information with computerised dosimetry from a remote afterloading machine may improve the accuracy of radiation delivery.

The development of high dose rate remote afterloading machines may allow single-fraction peroperative irradiation of tumour sites following surgery.

Newer afterloading machines (e.g. *microSelectron-HDR*) containing iridium-192 for interstitial implantation and cobalt-60 sources for gynaecological applications are able to use a single source which can be switched to different parts of the implant for differing periods of time. The sequence of switching channels will be chosen with the help of computer programmes designed to provide optimal dose distribution over the period of the implant.

20. Mouth, secondary nodes of neck, tonsil, nasopharynx, paranasal sinuses, ear, salivary glands

ORAL CAVITY

Anatomy

Cancers of the mouth or oral cavity fall into several anatomical groups with general similarities and some individual differences. They include the lips, the hard palate, the upper and lower alveolus, the buccal cheek, retromolar trigone, and anterior two-thirds of the mobile tongue. A view of the oral cavity is seen in Figure 20.1A.

The anterior limit of the mouth is the vermilion border of the lip. The posterior limits are the circumvallate papillae of the dorsum of the tongue and the anterior margin of the oropharynx (Fig. 20.1B).

The tongue and floor of mouth are the commonest sites.

Pathology

Epidemiology

Cancer of the oral cavity represents less than 1% of all cancer deaths. It is commoner in men, with a male:female ratio of 2:1. Its incidence is declining in males and rising in females. Oral cancer is much commoner in India, probably related to chewing the betel nut (with tobacco and caustic lime) and in France due to alcohol and smoking, often in combination.

Aetiology

Environmental irritants predispose—tobacco, chewing betel nut, alcohol, dental sepsis, poorly fitting dentures, syphilis, iron deficiency anaemia and leucoplakia. Improved hygiene, nutrition and dental care, and the decline in incidence of syphilis have lowered the incidence in many countries.

An increased risk has been found among textile workers, particularly if exposed to the dust from the 'carding' of raw cotton or wool.

Histology

Over 90% are squamous carcinomas. The majority are well differentiated. A few are adenocarcinomas or malignant mixed tumours from minor salivary submucosal glands. Soft tissue sarcomas and lymphomas occur rarely.

Spread

Early spread is local, e.g. to the gum, palate, cheek. Bone may be invaded, especially the mandible. There is a rich lymphatic network, predominantly to the submandibular and upper deep cervical nodes (Figs 20.2–20.4). The lymphatics of the oral cavity anastomose in the midline. Contralateral spread may therefore occur.

Blood spread is late and rare. It is mainly to lung, bone and liver.

Clinical features

Most lesions present as ulcers of variable depth and induration. Others are papillary growths or fissured forms. Infection may follow, causing halitosis and excessive salivation. There may be associated leucoplakia. Oral pain may be prominent in the later stages, often radiating to the ear. The tongue may become fixed, with difficulty in eating and speaking.

Diagnosis is usually straightforward on inspection, but a thorough local examination and palpation of the lesion are necessary to reveal the full extent of invasion. The neck is palpated for enlarged nodes. A biopsy should be taken to confirm the diagnosis.

Staging

Tumours of the oral cavity should be staged clinically, using the TNM classification (Table 20.1), by size and local extent. Full blood count and radiographs of the

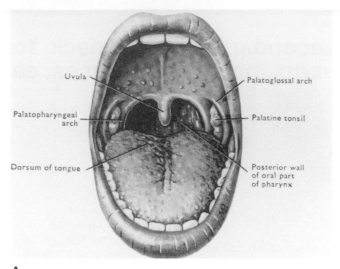

A

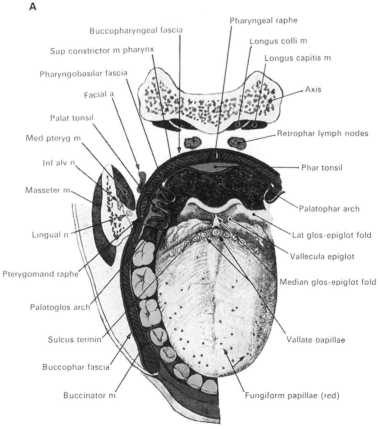

B

Fig. 20.1   A The fauces and its isthmus seen through the widely open mouth. (Reproduced with permission from Romanes G J 1971 Cunningham's Manual of Practical Anatomy, 13th edn, Oxford University Press, Oxford) **B** Horizontal section immediately above the tongue. (Reproduced with permission from Walmsley R & Murphy T R 1972 Jamieson's Illustrations of Regional Anatomy, 9th edn, Churchill Livingstone, Edinburgh.)

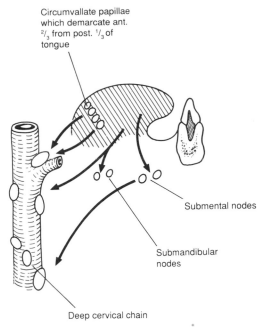

Fig. 20.2 Lymphatic drainage of the tongue. (Redrawn from Ellis H 1975 Clinical Anatomy, 5th edn, Blackwell Scientific, Oxford.)

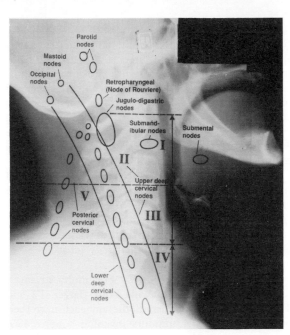

Fig. 20.4 Lymphatics of the head and neck from Figure 20.3, superimposed on lateral radiograph of the neck.

Table 20.1 TNM staging of mouth cancer

T stage	Clinical findings
T1	Tumour less than 2 cm
T2	Tumour 2–4 cm
T3	Tumour greater than 4 cm
T4	Invasion of neighbouring structures, e.g. mandible

chest and mandible (orthopantomogram) should be arranged.

Treatment of tumours of the oral cavity

Ideally the patient should be jointly assessed by a surgeon and a radiotherapist to decide on the choice of treatment. Surgery and radiotherapy can both be curative. The choice will depend on the aetiology and local extent of the disease, the age and general condition of the patient and the expertise available in radiotherapy and surgery. In general for early disease, radical radiotherapy or surgery may offer comparable local control. For advanced disease, the prospects of cure by local radiotherapy diminish substantially and radical surgery, if the patient is fit, is generally preferred. Chemotherapy is not curative but useful palliation can sometimes be achieved in advanced disease not controlled by surgery or radiotherapy.

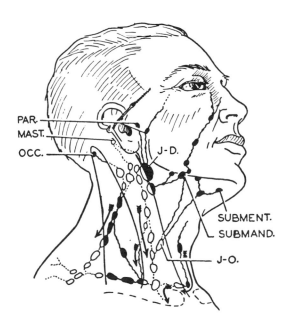

Fig. 20.3 The lymphatics of the head and neck. (After Rouvière; reproduced with permission from Basmajian J V, Grant's Method of Anatomy, 8th edn, © 1971 Williams & Wilkins, Baltimore.)

Radical radiotherapy

Radical irradiation of early tumours of the oral cavity should be by small beam-directed megavoltage fields using a full head shell and a mouth bite or by interstitial implantation or a combination of both. Afterloaded implantation using iridium wire is preferable to caesium needles because of the reduced radiation exposure to staff and its greater adaptability to the anatomy of the tumour (Ch. 19). Preparatory dental treatment (see below) should be carried out.

Early disease. Small superficial tumours (T1 and small T2) of the floor of mouth, tongue, lip and cheek in the absence of nodes are curable by implant (Fig. 20.5) alone (65–70 Gy), as long as the tumour can be completely encompassed by the sources in all planes and is not lying immediately adjacent to or invading bone.

More advanced tumours. For more advanced tumours which do not invade bone (larger T2 and T3), radical surgery and radiotherapy each have their proponents. For T4 tumours invading bone, radical surgery is preferred.

Dental treatment. The teeth may be damaged as a direct result of radiation ischaemia or, more importantly, as an indirect effect of a dry mouth (xerostomia) caused by inhibition of salivary secretion.

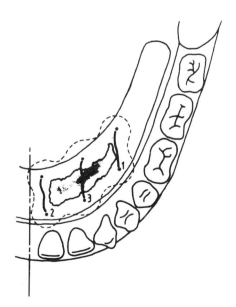

Fig. 20.5 Stage T2a (22 mm diameter) superficial squamous carcinoma, anterior floor of mouth. Implantation with hairpins (2.5 cm long, leg separation = 12 mm). Numbers indicate order in which guides were implanted. Reference isodose indicated by broken line around sources. (Reproduced with permission from Pierquin et al 1987.)

There is a reduction in the amount of saliva secreted and an increase in its viscosity. Both these factors predispose to bacterial growth and dental decay. In addition the reduction in the pH of the saliva assists bacterial enzymatic activity, with the production of acids which destroy tooth enamel. Even teeth not in the primary beam are subject to caries. Unless preventative measures are taken, all teeth may be destroyed within 1–2 years of treatment. If later extractions become necessary, osteomyelitis may follow, especially in the mandible, and even bone necrosis.

Before irradiation, the patient should be seen by an oral surgeon familiar with the management of patients undergoing irradiation for head and neck cancer. The current trend is towards trying to conserve the teeth since the risk of bone necrosis is reduced if extraction can be avoided. At the least, scaling and cleaning should be done. Any teeth which are non-viable or would require root filling or extensive restoration are extracted. The gums are sutured to encourage prompt healing. There is no fixed period necessary to allow healing of the socket. A week will usually suffice. However if urgent radiotherapy is required planning should not be delayed following an extraction.

Scrupulous attention to dental hygiene is essential during and after radiotherapy. A number of measures may help in minimising dental caries. They include:

1. Regular brushing of the teeth.
2. Corsodyl mouthwashes for 1 minute after each meal and in the evening before going to bed.
3. Any extractions required following radiotherapy should be carried out with an atraumatic technique under general anaesthesia and antibiotic cover. Multiple extractions should be staged.

Radical radiotherapy: carcinoma of the floor of mouth

1. T1 without nodes (N0)
Iridium hairpin implant alone (65–70 Gy to reference 85% isodose)

2. T2 without nodes (N0)

Target volume
Radical radiotherapy is given to the primary with at least 2 cm margin of normal tissue and to the submental and submandibular nodes (Fig. 20.6).

Technique
A right-angled wedged pair of fields (Fig. 20.8) or, for midline lesions of the anterior floor of the mouth, a lateral parallel pair of fields is used.

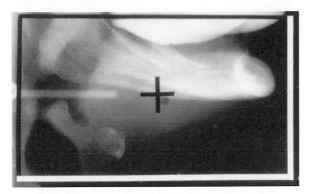

Fig. 20.6 Lateral field margins for early carcinoma of the floor of the mouth. (Courtesy of Dr D Radstone, Sheffield.)

If not fit for implant:

60 Gy in 25 daily fractions over 5 weeks (4–6 MV photons)

3. T1 and small T2, mobile nodes (N1)

Target volume
Palpable submental, submandibular or upper deep cervical nodes (level I and II (Table 20.2) can often be encompassed with the primary tumour within the radical irradiation field. If the nodes are mobile and ipsilateral (N1) but cannot be encompassed within a reasonable radical volume (e.g. up to 60 cm²), a block dissection of the affected side is followed by radical radiotherapy to the primary.

Technique
Parallel opposed pair of wedged lateral fields.

Dose and energy
48 Gy in 20 daily fractions over 4 weeks (4–6 MV photons), then boost with iridium hairpin implant (20–25 Gy)

Dose and energy
60 Gy in 25 daily fractions over 5 weeks to palpable disease or 50 Gy in 25 daily fractions over 5 weeks postoperatively if necessary

Table 20.2 Guidelines for cervical nodal* irradiation in squamous cell carcinoma of the head and neck

Indications	Irradiation
Oral cavity	
T2N0 with well lateralised primary	Levels I and II on same side
T2N1 with well lateralised primary	Levels I to V on same side
T2N0 with primary approaching midline, all T3N0 and T4N0	Levels I, II and III bilaterally
All others	Levels I to V bilaterally
Oropharynx	
T2N0 tonsil	Levels I and II on same side
T2N1 tonsil	Levels I to V on same side
T2N0 other sites	Levels I, II and III bilaterally
All others	Levels I to V bilaterally
Nasopharynx	
Squamous carcinoma T1N0	No neck irradiation
Squamous carcinoma T2–4N0	Level II, plus lateral pharyngeal and upper posterior triangle
All undifferentiated carcinoma and squamous carcinoma with node involvement	Levels 1 to V
Hypopharynx	
All	Levels I to V bilaterally
Paranasal sinuses	
Squamous carcinoma	Lateral pharyngeal nodes only
Squamous carcinoma N+ and undifferentiated carcinoma	Levels I to V bilaterally
Larynx	
T1–2N0 glottic	No nodal irradiation
T3–4N0 glottic	Levels II and III bilaterally
T2N0 supraglottic	Levels II and III bilaterally
All others	Levels I to V bilaterally

* Lymph node levels are defined as follows: level I, submandibular; level II, upper deep cervical; level III, middle deep cervical; level IV, lower deep cervical; level V, posterior triangle.
(Reproduced with kind permission of Dr M Henk and the CHART steering committee.)

Management of nodes. The principles of management of neck nodes are described on page 319.

The indications for irradiation of neck nodes in cancer of the oral cavity and the levels to be irradiated ipsilaterally or bilaterally are summarised in Table 20.2. In T1N0 tumours treatable by implant alone, no nodal irradiation is necessary.

Surgery

The general indications for surgery in tumours of the oral cavity are:

— Tumours attached to or invading the mandible where the risk of radionecrosis is high
— Tumours with widespread associated leucoplakia
— Radioresistant tumours such as melanoma
— Radiation induced tumours
— Very large tumours unlikely to be cured by radiotherapy because of their bulk (T3 and T4)
— Tumours of the tip of the tongue which are difficult to immobilise and therefore to irradiate accurately
— Tumours associated with syphilitic glossitis. Syphilis itself may cause ischaemia due to narrowing of small vessels (endarteritis). The addition of irradiation may precipitate necrosis.

Chemotherapy

A curative role has not been established for cytotoxic chemotherapy. It may improve local control in conjunction with surgery or radiotherapy. Tumour shrinkage and symptomatic improvement can occur with one or two courses of cisplatin containing combination chemotherapy prior to radiotherapy.

Palliative cytotoxic therapy should also be considered in symptomatic patients where surgery and/or radiotherapy have failed. The routine use of cytotoxic chemotherapy in advanced head and neck cancer cannot however be recommended. It is essential to ensure that the patient is fit since agents such as cisplatin and methotrexate, among the most active of drugs, have major toxicities. These are poorly tolerated by the elderly and those in poor general medical condition. Suggested palliative single agent chemotherapy for up to six courses subject to response and tolerance is:

1. Cisplatin 100 mg/m² i.v. infusion in 2 litres 0.9% saline over 6 hours repeated every 3–4 weeks (see Ch. 31 for guidance on management of cisplatin therapy), or:
2. Methotrexate 100 mg/m² i.v. bolus, with folinic acid 15 mg orally 6-hourly for six doses starting 24 hours

AFTER methotrexate injection. Repeated every 2–4 weeks.

CANCER OF THE TONGUE

This is the commonest cancer of the mouth. Approximately 70% occur on the anterior two-thirds, mainly on the lateral aspect. Tumours of the posterior third differ. They tend to be more anaplastic and are more likely to metastasise to the regional nodes. Lymphoepithelioma and lymphoma occur more commonly in the posterior third. In addition, tumours of the posterior third tend to present later since they are less accessible to examination by the patient or doctor than more anterior lesions.

Lymphatic spread (Fig. 20.2) from the tip of the tongue is to the submental nodes. The remainder of the tongue drains to the submandibular and deep cervical nodes; 30% of patients with cancer of the oral tongue will have palpable nodes at presentation. Since the lymphatics cross the midline, contralateral nodes may be palpable in patients where the tumour appears clinically confined to one side of the tongue.

Staging

This should include bimanual palpation of the tumour and examination of the neck for lymph nodes. An examination of the tumour and a biopsy should be carried out under general anaesthesia. Staging investigations are as for other oral cavity tumours (see above). A radiograph of the mandible (orthopantomogram) should be requested if there is clinical invasion of the floor of the mouth.

Treatment

Local cure and conservation of function of the tongue are guiding principles. Choice of treatment depends upon the site, stage and pathology and the general condition of the patient.

Tumours of the anterior two-thirds of the tongue are more easily accessible to implantation than the posterior third. Larger tumours (T3 and T4) are poorly controlled by radiation alone and best treated by radical surgery. If such patients are unfit for surgery, external beam alone is used.

Poorly differentiated and deeply infiltrating squamous carcinomas are more likely to be associated with palpable nodes. Lymphomas, usually of the non-Hodgkin type, occur more commonly in the posterior third of the tongue. They are best treated by external beam alone.

Anterior two-thirds of tongue

Except for small T1 (1 cm or less) tumours, initial surgery is best avoided because the loss of tissue is mutilating and likely to cause functional impairment (speech, swallowing). Surgery is commonly reserved for salvage of tumours not controlled by radiotherapy.

Both surgery and radiotherapy have an equal probability of curing early (T1) well-differentiated squamous cell tumours of the anterior two-thirds of the tongue.

Early disease. Wedge excision gives good functional results in small (1 cm or less) tumours of the tip or lateral border of the tongue.

For T1 and small, not deeply infiltrating T2 tumours on the lateral border of the anterior two-thirds of the tongue, interstitial implantation is recommended (Fig. 20.5 and Fig. 19.3) (see Ch. 19 for details of technique). For larger T2 and T3 tumours of the anterior two-thirds of the tongue which are too extensive for implantation, treatment should be by external beam irradiation initially or surgery.

More advanced tumours (T3–4). A hemiglossectomy is necessary for larger tumours (>4 cm) provided they do not involve the gingival margin or cross the midline. Tumours crossing the midline require more extensive resection. A myocutaneous flap can be used to replace the resected part of the tongue, permitting a reasonable quality of speech and swallowing. For T4 tumours, surgery is preferred to radiotherapy. Radical external beam irradiation to the primary and draining nodes (as for T2 and T3) is the alternative for inoperable T3 and T4 tumours.

External beam irradiation. This is appropriate as primary treatment for patients who are not fit for implantation or for larger T2 and inoperable T3 or T4 tumours. Larger T2 tumours should receive initial external beam followed by a boost with an iridium hairpin implant.

Target volume

This includes the primary tumour with at least a 2 cm margin and the submandibular and upper deep cervical nodes (Fig. 20.7).

Technique

A shell and mouth bite are required. The latter keeps the hard palate out of the field. For lateral tumours an anterior and lateral wedged pair of fields is suitable (Fig. 20.8.). If the lesion extends to the midline, a parallel opposed pair of fields is preferable.

Dose and energy

Implant or external beam alone (T1 and small T2)

Iridium implant (65–70 Gy to reference 85% isodose)

If unfit for implant:

60 Gy in 25 daily fractions over 5 weeks (4–6 MV photons)

Combined external beam and implant (larger T2)
48 Gy in 20 fractions over 4 weeks (4–6 MV

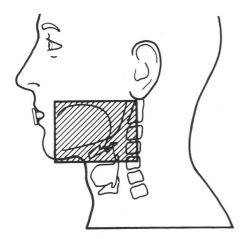

Fig. 20.7 Lateral field margins for localised carcinoma of the tongue. (Reproduced with permission from Dobbs et al 1992.)

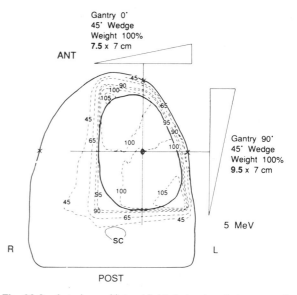

Fig. 20.8 Anterior and lateral fields to treat early tumours of the tongue and floor of the mouth. SC, spinal cord; X, laser reference point. (Reproduced with permission from Dobbs et al 1992.)

photons) to the primary and neck followed by boost by an implant (20–25 Gy)

External beam alone (inoperable T3 and T4)
60 Gy in 25 daily fractions over 5 weeks (4–6 MV photons)

Posterior third of tongue. For tumours of the posterior third of the tongue, which are usually extensive at presentation, external beam irradiation is recommended since surgery would involve a total glossectomy and major functional impairment. Implantation of the posterior third of the tongue with iridium hairpins is rarely practical because of difficulty of access. An iridium wire boost (30 Gy) can be given using the loop technique (Fig. 19.4B) following external beam (50 Gy in 20 daily fractions over 4 weeks; 4–6 MV photons). Implanting the posterior third of the tongue requires considerable experience.

Target volume

The primary tumour and upper and midcervical nodes are included (Fig. 20.9). In view of the high incidence of nodal involvement, some radiotherapists include all the lymphatics (levels I–V, see Table 20.2) from the base of the skull to the clavicles.

Technique

A parallel opposed pair of lateral wedged fields cover the primary and upper neck. The lower neck is treated by an open direct field with midline shielding of the spinal cord. A 0.5 cm gap is left at the junction of the upper and lower fields to avoid overlap, unless

asymmetric diaphragms are used (Fig. 21.19). If the latter are used, no gap is needed at the junction and the fields are simply matched to avoid any overlap. Wherever a junction between lateral and anterior fields occurs, the junction must lie at least 1 cm below any central disease.

Dose and energy

If nodal areas not overlying the spinal cord
60 Gy in 25 daily fractions over 5 weeks (4–6 MV photons)

If nodal areas treated overlie the cord. The volume of the upper neck field is reduced at 40 Gy to exclude the spinal cord and the dose to the reduced field continued to 66 Gy in 33 fractions. The anterior lower neck field has midline lead shielding throughout the course of treatment to protect the spinal cord. An additional 26 Gy in 13 daily fractions is given by electron fields to each side of the neck overlying the cord. The energy of electrons needed is chosen using the technique described in Figures 20.17 and 20.18.
66 Gy in 33 fractions over 6.5 weeks (4–6 MV photons or electrons)

Lymphomas. Lymphomas of the posterior third of the tongue are usually of high grade non-Hodgkin type. External beam irradiation should be the definitive treatment.

ALVEOLUS AND HARD PALATE

Treatment

The management of carcinoma of the alveolus and hard palate is controversial. There are proponents for both radical surgery and radiotherapy. Many of these tumours involve bone, although this may be difficult to demonstrate. If bone is involved, radical surgery is the treatment of choice.

It is essential to exclude a primary tumour arising in the maxillary antrum by tomography or CT scanning. Most lesions are treated by megavoltage irradiation using anterior and lateral wedged fields. However if the lesion extends to or beyond the midline, parallel opposed wedged lateral fields are required. Dosage and fractionation are the same as for the floor of the mouth.

BUCCAL CHEEK

Small superficial growths (less than 1 cm) are often best excised in addition to any associated areas of leucoplakia. Otherwise they can be adequately treated by a single plane iridium implant using the plastic

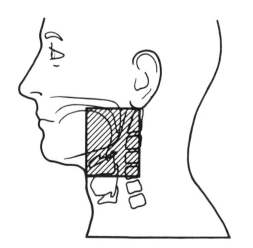

Fig. 20.9 Treatment volume for tumours of the posterior third of the tongue. (Reproduced with permission from Dobbs & Barrett, Practical Radiotherapy Planning, 1st edn, Edward Arnold, 1985.)

tube technique (65–70 Gy to reference 85% isodose) or by electrons.

Lesions, especially at the back close to the inter-maxillary commissure, are difficult to implant and are best treated by external beam or electrons.

For T1 and T2 lesions thicker than 1 cm, implantation alone is inadequate and should be combined with external beam or electrons. Initial electron or megavoltage irradiation to 40 Gy in 20 daily fractions over 4 weeks is followed by an iridium implant (40 Gy to 85% reference isodose).

For patients not fit for surgery or implantation external beam irradiation is an alternative. A direct electron field or anterior and lateral wedged pair at megavoltage can be used. Dosage and fractionation are as for the floor of mouth (p. 315).

For T3 and T4 lesions the probability of local control by radiotherapy is low. Disabling trismus due to severe fibrosis is common. Radical surgery with reconstruction is therefore preferred.

LYMPH NODE METASTASES IN THE NECK

Metastasis to the neck is the most serious aspect of mouth (and throat) cancer, being the commonest cause of death. Prognosis depends more on the presence or absence of secondaries in cervical nodes than on the primary growth.

As a generalisation, it may be said that *operable nodes in squamous carcinoma are best treated by surgery*, usually radical block dissection, while inoperable nodes must rely on radiation as a poor second best. In a radical neck dissection the submental, submandibular, anterior and posterior cervical nodes are removed in addition to the sternomastoid and omohyoid muscles. The internal jugular vein is divided and tied off above and below.

In squamous carcinoma, four clinical situations have to be discussed:

1. No nodes palpable (N0). At one time 'prophylactic' removal of nodes on the affected side was advised, to remove early microscopic secondaries. The operation of radical neck dissection is a major procedure with significant morbidity and some mortality. However, nine out of 10 cases proved to be free of secondaries, and it seemed unjustifiable to penalise the many for the sake of the few. Radical surgery is, of course, unsuitable for patients who are elderly or in poor condition.

'Prophylactic' or 'elective' neck irradiation has a low morbidity compared with radical neck dissection. However elective neck irradiation, while it does reduce the incidence of the development of subsequent nodal metastases, does not improve survival compared with a 'wait and see' policy. There are three situations where elective neck irradiation is advisable. First, where the likelihood of microscopic nodal metastases is high (e.g. supraglottic tumours); secondly, when the patient is unlikely to be a regular attender at follow-up; and thirdly, where the general condition of the patient would contraindicate a radical neck dissection.

Most therapists prefer a 'wait and see' policy, with regular follow-up at monthly intervals in the first year and every 2 months in the second year. However elective neck irradiation is becoming increasingly popular. It is within the first 2 years following treatment when lymph node spread is most likely to occur. Indeed, about 50% of block dissections are carried out within 3 months of completion of treatment of the primary. Fine needle aspiration of suspicious nodes can be carried out to obtain histological proof of involvement. Biopsy, however, is contraindicated since it increases the risk of subsequent recurrence. If lymphatic metastases are strongly suspected, the patient should be prepared for a block dissection and the suspicious node examined by frozen section before proceeding to a radical neck dissection.

2. Nodes palpable and operable (N1, N2). Mobile nodes confined to one side of the neck are described as N1 and bilateral mobile nodes as N2.

a. N1 nodes. There are several possibilities, each with its advocates. Some remove the nodes first, then irradiate the primary. Others prefer to irradiate the primary first, then excise the nodes 4–6 weeks later. Others prefer to remove the primary and the nodes in one extensive operation. Alternatively, if the nodes lie close to the primary, they may be included in a volume that is small enough to be treated to a radical dose. A 'wait and see' policy can then be adopted for the neck. If the nodes lie too far from the primary to be included in a radical volume, radical radiotherapy to the primary, followed by neck dissection, is generally the preferred sequence.

If the primary is treated first with irradiation and the nodes are enlarging and/or becoming fixed, a 'holding' single dose of 15 Gy to the involved node can be given. The block dissection can then be carried out as planned.

The local recurrence rate after radical neck dissection is high, of the order of 30%. There are three main risk factors for recurrence, of which extracapsular spread is the strongest predictor of recurrence.

— Invasion through the capsule of the nodes
(extracapsular spread)
— The size of the nodes (>3 cm)

— The number of nodes involved by tumour (more than three).

If one or more of these factors are present, postoperative radiotherapy is advisable to the involved side of the neck.

b. N2 nodes. Bilateral nodal metastases are associated with a poor prognosis. Complete radical neck dissection on both sides is not possible since the internal jugular vein has to be preserved on one side. In a bilateral block dissection, the operation on the second side is carried out at a later stage, with preservation of the internal jugular vein. The latter should be followed by postoperative radiotherapy. Because of the poor prognosis and morbidity of bilateral neck dissection, most patients are treated by bilateral radical neck irradiation.

3. Fixed nodes (N3). Fixed nodes are often regarded as inoperable. The interpretation of fixity is often difficult. Indeed nodes which appear fixed to the carotid sheath may sometimes be completely removed. Urgent joint assessment with a head and neck surgeon is essential to determine operability. Occasionally a fixed node may become mobile and operable after a course of radical irradiation. If the nodes are judged inoperable, the situation is almost invariably palliative.

4. Metastatic neck nodes (squamous carcinoma) of unknown primary site. In the upper and mid-cervical region the most likely primary sites are the nasopharynx, pyriform fossa and the vallecula. If the node is solitary and mobile, a radical neck dissection of the involved side should be considered. If the node is fixed and inoperable and the patient is fit, radical radiotherapy to both sides of the neck shielding the cord is recommended. If the nodes are large and multiple and biopsy shows undifferentiated carcinoma, the pharynx is a likely primary site. Radical radiotherapy should be delivered to the pharynx and nodes.

Five year survival for radical radiotherapy of metastatic neck nodes of unknown primary is poor (15%), but long-term survival is occasionally seen and justifies treatment.

Target volume and technique for neck irradiation

For irradiation of one side of the neck, the volume should be treated by a single anterior field extending from the mastoid process to the inferior border of the medial end of the clavicle (Fig. 20.10). The head is extended so that the submandibular and upper deep cervical nodes can be included while limiting dosage to the floor of the mouth. The medial margin of the field lies just lateral to the larynx and spinal cord. The neck nodes may be divided into five levels. The levels which need to irradiated are summarised in Table 20.2.

Avoidance of the spinal cord should be confirmed by simulator or port films. If verification is not available, the anterior field can be angled 10° laterally to ensure avoidance of the cord. The asymmetrical diaphragm technique is also useful. Bolus can be applied to the neck to compensate for the irregular contour of the neck and secure uniform dosage. This does however sacrifice the skin sparing effect of megavoltage irradiation.

For bilateral neck irradiation, a single anterior field is used to encompass the neck, with a 2 cm wide central lead strip protecting the midline structures. Bolus can be applied.

Dose and energy

48 Gy in 20 daily fractions over 4 weeks (4–6 MV photons)

Nodes which were palpable before irradiation are boosted to a further **12 Gy in 5 daily fractions over a week using electrons**. A technique for determining the energy for electrons to treat the nodes adequately without overdosing the spinal cord is shown in Figures 20.17 and 20.18.

Radiation reactions

Smoking and alcohol should be forbidden during the reaction period. About the third week of the course the mucosal reaction will begin (Fig. 20.11) and settle by 3 weeks after treatment. It is always a strain on any patient, with soreness, loss of taste and dysphagia.

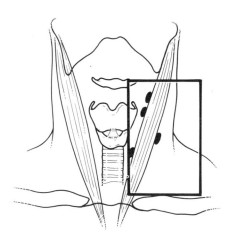

Fig. 20.10 Anterior field for irradiation of secondary neck nodes. A parallel posterior field can be added. The hyoid, thyroid and cricoid and upper tracheal cartilages are shown (from above downwards).

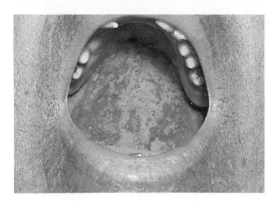

Fig. 20.11 Typical acute reaction on the hard palate during radical radiotherapy.

Patients need considerable moral support and reassurance from the treatment staff, and must be encouraged to take adequate nourishment and fluid. It is often advisable to admit to hospital during the acute phase, so that the nursing staff can ensure proper hygiene and nutrition. Mouthwashes should be frequently used, e.g. Difflam (a local analgesic and anti-inflammatory agent), sodium bicarbonate (a teaspoonful in a pint of warm water), or 0.01% chlorhexidine.

Complications of radiotherapy of cancer of the oral cavity

Late effects. After the acute reaction has passed, late effects follow which may be troublesome. Some degree of dryness of the mouth and throat is unavoidable, owing to inhibition of mucous glands. This will be particularly marked if the major salivary glands, especially the parotids, have been in the high dose region. It is important to leave at least one parotid gland in the low dose area if possible, and it is worthwhile adjusting field layouts with this in mind. Loss of taste is another unpleasant side-effect, but one which usually recovers.

Skin changes are generally mild with megavoltage radiation and give no trouble. Submental oedema sometimes occurs, due to lymphatic obstruction, giving a 'dewlap' appearance, but is seldom of sinister importance.

Fibrosis of the submandibular gland, often asymmetrical, may mimic nodal recurrence.

Radionecrosis of soft tissue and bone. Necrosis may occur in the soft tissues of the mouth and in the underlying mandible following both external beam and interstitial implantation. Soft tissue necrosis alone is commoner (15%) after implantation than after megavoltage external beam irradiation but usually heals with

conservative measures in a few weeks. Radionecrosis of the mandible (osteoradionecrosis) is more likely to occur if soft tissue necrosis develops on the overlying gingiva. Its incidence is much lower (2%) than soft tissue necrosis. With conventional fractionation radionecrosis is rarely seen under 60 Gy. The incidence is 1–2% up to 70 Gy and 9% above 70 Gy.

Osteoradionecrosis

Aetiology. Radiation causes damage both directly to bone and indirectly by impairing its vascular supply. The direct effect is considered the more important since the bone damage may occur without obvious vascular damage. Irradiation directly damages some of the bone cells, osteoclasts, which resorb bone and others, osteoblasts, which reconstruct it. These irradiated cells retain their function until some attempt to divide and then undergo mitotic death months or years after irradiation. Gradually the population of bone cells and thus the process of remodelling in the irradiated area diminish. As a result the mandible becomes thinner and loses its structural integrity.

Reduced vascular supply to the periosteum, due to damage to the endothelial cells that line the blood vessels, indirectly contributes to osteoradionecrosis.

Radionecrosis is seen much more frequently in the mandible than in the maxilla. This is because the mandible has denser bone than the maxilla and derives its blood supply only from the periosteum. By contrast the maxilla has a rich blood supply.

Infection may be introduced to the bone by local trauma, tooth extraction or dental infection. Infection stimulates cell division in bone and mitotic death. While tumour involvement may inhibit bone remodelling, it may also precipitate radionecrosis by stimulating the division of osteoblasts to remodel bone following the death of tumour cells. There is a threefold higher incidence of radionecrosis of the mandible in patients who have retained their teeth before radiotherapy compared with the edentulous. Patients with oral cancer are often alcoholic, with poor general medical state and oral hygiene. The latter predisposes to mucosal ulceration and ensuing osteoradionecrosis.

Diagnosis. Presentation is with a flat ulcer with bone visible at its base. It may be painless, even in the presence of a pathological fracture of the mandible. Pain, trismus and general ill health are, however, often present due to associated infection. A radiograph of the mandible (orthopantomogram) typically shows an area of rarefaction, sometimes with evidence of osteomyelitis or pathological fracture (Fig. 20.12).

Management of radionecrosis. Radionecrosis should be managed conservatively since surgical intervention

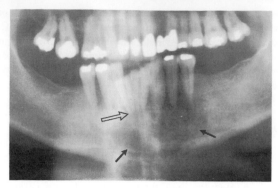

Fig. 20.12   Radiograph of the mandible (orthopantomogram) showing a radiolucent area of radionecrosis (small arrows) and an associated pathological fracture (large arrow). (Courtesy of Mr P McAndrew, Rotherham.)

may exacerbate the process of necrosis. Scrupulous attention should be paid to dental hygiene. Mouthwashes with 0.01% chlorhexidine should be carried out after each meal and the patient encouraged to remove food debris.

In most cases small areas of soft tissue necrosis heal within a few weeks with conservative local measures (antibiotics, steroids). If radionecrosis of the mandible occurs, a period of observation, often over months or several years, is worthwhile since spontaneous healing occurs in 50%. The dead bone (sequestrum) may separate spontaneously followed by healing. Once loose, the sequestrum can be carefully removed to avoid abrasion of the adjacent tongue. Surgical resection and reconstruction of the mandible may, however, be necessary to relieve the chronic pain and infection associated with mandibular radionecrosis. All the irradiated bone must be removed. Often both sides of the mandible are involved and require replacement, resulting in substantial deformity.

Results of treatment of oral cancer

About 90% of T1 and 75% of T2 tumours are controlled by radiotherapy. Salvage surgery is successful in approximately half of the failures. For T3 tumours the local control rate falls to 50% and few of the failures are successfully salvaged by surgery.

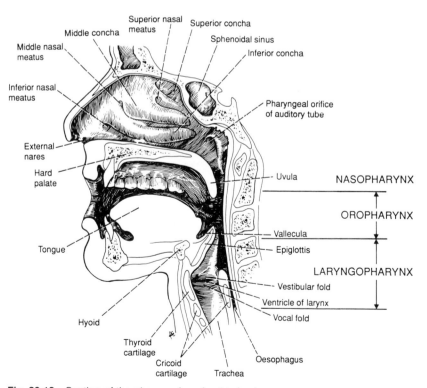

Fig. 20.13   Section of the pharynx, from front to back.

OROPHARYNX

Anatomy

The oropharynx (Fig. 20.13) extends from the junction of the hard and soft palate to the level of the vallecula. It contains the posterior third or base of the tongue, the soft palate, tonsils, and the posterior oropharyngeal wall.

The tonsil (Figs 20.1, 20.13 and 20.14) forms part of a protective ring (Waldeyer's ring), a more or less complete circle of lymphoid tissue at the entrance to the pharynx. It includes the two lateral tonsils, the nasopharyngeal tonsil (adenoids) on the roof and posterior wall of the nasopharynx, and lymphoid tissue on the posterior surface of the tongue (lingual tonsil).

The soft palate (Fig. 20.1A) is a mobile muscular flap which extends from the back of the hard palate. It divides the nasopharynx from the oropharynx. From the centre of the posterior border of the soft palate hangs the uvula which rests on the dorsum of the tongue.

CANCER OF THE TONSIL

Pathology

Tumours in this region are of two main types— squamous carcinoma from the epithelium (75%), and

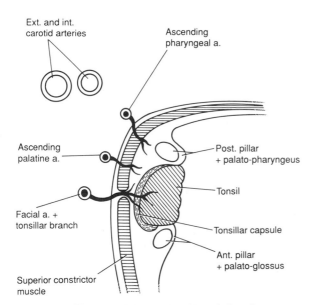

Fig. 20.14   Diagram of the tonsil and its relations in horizontal section. (Reproduced with permission from Ellis, Clinical Anatomy, 5th edn, Blackwells, 1975.)

Labels in figure:
Ext. and int. carotid arteries
Ascending pharyngeal a.
Ascending palatine a.
Post. pillar + palato-pharyngeus
Tonsil
Tonsillar capsule
Facial a. + tonsillar branch
Ant. pillar + palato-glossus
Superior constrictor muscle

non-Hodgkin lymphoma. Macroscopically they are either an exophytic mass protruding into the throat or infiltrative and ulcerating.

Spread

Local spread is early, beginning with the anterior and posterior pillars and the soft palate. The lower end of the anterior pillar extends to the posterolateral corner of the tongue, which may be invaded. Spread backwards involves the lateral wall of the oropharynx.

Lymphatic drainage of the anterior tonsillar pillar and fossa is to the jugulodigastric (tonsillar) node (Fig. 20.3) lying just behind the angle of the mandible and to the upper deep cervical nodes. If the soft palate is involved, spread may occur to the retropharyngeal nodes which lie between the pharynx and the pre-vertebral fascia on a plane just in front of the mastoid process.

Tumours confined to the posterior pillar are rare. They spread inferiorly to the posterior pharyngeal wall and, unlike tumours of the anterior pillar, may involve the spinal accessory nodes.

Careful local examination by inspection and palpation is essential since the technique and success of local treatment depend on it.

Clinical features

Symptoms are minimal at the start, with slight sore throat; in later stages, dysphagia and pain may be prominent. Often it is the secondary mass in the neck which brings the patient to the doctor, and the primary is only then discovered.

In general, tumours of the anterior tonsillar pillar are less aggressive and, like tumours of the retromolar trigone and soft palate, present less frequently with palpable neck nodes (40–50%) than tumours of the tonsillar fossa (75%). Overall 75% of tonsillar tumours are associated with palpable nodes and in 20% they are bilateral.

Treatment

In general radiotherapy is preferable to surgery since local cure can often be obtained without the functional and cosmetic impairment of radical surgery.

Radical radiotherapy is mainly by external beam since both primary and cervical nodes need to be treated. Some radiotherapists have obtained better local control in early T1 tumours without nodes by boosting the primary with an iridium implant using the 'loop' technique (Fig. 19.4 B). Surgery is, however, possible

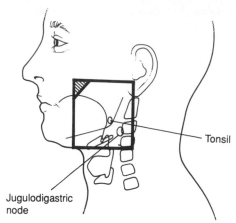

Fig. 20.15 Treatment volume for small tumours of the tonsillar fossa. Lead shielding as indicated for opposing lateral fields. (Redrawn from Dobbs & Barrett, Practical Radiotherapy Planning, Ist edn, Edward Arnold, 1985.)

and equally effective for early T1 and T2 tumours. Surgery involves a radical tonsillectomy, partial mandibulectomy and ipsilateral radical neck dissection. Loss of tissue is compensated for by a flap repair.

Radical radiotherapy

Epithelial tumours

Small tumours of the tonsillar fossa or anterior tonsillar pillar without nodes (N0)

Target volume
The primary site and the ipsilateral submandibular and upper deep cervical nodes are irradiated (Fig. 20.15). The superior margin includes the roof of the hard palate. The inferior limit is the lower margin of the hyoid bone. Anteriorly, the field extends through the middle third of the tongue. The posterior border lies just anterior to the spinal cord. The medial limit is the midline.

Technique
An anterior and lateral right-angled wedged pair is used or, for T1 tumours, an oblique lateral wedged pair with CT planning (Fig. 20.16A) .

Larger tumours involving the soft palate or base of tongue or crossing the midline

Target volume
These tumours have a higher propensity for bilateral nodal spread. The target volume should therefore include the primary site and the upper deep cervical nodes on both sides of the neck.

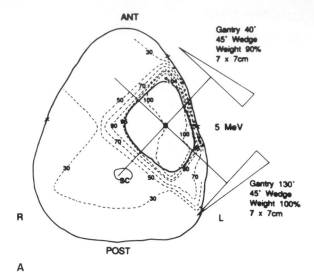

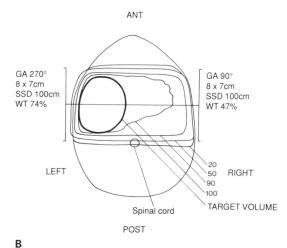

Fig. 20.16 Early carcinoma of the tonsil. **A** Anterior and posterior oblique wedged pair of fields. (Reproduced with permission from Dobbs & Barrett, Practical Radiotherapy Planning, Ist edn, Edward Arnold, 1985.) **B** Parallel opposed fields for treatment of early carcinoma of the left tonsil with 2:1 weighting.

Technique
Parallel opposed megavoltage fields are used with a 2:1 weighting on the side of the primary (Fig. 20.16B). The weighting enables a lower but prophylactic dose to the tonsil on the opposite side and the upper deep cervical nodes while limiting the dose to the contra-lateral oral mucosa and parotid gland. After 40 Gy, if involved nodes overlie the cord, that part of the volume is treated with electrons of suitable energy (Figs 20.17 and 20.18).

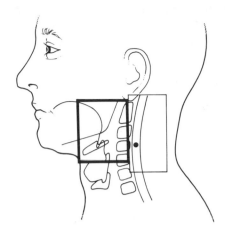

Fig. 20.17 Early tonsillar cancer with nodal involvement. Diagram showing field margins of megavoltage (bold) field to primary tumour and jugulodigastric node and electron beam (light) to posterior cervical nodes. Black dot marks thinnest point of the neck at which depth of spinal cord is measured for choice of electron energy.

Dose and energy

1. Nodal disease not overlying spinal cord
60 Gy in 25 daily fractions over 5 weeks (4–6 MV photons)

2. Nodal disease overlying spinal cord. As for tongue (p. 318).

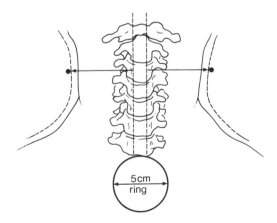

Fig. 20.18 Technique for measuring the minimum depth of the spinal cord in the neck within an electron field. A ball bearing is placed on each side of the shell at the narrowest point of the neck overlying the cord and within the electron field. The surface marking of the spinal cord is a line running inferior to the mastoid process. A simulator film is taken with a magnification ring. The distance from the ball bearing to the lateral border of the spinal cord is measured. Electron energy is chosen to minimise the dose to the spinal cord. (Courtesy of Dr I Manifold, Sheffield.)

Lymphomas. Lower doses are needed to treat lymphomas compared with squamous carcinomas of the head and neck, since lymphomas are more radiosensitive.

Target volume
Wide field regional radiotherapy is indicated. The volume includes Waldeyer's ring and the lymph nodes on both sides of the neck from the base of the skull to the clavicles.

Technique
There are two chief alternative techniques: (1) lateral opposed fields reaching high enough to include the nasopharynx, and (2) anterior and posterior opposed fields, making allowance for the irregular contour and varying thickness of the neck, either by using bolus on the neck or shielding the laryngeal region with lead for part of the course.

Dose and energy

Low grade non-Hodgkin lymphomas
35 Gy in 20 daily fractions over 4 weeks (4–6 MV photons)

High grade non-Hodgkin lymphomas
40–45 Gy in 20 daily fractions over 4 weeks (4–6 MV photons)

The primary lesion in the mouth can, if necessary, be raised to higher dosage locally by supplementary small fields after the main course, to give an extra 5–10 Gy. These must avoid the spinal cord and should be checked on the simulator or by portal films. Dosage to the spinal cord should not exceed 40 Gy.

Radiation reactions. Mucositis, especially in radical treatments, is inevitably troublesome, with sore throat, dysphagia, dryness and loss of taste. It is often desirable to admit the patient to hospital towards the end of the course for nursing care, mouth hygiene and nutrition, especially fluid intake. An aspirin–mucilage mixture before meals helps to make swallowing more comfortable.

Cervical nodes from squamous carcinoma of the oropharynx

The management has been discussed above (p. 319) and most of it is applicable here. The situation is similar to the posterior third of tongue, with a high proportion of anaplastic growths, and involvement of nodes of neck from the start. In such cases treatment should be directed to the primary and the whole of the neck

(40 Gy in 20 fractions over 4 weeks) and possible supplementary fields as outlined on page 318.

Results of treatment

The prognosis for growths with no evident secondaries is fairly good, with 5-year survival about 75%, falling to 40% in the presence of secondary nodes. The highest local control rates have been obtained in T1 and T2 tumours by combining external beam and interstitial implantation.

SOFT PALATE

Treatment

For squamous tumours of the soft palate radiotherapy is the treatment of choice. The target volume is similar to the tonsil, with the exception that the posterior margin should extend back to include the retropharyngeal nodes to which the soft palate drains.

For tumours <3 cm the choice is between external beam (60 Gy in 25 daily fractions over 5 weeks (4–6 MV photons), and implantation (65–70 Gy) using the loop technique (Fig. 19.4B); for tumours >3 cm, external beam to 48 Gy in 20 daily fractions with a boost by implant (20 Gy) to the primary site or external beam alone (60 Gy in 25 daily fractions over 5 weeks).

This is a very difficult site to implant successfully. For superficial lesions a permanent gold grain implant

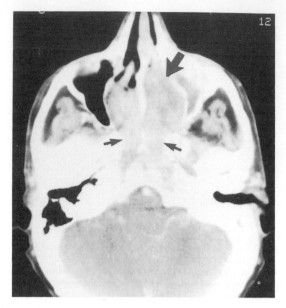

Fig. 20.20 CT scan showing carcinoma of the nasopharynx (back arrows) extending into the nasal cavity (front arrow). (Courtesy of Dr R Nakielny, Sheffield.)

or an iridium wire implant using the loop technique is possible. The latter technique includes excision of the uvula before implantation to avoid underdosage to this outcrop of the soft palate.

Prophylactic neck node irradiation should be considered according to the guidelines in Table 20.2 in view of common and bilateral involvement.

CARCINOMA OF NASOPHARYNX (POSTNASAL SPACE)

Anatomy

The nasopharynx is the nasal part of the pharynx (Fig. 20.13). It is pyramidal in shape. Its roof is the base of the skull, formed by the body of the sphenoid bone and the basiocciput. The roof curves backwards to become continuous with the posterior wall. The latter is formed by the upper cervical vertebrae. Anteriorly, the nasopharynx is continuous with the nasal cavity. On the lateral walls of the nasopharynx are the orifices of the auditory (eustachian) tube which leads to the middle ear. Immediately behind this tubal opening is a deep depression, the pharyngeal recess (Fig. 20.19) (fossa of Rosenmüller). This is a common site of origin for nasopharyngeal cancer (Fig. 20.20). The floor is the upper border of the soft palate. Lymphatic spread is to the node of Rouvière (Fig. 20.3) lying in the retropharyngeal space (Fig. 20.1B) in front of the atlas (first cervical

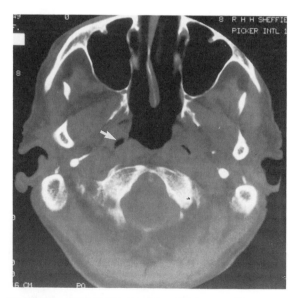

Fig. 20.19 CT scan showing normal anatomy of the nasopharynx. The fossa of Rosenmüller (pharyngeal recess) is arrowed. (Courtesy of Dr R Nakielny, Sheffield.)

vertebra) and to the posterior, upper and midcervical nodes.

Epidemiology

Nasopharyngeal cancer represents 0.1% of all cancers and of cancer deaths. Although rare in Western Europe, nasopharyngeal cancer is very common in parts of the Far East. In areas of Southern China it accounts for the majority of malignant disease. The strongest evidence for a causative agent is the presence of antibodies to a virus (Epstein–Barr) in the blood of patients with nasopharyngeal carcinoma and there is evidence that this virus can persist as a latent infection in nasopharyngeal epithelium. The smoking and curing of fish, a common practice in the Far East, have been postulated as sources of chemical carcinogens. The disease is commoner in men (sex ratio 3:1) and commonest between the ages of 40 and 60.

Pathology

The great majority are squamous carcinomas, often poorly differentiated with a florid lymphocytic infiltrate (lymphoepithelioma); they are difficult to distinguish from lymphoma. Some are lymphomas, almost invariably of the non-Hodgkin type. Adenocarcinomas of salivary type also occur but are rare.

Spread

The mode of spread is important and accounts for the great variety of presenting symptoms—to the posterior part of the nose (nasal obstruction, bleeding), eustachian tube (deafness), upper cervical vertebrae (pain), base of skull (double vision due to involvement of third, fourth and sixth cranial nerves from spread into the cavernous sinus through the foramen lacerum). The ninth, tenth, eleventh and twelfth cranial nerves may also be affected. This can be due to direct extension of tumour into the parapharyngeal space from the lateral wall of the nasopharynx or due to involvement of the node of Rouvière. Tumour may be visible in the nose or bulging behind the soft palate in the mouth. Growth is insidious, and the commonest presentation (50%) is an enlarged node in the neck just below the lobe of the ear (jugulo-digastric) or in the posterior cervical chain.

Diagnosis and investigation

The nasopharynx should be examined with a mirror or in theatre under anaesthesia and visible tumour biopsied. Even if no tumour is seen, biopsy is still worthwhile since a microscopic tumour may occasionally be revealed. Investigation includes a soft tissue lateral film to show the air cavities and irregularities of the nasopharyngeal wall and special projections to examine the base of the skull for bone erosion. A CT scan of the nasopharynx and neck should be carried out to detail the extent of local spread and nodal involvement. It is also a useful means of assessing the response to treatment.

Treatment

Surgery is quite impractical, and external irradiation is the treatment of choice for both epithelial tumours and lymphomas.

Radical radiotherapy

Epithelial tumours

Target volume
For squamous cell carcinoma, this should include the primary and the routes of spread, particularly the base of the skull. The primary site and the upper deep cervical, lateral pharyngeal and upper posterior triangle lymph nodes on both sides of the neck should be included (Fig. 20.21).

For all undifferentiated tumours and squamous

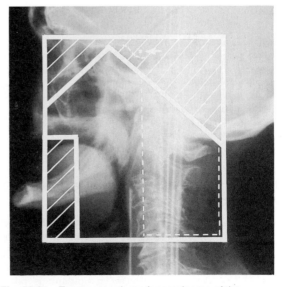

Fig. 20.21 Treatment volume for carcinoma of the nasopharynx (interrupted lines for electrons). Note the shielding of the anterior orbit, optic chiasm (arrowed) and of the brainstem. (Courtesy of Dr I Manifold, Sheffield.)

carcinoma with node involvement all the nodes on both sides of the neck (levels I–V) should be irradiated (see Table 20.2).

Technique

The patient lies supine with the head extended. A full head shell is required. A large lateral opposed pair of fields encompass the primary tumour and the nodes of the upper neck. The field includes the nasopharynx, the base of skull, the parapharyngeal space and the posterior half of the orbit (but ensuring full tumour dose is not given to the posterior retina) and any tumour extending into the nasal cavity or the oropharynx. An additional direct anterior field may be required if there is involvement of the nasal cavity. The front half of the orbit, brainstem and optic chiasm are shielded with lead (Fig. 20.21). The doses to the lens are calculated using thermoluminescent dosimetry (p. 78). Once a maximum safe dose to the spinal cord has been reached (40 Gy in 20 daily fractions), the volume is reduced by bringing the posterior margin of the field in front of the spinal cord. Involved nodes overlying and posterior to the spinal cord are boosted with electrons (Figs 20.17 and 20.18).

The lower neck is treated by a direct anterior field with midline shielding of the larynx and spinal cord.

Dose and energy

Primary tumour and palpable nodes
40 Gy in 20 daily fractions over 4 weeks (4–6 MV photons)

Reduced volume (lying in front of cord)
26 Gy in 13 fractions over 2.5 weeks (4–6 MV photons)

Electrons of suitable energy to the same dose to nodes overlying and posterior to the spinal cord.
Total dose: 66 Gy in 33 daily fractions over 6.5 weeks

Prophylactic nodal areas
50 Gy in 25 daily fractions over 5 weeks (4–6 MV photons or photons with electron boost)

The choice of electron energy for treating the nodes is based on the measurement of the depth of the spinal cord from the surface of the neck. A small ball-bearing is placed on the shell at the thinnest part of the neck (Fig. 20.18). An anteroposterior radiograph is taken with a 5 cm brass circle to calculate the magnification factor. The distance between the ball-bearing and the lateral margin of the cord (approximately 0.5 cm

lateral to the midline) is measured and adjusted for magnification.

Radiation reaction. Dysphagia due to oropharyngeal mucositis is accompanied by loss of taste. The former usually settles within a few weeks of the end of treatment but the latter may persist for several months.

Complications. The most troublesome long-term symptom is usually dryness of the mouth due to the total inhibition of the secretion of both parotid glands. The risk of dental caries is increased and good dental care is essential.

Secretory otitis media from fibrosis of the eustachian tube is very common. Treatment is by the insertion of grommets.

Damage to spinal cord, brainstem or optic nerves is rare with careful planning. Some dose to the lens may be unavoidable, with resultant cataract. Biochemical evidence of hypopituitarism is not uncommon but clinical hypopituitarism is rare.

Lymphomas. These are managed on the lines laid down for mouth and tonsil (p. 325).

Results of treatment

For squamous cell carcinoma, overall 5-year survival is about 60%. The lower the level of nodal involvement in the neck, the worse is the prognosis.

Non-Hodgkin lymphomas have a slightly better outlook.

PARANASAL SINUSES

Anatomy

The paranasal sinuses include the maxillary antrum, ethmoid, sphenoid and frontal sinuses.

The maxillary sinus (or antrum) lies in the cavity of the upper jaw (maxilla). It is related (Fig. 20.22) medially to the nasal cavity, inferiorly to the alveolus, superiorly to the orbit and ethmoid sinuses, laterally to the cheek and posteriorly to the pterygoid fossa. The maxillary antrum can be usefully divided into two parts. These are separated by an imaginary line (Ohngren's line) running from the medial canthus to the angle of the mandible. The upper part is known as the *suprastructure* and the lower as the *infrastructure*.

The ethmoid sinuses lie between medial walls of the orbits and upper nasal cavity and superiorly on each side of the cribriform plate below the frontal lobes of the brain.

The sphenoid sinuses lie in the body of the sphenoid bone beneath the pituitary fossa, one on each side of the midline. Each drains into the nasal cavity.

The frontal sinuses are related posteriorly to the

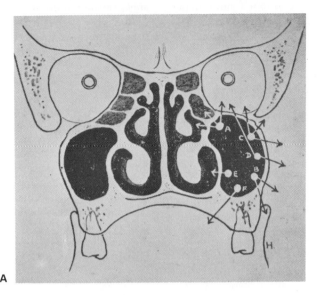

Fig. 20.22 **A** Coronal section through the orbit, nose and mouth. The arrows show various possible pathways of tumours arising in different parts of the maxillary antrum. (Reproduced with permission from Rock Carling, Windeyer & Smithers, British Practice in Radiotherapy, Butterworths, 1955.) **B** Coronal section through orbit, nose and mouth. (Reproduced with permission from Walmsley R & Murphy T R 1972 Jamieson's Illustrations of Regional Anatomy, 9th edn, Churchill Livingstone.)

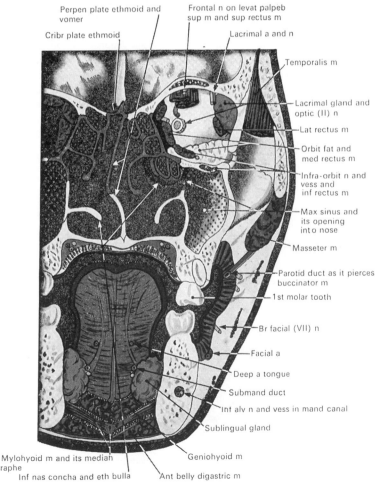

Perpen plate ethmoid and vomer

Cribr plate ethmoid

Frontal n on levat palpeb sup m and sup rectus m

Lacrimal a and n

Temporalis m

Lacrimal gland and optic (II) n

Lat rectus m

Orbit fat and med rectus m

Infra-orbit n and vess and inf rectus m

Max sinus and its opening into nose

Masseter m

Parotid duct as it pierces buccinator m

1st molar tooth

Br facial (VII) n

Facial a

Deep a tongue

Submand duct

Int alv n and vess in mand canal

Sublingual gland

Geniohyoid m

Mylohyoid m and its median raphe

Inf nas concha and eth bulla

Ant belly digastric m

B

frontal lobes. Inferiorly are the ethmoid sinuses, the roof of the nose and the orbits.

Epidemiology

Tumours of the nose and paranasal sinuses are uncommon. They account for 0.2% of all cancers and of cancer deaths. The maxillary antrum is the commonest site, followed by the ethmoids. Causative factors are obscure but exposure to wood dusts in the timber industry and furniture manufacture and leather dust in the shoe industry account for some tumours (adenocarcinoma), presumably due to a carcinogen. The maximum incidence is between the ages of 55 and 75. The male to female ratio is 1.7:1.

MAXILLARY ANTRUM

Pathology

Squamous carcinoma is the usual type. Adenocarcinoma, lymphoma and various sarcomas (e.g. osteosarcoma, fibrosarcoma) can occur.

Spread

The tumour usually begins in the lining of the membrane of the cavity and can therefore remain silent for a long time. Tumours in the antroethmoidal

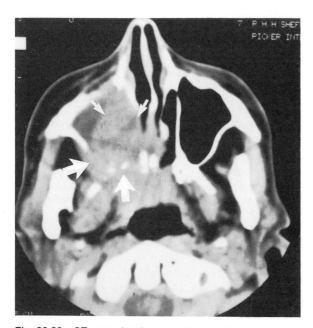

Fig. 20.23 CT scan showing a carcinoma of the maxillary antrum (small arrows) invading the pterygoid fossa (large arrows). (Courtesy of Dr R Nakielny, Sheffield.)

angle in the ethmoids (A in Fig. 20.22A) may spread to the nose and superficially into the subcutaneous tissues above or below the inner canthus. Tumours of the anterolateral wall (B in Fig. 20.22A), if lying inferiorly, cause swelling of the cheek with depression of the angle of the mouth. Tumours arising in the upper part of the anterolateral wall (C in Fig. 20.22A) may invade the zygoma and cause swelling below the outer canthus. The eye may be displaced upwards if the tumour invades the floor of the orbit. Tumours of the posterolateral wall may invade the orbit from behind, causing protrusion of the eye (proptosis), or the pterygoid region, presenting as a mass in the lower part of the temporal fossa. Tumours at the latter site often cause trismus. Spread to nodes in the neck is late.

Clinical features

Symptoms arise eventually from local spread—nasal blockage, discharge and bleeding, bulging of the cheek, or ulceration in the mouth. If the orbit is invaded, the eye may be pushed upwards, causing double vision (diplopia), or forwards (proptosis). Palpable nodes are uncommon at presentation (<10%).

Oral pain may at first be thought to be arising from the teeth. Tumour presenting in the mouth may be mistaken for a primary tumour of the gum. It is essential to exclude a tumour originating in the antrum in any patient with malignant disease presenting in the hard palate or upper gums.

Investigation

Plain radiographs or tomograms may show destruction of the antral walls. CT scanning is the most accurate means of assessing local spread (Fig. 20.23) and determining operability.

Treatment

Both surgery and radiotherapy yield poor results since these tumours are usually advanced at presentation.

Surgical excision is suitable for small well-differentiated tumours and may be curative. However it involves gross mutilation, with the removal of the upper jaw and any invaded structures. A dental prosthesis is necessary to compensate for the palatal defect. If the orbit is involved, removal of the orbital contents including the eye will be necessary. Post-operative radiotherapy is often given, based on the operative findings and histology. Residual disease or moderately or poorly differentiated histology favours the use of radiation.

Radical radiotherapy

Primary radiotherapy is appropriate for patients whose tumours are inoperable or who are unfit for or refuse surgery.

Before radiation begins, it is important to provide adequate drainage of the antral cavity because (1) it is always more or less infected from the start and (2) as radiation proceeds, fragments of growth and dead bone will become foci of further infection, leading to pent-up discharges, necrosis and pain during treatment. Surgical drainage is carried out, preferably by palatal antrostomy, i.e. removal of part of the hard palate and upper alveolus, thus permanently exposing the interior of the antrum. The surgeon removes any loose and decayed teeth, dead bone and necrotic debris and takes a biopsy. The opening has another advantage—the cavity can be inspected later for evidence of recurrence. The gap is closed by an individually made obturator worn like a denture, so the patient can eat and speak normally.

Target volume

The region is awkward for the therapist because of the irregular contours and the proximity of the eyes, both of which must be taken into account in the treatment plan. A full head mould with beam direction is desirable. This is an ideal site for CT planning.

1. If there is no suspicion of invasion of the orbits, the target volume encompasses the tumour, the whole of the maxillary antrum and potential pathways of spread. The lower margin includes the hard palate. The medial limit, the inner canthus of the opposite eye, extends across the midline to cover both ethmoid

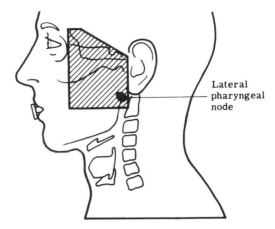

Fig. 20.25 Margins of the lateral field with lead shielding to the optic chiasm and hypothalamus. (Reproduced with permission from Dobbs and Barrett, Practical Radiotherapy Planning, Ist edn, Edward Arnold, 1985.)

sinuses and the nasal cavity. The lateral margin is the gingivobuccal sulcus. Anteriorly the limit is the cheek and posteriorly the pterygoid fossa and the lateral pharyngeal node (Figs 20.24 and 20.25).

2. If the overlying skin of the cheek is involved by tumour, wax bolus is used to overcome the skin sparing effect of megavoltage irradiation. The target volume is otherwise the same as above.

3. If invaded by tumour, the orbit must be included in the treatment volume.

Irradiation of the eye must be fully and carefully explained to the patient, so that he or she understands the vital necessity of irradiating the eye and the likelihood of deterioration of vision in later years.

The fields should extend to the roof of the orbit. The target volume is otherwise as above. No effort is made to spare the eye on the involved side, but every effort is made to avoid the other eye.

Technique

A full head mould with mouth bite is needed. A right-angled wedge pair is the commonest technique. The lateral field is angled about 5–10° posteriorly to avoid the contralateral lens. A third postero-oblique field may be needed from the contralateral side to compensate for the fall-off in dose at the posteromedial part of the target volume (Fig. 20.26).

The brain and optic chiasm are shielded. Whenever the orbit has to be included, the patient should be instructed to keep the eyes open during radiation exposure and look up into the X-ray beam, thus making use of the surface sparing effect of megavoltage irradiation. If wax bolus is used, cylindrical peep-holes

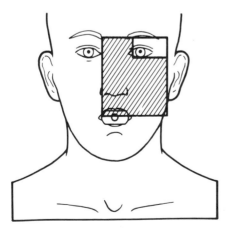

Fig. 20.24 Margins of the anterior field with lead shielding to the cornea, lens and lacrimal gland. (Reproduced with permission from Dobbs and Barrett, Practical Radiotherapy Planning, Ist edn, Edward Arnold, 1985.)

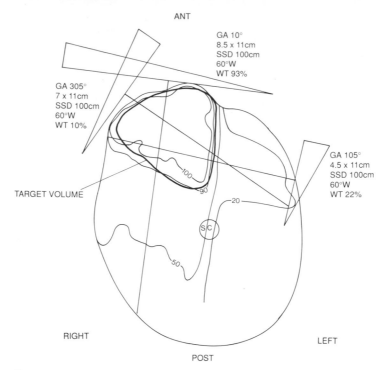

Fig. 20.26   Three field technique for treatment of carcinoma of the maxillary antrum. (Courtesy of Dr A Champion, Sheffield.)

1.5 cm in diameter should be cut out for this purpose. This minimises damage to the cornea.

Dose and energy
60 Gy in 25 daily fractions over 5 weeks (4–6 MV photons)

The dose to the optic chiasm should be measured and should not exceed 40 Gy.

Palliative radiotherapy

For advanced cases the technique is simpler and it is often adequate to apply a single direct anterior field.

An applied dose of 45 Gy in 15 daily fractions over 3 weeks (4–6 MV photons)

Radiation reactions. Skin and mucosal reactions develop in the usual way and are managed on similar lines.

Irradiation of the eye leads to conjunctivitis, beginning in the latter part of the course. Antibacterial eyedrops (Chloromycetin) should be instilled daily to counteract infection which might damage the cornea.

Late effects on the eye are described in Chapter 27. If full dosage has been given, degenerative changes on the lens (cataract) and retina are virtually certain, commonly about 3 or 4 years later. Vision will be impaired

and may be lost entirely. Sometimes a chronically painful eye has to be enucleated. If the eye has been irradiated, follow-up by an ophthalmologist is recommended.

Neck nodes

The management of neck nodes is summarised in Table 20.2. Unless involved, the cervical nodes need not be treated. If they are palpable, a radical neck dissection may be preferable to irradiation since their inclusion may make the target volume too large for a radical dose.

Results of treatment

The 5-year local control for tumours of the infrastructure is better than for the suprastructure (65% versus less than 50%). For more advanced disease it is about 30%. Failure is usually due to persistent or recurrent disease at the primary site.

CANCER OF THE ETHMOID SINUS

Since the ethmoids lie between the orbit, they are liable to be secondarily involved by tumours of the maxillary antrum and nasal cavity. It is often difficult to say exactly where a growth originated.

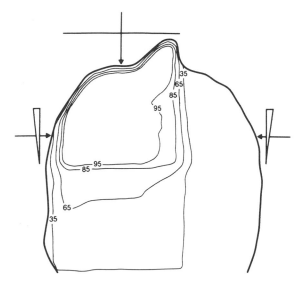

Fig. 20.27   Carcinoma of ethmoid and antrum—three field technique. (Reproduced with permission from Easson & Pointon, The Radiotherapy of Malignant Disease, Ist edn, Springer-Verlag, 1985.)

Clinical features

It may present at the side of the bridge of the nose, or more often with nasal blockage. The orbit is very liable to invasion and the eye may be pushed laterally.

Investigation and staging

The diagnosis is confirmed by biopsy. A CT scan is essential to assess the extent of bone destruction, especially posteriorly (Fig. 20.23).

Treatment

Surgical treatment is hardly ever practicable. Radiation is the usual method and the general principles are similar to those for carcinoma of the maxillary antrum.

Radical radiotherapy

Target volume
The target volume includes the ethmoid sinuses, the maxillary antrum and the nose, but avoiding the eye.

Technique
Figure 20.27 shows a technique for an early tumour, using a heavily weighted anterior field, with supplementary dosage (approximately 10% of the total) from two wedged lateral fields directed behind the lens of each eye, to boost the dosage in the posterior part of the sinus. The front border of the lateral fields lies behind the orbit to avoid the eye. The dose to the optic chiasm must not exceed 40 Gy.

Results of treatment

The 5-year survival for carcinoma of the ethmoid sinus is about 30%.

CANCER OF THE NOSE AND NASAL SINUSES

Tumours of the nose and nasal cavity are rare. Squamous cell carcinoma is the commonest histological type (though its nomenclature has been confusing over the years, and it is often called transitional cell carcinoma). The aetiology of most tumours at these sites is unknown. However workers in the furniture and timber industries (wood dust) and the leather footwear industry are at increased risk of adenocarcinoma. Adenoid cystic carcinoma, malignant melanoma and olfactory neuroblastoma are rare.

Clinical features

Symptoms are of nasal bleeding, discharge or obstruction. Tumours may be visible on inspection of the nasal cavity. Lymph node involvement is uncommon.

Diagnosis and staging

An examination under anaesthesia of the nasal cavity and a biopsy are required. A CT scan is essential to determine the posterior extent.

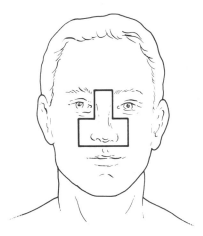

Fig. 20.28   Carcinoma of the nasal cavity—single anterior field. (Redrawn from Easson & Pointon, The Radiotherapy of Malignant Disease, Ist edn, Springer-Verlag, 1985.)

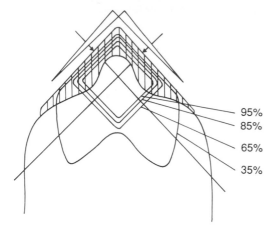

Fig. 20.29 Carcinoma of nasal cavity—wedge pair (5 × 5 cm). (Redrawn from Easson & Pointon, The Radiotherapy of Malignant Disease, Springer-Verlag, 1985.)

Treatment

Radical radiotherapy is the treatment of choice.

Radical radiotherapy

Target volume and technique

For anterior lesions of the nasal cavity a direct anterior field may suffice (Fig. 20.28) to cover the nose. For more posterior lesions an anterior oblique wedged pair is recommended (Fig. 20.29). The eyes should be shielded with lead. The optic chiasm must not be overdosed.

Dose and energy

60 Gy in 25 daily fractions over 5 weeks (4–6 MV photons or 12–16 MeV electrons)

Results of treatment

Overall 5-year local control is 70%.

THE EAR

CANCER OF THE EXTERNAL AND MIDDLE EAR

Anatomy

The three parts of the ear are the external ear, the middle ear and the inner ear (Fig. 20.30).

The *external ear* consists of the pinna or auricle, the external auditory meatus and the tympanic membrane. The external auditory meatus is the passage leading from the tympanic membrane to the exterior.

It is important to distinguish tumours arising from the anterolateral and posteromedial parts of the ear, particularly if electron beam therapy is not available. In the anteromedial part of the ear the skin is closely adherent to the underlying cartilage. Radionecrosis is likely if superficial or orthovoltage irradiation is employed due to the higher absorption in cartilage (see below). In the posteromedial part, the blood supply is richer due to a thin layer of subcutaneous tissue between skin and cartilage. The risk of radionecrosis is less.

The *middle ear* is a narrow cavity in the petrous part of the temporal bone. It contains the auditory ossicles.

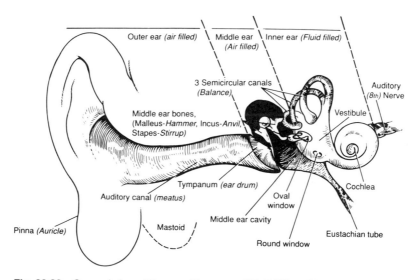

Fig. 20.30 General view of the ear. (Courtesy of Mr P Elliott, Sheffield.)

The lateral wall of the middle ear is the tympanic membrane. The medial wall separates it from the inner ear. Anteriorly it is connected to the pharynx by the eustachian tube. Posteriorly it communicates with the tympanic antrum and the mastoid air cells. Behind the tympanic antrum lie the sigmoid sinus and cerebellum. Inferiorly lies the jugular vein and superiorly the middle cranial fossa and the temporal lobe of the brain.

The *inner ear* is contained in the petrous part of the temporal bone. It contains the cochlea, the organ of hearing.

The lymphatic drainage of external ear is to the parotid and preauricular nodes anteriorly and to the postauricular and external jugular nodes posteriorly.

CANCER OF THE PINNA

The majority of tumours of the pinna arise from the skin. Basal cell carcinomas are more common than squamous cell carcinomas.

Treatment

These tumours may be treated by both surgery and radiotherapy. Before the advent of electron beam therapy, tumours of the anterolateral part of the ear were treated by excision. This was because of the risk of cartilage radionecrosis resulting from the attenuation of superficial or orthovoltage X-rays in tissues of high atomic number due to the photoelectric process (p. 64). With electrons, as with other forms of megavoltage irradiation of high photon energy, attenuation is largely by pair production (p. 61). Absorption in cartilage and bone is therefore much lower than with lower photon energies.

The majority of tumours of the pinna can be treated satisfactorily with electron beam therapy. The energy chosen is suited to the thickness of the lesion. Surgery is recommended for tumours of the external auditory meatus and retroauricular sulcus if they have invaded cartilage or bone.

Radical radiotherapy

Target volume
This should include the tumour with a 0.5 cm margin for basal cell carcinomas and a 1 cm margin for squamous cell carcinomas.

Technique
The ideal treatment is with a direct single field using electrons because of their sharp fall-off in dose at depth and limited absorption in cartilage or bone. In general

6–10 MeV electrons are adequate, depending on the thickness of the lesion. The patient is treated supine with the head turned away from the affected side. A margin of 1 cm of normal tissue around the tumour is included. An impression is taken for a lead cut-out. To compensate for the air gap the ear is filled with wet bolus or a wax cast to the level of the top of the ear. If electrons rather than superficial or orthovoltage are used, the surface of the treated area is boolused to an appropriate thickness to overcome the skin sparing effect and bring the maximum dose to the surface.

For tumours of the posterior part of the pinna, the skin of the mastoid region can be shielded from the exit dose with a small wedge of wax to absorb the electrons.

Dose and energy

Tumours <3 cm
50 Gy in 10 daily fractions over 2 weeks (6–10 MeV electrons)

Tumours >3 cm
55 Gy in 15 fractions over 3 weeks (6–10 MeV electrons)

Reaction and complications. The skin reaction and its management are as for other sites (see p. 298). However, perichondritis may occur, especially if the cartilage is invaded. The clinical features of perichondritis are pain and exquisite local tenderness, often with evidence of local infection. It is important to start antibiotic therapy early to prevent radionecrosis.

Results of treatment

The results of treatment are excellent, with an overall cure rate of 90%.

CANCER OF THE EXTERNAL AUDITORY CANAL AND MIDDLE EAR

Pathology

These tumours are rare. They occur mainly in middle age. Squamous carcinoma is the usual type. Other tumours include adenoid cystic carcinoma and sarcomas. There is an association with chronic ear infection (otitis media) and a discharging ear in most cases. Because of this, malignant change is insidious and apt to be overlooked.

Spread

Tumours of the cartilaginous part of the canal tend

to be expansive while those of the bony part are confined by the bony walls. Spread to the auricle and middle ear is common.

With tumours of the middle ear, local spread with accompanying sepsis occurs early. It may be backward into the mastoid bone, forward towards the naso-pharynx, outward to the external auditory meatus, upward to the cranial cavity, downward to the jugular region, inward to the inner ear and petrous part of the temporal bone. The facial nerve is often invaded, causing facial palsy (weakness or paralysis of the muscles of the face). The temporomandibular joint and parotid gland may also be invaded.

Clinical features

The clinical picture is usually of infection, with even-tual blood-stained discharge. Examination may show granulation tissue and polypoid fragments. Pain is absent at the start. Later there will be facial palsy and deafness.

Diagnosis and investigation

The ear, parotid and mastoid regions must be ex-amined and the neck palpated for nodes. The integrity of the cranial nerves (especially the seventh) is checked. The nasopharynx should be inspected to exclude anteromedial spread. When suspicion is aroused, examination under anaesthesia is necessary to obtain a biopsy. Most tumours are advanced at the time of

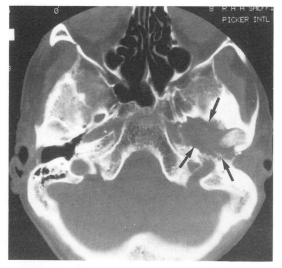

Fig. 20.31 CT scan showing a carcinoma of the middle ear eroding the petrous temporal bone. (Courtesy of Dr R Nakielny, Sheffield.)

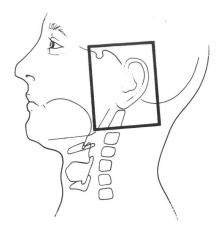

Fig. 20.32 Field margins for carcinoma of the middle ear. (Redrawn from Dobbs & Barrett, Practical Radiotherapy Planning, lst edn, Edward Arnold, 1985.)

diagnosis. Skull X-ray, tomograms, CT (Fig. 20.31) and MRI scanning may help in assessing the degree of bony (base of skull and petrous temporal bone) and soft tissue (mastoid and parotid) spread.

Treatment

The results of both surgery and radiotherapy are equally poor for cancer of the middle ear. Mastoidectomy is appropriate for early tumours. For more advanced tumours (1) biopsy followed by radical radiotherapy or (2) radical surgery followed by postoperative radiotherapy are recommended.

Radical radiotherapy

Target volume
This includes the primary tumour, the mastoid process and the pre- and postauricular nodes (Fig. 20.32). The pre- and postauricular nodes define the anterior and posterior limits respectively. The superior margin lies below the eye. The inferior margin is the tip of the mastoid bone. The wedge-shaped volume with its apex towards the brainstem is illustrated in Figure 20.33.

Technique
A head shell is needed, with the patient lying supine with the head rotated 90° away from the treated side so that the treated ear faces upwards. The head is extended to avoid irradiation of the eye from the exit beam of the posterior field. Anteroposterior and lateral radiographs are taken and the target volume marked. Anterior and posterior oblique fields are used. Care is taken to ensure the posterior beam exits below the

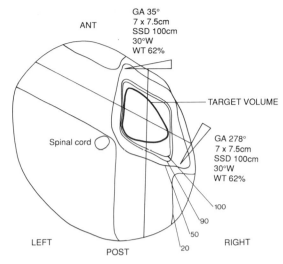

Fig 20.33 Anterior and posterior wedged pair of fields for carcinoma of the middle ear.

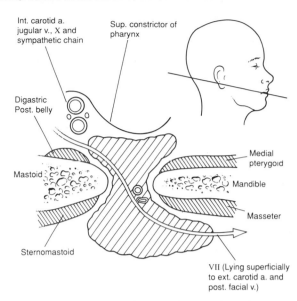

Fig. 20.34 Parotid and its surrounds in a schematic horizontal section — the facial nerve is the most superficial of the structures traversing the gland. (The line of section is shown in the inset head.) (Redrawn from Ellis, Clinical Anatomy. 5th edn, Blackwell Scientific, 1975.)

eyes. CT reconstruction of the oblique plane is helpful in confirming this (Plates 14 and 15). An outline is taken through the centre of the volume, on which the target volume brainstem and lens are drawn. The treated fields can be cut out from the shell if there is no superficial involvement of the ear.

Dose and energy

Primary or postoperative radical radiotherapy:

60 Gy in 25 daily fractions over 5 weeks (4–6 MV photons)

Care should be taken to limit the dose to the brainstem to 40 Gy.

Reaction. The acute reaction is usually not troublesome but hearing may be impaired due to secretory otitis media.

Results of treatment

The outcome of treatment is poor. Radical surgery with postoperative radiotherapy has a better 5-year survival (40%) than primary radiotherapy (15–20%). Bony invasion confers a poor prognosis.

SALIVARY TUMOURS

Tumours of the salivary glands are uncommon and only represent 0.3% of cancers and 0.1% of all cancer deaths. The parotid gland is by far the commonest site (80%). Tumours mainly occur both in the major glands (parotid, submandibular and sublingual) and in the small mucous glands of the mouth and upper air passages, including the nasopharynx, trachea and bronchi.

Anatomy

The *parotid* gland lies in its own fascial compartment in the space between the mandible and the mastoid process. It has both superficial and deep lobes (Fig. 20.34). Its superficial lobe overlies both the masseter muscle anteriorly and the sternomastoid muscle posteriorly. Anteroinferiorly, it is separated from the submandibular gland by a thickening of the parotid fascia, the stylomandibular ligament. Its deep lobe, lying at the level of the transverse process of the second cervical vertebra, is related medially to the styloid process and its muscles which separate it from the internal carotid artery, internal jugular vein, the lower four cranial nerves and the lateral pharyngeal wall. The superficial part is limited above by the zygomatic arch.

The main anatomical point to note is the relation of the parotid gland to the facial (seventh cranial) nerve which traverses it. Malignant tumours, unlike benign ones, often cause a facial palsy. The facial nerve may also be damaged when a tumour is surgically removed.

The parotid drains to the preauricular and deep parotid nodes and thence to the upper deep cervical nodes.

Table 20.3   Pathological classification of primary salivary tumours

Benign	Malignant
Pleomorphic adenoma	Pleomorphic adenocarcinoma
Monomorphic adenoma	Adenoidcystic carcinoma
Adenolymphoma	Mucoepidermoid carcinoma
	Adenocarcinoma
	Acinic cell carcinoma
	Non-Hodgkin lymphoma

The *submandibular* gland also has superficial and deep lobes. It lies at the angle of the jaw. The superficial lobe is wedged between the mylohyoid muscle and the mandible. The deep lobe is adjacent to the mylohyoid, and posteriorly lies against the hyoglossus muscle. The gland is limited above by the mucous membrane of the tongue and below by the hyoid, to which it has a fascial attachment. The submandibular duct arises from the deep lobe and opens adjacent to the frenulum of the tongue.

The submandibular gland drains to the submandibular nodes and thence to the upper deep cervical nodes.

The *sublingual* gland (Fig. 20.22B) lies just below the mucosa of the floor of the mouth and in front of the submandibular gland. Medially it is related to the submandibular duct and the lingual nerve, which separate it from the base of the tongue.

The gland drains into the floor of the mouth through a number of ducts.

Pathology

About a quarter of parotid tumours and a half of submandibular tumours are malignant. The average age for benign tumours is 40 years and for malignant tumours 55 years. The clinical behaviour of some tumour types is very variable, even among tumours of similar microscopic appearance. Thus attempts at predicting behaviour are in practice of limited use. Table 20.3 shows the pathological classification of salivary tumours.

Benign tumours

The commonest benign tumour is the *pleomorphic salivary adenoma*. It is often called 'mixed parotid tumour'. Though of epithelial origin, it often contains material that stains like cartilage. To the naked eye, the tumour looks well encapsulated. Microscopically, however, there are outgrowths at the periphery of the tumour protruding into the surrounding tissue. Simple enucleation of the tumour is very likely to leave these peripheral remnants of tumour behind and give rise to local recurrence.

Adenolymphoma or *Warthin's tumour* is a rare tumour, almost exclusively occurring in the parotid gland. It probably arises from lymphoid elements. It is the parotid tumour most likely to be bilateral (5–10%).

Pleomorphic salivary adenoma

Clinical features. This tumour presents as a firm swelling, usually near the angle of the jaw. The facial nerve is almost always unaffected.

Treatment. The treatment of choice is a superficial parotidectomy with conservation of the facial nerve. Care should be taken to excise beyond the 'false capsule', otherwise remnants of tumour will be left behind and seed recurrence. If removal is complete postoperative radiotherapy is not required. If the removal of the tumour is incomplete, postoperative irradiation is advised since there is otherwise a 30–40% risk of local recurrence and further surgery may result in damage to the facial nerve. If recurrence occurs after initial complete excision, further surgical excision should be attempted while preserving the facial nerve. If further excision is inadequate, then postoperative radiotherapy is given.

Technique and dosage are the same as for malignant tumours (see below).

Results of treatment. With adequate excision alone less than 5% of pleomorphic salivary adenomas will recur. Incomplete excision followed by postoperative radiotherapy yields similar results. The success of further surgery for local recurrence depends upon the number of previous operations and the size and local extent of the recurrence.

Malignant tumours

Pleomorphic adenocarcinomas or *mixed malignant tumours* typically present with a history of a previously slow growing painless parotid swelling which has suddenly increased in size and become painful. This is an example of malignant transformation within a benign tumour. Sometimes this occurs in a recurrence from previous inadequate excision of a pleomorphic adenoma.

Adenoidcystic carcinomas account for 15% of malignant salivary tumours. They arise in both the major and minor salivary glands (for example in the hard palate). They have a marked tendency to infiltrate along nerves. Primary *squamous cell carcinomas* and *anaplastic carcinomas* of the parotid gland do occur very occasionally and are highly malignant. However the possibility that they may represent secondary spread from a primary tumour elsewhere in the head and

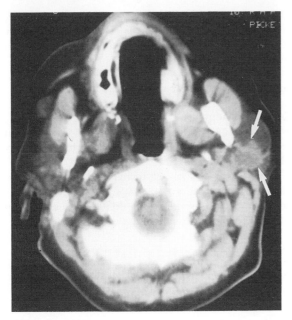

Fig. 20.35   CT scan showing parotid tumour (arrowed). (Courtesy of Dr R Nakielny, Sheffield.)

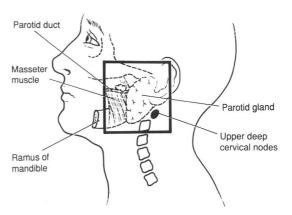

Fig. 20.36   Field margins for treatment of a parotid tumour, in relation to the underlying anatomy. (Redrawn from Dobbs & Barrett, Practical Radiotherapy Planning, Ist edn, Edward Arnold, 1985.)

neck should be considered. *Mucoepidermoid carcinomas* contain a spectrum of malignancies ranging from the histologically relatively low grade and benign in behaviour to the high grade and clinically aggressive. *Acinic cell carcinomas* are relatively slow growing. Both Hodgkin's and non-Hodgkin lymphoma may arise in the parotid gland. However it is often difficult to be certain that the true origin is not in the adjacent parotid nodes.

Clinical features. Malignant tumours are more likely to present with pain and a facial palsy. Lymph node involvement is uncommon. Most malignant tumours do not metastasise to distant sites, with the exception of adenoid cystic carcinoma which may involve the lungs and liver. Lung metastases are often slow growing over many years without giving rise to symptoms.

Diagnosis and investigation. The parotid lump is examined for mobility and the integrity of the facial nerve is tested. The neck is palpated for lymph nodes. Staging investigations should include a chest X-ray and a CT scan (Fig. 20.35) to assess the local extent, particularly medially.

Treatment. Surgical biopsy and excision followed by radical postoperative radiotherapy is the treatment of choice for most malignant salivary tumours. However low grade carcinomas which have been adequately excised do not require further treatment. Lymphomas of the minor salivary glands in the nasopharynx are treated by radical radiotherapy, but surgery or surgery

and postoperative radiotherapy are appropriate for minor salivary gland tumours in operable sites.

Indications for radical radiotherapy may be summarised as:

— Inadequate surgical excision
— High grade malignancy
— Lymphomas

Palliative radiotherapy is indicated to relieve pain and fungation from advanced disease in patients not fit for radical radiotherapy or in the presence of distant metastases.

PAROTID TUMOURS

Radical radiotherapy

Target volume

This should include the whole of the parotid bed. The upper limit should be the zygomatic arch. The lower border should lie below the inferior pole of the gland and incorporate the upper deep cervical nodes (Fig. 20.36). Anteriorly the field should extend to include the masseter muscle and posteriorly the mastoid process. The medial limit for malignant tumours should cover the whole of the parapharyngeal space. A less generous medial limit is required for pleomorphic adenoma. The lateral margin should cover all the palpable disease and the surgical scar. For squamous or anaplastic tumours, where the risk of lymphatic metastases is high, and in patients with palpable nodes, the ipsilateral neck node groups are treated in addition to the primary.

The target volume is triangular in shape with the apex towards the brainstem. It should allow at least

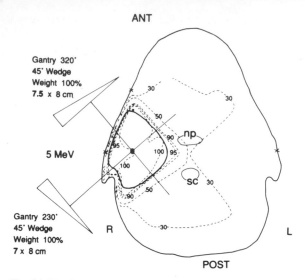

Fig. 20.37 Anterior and posterior oblique wedged fields for treatment of a parotid tumour. (Reproduced with permission from Dobbs & Barrett, Practical Radiotherapy Planning, Edward Arnold, 1st edn, 1985.)

a 1 cm margin of normal tissue around the tumour. This margin may have to be less generous medially to avoid excessive irradiation of the brainstem.

Technique

The choice of technique will depend upon whether the intention is radical or palliative. Uniform irradiation of the parotid region is difficult to achieve due to the changing contour of the neck. The proximity of critical structures such as the brainstem and the eye require very careful planning and verification.

The best field arrangement is a wedged pair of anterior and posterior oblique fields (Fig. 20.37). A shell is required with the patient supine and the head extended and rotated 90° away from the affected side so that the parotid region faces upward. No mouth bite is necessary. It may be necessary to incline the plane downwards by 10–15° for the posterior beam to exit below the eyes, if the patient is unable to extend the neck adequately or if the target volume needs to include the base of the skull.

The scar and any palpable disease are marked with wire. Anteroposterior and lateral films are taken on the simulator. An outline is taken through the centre of the volume. CT planning, with reconstruction, if necessary, of CT images in the inclined plane (Plates 14 and 15), is helpful in ensuring adequate coverage of the tumour and avoidance of the brainstem and the eyes.

If the lower ipsilateral neck is treated, a direct electron field is used. The energy is chosen according to the depth of the tumour as assessed on CT scan. The target volume should be encompassed within the 90% isodose.

Bolus is applied to overcome the skin sparing effect of electrons if there is superficial disease or scars.

Dose and energy

60 Gy in 25 daily fractions over 5 weeks at megavoltage (4–6 MV photons or high energy electrons)

Acute reaction. Skin erythema and mucositis, xerostomia, alopecia and loss of taste occur during treatment. Oral hygiene and dental care are as for other head and neck sites.

Palliative radiotherapy

A simple direct field using orthovoltage, electrons or cobalt is adequate. Bolus is applied for electron or cobalt fields if there is skin infiltration.

Dose

30 Gy in 10 daily fractions or, in fitter patients, 45 Gy in 20 daily fractions

SUBMANDIBULAR TUMOURS

Radical radiotherapy

Target volume

This should include the whole of the submandibular gland and at least a 1 cm margin of normal tissue.

Technique

Small tumours not extending to the midline may be treated by anterior and lateral wedged fields. Larger tumours reaching the midline should be treated by a parallel opposed pair of fields. Wedges may be required.

Dose is as for malignant parotid tumours.

Palliative radiotherapy

Technique, dose and energy are as for malignant parotid tumours.

Results of treatment of malignant salivary tumours

Prognosis is good for low grade mucoepidermoid and acinic cell tumours (80–90% 5-year survival), intermediate for adenocarcinoma (50%) and adenoid cystic (60%) and poor for high grade mucoepidermoid (20%) and squamous cell carcinoma.

21. Larynx, lower pharynx, postcricoid, thyroid

It is convenient to deal with these sites together.

Anatomy

Lower pharynx

The lower pharynx (hypopharynx or laryngopharynx) extends from the tip of the epiglottis (just above the level of the hyoid bone) to the lower end of the cricoid cartilage, at the junction of the hypopharynx and oesophagus. The anatomy is complicated. Details are given in Figure 21.1.

The larynx

This is best considered as consisting of three sections:

1. The *glottis*—the gap framed by the vocal cords. These are joined at the front and at the back by tendons, the anterior and posterior commissures. Tumours of the anterior commissure have a worse prognosis since at the point of insertion of this tendon there is no perichondrium to act as a barrier to spread. Similarly, tumours of the posterior third of the vocal cords can spread through the posterior commissure into the pyriform fossa. Tumours of the glottis are illustrated in Figures 21.2–21.5.

2. Above the glottis, or *supraglottic*. This includes the epiglottis, the aryepiglottic folds, the arytenoids, the ventricular bands (false cords) and the ventricular cavities. Typical tumours are illustrated in Figures 21.6, 21.9 and 21.10.

3. Below the glottis, or *subglottic*.

It can be seen that the boundaries of the various compartments are not sharply demarcated, and it is often difficult to say where a growth really originated. Overall, 60–70% of laryngeal tumours arise from the

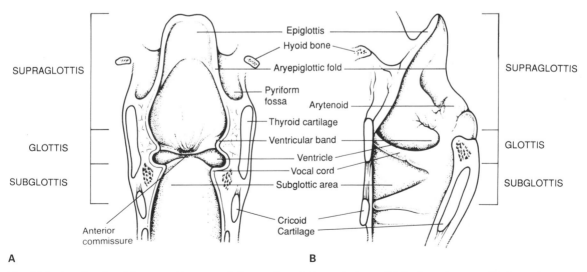

Fig. 21.1 Landmarks of the normal larynx and pharynx from **A** the posterior and **B** the lateral aspect. (Redrawn from Robinson, Surgery, Longmans.)

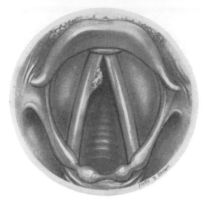

Fig. 21.2   Cordal lesion. Involvement of anterior third of vocal cord. Lymph node metastases rare. (Reproduced from Kunkler and Rains, Treatment of Cancer in Clinical Practice, Livingstone, 1959.)

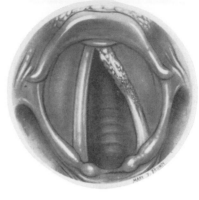

Fig. 21.3   Cordal lesion. Involvement of free edge and upper surface of anterior third of vocal cord. Spread to the anterior commissure. (Reproduced from Kunkler and Rains, Treatment of Cancer in Clinical Practice, Livingstone, 1959.)

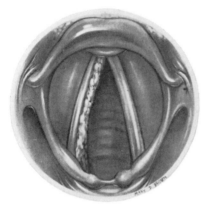

Fig. 21.4   Cordal lesion. Full length of edge of cord involved with slight impairment of mobility. (Reproduced from Kunkler and Rains, Treatment of Cancer in Clinical Practice, Livingstone, 1959.)

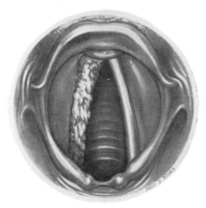

Fig. 21.5   Cordal lesion. Full length of edge and upper surface of cord involved by proliferating and infiltrating growth. Cord fixed. (Reproduced from Kunkler and Rains, Treatment of Cancer in Clinical Practice, Livingstone, 1959.)

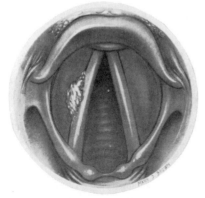

Fig. 21.6   Supraglottic carcinoma. (Reproduced from Kunkler and Rains, Treatment of Cancer in Clinical Practice, Livingstone, 1959.)

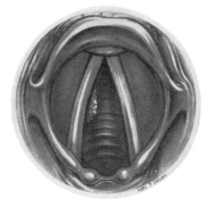

Fig. 21.7   Subglottic carcinoma. (Reproduced from Kunkler and Rains, Treatment of Cancer in Clinical Practice, Livingstone, 1959.)

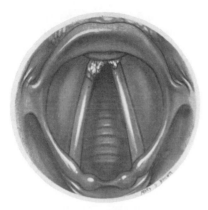

Fig. 21.8   Tumour of the vocal cords. Bilateral or commissural lesion. (Reproduced from Kunkler and Rains, Treatment of Cancer in Clinical Practice, Livingstone, 1959.)

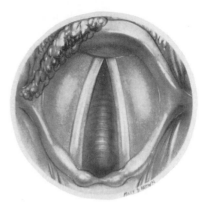

Fig. 21.9   Epilaryngeal carcinoma. Lesion of the epiglottis. (Reproduced from Kunkler and Rains, Treatment of Cancer in Clinical Practice, Livingstone, 1959.)

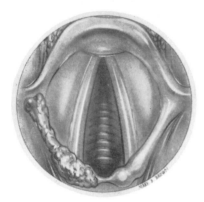

Fig. 21.10   Epilaryngeal carcinoma. Lesion of the aryepiglottic fold. (Reproduced from Kunkler and Rains, Treatment of Cancer in Clinical Practice, Livingstone, 1959.)

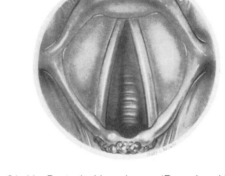

Fig. 21. 11   Post-cricoid carcinoma. (Reproduced from Kunkler and Rains, Treatment of Cancer in Clinical Practice, Livingstone, 1959.)

vocal cords, 30% from the supraglottic region and less than 5% from the subglottic area. Figure 21.7 shows a typical subglottic tumour.

Lymphatic drainage

The true vocal cords do not have any lymphatic drainage. This explains the absence of nodal metastases in tumours confined to cords (T1). For T2 and small T3 tumours arising from the vocal cords the incidence is 2–5%. Tumours of the anterior commissure and anterior subglottis may involve the pretracheal nodes in the midline.

The supraglottic region, by contrast, has a rich lymphatic supply, draining principally to the upper deep cervical nodes. Up to 40% of patients with supraglottic tumours have palpable nodes and a higher proportion (70%) have microscopic nodal deposits

at the time of surgery. The subglottic region drains to the pretracheal, lower cervical and mediastinal nodes. Nodal metastases in subglottic tumours occur late.

Pathology

Laryngeal cancer accounts for 0.9% of all cancers and 0.6% of cancer deaths. The yearly incidence is about 4 per 100 000 in the UK. In Northern Europe it constitutes 20% of tumours of the head and neck. The highest incidence is reported in Brazil and India. Most of these tumours occur in the fifth to seventh decades. The male: female sex ratio is 5:1. Smoking is an important aetiological factor. The mortality from laryngeal cancer in smokers is five times that of non-smokers. Some tumours may be related to human papilloma virus infection.

Ninety-five per cent of laryngeal tumours are invasive

squamous carcinomas, usually well differentiated. Verrucous carcinoma is an uncommon variant of squamous carcinoma, which resembles a viral wart and consequently can be difficult to diagnose microscopically. Another variant is spindle cell carcinoma—a squamous tumour mimicking sarcoma; it usually presents as a rounded nodule. Similar tumours arise elsewhere, particularly in the upper aerodigestive tract. Other varieties of tumour are all rare.

Premalignant lesions may be seen—hyperkeratosis, dysplasia and carcinoma-in-situ. These may follow a prolonged course and be difficult to separate from carcinoma, with repeated biopsies and recurrences.

Local spread

On the vocal cord the lesion commonly begins near the centre and spreads along the cord, later involving the junction of the cords (anterior commissure—Figs 21.3 and 21.8) and then spreading across to the other cord. It is usually slow growing and confined to the cord for a long time. The cords move (apposition and separation) in normal respiration and phonation, and their mobility is maintained until infiltration of the intrinsic muscles of the larynx impairs it and causes some degree of fixation. Late local spread involves the supraglottic region and the laryngeal cartilages; subglottic invasion is less common. Tumours of the epilarynx (epiglottis, arytenoid and aryepiglottic fold) spread locally to the opposite side, to the pre-epiglottic space and the thyroid cartilage. Tumours of the ventricular bands (false cords) spread superiorly to the aryepiglottic folds and arytenoids and anteriorly to the anterior commissure. Tumours arising from the laryngeal ventricle spread to the supraglottis or the contralateral vocal cord and may be transglottic. Subglottic tumours tend to spread circumferentially and invade the cricothyroid membrane. Posteriorly they may spread to the hypopharynx via the cricoid cartilage.

Clinical features

Tumours of the vocal cords tend to present early, with a hoarse voice, since even tiny irregularities of their margins cause enough changes in the vibrating air column to produce hoarseness. Prompt attention to this favours early diagnosis. Advanced growths will narrow the airway 'chink' of the glottis and produce stridor, i.e. audible wheezing on inspiration. Neglect results in increasing dyspnoea, and impending suffocation may have to be relieved by an emergency operation (tracheostomy) whereby an opening is made in the trachea lower down in the neck, and a tube inserted through which the patient can breathe.

Growths in the rest of the larynx or pharynx tend to remain silent for many months. A mass may reach considerable size (3–4 cm) before causing really troublesome symptoms. Lesions in the pyriform fossa are particularly liable to long latency. There may be intermittent vague discomfort or sore throat at first, followed later by interference with speaking (hoarse-

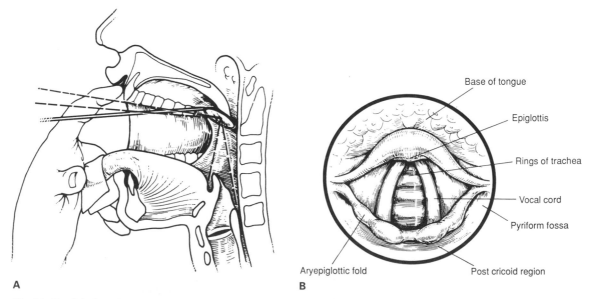

Fig. 21.12 **A** Indirect laryngoscopy and **B** the mirror view of the larynx.

ness, dysphonia), swallowing (dysphagia) or breathing (dyspnoea), depending on the exact site of the growth and the extent of local invasion. By this time—or very often before—there may be secondary cervical nodes, and a lump in the neck is all too commonly the presenting complaint, leading to the discovery of the primary in the throat.

Diagnosis and staging

Preliminary clinical examination is by indirect endoscopy (laryngoscopy) using a long-handled mirror (Fig. 21.12). Except for very early cases, especially on

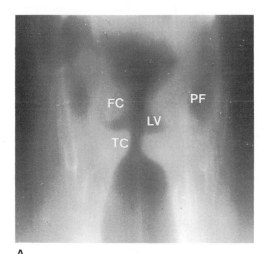

A

B

Fig. 21.13 Laryngeal tomograms: **A** normal appearance of vocal cords (TC), laryngeal ventricle (LV), false cords (FC), pyriform fossa (PF); **B** large mass involving the right vocal cord, false cord with obliteration of the ventricle (long arrow) and subglottic extension (short arrows).

the cords, it is not usually possible to see the whole of the tumour, but only the upper part, or the edge of an ulcer, or an abnormal bulge.

Futher detail, to outline the full extent of the mass, is obtainable by radiography. Soft tissue lateral films of the neck are taken and in addition, tomograms which will reveal the cords, impairment of their movement and any masses distorting the normal air spaces. Tomograms are helpful in the assessment of local spread (Fig. 21.13), particularly subglottic extension. CT scanning may provide information on the exact size and site of the tumour, but is not usually necessary for planning radiotherapy.

In most cases it is desirable to carry out direct endoscopy, under general anaesthesia, to inspect the whole of the growth and to take a biopsy.

Tumours are staged using the UICC classification (Table 21.1).

Treatment

Preliminary attention is to the patient's general condition, nutrition, and correction of anaemia. Oral hygiene is important, and any dental sepsis should be dealt with at the start.

Table 21.1 UICC staging of laryngeal cancer

Stage	Clinical findings
Supraglottis	
T1	Tumour confined to the region with normal mobility
T2	Tumour confined to the larynx with extension to adjacent site or sites or to the glottis without fixation
T3	Tumour confined to the larynx with fixation and/or other evidence of deep infiltration
T4	Tumour with direct extension beyond the larynx
Glottis	
T1	Tumour confined to the region with normal mobility
T2	Tumour confined to the larynx with extension to either the supraglottis or the subglottic regions with normal or impaired mobility
T3	Tumour confined to the larynx with fixation of one or both cords
T4	Tumour with direct extension beyond the larynx
Subglottis	
T1	Tumour confined to the region
T2	Tumour confined to the larynx with extension to one or both cords with normal or impaired mobility
T3	Tumour confined to the larynx with fixation of one or both cords
T4	Tumour with destruction of cartilage and/or with direct extension beyond the larynx

Glottic carcinoma

The choice of treatment is influenced by the stage of the tumour, likelihood of local control, general medical condition and treatment-related morbidity. As with other head and neck cancers, patients with advanced disease are often in poor general condition and this influences whether treatment is radical or palliative in intent.

The main treatments are surgery and radiotherapy. In general, the best treatment of T1 and T2 tumours is radical radiotherapy, since the cure rates are comparable with surgery and there is normally restoration of a good quality voice.

There is less agreement about the treatment of T3 and T4 tumours. In general, radical radiotherapy is advised as initial treatment for T3 tumours since this will cure about 30% of such patients. Salvage laryngectomy will cure a further 30% of those with persistent tumour. Radical radiotherapy for failures of primary surgery is rarely successful. For T4 tumours where there is invasion of the cartilage, the risk of radiation induced necrosis of the cartilage is high after a radical dose and local control rates are poor. Primary surgery is therefore advised for patients with T4 tumours who are in adequate general medical condition.

Secondary nodes of the neck appearing after radical radiotherapy are managed by radical neck dissection if possible.

Radical radiotherapy

Target volume
The target volume for T1 and T2 tumours should be centred on the vocal cords, which lie just below the laryngeal ventricle (Fig. 21.14) and 1 cm below the laryngeal promontory (Adam's apple). The volume should include the thyroid and cricoid cartilages. If there is supraglottic extension the upper margin should extend up to cover the hyoid bone and the upper deep cervical nodes (as supraglottic cancer, Fig. 21.17A). A generous margin should be allowed below any subglottic extension.

Technique
A head shell is needed with the mouth closed. A parallel opposed pair of lateral wedged fields is recommended for most patients. Wax build-up is recommended for tumours involving the anterior commissure to ensure adequate dosage to this region (Fig. 21.15). If the patient has a short neck and lateral fields would pass through the shoulder, a wedged pair of anterior oblique fields as in Figure 21.16 is recommended. The dose to the spinal cord is however greater than with lateral opposed wedged fields.

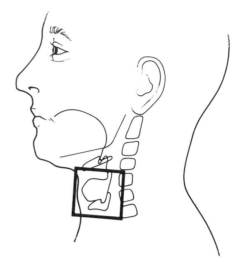

Fig. 21.14 Treatment volume for T1 and T2 glottic carcinoma. (Redrawn from Dobbs & Barrett, Practical Radiotherapy Planning, 1st edn, Edward Arnold, 1985.)

Dose and energy
60 Gy in 25 daily fractions over 5 weeks (4–6 MV photons)

Supraglottic carcinoma

Radical radiotherapy is indicated for supraglottic carcinoma (T1–3) with or without nodes (N0, N1). Laryngopharyngectomy is reserved for recurrence or persistent disease or for T4 tumours.

Target volume
When there is early disease and there are no palpable

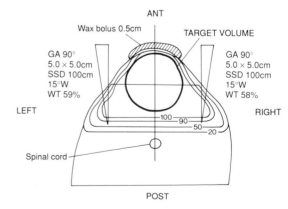

Fig. 21.15 T1 glottic tumour involving the anterior commissure. Isodose distribution for parallel opposed lateral fields. Note wax build-up to ensure adequate dosage to the anterior commissure.

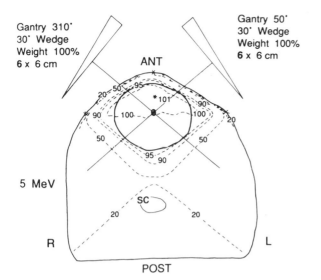

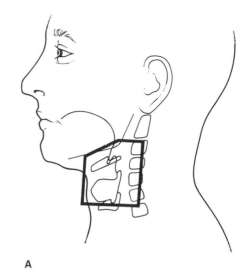

Fig. 21.16   T1 glottic tumour in a patient with a short neck. Isodose distribution for anterior oblique fields. (Reproduced with permission from Dobbs et al 1992.)

nodes, the volume (Fig. 21.17) encompasses the primary tumour and the upper deep cervical nodes. The mouth is closed during treatment. The upper margin of the field extends above the hyoid bone and includes the tonsillar region. The posterior border should extend half way across the vertebral bodies.

If the primary tumour is advanced or there are palpable neck nodes, the cervical node chains should be covered on both sides (Table 20.2).

Technique

A head shell is needed with the mouth closed. In the absence of nodes, a parallel opposed pair of wedged fields is used. The floor of the mouth is shielded with lead. In the presence of nodes the lower half of the neck is treated by an anterior 'split neck' field (Fig. 21.18). A lead strip should shield midline structures. The nodes are outlined by lead wire at the time of simulation. The junction of the upper and lower neck fields should be matched using asymmetric diaphragms (Fig. 21.19). If these are unavailable a small gap is left between the two fields to avoid overdosage due to overlap. If the nodes overlie the spinal cord, the posterior margin of the upper neck field is moved anterior to the cord after a dose of 40 Gy. The rest of the posterior part of the field is then treated with electrons of appropriate energy. The choice of energy of electrons is based on measurement of the distance between the thinnest part of the neck and the spinal cord (Fig. 20.18).

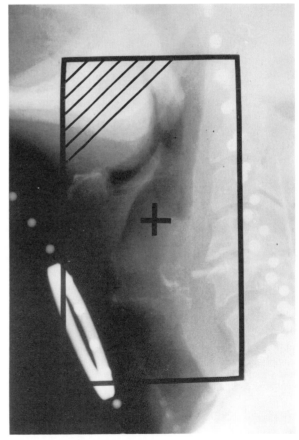

Fig. 21.17   Supraglottic carcinoma. **A** Treatment volume for supraglottic carcinoma. (Redrawn from Dobbs & Barrett, Practical Radiotherapy Planning, 1st edn, Edward Arnold, 1985.) **B** Typical lateral simulator film.

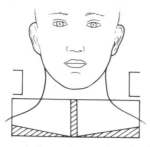

Fig. 21.18 Supraglottic carcinoma. Anterior field to treat lower neck and supraclavicular fossae. (Modified from Dobbs & Barrett, Practical Radiotherapy Planning, 1st edn, Edward Arnold, 1985.)

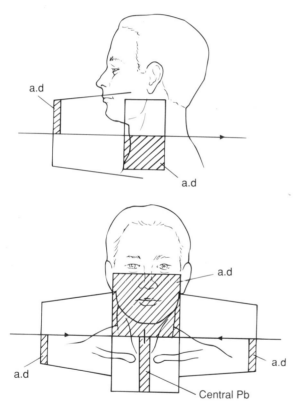

Fig. 21.19 Diagram showing the use of asymmetric diaphragms (a.d) to match adjacent fields at the centre of each beam where there is no divergence. (Courtesy of Dr I Manifold, Sheffield.)

Dose and energy

T1–T2, N0

Primary tumour and, prophylactically, the upper and midcervical nodes in front of the spinal cord
48 Gy in 20 daily fractions over 4 weeks (4–6 MV photons)

Reduced volume to primary and midcervical nodes
12 Gy in 5 daily fractions (4–6 MV photons)
Total dose: 60 Gy in 25 fractions over 5 weeks

More advanced
The volume encompasses the primary and all nodes, including those of the posterior triangle (see Table 20.2).
40 Gy in 20 daily fractions over 4 weeks (4–6 MV photons)

Reduced photon volume to the area in front of the spinal cord. Continue at dose rate of 2 Gy per fraction, 5 days a week, to give:
66 Gy in 33 fractions over 6.5 weeks to primary and palpable nodes
and
50 Gy in 25 fractions over 5 weeks to prophylactic areas

Electrons of suitable energy are used to treat nodal areas overlying and posterior to the spinal cord after 40 Gy, matched to adjacent photon fields.

Subglottic carcinoma

Target volume and technique
The primary tumour and first station draining lymph nodes, using an 'angled down' wedged pair, possibly with wax blocks to compensate for curvature, or the 'twisted wedge' technique is used (Fig. 21.31). The volume is anterior to the spinal cord. Matching posterior electron fields or an inferior field treating the mediastinum anteriorly is difficult and often unsatisfactory. However lesions at this site with nodal metastases carry a very poor prognosis.

Dose and energy
60 Gy in 25 daily fractions over 5 weeks (4–6 MV photons or electrons)

Radiation reactions
Acute. These are managed on the same lines as for the mouth (p. 321). Huskiness may persist for months before improving. Occasionally, especially with large tumours, there may be reactionary oedema very early on, even after the first or second dose, which can be dangerous if the airway is already narrowed. Acute obstruction may be precipitated, calling for emergency tracheostomy to prevent suffocation. If this possibility is anticipated, an elective tracheostomy may be advisable.

If tracheostomy has been carried out, the metal tube must be replaced by a plastic tube before the start of the radiation, otherwise the soft secondary X-rays from the metal will cause excessive reaction in the adjacent skin.

For weeks or months following radical radiotherapy there may be persistent oedema of the laryngeal region and maybe patches of ulceration with infection. It is often difficult to distinguish this from persistent or recurrent growth, and even biopsies may not do so with certainty. Such cases may require laryngectomy to rescue the patient from an intolerable existence, even if there is no residual malignancy.

Late (late cartilage necrosis). Necrosis of laryngeal cartilages is a serious reaction, developing several months after radical radiotherapy. It is rarely seen after megavoltage, but occurred in the orthovoltage era since 200 kV radiation deposits much more energy in calcified cartilage due to attenuation by the photo-electric process (p. 64). It is characterised by pain and local tenderness. Infection is likely to follow, with dyspnoea and dysphagia. Tracheostomy may be necessary, or even laryngectomy. The danger of necrosis is a good reason for preferring surgery in cases where cartilage is already invaded by tumour.

Results of treatment

Radical radiotherapy cures about 85% of T1 and 70% of T2 glottic cancer. The rates are lower, at 50–60%, for T3 and T4 tumours.

The equivalent cure rates for supraglottic cancer are poorer for early disease: about 70–80% for T1N0 and T2N0. For T3N0/1 and T4N0/1 about 55% are cured. When the nodes are fixed (N3) only 40% are cured.

For early subglottic carcinoma, overall survival with radiotherapy is 30–40%.

HYPOPHARYNX

Anatomy

The hypopharynx (Fig. 21.1) lies posterolateral to the larynx and anterior to the fourth and fifth cervical vertebrae. It extends downwards from the aryepiglottic fold at the level of the hyoid bone to the inferior border of the cricoid cartilage. It comprises three areas: the pyriform fossa, the postcricoid region and the posterior pharyngeal wall. Lymphatic drainage of the hypopharynx is to deep cervical chains.

The pyriform fossae are shaped like gutters on either side of the larynx (Fig. 21.20). Behind the larynx lies the postcricoid region which extends from the arytenoid cartilages to the inferior margin of the cricoid cartilage. The posterior pharyngeal wall runs from the floor of the vallecula to the cricoid cartilage.

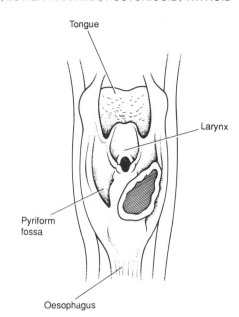

Fig. 21.20   Carcinoma of the hypopharynx (right pyriform fossa). Reproduced with permission from Macfarlane, Textbook of Surgery, Churchill Livingstone.

PYRIFORM FOSSA
Pathology

Cancer of the pyriform fossa is the commonest of hypopharyngeal cancers in most parts of the world; 90% of patients are males, principally in the 5th–7th decades. Alcohol and tobacco are thought to be the main aetiological factors. In contrast to postcricoid carcinoma, iron deficiency is not an important aetiological factor. Macroscopically the tumour appears as a fungating mass or deep ulcer. It often extends to other regions of the hypopharynx and to adjacent structures such as the aryepiglottic fold and ventricular bands, so fixing the hemilarynx. Microscopically it is normally a moderately differentiated squamous carcinoma.

Clinical features

The primary is often symptomless and presentation is normally with a lump in the neck from secondary lymph node spread. Nodes are palpable in 50% of patients at presentation. The primary is normally advanced (T3 or T4). The upper deep cervical nodes may become very large, fungate and become fixed. Symptoms include a sensation of something sticking at the back of the throat, dysphagia, pain and weight loss.

Investigation and diagnosis

Indirect laryngoscopy may show an exophytic tumour associated with pooling of saliva. Direct laryngoscopy and biopsy is required. Tomograms of the larynx may help define the local extent of the tumour and show distortion and obliteration of the affected pyriform fossa. CT scanning is particularly helpful.

Staging

T1 is a tumour limited to one site. T2 extends to an adjacent site or region without fixation of the hemilarynx. T3 is a tumour extending to an adjacent site or region with fixation of the hemilarynx. T4 is a tumour extending to bone, cartilage or soft tissues.

Treatment

Unfortunately the majority of patients are incurable. However radical radiotherapy is the primary treatment of choice for early tumours and locally advanced tumours with or without ipsilateral lymphadenopathy. When nodes are bilateral the prospect of cure is negligible and only palliative radiotherapy is worth attempting.

Radical radiotherapy

Target volume
Early tumour (T1–2 N0 or small volume nodes (N1)). The target volume should include the primary tumour and upper deep cervical nodes from the angle of the jaw to the inferior border of the cricoid cartilage (Fig. 21.21).

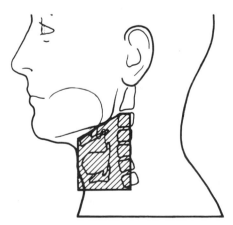

Fig. 21.21 Field margins for early carcinoma of the pyriform fossa. (Redrawn from Dobbs & Barrett, Practical Radiotherapy Planning, 1st edn, Edward Arnold, 1985.)

T3 with large nodes (N2). A larger volume includes the primary tumour and the nodes on both sides of the neck extending up to the base of the skull (Fig. 21.22A).

Technique
A head shell is needed in the supine position, the neck straight and the mouth closed.

For early tumours with no or small volume nodes a parallel opposed pair of lateral wedged fields is used. For more advanced tumours with bulky ipsilateral cervical nodes on one side, a lateral field on the side of the node and an anterior oblique field on the opposite

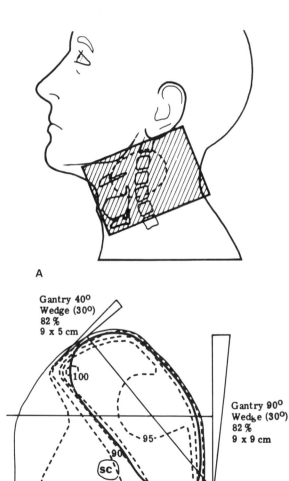

Fig. 21.22 A T3 pyriform fossa tumour with large node mass. **A** Lateral field margins on inclined plane; node mass is indicated by dotted line. **B** Isodose distribution. (Reproduced with permission from Dobbs et al 1992.)

side are used to limit the dose to the spinal cord (Fig. 21.22). Care is taken to limit the spinal cord dose to 40 Gy. Nodal masses overlying the cord, as for tonsillar cancer, can be boosted by electrons of appropriate energy (Fig. 20.17). If there are bilateral nodes, parallel opposed fields are needed for palliation.

Dose and energy

Radical
60 Gy in 25 daily fractions over 5 weeks (4–6 MV photons)

More prolonged fractionation with dose modification is needed when including the spinal cord and using electrons (see supraglottic laryngeal cancer, p. 348).

Palliative
30 Gy in 10 daily fractions over 2 weeks (4–6 MV photons)

Radiation reaction. This is as in laryngeal cancer and is managed on the same lines.

Results of treatment

The results of treatment for cancer of the pyriform fossa are poor. In patients suitable for surgery, 35% 5-year survival may be obtained. Following radical radiotherapy 5-year survival is about 20%.

POSTCRICOID AND POSTERIOR PHARYNGEAL WALL

These regions are considered together since they have similar epidemiology, pathology and management. Postcricoid cancer is a special variety of hypopharyngeal growth, just behind the larynx and above the oesophagus (Fig. 21.11).

Pathology

The highest incidence of cancer of the postcricoid and posterior pharyngeal wall cancer is in Egypt and Iraq, affecting principally farm labourers in the fifth decade. Cancer of the posterior pharyngeal wall is commoner in men and postcricoid cancer in women. The precise aetiology in most patients is unknown. However a small number of cases of hypopharyngeal cancer are radiation induced, occurring after a latency of 20 years following radiation given for thyrotoxicosis. The incidence of postcricoid cancer is falling in the UK as a result of correcting dietary deficiencies. Carcinoma of the postcricoid region is associated,

although not invariably, with chronic iron deficiency anaemia and other signs which include a smooth tongue (superficial glossitis) and hollow spoon-shaped nails (koilonychia). This is known, after the workers who described it, as the Plummer–Vinson syndrome in Britain and as the Paterson–Brown–Kelly syndrome in America. About 50% of patients with carcinoma of the postcricoid region have an associated postcricoid web (a small web-like projection of atrophic epithelium projecting in the entrance of the oesophagus). The whole of the epithelium of the upper digestive tract is atrophic, unstable and premalignant, and there may be malignant degeneration in the mouth, pharynx or oesophagus at any time.

Tumours of the postcricoid or posterior pharyngeal wall have usually spread to other areas of the hypopharynx. Macroscopically they appear as a fungating growth or ulcer. This may spread to the pyriform fossa, larynx, oropharynx, cervical oesophagus and thyroid gland. Microscopically it is normally a moderately differentiated squamous cell carcinoma. Spread to lymph nodes (paratracheal, upper and lower deep cervical) occurs in 40% of cases and is late. Nodal involvement is commonly bilateral when the tumour crosses the midline, especially with annular postcricoid tumours.

Clinical features

The cardinal symptom is progressive dysphagia. Indirect laryngoscopy may show only slight oedema or a suspicious pool behind the larynx. The edge of the tumour may be seen in advanced cases (Fig. 21.11).

Diagnosis and investigation

Direct endoscopy should be done, to see the full extent and for biopsy. Soft tissue films of the neck may show widening of the retrolaryngeal and retrotracheal space. A barium swallow shows an irregular filling defect. CT scanning is useful to show invasion of the pre-epiglottic space and the thyroid cartilage.

Treatment

If there is no lymphatic involvement and the primary is resectable, radical surgery gives the best chance of cure. The operation requires the removal of the larynx, hypopharynx and the oesophagus (laryngopharyngectomy). The alimentary tract has to be restored, usually by bringing up the stomach and joining it to the pharynx. Postoperative radiotherapy is not advised in view of the poor radiation tolerance of the stomach, which would lie within the field.

Radical radiotherapy is indicated in patients with an unresectable localised tumour. The prognosis of patients with nodal or mediastinal spread is so poor that radical radiotherapy is not worthwhile.

Radical radiotherapy

Postcricoid

Target volume
This should include the primary tumour and lower cervical nodes (Fig. 21.23). A 2–3 cm margin should be allowed inferior to the macroscopic limit of the tumour to cater for submucosal spread.

Technique
The patient is treated in a head shell extended below the clavicles, in the supine position with the neck straight and the mouth closed. A 'twisted' wedge technique is used. Two lateral fields are used, with wedges in the vertical and horizontal (one of which is therefore non-coplanar) planes and angled downwards using a couch twist of approximately 25° (Fig. 21.31).

Dose and energy
60 Gy in 25 daily fractions over 5 weeks (4–6 MV photons)

Posterior pharyngeal wall

Target volume
This includes (1) the entire hypopharynx with a 2 cm

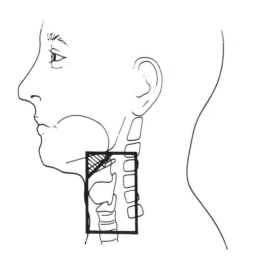

Fig. 21.23 Treatment volume for postcricoid carcinoma. (Redrawn from Dobbs & Barrett, Practical Radiotherapy Planning, 1st edn, Edward Arnold, 1985.)

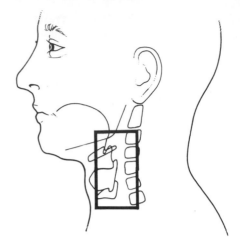

Fig. 21.24 Treatment volume for carcinoma of the posterior pharyngeal wall. (Redrawn from Dobbs & Barrett, Practical Radiotherapy Planning, 1st edn, Edward Arnold, 1985.)

margin above and below macroscopic tumour and (2) the upper deep cervical nodes on both sides (Fig. 21.24). The posterior margin lies in front of the spinal cord.

Technique
Parallel opposed lateral fields, wedged if necessary.

Dose and energy are as for postcricoid cancer.

Results of treatment

The outlook is poor for postcricoid and posterior pharyngeal wall cancer, with 15–20% 5-year survival for patients with involved nodes and 35% in rare early cases with negative nodes.

CANCER OF THE THYROID GLAND
Anatomy

The thyroid gland is composed of two lobes joined by a narrow isthmus, overlying the trachea (Fig. 21.25). To the left side between the trachea and the oesophagus runs the recurrent laryngeal nerve. The lymphatic drainage is to the deep cervical nodes, the pre- and paratracheal lymph nodes and downwards to the mediastinum.

Epidemiology

Thyroid cancer is rare, accounting for 0.4% of all cancers and 0.3% of cancer deaths. The incidence in the UK is 1 in 100 000. It can occur at any age but there is a minor peak between 5 and 20 years and a

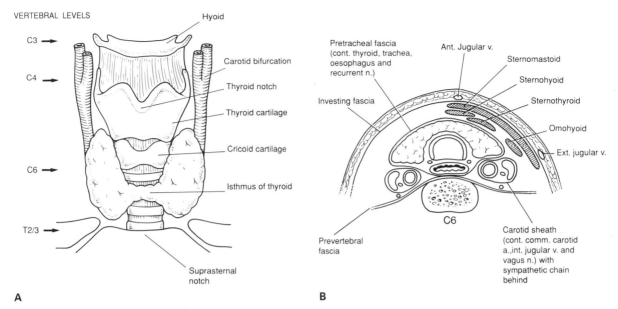

Fig. 21.25 **A** Structures palpable on the anterior aspect of the neck, together with corresponding vertebral levels. (Redrawn from Ellis, Clinical Anatomy, 5th edn, Blackwells. 1975.) **B** Transverse section of the neck through C6 showing the relations of the thyroid gland. (Reproduced from Ellis, Clinical Anatomy, 5th edn, Blackwells, 1975.)

major peak between 40 and 65 years. It is commoner in women, with a 2:1 sex ratio.

Tumours of the thyroid gland may be benign nodules (adenomas) or malignant. There are five malignant histological types:

— Papillary carcinoma
— Follicular carcinoma
— Anaplastic carcinoma
— Medullary carcinoma
— Lymphoma.

Papillary carcinoma is the most common. The incidence of thyroid cancer, particularly follicular carcinoma, is higher in areas of endemic goitre where iodine levels are low. By contrast, papillary carcinoma is commoner in areas rich in iodine (e.g. Iceland).

Papillary carcinoma is the commonest histological type induced by irradiating the neck in childhood. There is an increased incidence of thyroid cancer following mantle irradiation for Hodgkin's disease. Compensated hypothyroidism (normal serum thyroxine and free thyroxine index but elevated thyroid stimulating hormone (TSH)) is common in these patients. It may be the persistent TSH drive that assists the carcinogenic properties of irradiation. Hashimoto's thyroiditis predisposes to thyroid lymphoma. The cause of anaplastic (undifferentiated) cancer is unknown but there is some evidence that it may arise from a differentiated form of cancer.

Genetic factors are important in the genesis of medullary carcinoma of the thyroid. It is inherited as an autosomal dominant; 20% of cases are familial. The familial form may occur in isolation, in association with a phaeochromocytoma or as part of multiple endocrine neoplasia.

Pathology and clinical features

The main clinical features differentiating the various histological types are summarised in Fig. 21.26 and Table 21.2.

Papillary carcinoma is so-called because the characteristic microscopic picture has delicate finger-like cores of stroma lined by tumour cells. However it is the cytology (and behaviour) of these cells that is the defining feature for diagnosis; they can be arranged in follicles in part or all of the tumour. There are often small specks of calcium (psammoma bodies) in the stroma. It is the commonest type of thyroid tumour, accounting for 60% of cases, including almost all of those in childhood and adolescence. Some cases present as a solitary mass in one lobe of the thyroid, but many show multiple foci throughout the gland. Metastasis is characteristically to nearby lymph nodes, and enlargement of the latter is a frequent first symptom. However growth is usually very slow, and the long-term outlook remains good, even with established metastases.

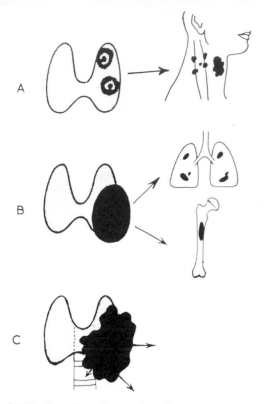

Fig. 21.26 Thyroid carcinoma: **A** papillary, metastases to lymph nodes, **B** follicular, metastases to lungs and bones, **C** anaplastic, local infiltration. (Reproduced with permission from Macfarlane, Textbook of Surgery, Churchill Livingstone.)

Sometimes a tiny tumour is discovered incidentally during examination of a thyroid removed for other purposes (e.g. thyrotoxicosis). This occult sclerosing papillary carcinoma is usually ignored, and no treatment is necessary.

Follicular carcinoma is more variable in its behaviour; it characteristically spreads via the bloodstream to give metastases in bone and lung. It is usually a solitary, circumscribed mass; a very well-differentiated follicular carcinoma can be mistaken for a benign adenoma, the true diagnosis becoming apparent many years later when a metastasis is found. Moderately and poorly differentiated follicular carcinomas are more aggressive, and may show metastases at the time of diagnosis. Up to 10% of patients present with, for example, pathological fracture or dyspnoea from lung deposits.

An important feature of any well-differentiated thyroid tumour (papillary or follicular) is that some (about 50%) are capable of synthesising and secreting thyroid hormones. This feature is commoner in the follicular than the papillary type. Even more striking is the fact that this capacity is also shown by their metastatic deposits. As in normal thyroid tissue, the hormones are built up from iodine removed from the blood and this enables radioactive iodine to be used in the treatment of these particular tumours. It is demonstrable in the metastases after oral administration of radioactive iodine, if all the normal thyroid tissue has been ablated (p. 357)

Anaplastic carcinoma. This undifferentiated tumour, often composed of giant or spindle cells, occurs typically in the elderly. Histologically it may be difficult to distinguish from a sarcoma or a high grade non-Hodgkin lymphoma. In the absence of definitive histology, the distinction may only ultimately be made by the response to radiotherapy. Lymphoma usually responds quickly (often within 24 hours). Anaplastic carcinoma is relatively radioresistant. It grows rapidly, locally compressing the trachea, and may cause stridor and dyspnoea. The oesophagus may also be involved causing dysphagia. Invasion of nerves may cause pain and, if the recurrent laryngeal nerve is involved, vocal cord palsy. It metastasises early to lung, bone and liver, but local growth in the neck is the main problem.

Medullary carcinoma. This arises from the para-follicular C cells which make the hormone calcitonin. It is normally slow growing and may have amyloid in its stroma. Calcium may be present in the tumour and may be visible on X-ray. However the absence of calcium, numerous mitoses, necrosis and spindle cells suggest more aggressive behaviour. Spread to lymph nodes and the mediastinum is common. Serum levels of calcitonin may be elevated but these are not specific to medullary carcinoma since calcitonin is secreted by non-thyroid tumours (e.g. lung, breast, colon and gastric cancer).

Malignant lymphomas. These are non-Hodgkin lymphomas of mucosa associated lymphoid tissue (MALT) pattern, ranging from low to high grade malignancy. Many arise in association with Hashimoto's thyroiditis. Initially confined to the thyroid, they may spread to local lymph nodes or recur in the gastrointestinal tract.

Staging

T1 is a mobile unilateral tumour. T2 is a mobile bilateral tumour. T3 is a unilateral or bilateral tumour fixed to surrounding structures. N and M stages are as for other head and neck sites.

Diagnosis and assessment

Management depends very much on history, exami-

Table 21.2   Clinical features of thyroid cancer

Feature	Papillary	Follicular	Anaplastic
Typical age (years)	Under 40 including children and adolescents	40–50	60+
Growth rate	Slow (years)	Intermediate	Rapid
Presenting signs	Nodule in one lobe or secondary	Thyroid nodule for years or recent enlargement or secondary, e.g. pathological fracture	Large diffuse fixed swelling
Spread	Neck nodes	By blood, e.g. lung, bone	Lymphatic and blood
Primary treatment of choice	Total thyroidectomy or lobectomy	Total thyroidectomy	External radiation
Thyroxine therapy	Full (for TSH suppression)	Full (for TSH suppression)	Full (for replacement)
Radiosensitivity	Moderate	Low	?High
Radioactive iodine uptake	?Limited	Yes, ablation doses for residual thyroid tissue and functioning secondaries	None
Treatment of secondary neck nodes	Operable: surgery; inoperable: external irradiation	Ablation if iodine-131 uptake; if no uptake, surgery; if operable, external irradiation	External irradiation
Prognosis and 5-year survival	Good (80–90%); can be >20 years (local or metastatic)	Intermediate (70%)	Poor (20%)

nation and special investigations. The histological type strongly influences management so that a histological diagnosis is virtually essential for rational treatment.

A history should include a family history of thyroid or other endocrine disease, previous thyroid disease

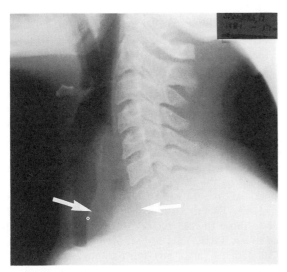

Fig. 21.27   Lateral radiograph of the neck showing widening of the prevertebral space (arrowed) due to carcinoma of the thyroid. (Courtesy of Dr R Nakielny, Sheffield.)

and irradiation of the neck. The neck should be examined for a scar from previous thyroid surgery, which may have been carried out many years previously. An indirect laryngoscopy should be performed to look for evidence of vocal cord paresis from involvement of or damage to the recurrent laryngeal nerve. X-ray of the neck may show (1) calcium as large irregular deposits or as a fine speckling (psammoma bodies in papillary carcinoma) in medullary thyroid cancer, and (2) widening of the prevertebral space (Fig. 21.27) or tracheal compression. Ultrasound of the neck may differentiate cystic areas from solid areas.

As a general rule, one of the first steps in all thyroid masses is a radioactive iodine uptake test and scintiscan of the neck (p. 188). 'Cold' areas (Fig. 21.28A) are suspicious but not diagnostic of cancer; 'hot' areas (Fig. 21.28B) rarely prove malignant (see below).

There is least diagnostic difficulty in rapidly-growing anaplastic tumours of the elderly, where the diagnosis is usually obvious. Benign enlargement of the thyroid can result in tracheal deviation. However marked tracheal compression with symptoms of airway obstruction is usually due to malignancy. Tomograms of the larynx or trachea and a barium swallow may help to distinguish a tumour arising in the thyroid from one invading from an adjacent region such as the hypopharynx.

The only lesion with which it might be confused is

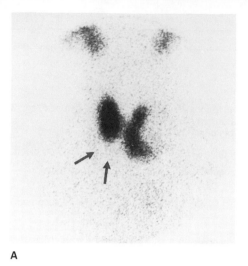

A

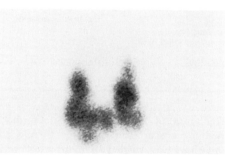

B

Fig. 21.28 Radioiodine scans (anterior view) showing **A** a 'cold' nodule in the right inferior pole of the thyroid gland and **B** toxic multinodular goitre. (Courtesy of the Department of Medical Physics, Sheffield.)

one of the forms of thyroiditis (associated with the names of Riedel and Hashimoto); raised serum thyroglobulin and microsomal antibodies confirm thyroiditis. If medullary carcinoma is suspected, serum calcitonin should be measured.

Treatment

Surgery

If the patient is in good general condition and malignancy has been confirmed histologically, as much of the thyroid gland should be removed as possible, ideally a total thyroidectomy. The only exception to this principle is lymphoma. Some have argued for carrying out a complete lobectomy on the affected side and a subtotal removal on the other side to preserve one of the parathyroid glands. If all the parathyroid glands are removed, the production of parathormone is abolished. Hypocalcaemic tetany may result postoperatively.

Often enough the diagnosis of malignancy and its type has to be awaited after partial thyroidectomy. It may even come as surprise. If it is of *papillary* type, a decision must be made as to whether to proceed to a further operation for complete removal of the thyroid gland. In favour of this is the fact that multiple foci are common. Arguments against further surgery are (1) papillary carcinomas grow very slowly and metastasise late; (2) second operations are always hazardous and carry increased danger of damage to laryngeal nerves and parathyroid glands. Practice varies. In the UK surgeons are commonly recommended to carry out a near total or subtotal thyroidectomy. Lymphatic invasion in the thyroid specimen (as opposed to lymph node involvement) does not worsen the prognosis of papillary carcinoma. Hence prophylactic nodal dissection is not required. This operation can be carried out as and when nodal recurrence occurs.

If the nodule proves to be *follicular* carcinoma, the case for complete removal of the thyroid is stronger, since this type, in addition to being possibly multifocal, is more aggressive and more liable to metastasise, as well as being less radiosensitive. A second operation is therefore fully justified, even if there are metastases at presentation. Even if the decision is against a second operation, thyroid ablation by iodine-131 is carried out, as described below, to remove any remaining thyroid tissue. Prophylactic dissection of the lymphatics of the neck is not necessary, since the risk of recurrence following postoperative radioiodine treatment is low.

Urgent surgical relief of airway obstruction is commonly required for anaplastic tumours.

Hormone therapy

The activity of the thyroid gland, and therefore the production of the thyroid hormones, thyroxine (T4) and tri-iodothyronine (T3), is dependent on pituitary TSH. The production of TSH is in turn under the control of thyrotrophin releasing hormone (TRH) from the hypothalamus. The amount of TSH produced is itself regulated by the amount of thyroid hormone produced by the thyroid, i.e. T4, T3 and TSH are in mutual adjustment by a feed-back mechanism. Low circulatory T3 and T4 provoke more TRH, more TSH and so more thyroid activity. High T3 and T4 levels lead to less TRH, TSH and reduced thyroid activity.

All patients, after any form of thyroidectomy for malignancy (or even failing operation in anaplastic growths), should be given thyroxine tablets by mouth for the rest of their lives. The usual dose is 0.2–0.3 mg/day. This is for two good reasons: (1) after removal of the thyroid, replacement of the missing hormones is necessary, otherwise the patient would suffer all the effects of hypothyroidism (p. 484); (2) if there is any thyroid tissue remaining, it will be subject to stimulation by TSH, as will some well-differentiated thyroid cancers. Thyroxine in large doses removes the normal stimulus to the pituitary to secrete TSH. Low TSH results in low activity of thyroid cells, normal and malignant, and thus favours quiescence of any residual foci of tumour tissue in the neck or elsewhere.

In the case of anaplastic and medullary tumours, sufficient thyroxine should be given for replacement therapy, since this type of cell is unresponsive to hormonal factors.

Treatment of neck nodes

Here again, treatment depends on the histological type. In *anaplastic* tumours, surgery is not helpful even if the nodes are operable, since distant metastases are virtually certain to be present. External irradiation is therefore the best option.

In *papillary* carcinoma, operable nodes may be removed but a full block dissection of the neck with its attendant morbidity is not necessary. This is because, although neck dissection may reduce the recurrence rate, there is no evidence that it improves survival. Inoperable nodes are treated by radiation.

In *follicular* carcinoma, treatment again will depend on the ability of the nodes to take up iodine-131, as described below. If they cannot be induced to do so, block dissection is justified for operable nodes. If the nodes are not operable, external beam irradiation is given.

Radioactive iodine and functioning differentiated carcinomas

The differential uptake of iodine by the thyroid is described on page 522. Radioactive iodine, being clinically indistinguishable from stable iodine, is taken up in the same way, and thus is an ideal tool for internal—even intracellular—radiation. Well-differentiated carcinomas take up iodine not only microscopically but functionally, follicular more so than papillary. Iodine uptake occurs in about half of well-differentiated carcinomas. The degree of uptake may not be adequate for the purposes of radioiodine treatment. For this reason a tracer dose of iodine-131 is given and a scintiscan is taken 24 hours later (p. 522), which will reveal any functioning thyroid tissue. The scan can be extended to the rest of the body, and a 'profile' count obtained, with peaks opposite areas of above-normal

uptake elsewhere, i.e. any functioning metastases. In practice it is very difficult to achieve complete surgical removal of the thyroid gland and some residual tissue in the neck is usually found on postoperative scan since some thyroid tissue is inevitably left behind by the surgeon to conserve the parathyroid glands. Only when an ablation dose has been given, destroying all normal thyroid tissue, can residual uptake in the neck or at distant sites be assumed to be due to presence of tumour. The decision to use radioiodine should therefore not be taken purely on histological grounds.

Any remaining thyroid tissue after thyroidectomy of any degree, as revealed by the scan, should be eliminated as a potential danger. A *therapeutic ablation* dose of 3 GBq is given. The patient should be in a separate side-ward and full precautions taken against radiation hazards (Ch. 12). This dose will destroy remaining thyroid tissue. About 50% of follicular carcinomas will also take up iodine in the same way but if normal thyroid tissue is also present, then, as a rule, the normal tissue will take it up preferentially from the circulation, as it will be the successful competitor for whatever iodine is available in the circulation. The purpose of the ablation is to remove this competition. When all normal thyroid tissue has been destroyed by the iodine-131, the malignant tissue, stimulated by TSH, begins to function, to replace the missing thyroid.

Following the first ablation dose, a follow-up tracer scan should be carried out at intervals of 3–4 months, to detect any functioning tissue in the neck or elsewhere. Such tissue may be the focus for recurrence or metastases. If they take up worthwhile amounts of iodine-131 (i.e. 0.1% per gram of functioning tumour at 24 hours), they can now be destroyed by large therapeutic ablation doses of about 7 GBq. Assuming a biological half-life of 3 days, this will deliver a dose of 60 Gy to areas of tumour. If the degree of uptake is borderline, TSH (10 units intramuscularly) can be given daily for 3–5 days, before a therapeutic dose of iodine, to stimulate greater iodine uptake by the tumour. As long as there is adequate uptake, further therapeutic doses are given (bearing in mind the dose that can be given by external beam), unless there is a contraindication, such as low white cell count, or a maximum dose of 37 GBq has been reached. Beyond this dose, the risks of pancytopenia, aplastic anaemia and leukaemia increase. The investigation and treatment of patients with well-differentiated thyroid cancer is summarised in Figure 21.29.

Patients under the age of 35 with well-differentiated papillary or follicular carcinoma not penetrating the capsule (T1 or T2) and without lymph node or distant

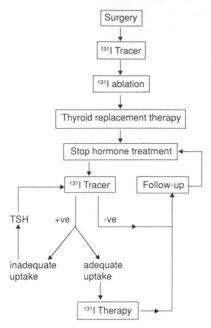

Fig. 21.29　Use of iodine-131 in thyroid cancer.

metastases have a particularly good prognosis. For this group of patients radioiodine therapy can be avoided.

Reactions to radioiodine. These large ablation doses can produce local and general reactions but these are usually mild.

In the gland itself there may be an inflammatory reaction with painful swelling and tenderness the next day, subsiding in the following week. If the swelling is severe, it may require a short course of oral or parenteral steroid therapy. There is also some excretion via the salivary glands (e.g. parotid) and a similar reaction may occur here. Symptoms and signs of hypothyroidism do not usually develop until at least a month later and are usually mild.

General effects such as radiation sickness and lassitude are seldom troublesome and leucopenia is short lived (lowest at 3–6 weeks). The gonads (ovaries and testes) will be affected, with menstrual disturbances and temporary inhibition of sperm formation. These are unlikely to be of practical importance. The dose to the gonad is normally about half of the plasma dosage and sterility is unlikely to occur unless there is a pelvic bone metastasis close to the testis or an ovary. Pregnancy is an absolute contraindication to isotope therapy because of the risk of radiation damage to the fetus. There is a theoretical risk of mutagenic effects.

The risk of leukaemia and aplastic anaemia is largely avoidable if the total administered dose is limited to

37 GBq or if therapeutic doses are not repeated more frequently than once a year.

Painful swelling of the parotid glands may occur if the parotid duct becomes narrowed but this usually resolves spontaneously. Lung fibrosis may occur due to radioiodine uptake in lung metastases.

Radical external beam irradiation

Indications

— All anaplastic tumours (regardless of any surgery performed).
— Inoperable thyroid tumour or neck nodes where iodine-131 is not appropriate.
— After incomplete thyroidectomy for papillary or follicular carcinoma (the alternative is a second operation to complete the thyroid removal) where iodine-131 has failed or is not appropriate.
— Lymphoma.

Target volume

This will depend on the pathological type, the loco-regional extent of the tumour and whether the nodes are involved. If all the regional nodes are included, the volume then extends from the hyoid bone above to the division of the trachea (carina) below. However for well-differentiated cancers, only the thyroid bed and adjacent lymphatics need to be included. In this case the volume extends from the hyoid bone to the sternal notch. The posterior border lies parallel to the spinal cord and incorporates the anterior margin of the vertebrae. The anterior margin includes the skin of the neck.

Technique

External radiation of the thyroid presents technical

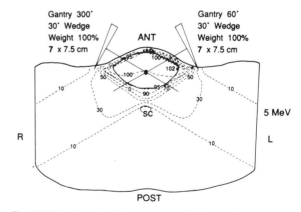

Fig. 21.30　Anterior oblique wedged fields used to treat localised carcinoma of the thyroid. (Reproduced with permission from Dobbs et al 1992.)

difficulties. The contours are irregular, with rapidly changing dimensions from point to point. The treatment volume curves around the spinal cord. Careful planning is required to avoid exceeding the radiation tolerance of the spinal cord. A shell is necessary to immobilise the neck. The patient is treated supine with the head extended. Bolus is applied to the scar and any superficial tumour.

No nodes palpable. If only the thyroid bed and adjacent lymph nodes are treated, two anterior oblique wedged fields usually suffice (Fig. 21.30). Contours for computer planning are taken through the centre, top and bottom of the fields. Alternatively two lateral wedged oblique fields, angled down, are used. To compensate for the oblique incidence in the antero-posterior plane, a horizontal wedge is used for one field (Fig. 21.31). A vertical wedge is used for the other field. The wedges are interchanged after half the

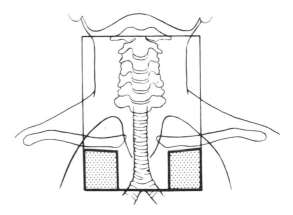

Fig. 21.33 Anterior and posterior fields used to treat anaplastic tumours. (Reproduced with permission from Dobbs & Barrett, Practical Radiotherapy Planning, 1st edn, Edward Arnold, 1985.)

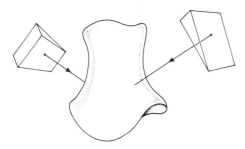

Fig. 21.31 Twisted wedge technique for treatment of postcricoid and thyroid carcinoma showing horizontal and vertical positions of the wedges. (Courtesy of Dr I Manifold, Sheffield.)

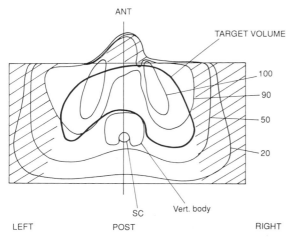

Fig. 21.32 Isodose distribution from an anterior 20 MeV electron field with additional bolus.

treatment to obtain homogeneous irradiation of the treatment volume.

Palpable nodes. Where the nodes are affected, a single direct anterior 20 MeV electron field with wax gives a suitable dose distribution (Fig. 21.32). An additional thickness of wax bolus can be placed over the central part of the field to bow the isodoses forward in front of the spinal cord.

For large anaplastic tumours and for lymphomas of the thyroid simple anterior and posterior fields including all or most of the neck are satisfactory, with a downward tongue for the mediastinum (Fig. 21.33). The spinal cord dose should not exceed 40 Gy in 4 weeks.

Dose and energy

Carcinoma
Full tolerance dose depending on the volume indicated

Electrons may be used to boost residual masses.

Non-Hodgkin lymphoma

High grade
40 Gy in 20 daily fractions over 4 weeks (4–6 MV photons)

Low grade
35 Gy in 20 daily fractions over 4 weeks (4–6 MV photons)

Palliative radiotherapy

The indications for palliative external radiation are: (1) symptomatic neck nodes in patients not suitable for radical radiotherapy or surgery, and (2) bony metastases.

Dose and energy
22.5 Gy in 5 daily fractions (cobalt-60 or 4–6 MV photons)

The treatment of secondaries which take up iodine is described below.

Results of treatment

Survival times are extremely variable, as shown in Table 21.2. The anaplastic types fare worst and papillary best. Patients with papillary tumours may have strikingly long survival over many years, even in the presence of secondaries. Follicular carcinoma is not nearly as favourable. Radioactive iodine-131 offers excellent palliation in those patients who take it up in adequate concentration, including in secondary deposits.

Follow-up

Long-term follow-up is necessary and may include clinical assessment, and thyroglobulin (for well-differentiated carcinoma after complete ablation of the normal thyroid) or calcitonin as markers. The adequacy of thyroid hormone suppression should be monitored. Iodine-131 tracer scanning should be repeated as necessary. Hypocalcaemia may need treatment.

22. Oesophagus, gastrointestinal tract, lung, thymus, pancreas, liver

CANCER OF THE OESOPHAGUS

Anatomy

The oesophagus is a muscular tube which runs from the lower border of the cricoid cartilage at the level of the 6th cervical vertebra to the origin of the stomach at the level T10. For clinical purposes the oesophagus is divided into thirds: upper, middle and lower (Fig. 22.1).

The upper third (or cervical part) extends from its origin to the level of the bifurcation of the trachea at the junction of T4 and T5. At its origin the oesophagus is in the midline and veers to the left as it descends. It is related to the trachea and thyroid gland anteriorly and the lower cervical vertebrae posteriorly. Laterally lie the common carotid arteries and the recurrent laryngeal nerves.

The middle third (or thoracic part) runs from the bifurcation of the trachea to the junction of T7 and T8. From lying slightly towards the left, it returns to the midline at T5 and then passes downwards forwards and to the left. In front it is crossed by the trachea, the left main bronchus and the pericardium. Behind lie the thoracic vertebrae.

The lower third extends from the junction of T7 and T8 and passes forwards through the diaphragm to the opening of the stomach.

Lymphatic drainage. There is a rich lymphatic plexus around the oesophagus (Fig. 22.1), which drains into

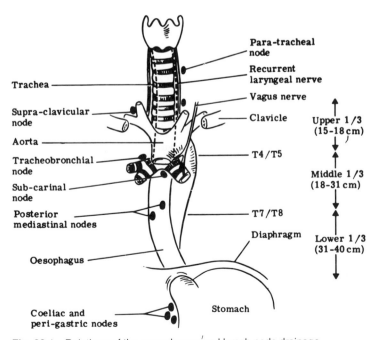

Fig. 22.1 Relations of the oesophagus and lymph node drainage. (Reproduced with permission from Dobbs & Barrett, Practical Radiotherapy Planning, Ist edn, Edward Arnold, 1985.)

the posterior mediastinal nodes which in turn drain upwards to the supraclavicular nodes and downwards to the coeliac nodes close to the stomach. The importance of this interconnecting network of lymphatics is that cross-regional drainage is common. This explains why tumours of the upper third of the oesophagus frequently have abdominal nodal metastases at presentation. Overall, 70% of all patients have nodal metastases at the time of diagnosis.

Pathology

Cancer of the oesophagus accounts for about 1.9% of all cancers and 3.1% of cancer deaths. It is a disease of the elderly, usually over the age of 60. Overall it is commoner in men than women, with a sex ratio of 1.8:1. Cancer of the upper oesophagus is, however, commoner in women. There are areas of the world where the incidence is substantially higher, for example on the east coast of the Caspian sea in Turkmenistan and Iran, in Japan and parts of northern China. The reasons for the increased incidence are probably multiple. Dietary contaminants such as the nitrosamine group of chemicals and certain toxins from fungi (mycotoxins) have been postulated as aetiological factors. Alcohol and tobacco combine to increase the risk of oesophageal cancer. Conditions predisposing to the development of oesophageal cancer include: tylosis palmaris et plantaris, a scaling skin disorder of the palms and soles of the feet; Plummer–Vinson syndrome (upper third); achalasia of the cardia (mainly middle third); malnutrition; and oesophageal acid reflux.

Fifteen per cent of tumours arise in the upper third. The majority occur in the middle and lower thirds. Ninety per cent are squamous cell carcinomas. About 10% are adenocarcinomas, mainly in the lower third where they arise in the context of gastric reflux and glandular metaplasia (Barrett's oesophagus). The degree of differentiation of the tumour is variable. Oat cell carcinoma (similar to oat cell carcinoma of the lung in its behaviour), adenoid cystic carcinoma and sarcomas of the oesophagus are rare.

It is important to appreciate that submucosal spread upwards and downwards is common and may extend several centimetres beyond the macroscopic limits of the tumour. 'Skip' lesions may occur elsewhere in the oesophagus several centimetres away from the primary tumour, due to submucosal lymphatic and vascular spread. The oesophageal wall is thin and extra-oesophageal spread to the aorta, trachea, pleura, pericardium and even vertebral bodies may soon follow. Blood-borne spread occurs early to the liver, and subsequently lungs and bones; 30% of patients have distant metastases at the time of diagnosis.

Clinical features

The cardinal symptom is progressive dysphagia, first for solids and later for fluids as well. There may be regurgitation and vomiting. If the oesophagus is obstructed, it can still cope with a large amount of contents, propelling small quantities of food past the obstruction in a series of waves of muscular contraction. Once the lumen of the oesophagus is reduced to a critical size, dysphagia becomes absolute. Discomfort and chest pain from extraoesophageal spread may follow. Malnutrition, loss of weight and dehydration will become serious if not relieved. As a result the patient's general medical condition is often too poor to undertake either radical surgery or radiotherapy.

Diagnosis and staging

It is necessary to establish the site of the tumour and obtain a biopsy.

The first investigation is a barium swallow. This may show the level of obstruction and narrowing. The upper level of the growth can be determined in this way, but the lower end may be difficult to discern. The movement of the diaphragm should be screened. Paralysis suggests compression of the phrenic nerve in the mediastinum.

Next, instrumental oesophagoscopy is carried out under general anaesthesia. The tumour is inspected. Multiple biopsies are taken to give a good chance of establishing a histological diagnosis. The oesophagoscope should be passed downwards, if possible, to assess the length of the tumour. Temporary relief of dysphagia may be achieved by gentle dilatation to widen the lumen.

A bronchoscopy should be carried out at the same time as oesophagoscopy to exclude compression of the bronchi by the primary tumour or from involved mediastinal nodes.

A chest radiograph may show metastases in the lung fields or widening of the mediastinum due to nodal metastases. Liver ultrasound is done to detect liver metastases. CT scanning of the chest and upper abdomen is often helpful in demonstrating nodal involvement (mediastinal and coeliac) and liver metastases.

Treatment

The situation is similar to lung cancer—surgery is possible for a minority. Surgery is contraindicated in many patients because of poor medical condition, invasion of the mediastinum, mediastinal nodes or distant metastases.

In general, adenocarcinomas, usually of the lower third, are best treated by radical surgery. Adenocarcinomas are relatively radioresistant. For this reason radical radiotherapy is not recommended. For squamous carcinomas of the upper third, radical radiotherapy is preferred, since laryngopharyngectomy can be avoided. For the middle third either radical surgery or radical radiotherapy may be feasible. Attention to maintenance of general medical condition, e.g. correction of nutritional deficiencies and anaemia, is particularly important in patients undergoing radical treatment.

Surgery

Radical. Apart from age, poor general condition and evidence of spread beyond the oesophagus, radical surgery is contraindicated if the tumour is poorly differentiated or judged to be over 5 cm in length. The chances of finding a genuinely localised tumour are remote. Only about 40% of squamous cell carcinomas are operable.

Following oesophagectomy, the defect is replaced by transplanting part of the colon with its vascular supply between the proximal remnant of the oesophagus and the stomach. Operative mortality is still high at 10–15%.

Palliative

Dilatation. Dilating the oesophageal lumen can provide short-term improvement in swallowing where only short lengths of the oesophagus are occluded. It can be carried out during diagnostic endoscopy and is repeatable.

Intubation. A very useful method when radical treatment is contraindicated is to insert a tube to maintain a free passage past the tumour and so ensure adequate swallowing for the remainder of life. Various types of tube are available. There are two main types, 'push-through' and 'pull-through'. Push-through types, such as the Souttar tube composed of flexible metal coils, are pushed blindly through the obstruction and are suitable for obstructions up to 10 cm in length in the upper or middle thirds of the oesophagus. Pull-through types, such the Mousseau–Barbin plastic tube or the soft rubber Celestin tube, are so called because they are pulled through the obstruction using a guide wire or string from above into the stomach where they are secured by a suture. They are most suited for tumours of the middle or lower thirds. The success rates for intubation vary from 40 to 85%, with an average duration of benefit of 4 months.

Intubation is not without hazard, carrying a mortality of up to 20%, usually from oesophageal perforation occurring during the procedure.

Gastrostomy and cervical oesophagostomy. This involves opening the stomach to insert a feeding tube which is brought out on the anterior abdominal wall. An opening is made in the cervical oesophagus to aspirate secretions from the upper airway and prevent aspiration. It may be valuable as a temporary measure while radical radiotherapy is carried out, but as a permanent procedure it is clearly objectionable. The patient is unable to eat or drink and personal hygiene is difficult to maintain.

Laser therapy. Debulking of the tumour by laser therapy can provide rapid relief of relatively short obstructing lesions. It is, however, only available in a limited number of centres in the UK.

Radical radiotherapy

Radical radiotherapy is applicable to a small proportion of patients with localised tumours of limited length in the middle and upper thirds of the oesophagus. Preoperative radiotherapy is an attractive concept with a view to sterilising the tumour and then resecting it but there is no convincing evidence that it improves survival compared with surgery alone.

There is little information on the value of postoperative radiotherapy following oesophagectomy. Surgeons are understandably reluctant to submit a patient to an additional major treatment procedure. Again, no convincing survival benefit over surgery alone has been demonstrated.

Criteria for selection

1. Squamous cell carcinoma not greater than 5 cm in length
2. No mediastinal spread
3. No lymph node or distant metastases
4. Adequate general medical and nutritional state
5. Under the age of 70.

Advanced age is a relative contraindication. The prognosis for women with squamous cell carcinoma of the oesophagus is better than that for men. For this reason, if the first four criteria are fulfilled, a woman over the age of 70 with a squamous carcinoma may be treated radically. A man of the same age would be better treated by palliative radiotherapy.

Target volume
This should include the primary tumour, as defined

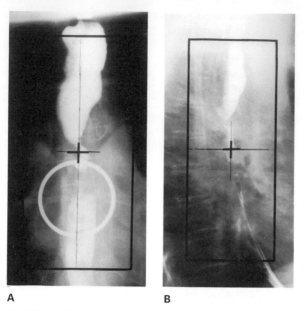

A **B**

Fig. 22.2 Simulator radiographs showing field margins for carcinoma of the middle third of the oesophagus. **A** Anteroposterior, **B** lateral. (Courtesy of Dr I Manifold, Sheffield.)

by barium swallow and oesophagoscopy, with a margin of 5 cm above and below (Fig. 22.2). The length of the volume should not exceed 18 cm. The lateral margins should be sufficient to encompass the soft tissues of the oesophageal wall (usually 6 cm) or 8 cm if the adjacent nodes liable to invasion are included. In the older patient a reduction of a few centimetres in the margin above and below the tumour is advisable to limit the severity of the acute radiation reaction.

Technique

Anatomical factors constrain the delivery of a homo-

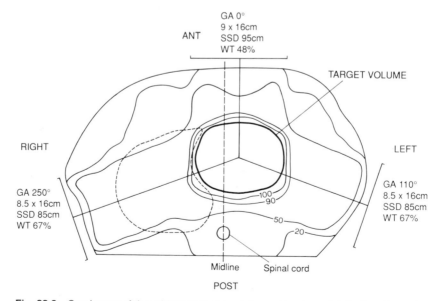

Fig. 22.3 Carcinoma of the middle third of oesophagus. Isodose distribution of anterior and two posterior oblique fields. (Courtesy of Dr J Bolger, Sheffield.)

geneous dose of radiation to the oesophagus. The changing position of the oesophagus during its course and the variation in the contour of the body often require the plane of treatment to be inclined rather than parallel to the couch. It should be noted that the treated volume is cylindrical in shape. In addition, overdosage to the spinal cord and the lung must be avoided.

The technique for the upper third is described in Chapter 21 (p. 352). For middle and lower third lesions a three field isocentric technique of an open anterior field and two wedged posterior oblique fields is used (Fig. 22.3). A CT planning scan is helpful in optimising the positioning of the fields and avoiding the spinal cord.

The patient is simulated supine with the hands resting behind the head. Thin barium is swallowed to identify the tumour and to choose the upper and lower limits of the field. Having defined the upper and lower limits and the width of the volume, the patient is simulated from the side to define the depth in the anteroposterior plane. Some inclination may be required to avoid inclusion of the spinal cord. Sometimes it is impossible to avoid the cord completely, if the tumour is to be adequately covered. However not more than a 1 cm length should be included in the treated volume. The posterior oblique fields are viewed to confirm adequate coverage. Contours are taken through the top, middle and bottom of the volume. The positions of the target volume, spinal cord, heart and lungs are marked. A correction should be made for the greater transmission of radiation through the lungs (usually 3% per centimetre of lung traversed). A beam passing through the lung may give a 30–40% higher radiation dose to the oesophagus than the same beam through solid tissue. The dose to the spinal cord should not exceed 40 Gy in 20 daily fractions over 4 weeks.

Dose and energy
52.5 Gy given in 20 daily fractions over 4 weeks (9–10 MV photons)

Radiation reactions
Acute. Radical radiotherapy can be a severe strain and hospital admission, particularly for the second half of treatment, is recommended when symptoms of the acute reaction become more marked. General reactions with nausea and anorexia may occur and even interrupt treatment for a few days. Adequate fluid intake and nutrition must be watched. Radiation oesophagitis develops midway through the course and makes feeding even more difficult. Soft diet, high calorie fluid supplements and mucaine are helpful. Nasogastric feeding with a fine-bore (Clinifeed) tube may be necessary if oral intake of calories is insufficient. Fungal infection of the oesophagus with candida is frequent and should be treated with antifungal therapy such as nystatin suspension.

Because of the thinness of the oesophageal wall, infiltration by the tumour in depth can soon occur and lead to perforation. This may even be precipitated by destruction of the tumour under radiation. Infective mediastinitis will follow, usually fatal. Similarly, a major blood vessel may be eroded, with rapidly fatal haemorrhage. Aspiration pneumonia is not uncommon and often fatal despite antibiotic therapy. Radiation pneumonitis (p. 379) is rare.

Late. Late complications are mainly oesophageal strictures. These can occur as early as 3 months after treatment, but patients rarely survive long enough to develop this complication. Treatment is by dilatation, repeated if necessary.

Palliative radiotherapy

Palliative radiotherapy is worthwhile considering to relieve dysphagia in patients for whom radical radiotherapy is contraindicated. This may be by external beam or single-dose intraoesophageal irradiation using a 'Selectron' containing a cobalt source. Suspected or proven tracheo-oesophageal fistula, a communication between the oesophagus and the trachea from tumoral invasion, is a contraindication to palliative radiotherapy.

External beam
Target volume
A small margin of 1–2 cm above and below the tumour is recommended to limit the severity of the acute reaction.

Treatment technique
A simple pair of parallel opposed anterior and posterior fields is used.

Dose and energy
30 Gy given in 10 daily fractions or 22.5 Gy in 5 daily fractions (cobalt-60 or 4–6 MV photons)

Selectron
A single treatment of 15 Gy at 1 cm from the central axis of the cobalt-60 source.

Chemotherapy

Oesophageal cancer responds poorly to currently available chemotherapy. Agents such as cisplatin, bleomycin, methotrexate, 5-fluorouracil and Adriamycin have been used as single agents or in combination. Their toxicity makes their use difficult to justify since short-term partial responses in a minority of patients are all that can be achieved at present.

Results of treatment

The results of both radical surgery and radical radiotherapy in the UK are poor, with an overall 5-year survival of 5–10%. The best results of radical radiotherapy have been a 22% 5-year survival in a series from Edinburgh. Most series have been unable to match this. The prognosis is better in the upper third of the oesophagus (5-year survival 10–20%). Lower third tumours fare best with surgery, with a 30% 5-year survival.

CARCINOMA OF THE STOMACH
Pathology

Epidemiology and aetiology

The incidence of carcinoma of the stomach is declining in most countries including Britain but it still accounts for 10 000 deaths per year in England and Wales. It represents 7% of all cancers and 7.9% of all cancer deaths. It is the third commonest cause of death from cancer in men and the fourth most common in women. It is commoner in men than women, with a sex ratio of 2.2:1, and more common amongst manual workers than in professional groups. Its maximum incidence is in the sixth decade. There is a wide variation in the incidence in the UK. For example it is three times more common in the north-west of England than in the south-east. The highest incidence is in Japan (80 per 100 000), more than double the incidence in Britain.

The epidemiology of gastric cancer suggests diet as the main influence; Japanese who emigrated to the USA take on the local lower incidence. The precise factors are not clear; it is more frequent with higher carbohydrate consumption, and less with higher amounts of green vegetables. Bacterial action on nitrates could produce nitrosamines, a carcinogen; this reaction is inhibited by vitamin C. Bacteria may be more plentiful if gastric acid secretion is defective, and nitrites in the soil can enter the food chain.

Precursor lesions are rarely diagnosed, though cancer is more frequently seen in the context of chronic gastritis, or atrophy (as in pernicious anaemia). Occasionally *dysplasia* can be identified as a precursor; in Japan, with its high incidence of gastric cancer, many tumours are picked up as early gastric cancer, i.e.

superficial tumours with a good prognosis. Genetic factors may have a minor role, as the tumour is more common in blood group A than in group O.

The diffusely infiltrating (*linitis plastica*) variant of gastric cancer varies less between cultures, so presumably has a different aetiology.

Macroscopic and microscopic features

Most stomach cancers are diffuse and infiltrating with a rolled edge and central ulceration; 95% are adenocarcinomas. They occur mainly in the antrum (60%), or body, with 10% at the cardia. Local spread occurs through the stomach wall to the pancreas and omentum. Lymphatic spread, present in 50% of cases, is to the regional nodes on the lesser and greater curve of the stomach, the coeliac and other abdominal nodes. From the coeliac nodes metastases may reach the supraclavicular nodes via the thoracic duct. Spread may cross the peritoneum (transcoelomic) to the omentum and abdominal organs including the ovaries (the so-called Krukenberg tumour). Blood-borne spread to the liver, lungs and bone is common.

Clinical features

The commonest symptoms are loss of appetite, weight loss and non-specific upper abdominal pain. If there is obstruction to the outflow of the stomach at the antrum, vomiting may occur. There may also be dysphagia, particularly if the tumour lies at the gastro-oesophageal junction. Common physical findings are a palpable upper abdominal mass and an enlarged left supraclavicular node (Virchow's node). The liver may be enlarged and masses palpable in the abdomen and pelvis.

Diagnosis and investigation

Barium meal or gastroscopy of the stomach are the initial investigations. Typically a barium meal shows a malignant ulcer with irregular walls. The stomach, if diffusely infiltrated, appears small and contracted (linitis plastica). The ulcer should be biopsied and gastric washings examined for malignant cells. An apparently normal barium meal or gastroscopy does not exclude gastric cancer. Gastroscopy should be considered if the barium meal is normal, or vice versa, since both investigations have a false negative rate of 20–30%. Additional investigations should include a full blood count and chest radiograph and liver ultrasound for lung and liver metastases respectively. In Japan, where the disease is common, it has been shown that earlier detection by screening, by means of a barium meal and gastroscopy, has increased the proportion of patients in whom surgical resection is possible. The mortality from the disease in Japan has fallen. The low and declining incidence of the disease in the UK would not justify a large screening programme for the disease but limited screening can successfully identify those at high risk of developing the disease. These would include patients with a history of previous gastric surgery, pernicious anaemia or blood group A.

Treatment

Surgery

The only curative treatment is surgical resection. Total gastrectomy is the most radical kind. A more limited procedure of partial gastrectomy may be possible for localised tumours. Unfortunately the majority of tumours are too advanced for curative resection. Often some kind of palliative resection or bypass procedure can be undertaken to relieve symptoms of obstruction.

Radiotherapy

Opinion is divided on the role of radiotherapy. Most radiotherapists feel that it has no useful role since stomach cancer is relatively radioresistant. Others believe useful palliation can be achieved in relieving dysphagia and haemorrhage, at least in proliferative tumours. Infiltrative tumours, however, tend not to respond and should not be treated.

Palliative

Technique
Parallel opposed anterior and posterior fields are used.

Dose and energy
30 Gy in 10 daily fractions over 2 weeks (4–6 MV photons)

Intraoperative

Intraoperative radiotherapy (IORT), in which the residual disease is irradiated peroperatively, following tumour debulking, with high energy electrons from a linear accelerator, is being evaluated. Sensitive surrounding structures are moved out of the radiation field to limit the morbidity of IORT. Initial results from Japan claim an improvement in 5-year survival in more advanced stages of disease. Late small bowel and neurological damage does, however, occur. It seems unlikely that this form of treatment will be widely practised because of logistical difficulties. Too few patients have been treated and followed up long enough to assess its real worth.

Chemotherapy

Chemotherapy has only a limited role in the treatment of stomach cancer. There is no evidence that it improves survival. Short-term palliation can be achieved in a few patients. The most suitable agent is probably 5-fluorouracil which has a response rate of about 20% in advanced tumours. It has the advantage of limited toxicity. The optimum method of administration is uncertain. However a continuous 5-day infusion of 750 mg/m^2 per 24 hours has the advantage of less toxicity than weekly injections. Acute stomatitis, joint pains and scaling of the skin may still occur.

Results of treatment

The best results have been achieved in Japan where 5-year survival of 80% has been obtained for tumours confined within the serosa and without nodal metastases. It is not clear to what extent these excellent results are due to earlier diagnosis or better screening. Sadly, results in the UK remain poor with a 5-year survival of 4%. This only increases to 17% if a surgical resection can be carried out.

COLORECTAL CANCER
Pathology

Epidemiology and aetiology

Tumours of the colon and rectum are the second commonest cause of death from cancer in the UK, causing 20 000 deaths per year. The incidence is stable. They represent 12.4% of all cancers and 12.5% of cancer deaths. The overall male to female sex ratio is 1.3:1. Colonic cancer, especially on the right side, is slightly commoner in women. However males exceed females with rectal cancer by 2:1. Tumours of the colon outnumber those of the rectum in a ratio of 3:2. Sites in order of frequency are rectum, pelvic colon, descending colon, caecum, transverse colon, hepatic and splenic flexures. The majority of colorectal cancers are thought to develop from pre-existing benign polyps (adenomas) arising in the mucosa of the bowel. The size and number of the polyps are important in the relative risk of malignant change. Polyps less than 1 cm in diameter have a 1% risk of containing carcinoma. Polyps over 2 cm in diameter have a 30% risk. Multiple polyps have an eightfold higher risk than single polyps.

Genetic and dietary factors are thought to play an important role in the aetiology of colorectal cancer.

The disease is commonest in Western countries and lowest in Africa, South America and Asia. It is thought that these differences are mainly explained by dietary factors. Western diets are low in fibre content and rich in animal fats and meat. By contrast, the African diet is higher in fibre and lower in animal fats and meat, and is associated with a more rapid bowel transit time. The exposure time of the bowel to carcinogens is therefore shorter. The exact mechanism by which animal fats bring about the development of cancer is unknown. One hypothesis is that a change in the microbial flora of the bowel is brought about by the ingestion of fat. This results in a higher concentration of bile acids from the degradation of bile acids and cholesterol. Bile acids are known to promote the action of carcinogens such as dimethylhydrazine under experimental conditions. Other evidence has not supported this hypothesis.

The incidence of colorectal cancer is much lower in populations with a high proportion of vegetables in their diet. The explanation for this may be due either to the presence of vitamin A or to the high fibre content.

A minority of cases arise in cancer families; this implies a genetic contribution from a tumour suppressor gene (p. 245). The most striking is the malignant transformation of one or more intestinal polyps in the inherited condition of familial polyposis coli. Multiple polyps occur throughout the large bowel. There is an autosomal dominant inheritance of a tumour suppressor gene on chromosome 5. Affected individuals develop polyps from teenage years onward, with subsequent malignant change from 5–20 years later, reflecting further genetic events in the polyps. Other bowel diseases which predispose to colorectal cancer are two forms of inflammatory disease: ulcerative colitis and Crohn's disease. The risk in ulcerative colitis is highest if the disease has been present for 10 years (10% risk) or has been present since birth. Other risk factors are schistosomiasis (a parasitic disease) and previous surgery in which a ureter has been transplanted into the sigmoid colon (ureterosigmoidostomy).

Macroscopic and microscopic features

Colorectal cancers are usually polypoid masses, often with central ulceration and bleeding. Nearly all are adenocarcinomas. Direct spread may occur through the bowel wall into the pericolic and perirectal fat. The degree of penetration of the bowel wall is the basis of the Dukes' classification system (see below). Lymphatic spread is to the regional nodes. These are involved in 50% of cases at the time of surgery. Blood-borne spread to the liver via the portal system is common (15% at the time of surgery).

Clinical features

Common symptoms are a change in bowel habit (constipation or diarrhoea), rectal bleeding, tenesmus (a feeling of incomplete evacuation of the bowel), mucoid discharge, unexplained anaemia and weight loss. Tumours of the right side of the colon rarely obstruct the bowel and tend to present with anaemia. Tumours of the sigmoid are more likely to cause obstruction. Rectal cancer typically presents with bleeding and tenesmus.

An abdominal or rectal mass may be palpable. Over 50% of tumours are palpable on rectal examination. The liver may be enlarged by secondary deposits, with or without jaundice. Presentation may be with acute intestinal obstruction or perforation.

Diagnosis and staging

This should include inspection of the mucosa of the final 25 cm of the bowel by proctosigmoidoscopy. A flexible colonoscope can be used to look further down the lumen of the bowel. This should be followed by radiography of the bowel (barium enema). Contrast medium and air are instilled into the rectum. This provides a double contrast image which helps identify small tumours. Tumours may appear as strictures or masses indenting the contrast. If the result is equivocal, the examination should be repeated or a colonoscopy performed. Accessible tumours should be biopsied. For inaccessible tumours the histological diagnosis is made at laparotomy.

Staging

The most commonly used staging system is the Dukes' system based on the degree of invasion through the bowel wall and of lymphatic spread:

Dukes' classification
A—confined to the bowel wall
B—penetration beyond the muscularis propria to perirectal fat
C—draining nodes involved

Treatment

Surgery is the main curative treatment of colorectal

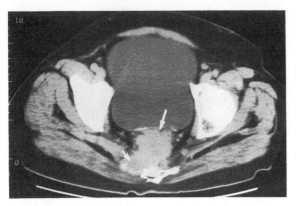

Fig. 22.4 CT scan showing invasion of the sacrum (small arrow) by recurrent carcinoma of the rectum (large arrow). (Courtesy of Dr R Nakielny, Sheffield.)

cancer. However radiotherapy has been shown to have a useful role as an adjuvant treatment to surgery in rectal cancer and for palliation of recurrent (Fig. 22.4) or inoperable disease. Apart from palliation, there is no established role for radiotherapy in colonic cancer.

Surgery

Radical surgical resection should include the affected segment of bowel and its local lymphatic drainage. This is followed where possible by anastomosis of the proximal and distal remnants of the bowel.

In rectal cancer the type of operation will depend on the site of the tumour. The classical operation for rectal cancer is excision of the anus and rectum (abdominoperineal excision). In about 10% of rectal tumours the primary tumour can be removed and the continuity of the bowel restored (anterior restorative resection) if at least 5 cm of clearance below the tumour can be achieved. This avoids the need for a permanent colostomy and has a similar local recurrence rate to abdominoperineal resection.

Radiotherapy for rectal cancer

For many years it was considered that rectal cancer was resistant to radiation. Recent studies have demonstrated that responses, though usually only partial, do occur. Both radical and palliative radiotherapy have a role. Radical dosage should be attempted where possible since it gives the best chance of good palliation.

There is some evidence that preoperative low dose irradiation e.g. 40 Gy in 20 daily fractions over 4 weeks, followed a month later by surgery, may increase the chances of rendering some initially fixed tumours sufficiently mobile to be operable.

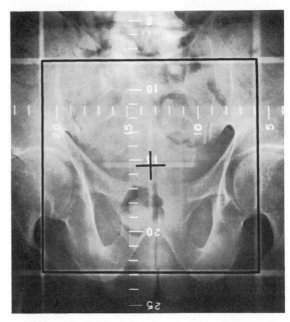

Fig. 22.5 Simulator radiograph (antero-posterior) showing radical treatment volume for carcinoma of the rectum. (Courtesy of Dr J Bolger, Sheffield.)

The value of postoperative radiotherapy is also unclear despite the fact that patients are frequently referred. It does appear to reduce the incidence of local recurrence but no improvement in survival has been demonstrated.

Radical radiotherapy

The indications are:

1. Primary
   a. Inoperable localised disease
   b. Local recurrence of disease following surgery
2. Postoperative
   a. Peroperative tumour spillage
   b. Macroscopic residual disease
   c. Tumour at the resection margins (microscopic).

Target volume

This includes the primary tumour or its bed, the local lymphatics and the presacral area (Fig. 22.5). The upper limit of the field is the top of the sacrum. Extending the upper margin beyond this level will include more small bowel in the field and increase the morbidity. Laterally the pelvic side walls and internal iliac nodes should be included. The inferior margin should be 4–5 cm below the tumour or its bed. The posterior limit should encompass the presacral nodes and the sacral hollow. Anteriorly a margin should be allowed in front of the anastomosis or the tumour and include, in women, the posterior vaginal wall.

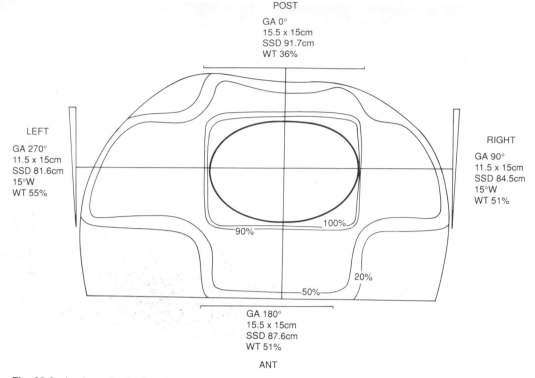

POST
GA 0°
15.5 x 15cm
SSD 91.7cm
WT 36%

LEFT
GA 270°
11.5 x 15cm
SSD 81.6cm
15°W
WT 55%

RIGHT
GA 90°
11.5 x 15cm
SSD 84.5cm
15°W
WT 51%

90%   100%
20%
50%

GA 180°
15.5 x 15cm
SSD 87.6cm
WT 51%

ANT

Fig. 22.6 Isodose distribution of posterior and two lateral wedged fields for radical radiotherapy of carcinoma of the rectum. (Courtesy of Dr J Bolger, Sheffield.)

Technique

The patient is simulated in the prone position with the toes together and the heels apart, the head resting on the hands. A four field box or three field (direct posterior field and two lateral or posterior oblique fields) technique is recommended (Fig. 22.6). These have the advantage over a parallel opposed pair of anterior and posterior fields that the dose to the bladder and small bowel is reduced. Lateral fields give a much sharper fall-off in dose anteriorly compared with posterior oblique fields. The latter give a more rounded dose distribution anteriorly. If the bladder or anterior abdominal wall is infiltrated, an anterior and posterior opposed pair of fields should be used.

For perineal lesions, a direct posterior field is preferred.

Dose and energy
50 Gy in 20 daily fractions over 4 weeks (9–10 MV photons)

Acute and late reactions. Proctocolitis and cystitis occur as described on page 411.

Palliative radiotherapy
The indications for palliative radiotherapy are:

— Bleeding
— Pain
— Rectal discharge.

Target volume
This should include the primary tumour and the whole pelvis.

Technique
A parallel opposed pair of anterior and posterior fields is used.

Dose and energy
20 Gy in 5 daily fractions or 30 Gy in 10 daily fractions (9–10 MV photons)

Chemotherapy

Adjuvant. The role of adjuvant chemotherapy following surgery to reduce the likelihood of recurrence is controversial. There is evidence that 5-fluorouracil, given for a year, and postoperative radiotherapy reduce local recurrence (33%) from the disease in patients who have undergone 'curative' resection for Dukes' B and C carcinoma of the rectum compared with surgery alone (55%). However no survival benefit has been shown.

Following curative resection, histological grade, Dukes' classification and venous spread are the main prognostic factors predictive of recurrence. It would seem logical to select high risk patients for adjuvant therapy if the early promise of 5-fluorouracil is fulfilled.

There is evidence that adjuvant 5-FU + Levamisole improves local control and survival in Dukes' C colonic cancer.

For locally advanced and metastatic disease. There is little effective chemotherapy for colorectal cancer. 5-Fluorouracil is currently the best choice since it is the least toxic and has a response rate of about 20%, which is as good as more toxic single agent or combination chemotherapy.

Results of treatment

Five-year survival is 80% for Dukes' A, 60% for Dukes' B and 25% for Dukes' C cancers of the colon and rectum.

About 30% of patients will obtain complete relief of their symptoms from palliative radiotherapy and a further 45% partial relief. Average duration of relief is 6–12 months.

ANAL CANCER

Anatomy

The anal canal (Fig. 22.7) runs downwards and backwards to the anal orifice and is 3–4 cm long. The lower half is lined by squamous epithelium and the upper half by columnar epithelium. The walls are composed of an internal sphincter of involuntary muscle and an external sphincter of voluntary muscle.

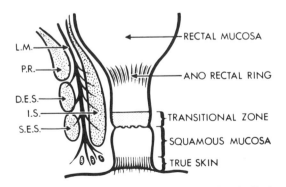

Fig. 22.7 Anatomy of the anal canal. L.M. = longitudinal muscle, P.R. = pubo-rectalis, D.E.S. = deep part of the external sphincter, I.S. = internal sphincter, S.E.S. = superficial part of the external sphincter. (Reproduced with permission from Scott, An Aid to Clinical Surgery, Churchill Livingstone, 1977.)

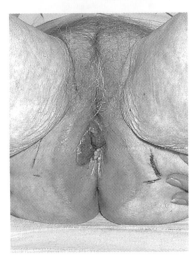

Fig. 22.8 Exophytic squamous cell carcinoma of the anal margin.

Carcinomas of the upper half are adenocarcinomas and of the lower half squamous carcinomas. The lymphatic drainage of both halves is also different. The upper half drains to the lumbar nodes and the lower half to the inguinal nodes.

Pathology

Anal cancer only accounts for about 5% of large bowel cancer. The incidence seems to be rising in the UK. Although most cases occur without any obvious predisposing factors, a few develop in association with AIDS. There is a higher incidence in homosexual men, probably related to human papilloma virus infection. Most occur between the ages of 55 and 65. The majority of tumours of the anal margin are in men and of the canal in women. The tumour appears as an ulcer. It may extend up into the rectum or below to the perineal skin. The majority are squamous cell carcinomas (Fig. 22.8). A distinctive tumour of this area is the cloacogenic carcinoma; it has a lower metastatic potential than squamous carcinoma.

Clinical features

The commonest symptoms are bleeding, anal pain and itching (pruritus ani). Benign fistulae, warts and leucoplakia are commonly also present.

Diagnosis and investigation

An examination of the anus and pelvis under general anaesthesia determines the local extent of the tumour.

Table 22.1   TNM staging of anal cancer

Stage	Clinical findings
Anal canal	
Primary tumour	
T1	Tumour extending not more than one-third of the circumference or length of the anal canal and not infiltrating the external sphincter muscle
T2	Tumour occupying more than one-third of the circumference or length of the anal canal or infiltrating the anal sphincter
T3	Tumour extending to the rectum or skin but not to other neighbouring structures
T4	Tumour infiltrating neighbouring structures
Nodes	
N0	No involvement of regional nodes
N1	Involvement of mesorectal and/or inguinal nodes
Anal margin	
Primary tumour	
T1	Tumour 2 cm or less in greatest dimension, strictly superficial or exophytic
T2	Tumour greater than 2 cm and up to 5 cm in largest dimension or tumour with minimal infiltration of the dermis
T3	Tumour more than 5 cm in its greatest dimension or tumour with deep infiltration of the dermis
T4	Tumour with extension to muscle or bone, etc.
Nodes	
N0	No evidence of regional lymph node spread
N1	Mobile unilateral regional nodes
N2	Mobile bilateral regional nodes
N3	Fixed regional nodes

A biopsy is taken. A CT scan of the pelvis is helpful in determining the local extent and whether or not the presacral and iliac nodes are involved.

Staging

Staging is according to the UICC TNM classification (Table 22.1).

Treatment

The main treatments are radical surgery or radiotherapy, and, more recently, adjuvant chemotherapy. The management of this condition is controversial. Radical surgery (abdominoperineal excision) was the treatment for all squamous cell carcinomas except for superficial ones which could be implanted. It is increasingly appreciated that external beam irradiation and interstitial irradiation, alone or in combination, can be curative.

Surgery

Local excision is possible for superficial tumours less than 2 cm in diameter (10%). The local recurrence rate is, however, high at 40%. Abdominoperineal excision with a permanent colostomy is then required. Radical surgery can be used to deal with persistent or locally recurrent tumour following radical radiotherapy.

Radiotherapy

Radical radiotherapy using external beam with or without interstitial implantation offers a good alternative curative technique for selected tumours. It has the advantage over radical surgery that the anal sphincter can be preserved, with much lower morbidity and mortality. Treatment technique is influenced by the site, local extent and presence of regional lymph node spread.

Implantation alone is recommended for superficial T1 and T2 tumours fulfilling the following criteria:

1. Lie below the anorectal ring
2. Occupy less than 50% of the anal circumference
3. Are 1 cm or less in thickness
4. No involvement of regional nodes.

Because of the poor tolerance of the perineal region to radical doses (e.g. 50 Gy), a good compromise is to give a preliminary subradical course of external beam irradiation to the primary and posterior pelvis, followed by an interstitial implant 2 months later. This approach is well tolerated. The long gap between the end of the course of external beam therapy and the implant is to allow maximal resolution of the tumour. This leaves a smaller residue of tumour to be boosted by implant.

An alternative is to give external beam alone to a radical dose, but there is a greater risk of causing an anal stricture (10–20%) requiring surgery than with implant alone.

Palliative radiotherapy for advanced anal carcinoma is not recommended since it is rarely effective.

External beam

Target volume
This should cover the primary tumour and the anal canal, the pararectal, hypogastric and obturator nodes (Fig. 22.9). The inferior margin should lie below the anal verge. The superior margin should be at the level of the bottom of the sacroiliac joints. The lateral margins allow coverage of the internal iliac nodes. The posterior margin includes the sacrum and the disease anterior to it.

Technique
The patient is simulated prone. Some barium is instilled

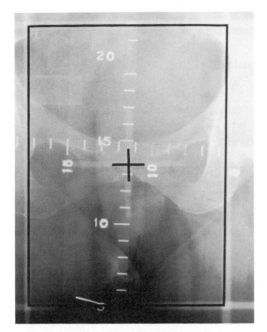

Fig. 22.9 Simulator radiograph (anteroposterior) showing radical treatment volume for carcinoma of the anal canal. (Courtesy of Dr J Bolger, Sheffield)

into the rectum to outline the anus and lower rectum. A direct posterior perineal and two wedged posterior oblique fields are used (Fig. 22.10). Angles of less than 45° for the posterior oblique fields should not be used to avoid excessive skin reaction in the natal cleft. Bolus is applied over the perineum to bring up the dose to the skin. This technique gives less dose to the small bowel than would be the case with an anterior and posterior parallel opposed pair of fields.

Dose and energy

Preimplant
30 Gy given in 15 fractions over 3 weeks (9–10 MV photons)

External beam alone
50 Gy in 20 daily fractions over 4 weeks (9–10 MV photons)

Interstitial implantation. Interstitial implantation alone with iridium-192 (Figs 19.9 and 19.11) wire is recommended for patients with T1 or T2 tumours of the anal margin or canal. The technique for implantation is described on page 308. The boost dose is 20–25 Gy.

Radiation reaction

External beam. The acute reaction of moist desquamation is very uncomfortable. Analgesia is often

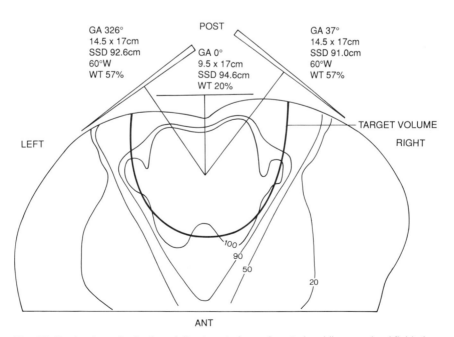

Fig. 22.10 Isodose distribution of direct posterior and posterior oblique wedged fields for radical radiotherapy of carcinoma of the anus. (Courtesy of Dr J Bolger, Sheffield.)

required. Mucous rectal discharge is frequent. An anti-diarrhoeal agent such as loperamide normally controls this. The acute reaction has normally settled by the third week after the end of treatment.

Implant. The acute local reaction of moist desquamation is mild and has normally settled within 3 weeks.

Complications

Radiation necrosis. Soft tissue necrosis usually settles with conservative measures such as the daily application of gentian violet. Excision is required for persistent necrosis. Anal stricture occurs rarely.

Inguinal nodes. If inguinal nodes are enlarged and mobile, the treatment is block dissection. Fixed nodes are inoperable and respond poorly to radiotherapy. Palliative radiotherapy should be reserved for pain and ulceration.

Technique

A direct field to the groin(s) with skin bolus.

Dose and energy

30 Gy in 10 daily fractions (cobalt-60 or 4–6 MV photons)

Chemotherapy

Combining radiotherapy with chemotherapy (intravenous 5-fluorouracil and Mitomycin C) improves the local tumour response compared with radiotherapy alone. Further confirmation of this is required and it would be premature to advocate routine adjuvant chemotherapy.

Results of treatment

The 5-year local control rate achieved by radical radiotherapy and radical surgery are similar. The results of radiotherapy are better in the anal canal, with a 5-year local control rate of 80%. Five-year survival following surgery is 50–60% for the anal canal and 65–75% for the anal margin.

CANCER OF THE LUNG

Lung cancer (bronchogenic carcinoma) is the commonest cause of death from cancer in men and the second commonest in women. The annual death rate of 40 000 indicates the scale of the problem. Overall it accounts for 35% of male and 15% of female cancer deaths. There has been a modest fall in the mortality in men but a continued rise in women. This rise is related to an increase in smoking among women. The highest age incidence is 45–65 years. The male:female ratio is 5:1.

Pathology

Aetiology

In the early part of this century lung cancer was relatively rare. Environmental factors (Ch. 13) are clearly at work in industrial situations, e.g. mining and factories with exposure, for example, to asbestos, nickel and chrome. There is overwhelming evidence that cigarette smoking is the main cause in up to 90% of cases of lung cancer. Cigars and pipes are much less dangerous. The risk is related to the number of cigarettes smoked. For example the risk of developing lung cancer in a person who smokes 25 or more cigarettes per day is 25–30 times that of a non-smoker. It is encouraging that if a smoker gives up the habit, the risk of developing lung cancer diminishes markedly but the risk after stopping smoking for 20 years is still 2–3 times that of someone who has never smoked. Early onset of smoking, high tar content of the cigarettes and long duration of smoking all increase the risk of lung cancer. Passive smoking also increases the risk of lung cancer, albeit to a lesser degree, for example in the non-smoking wives of husbands who smoke.

Macroscopic and microscopic features

The majority of cancers (55%) arise near the root of the lung, close to a main bronchus; 40% are peripheral; about 5% are multifocal or indeterminate. If a bronchus becomes completely blocked, the lung beyond the obstruction will collapse and is prone to infection.

There are four main histological types. The commonest is squamous carcinoma (50%), with varying degrees of anaplasia. A special variety is oat cell carcinoma (20%): small slightly elongated, darkly staining cells with a fanciful resemblance to oat grains. In other respects these cells are anaplastic. Twenty per cent are large cell carcinomas (an unsatisfactory designation of undifferentiated tumours) and 10% adenocarcinomas.

Spread

Spread is local, lymphatic and blood-borne. Direct extension can occur to adjacent lung, pericardium and heart, oesophagus and chest wall including ribs. Pleural involvement may cause a pleural effusion, often blood-stained. Lymphatic spread is to adjacent nodes (Fig. 22.11) and later to nodes above the clavicle and occasionally to the axilla. Blood spread may be early and

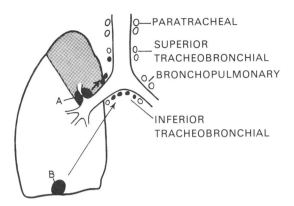

Fig. 22.11 Carcinoma of the lung, with lymph node distribution. **A**, Central tumour causing bronchial occlusion and peripheral pulmonary collapse. **B**, Peripheral tumour. (Reproduced with permission from Jayne, in Macfarlane, Textbook of Surgery, Churchill Livingstone.)

wide, to liver, skin, bone and brain. Metastatic spread is particularly common in small cell (oat cell) lung carcinoma, occurring in up to 80% at presentation.

Clinical features

The tumour may be silent for years and may only be discovered incidentally when a chest radiograph is taken for some other reason, or at mass radiography. Symptoms arise in various ways.

Respiratory

The commonest symptom is persistent cough. When the tumour ulcerates through the bronchial wall, the sputum becomes blood-stained (haemoptysis). Shortness of breath (dyspnoea) arises due to obstruction of the large or small airways, impairing lung function. Very severe dyspnoea and noisy main airway obstruction (stridor) may occur. Occasionally lung cancer may present as a chest infection which fails to resolve with antibiotic therapy. This is because infected material cannot be adequately cleared from beyond the blocked bronchus.

Invasion of adjacent structures

Pain may arise from invasion of the mediastinum or chest wall. Growths at the apex of the lung may cause pain radiating to shoulder and arm, classically in the distribution of the first thoracic nerve (T1) from involvement of the brachial nerve plexus. This clinical variety is the superior sulcus or Pancoast tumour (Fig. 22.12). This causes weakness of the hand grip

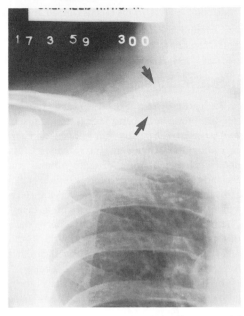

Fig. 22.12 Chest radiograph showing a Pancoast of the right apex destroying the 1st rib (arrows). (Courtesy of Dr R Nakielny, Sheffield.)

and Horner's syndrome due to involvement of the sympathetic chain.

Involvement of the recurrent laryngeal nerve may cause vocal cord palsy with hoarseness.

Pressure on the great veins in the upper mediastinum, including the superior vena cava, leads to *mediastinal obstruction* (Fig. 22.15), with swelling of the head, neck and upper limbs, and engorgement of the veins of the neck. The veins of the chest wall become dilated due to the development of a collateral circulation. Pressure on the oesophagus can cause dysphagia.

Lymphatic and distant metastases

The first sign may come from a metastasis while the primary lung lesion is silent. Supraclavicular and axillary nodes may be palpable. Common sites of distant metastases are the brain (raised intracranial pressure, change of personality), bone (pain, pathological fracture), liver (anorexia, weight loss, jaundice), skin (subcutaneous nodules). Metastases occasionally occur in the choroid of the eye (Plate 20).

General and non-metastatic effects

These include anaemia and lassitude. In addition certain non-metastatic effects may occur due to ectopic production from the tumour of chemical substances with endocrine effects. This occurs in all histological types but particularly with small cell lung cancer. These non-metastatic effects are described in Chapter 36.

Diagnosis and staging

Basic investigations include a chest radiograph, sputum cytology, full blood count and liver function tests.

Chest radiograph. After full clinical examination, a chest radiograph almost always provides suggestive evidence. This may show a discrete tumour mass or enlarged nodes at the lung hilum (Fig. 22.12) or in the mediastinum. There is often a varying degree of lung collapse. Pleural effusions, rib metastases or a raised hemidiaphragm (due to phrenic nerve paralysis) are common. Central necrosis within the tumour is particularly associated with squamous cell carcinoma.

Tomography and CT scanning (see below) often define the tumour more precisely where the chest radiograph is equivocal.

Sputum cytology. Microscopy of the sputum (cytology) may show malignant or atypical cells. The latter are inadequate for a firm diagnosis of lung cancer.

Bronchoscopy. Flexible bronchoscopy under local anaesthesia is the next step. Tumour is visible in 60% of cases and a biopsy should be obtained. Bronchial washings from abnormal areas of the bronchial mucosa may show malignant cells.

Percutaneous biopsy. A direct percutaneous biopsy under radiological control may yield the diagnosis if

bronchoscopy does not, particularly in peripheral tumours.

Mediastinoscopy. If there is a mediastinal mass and bronchoscopy is negative or radical surgery is contemplated a mediastinoscopy to obtain tissue is advised. Involvement of mediastinal glands contra-indicates radical surgery.

CT scanning and ultrasound. CT scanning may help establish the diagnosis when there are equivocal appearances on chest radiograph (e.g. distinguishing a hilar mass from pulmonary vessels). It may also demonstrate mediastinal nodes. Nodes larger than 1.5 cm are likely to be malignant. Pulmonary deposits not visible on plain radiography may be demonstrated. Abdominal scanning may show lymphadenopathy, liver and adrenal metastases. When brain metastases are suspected, particularly in small cell lung cancer, CT is more reliable than isotope scanning.

Abdominal ultrasound is useful for the detection of liver metastases. If liver function tests are abnormal but a liver ultrasound is negative, a CT scan should be requested to exclude liver metastases.

Ultrasound is also helpful in determining the site of pleural effusions, especially if loculated, if initial aspiration has been unhelpful.

Staging

The TNM staging system (Table 22.2) is used for pathological types other than small cell (non-small cell lung cancer). These TNM stages are also grouped into the following stages:

Stage I:	T1N0M0
	T1N1M0
	T2N0M0
Stage II:	T2N0M0
Stage III:	Any T3
	Any N2
	Any M1

Small cell lung cancer. A separate and simpler staging system is widely used for small cell lung cancer since the survival of stages I–III on the TNM system is the same. Patients are divided into two categories: limited and extensive disease. Limited disease is defined as tumour confined to one hemithorax, mediastinum and ipsilateral supraclavicular nodes. Extensive disease is tumour more extensive than the limited stage, with distant metastases, e.g. liver, bone, bone marrow and brain.

Treatment

An important division is made between small cell and

Table 22.2 TNM staging of non-small cell lung cancer

Stage	Clinical findings
Primary tumour	
T0	Primary tumour not demonstrable
TX	Positive cytology but tumour not demonstrable
T1	Tumour less than 3 cm diameter without proximal invasion
T2	Greater than 3 cm or invading pleura or with collapse of less than a whole lung, more than 2 cm from the carina
T3	Tumour of any size with invasion of the chest wall; or less than 2 cm from the carina; or causing collapse of a whole lung or effusion
Regional nodes	
N0	No demonstrable metastases
N1	Ipsilateral hilar node metastases
N2	Mediastinal metastases
Distant metastases	
M0	No metastases
M1	Metastases present

non-small cell lung cancer since their treatments are different. The choice of treatment is based on histology, general condition and extent of disease.

Small cell lung cancer. Chemotherapy is the treatment of choice for fit patients with small cell lung cancer. Palliative radiotherapy to the primary reduces the incidence of local recurrence but does not increase survival. Surgery is not recommended because of the very high incidence of metastatic disease.

Non-small cell lung cancer. For non-small cell lung cancer, the choice is between radical surgery and radical or palliative radiotherapy. Non-small cell lung cancer is relatively resistant to chemotherapy. Chemotherapy is therefore not recommended for routine treatment.

After full assessment, two vital decisions have to be made:

1. Is the tumour operable?
2. If inoperable is the patient suitable for radical or palliative radiotherapy or laser therapy?

Surgery

Radical. For non-small cell lung cancer radical surgery offers the best prospect of cure, but is only applicable to about 30% of patients. It should be considered for stage I disease. Removal of the whole lung (pneumonectomy) is necessary if the tumour arises in a mainstem bronchus, if the tumour involves more than one lobe or if the hilum is involved. A more limited removal of a lobe (lobectomy) may otherwise be performed. Adequate general medical condition and pulmonary function is required. Contraindications are mediastinal or distant metastases, pleural effusion, vocal cord or phrenic nerve paresis, mediastinal obstruction or tumours within 2 cm of the carina. Patients over the age of 70 are rarely operated on unless they are in very good medical condition.

The operative mortality for pneumonectomy is about 5% and for a lobectomy 2%.

Palliative. Palliative laser therapy can provide rapid relief of dyspnoea and haemoptysis if due to disease in the trachea or main bronchi. The patient is injected with a haematoporphyrin derivative 3 days before the laser source is applied. Local tumour destruction follows rapidly.

Radical radiotherapy

Radical radiotherapy should be considered in patients with localised disease if surgery is contraindicated or refused. It is suitable for less than 5% of patients. Criteria for eligibility are as follows:

— Tumour 5 cm or less in maximum dimension
— Age less than 70 years
— Good general medical condition
— Adequate pulmonary function (forced expiratory volume in 1 second greater than 1 litre)
— Non-small cell histology.

Contraindications are:

— Recurrent laryngeal or phrenic nerve palsy
— Mediastinal nodes.

Target volume

Split-course radiotherapy is recommended. The initial treatment volume should include the primary, with a 2 cm margin all round, and the whole of the mediastinum. The patient is rested for a month. Any patient who shows evidence of local progression, regional spread or metastases during the rest period is excluded from further treatment. In the second half of treatment, the treatment volume is reduced to cover the primary tumour and ipsilateral hilar nodes. For right-sided tumours the volume should include the lymphatics close to the right intermediate bronchus. The field should cross the midline to include the left paratracheal nodes, 1–1.5 cm lateral to the trachea. Left-sided tumours can spread to the contralateral paratracheal nodes, which therefore need to be included in the field.

Technique

The choice of technique will depend on the site of the tumour within the lung. A CT planning scan is helpful in accurate tumour localisation. Otherwise conventional simulation is carried out.

Central tumours. For centrally placed tumours a three field technique is used (Fig. 22.13) to reduce the dose to the spinal cord. The patient is simulated in the supine position, with the hands behind the head and elbows flexed. The anterior field is simulated and a radiograph taken (Fig. 22.13); the patient is then screened from the side to determine the depth of the field and a lateral radiograph is taken. Care is taken to avoid the spinal cord. The posterior oblique fields are then viewed.

Peripheral tumours. Peripheral tumours in the mid and lower zones of the lung may be treated with a wedged pair of fields (Fig. 22.14).

Tumours at the lung apex can be treated by a parallel opposed pair of anterior and posterior fields. The volume should include the tumour and a 2 cm margin.

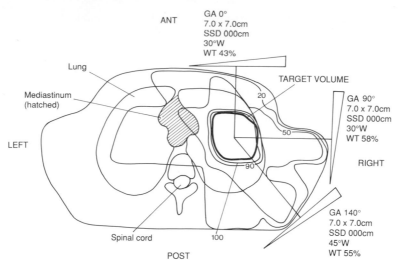

Fig. 22.13 Carcinoma of the right lung. Isodose distribution of three field technique (9 MV photons). (Courtesy of Dr A Champion, Sheffield.)

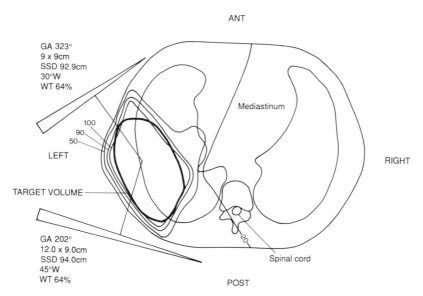

Fig. 22.14 Peripheral carcinoma of the lung. Isodose distribution of a wedged pair of fields for peripheral carcinoma of the lung (6 MV photons). (Courtesy of Dr A Champion, Sheffield.)

The whole of the adjacent vertebral body should be included in the initial volume since subclinical infiltration of the neural canal is common. The volume is reduced to exclude the spinal cord after a dose of 40 Gy.

Planning proceeds in the normal way (Ch. 6) with an outline drawing on which the target volume, heart, lungs and spinal cord are plotted. The presence of air in normal lung is a complicating factor in dosage calculation, since depth–dose tables and isodose curves are based on solid tissue. The presence of air decreases the absorption and scatter of radiation and increases the depth dose (on average 3% greater dose per centimetre of lung traversed) compared with solid tissue. If a beam passes through much aerated lung tissue, a correction has to be made to arrive at the true tumour dosage (see radical radiotherapy of the oesophagus, Ch. 22). For beams passing through the mediastinum, no correction is necessary.

Dose and energy

Large volume

30 Gy in 10 daily fractions over 2 weeks (6–10 MV photons)

Small volume

20 Gy in 10 daily fractions over 2 weeks (6–10 MV photons)

Acute reaction. Both general and local reactions occur. They usually subside within 3–4 weeks of the end of treatment. General reactions are anorexia, nausea and vomiting. The last two symptoms can usually be controlled with simple antiemetics.

Local reactions include tracheitis causing a sore throat and expectoration of mucus and oesophagitis causing dysphagia.

Late reactions. An oesophageal stricture may occur several months after treatment. These rarely occur in patients with a previously normal oesophagus.

Radiation pneumonitis can occur 4–6 weeks after the end of treatment. There is the acute onset of dyspnoea, non-productive cough and chest tightness. There is commonly nothing abnormal to hear on auscultation of the lung fields. Chest X-ray may show a hazy appearance in the treated area. Treatment is with oxygen, broad spectrum antibiotics and with steroids (prednisolone 60 mg per day). The dose of steroids can be tailed off gradually if there is a response or if there is no improvement within a fortnight. The outcome largely depends on the region and volume of lung irradiated. If the volume is large, the condition may be fatal. The apices of the lung tend to give rise to fewer symptoms since the ventilation and vascular perfusion of the upper lobes is normally less than that of the lower lobes.

Lung fibrosis within the treated volume occurs in virtually all patients but usually does not give rise to symptoms. The degree of fibrosis and the likelihood of dyspnoea is related to the total dose, secondary infection and pre-existing lung disease (e.g. chronic obstructive airways disease or industrial lung disease).

Occasionally there is transient radiation myelitis (Lhermitte's sign, see p. 449) but this usually recovers completely.

Palliative radiotherapy

External radiotherapy is helpful in relieving symptoms from local and metastatic disease. An alternative is endobronchial irradiation with a single fraction of high dose rate brachytherapy from an afterloading machine (*microSelectron*, see p. 303). This seems to have

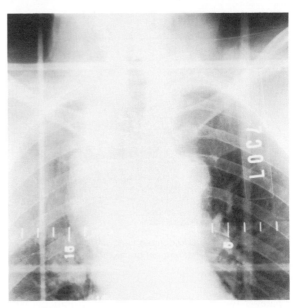

Fig. 22.15 Simulator radiograph showing field margins for palliative radiotherapy of superior mediastinal obstruction. Note widening of the superior mediastinum.

equivalent efficacy to external beam but is currently available in only a limited number of centres.

In general, treatment should be withheld until symptoms develop since there is no evidence that palliative radiotherapy alters survival in non-small cell lung cancer. In practice some asymptomatic patients may find it difficult to accept that they will not immediately receive treatment. In these circumstances it may be helpful to reassure the patient that he or she can be seen at short notice if symptoms develop, and treatment promptly instituted, if appropriate.

Symptoms of local disease such as dyspnoea, haemoptysis, dysphagia and mediastinal pain usually improve during or within a few weeks of treatment. Haemoptysis is relieved in 80% of cases and in 50% of cases of cough, dyspnoea and chest pain. Pleural effusions and laryngeal and phrenic nerve palsy rarely respond. The treatment of pleural effusion is described in Chapter 36.

Mediastinal obstruction (Fig. 22.15) completely resolves in 50% of cases and partially in an additional 30%. No response is obtained in 20%.

Good symptomatic responses to external beam therapy can be obtained in most patients with bone, skin or brain metastases.

The response of *spinal cord compression* (p. 492) is influenced by the histological type and the degree and duration of pretreatment neurological deficit. Complete paraplegia with loss of bladder function,

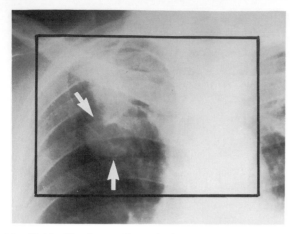

Fig. 22.16 Simulator radiograph showing typical field margins for palliative treatment of carcinoma of the right upper lobe.

whatever the histology, rarely responds. Patients with small cell lung cancer respond better than those with non-small cell disease as long as there is moderate retention of motor power.

Target volume

For local disease, the tumour plus a generous margin of several centimetres should be included (Fig. 22.16). Typical field sizes are 12×10 cm. For treatment of bone metastases, see page 512; brain metastases, see page 488; spinal cord compression, see page 491; and skin nodules, page 301.

Technique

For locoregional disease, anterior and posterior opposed fields are used. The techniques for brain and bone metastases are described on pages 488 and 512.

Dose and energy

17 Gy in two fractions a week apart (4–6 MV photons)

Radiation reaction. Radiation oesophagitis develops after treatment. It is usually mild and has normally settled within 3 weeks of the end of treatment.

Results of treatment

The results of treatment of non-small cell lung cancer are poor. The best results are obtained with surgery. Results of 'curative' resection are largely influenced by criteria for selection. Overall 5-year survival is 25–30%. For stage I disease it is about 55%, for stage II 25% and for stage III 15%.

Table 22.3 Chemotherapy regimes for small cell lung cancer

ECMV	
Etoposide 120 mg/m² i.v. infusion in 250 ml 0.9% saline over 30 mins	Day 1
Cyclophosphamide 1 g/m² i.v bolus	Day 1
Methotrexate 35 mg/m² i.v bolus	Day 1
Vincristine 1.3 mg/m² (max 2 mg) i.v bolus	Day 1
Etoposide 240 mg/m² orally	Day 2

Repeated every 21 days. Prophylactic antibiotics recommended

EV	
Etoposide 120 mg/m² i.v infusion	Day 1
Vincristine 1.3 mg/m² (max 2 mg) i.v bolus	Day 1
Etoposide 240 mg/m² orally	Day 2
Etoposide 240 mg/m² orally	Day 3

Repeated every 21 days. Prophylactic antibiotics recommended

For radical radiotherapy the 5-year survival is 6%. Average survival of patients treated palliatively is about 8 months.

SMALL CELL LUNG CANCER

Chemotherapy

Chemotherapy is the treatment of choice for small cell lung cancer. Combination chemotherapy (2–4 drugs) is more effective than single agents in obtaining complete, though usually temporary, remissions, and in prolonging survival. Overall (complete and partial) response rates of 75–90% can be achieved. It must be stressed that these responses are normally of limited duration (about 10 months). No particular combination is optimal. Typical combinations with response rates of the order of 75% are shown in Table 22.3.

Factors which influence the choice between no treatment, single agent and combination chemotherapy are prognostic factors such as age, general medical condition and performance status (Table 22.4). A balance has to be struck between the toxicity and clinical benefit of chemotherapy. Patients with extensive disease

Table 22.4 Poor prognostic factors in small cell lung cancer

Extensive disease
Poor performance status
Brain metastases
Marrow infiltration/anaemia
Abnormal liver function tests
Low serum sodium and albumin

and low performance status may be suitable for single agent oral or intravenous etoposide. Combination chemotherapy should be attempted in younger patients of good performance status.

It is recommended that three courses are given initially. Any useful clinical response usually occurs after one or two courses. Toxicity is cumulative and treatment beyond six courses is not recommended. If no response occurs after three courses, it is unlikely that a different combination is likely to be beneficial.

Symptoms such as anorexia, weight loss, haemoptysis, bone pain, cough, dyspnoea and dysphagia are relieved in 75% of cases after four courses of combination chemotherapy.

Radiotherapy

Radiotherapy to the primary tumour following chemotherapy is sometimes given in patients with limited disease. There is some evidence that relapse in the chest is reduced, with modest increases in survival, compared with radiotherapy alone. However no firm conclusions can be drawn and routine thoracic irradiation is not recommended. Palliative radiotherapy may be needed for symptomatic relief of symptoms of locoregional and metastatic disease (see Non-small cell lung carcinoma).

In patients who have obtained a complete response to chemotherapy, prophylactic cranial irradiation reduces the incidence of brain metastases to 8% compared to 22% following chemotherapy alone. It should only be given under these conditions. It is contraindicated in extensive disease. However to date there is no evidence that prophylactic cranial irradiation prolongs survival. Late side-effects such as dementia and cerebellar dysfunction may occur in some of the few patients who survive beyond 3 years.

Results of treatment

Untreated, the median survivals of limited and extensive disease are about 3 months and 6 weeks respectively. Combination chemotherapy increases these to 9–12 months and 3 months respectively. The addition of radiotherapy to the site of the primary disease reduces the local recurrence rate and may increase survival.

Despite high response rates to combination chemotherapy, relapse at the primary site or at distant sites occurs in 75% within 2 years. In limited disease 15–20% of patients who obtain a complete response survive 2–3 years. Less than 5% survive 5 years and can probably be regarded as cured.

THYMOMA

Thymomas are rare epithelial neoplasms of the thymus gland in the anterior mediastinum. Mean age at presentation is 45–50 years. The aetiology is unknown. In 50% of cases there is an associated systemic disease, of which the commonest is myasthenia gravis. Presentation in 40–50% is with an abnormal chest radiograph in an otherwise asymptomatic individual, and in 30% with myasthenia gravis. Chest symptoms are uncommon. About 60% of thymomas are visible on plain radiographs. CT scanning can help identify the tumour but cannot distinguish it from other mediastinal tumours (e.g. teratoma, seminoma).

Treatment

Surgery

The treatment of choice is total surgical removal. Whether complete clearance is essential is uncertain.

Radiotherapy

Thymoma is relatively radiosensitive and long-term control with inoperable disease is common. Preoperative radiotherapy should be avoided to prevent unnecessary irradiation of the mediastinum.

The role of postoperative radiotherapy is not well defined. The local recurrence rate for encapsulated non-invasive thymoma is only 2%. In this circumstance, a policy of surveillance can be adopted, using radiotherapy for recurrence. If the resected tumour is found to be invasive, postoperative radiotherapy should be given.

Primary radical radiotherapy is also recommended to delay tumour progression and to relieve local symptoms in inoperable disease.

Dose and energy
45 Gy in 20 daily fractions over 4 weeks is given (4–6 MV photons)

Technique
An anterior oblique wedged pair of fields is used, limiting the spinal cord dose to 40 Gy.

Chemotherapy

Thymoma is also chemosensitive. Short-term responses have been obtained with cisplatin, Adriamycin and prednisolone as single agents. Higher doses of cisplatin as a single agent and in combination have yielded better results (25–30% 5-year survival). Preoperative chemotherapy followed by surgical debulking of the residual disease is logical. Postoperative mediastinal irradiation can be limited to non-responders.

Results of treatment

Ten-year survival for non-invasive thymoma is 65% and for invasive tumour 30%.

CARCINOMA OF THE PANCREAS

The incidence of carcinoma of the pancreas has doubled over the last four decades. Its incidence increases with age, reaching 100 per 100 000 between the ages of 80 and 84 years. The aetiology is unknown but the incidence is doubled in cigarette smokers. Most (60%) of tumours occur in the head, 25% in the body and 15% in the tail of the pancreas; 90% are adenocarcinomas.

The tumour spreads locally to obstruct the common bile duct, causing jaundice, and to the duodenum, causing frank or occult gastrointestinal bleeding. Obstruction of the portal vein gives rise to ascites and portal hypertension.

Presentation is normally with jaundice, epigastric pain, diabetes mellitus, thrombophlebitis, anorexia and weight loss. In the presence of jaundice, 50% have a palpable gallbladder (unlikely to be due to stones, according to Courvoisier's law).

Ultrasound may show a pancreatic mass and can be used to guide a needle biopsy. Endoscopy is useful in showing extrinsic compression of the stomach or duodenum by a mass in the head of the pancreas and detecting tumours of the ampulla of Vater.

Treatment for most pancreatic cancer remains palliative since the disease is usually unresectable and is resistant to both chemotherapy and radiotherapy.

In' many advanced cases a palliative bypass procedure between the distended gallbladder and the jejunum is performed to relieve jaundice. A coeliac axis nerve block may help control pain uncontrolled by opiates.

The prognosis is very poor with virtually all patients dying within a year of the diagnosis.

LIVER

Primary liver cancer is rare. The vast majority of liver tumours are secondary deposits, particularly from cancers of the gastrointestinal tract and lung. The management of liver metastases varies with the extent of involvement and the chemosensitivity of the tumour. Surgical resection is rarely appropriate since isolated liver metastases are extremely uncommon. The role of chemotherapy is discussed under individual tumour sites.

Palliative radiotherapy can relieve the pain of hepatic distension in 80% of cases. A parallel opposed pair of fields is used. If any part of the liver is irradiated, the dose is 30 Gy in 10 fractions over 2 weeks. If the whole liver is irradiated the same dose is given in 15 fractions over 3 weeks (cobalt-60 or 4–6 MV photons).

HEPATOCELLULAR CARCINOMA

Primary hepatocellular carcinoma is an aggressive disease, usually presenting with abdominal pain, weight loss and anorexia. A tumour marker, serum alpha-fetoprotein, is elevated in 80% of cases. Surgical resection or liver transplantation is the only curative treatment. Unfortunately few patients are suitable for surgery due to cirrhosis of the liver, diffuse liver infiltration or metastatic disease. Radiotherapy and chemotherapy have no useful role. Five-year survival is poor (5–10%).

23. Breast

ANATOMY

The female breast overlies the second to the sixth ribs. The medial limit is the sternum. The lateral limit is the anterior axillary line. It is composed of lobules of glandular tissue lying in fat. The lobules are divided by fibrous ligaments (Cooper's ligaments) which run between the superficial fascia of the breast and the deep fascia overlying pectoralis major.

Lymphatic drainage

A knowledge of the lymphatic drainage of the breast (Fig. 23.1) is important since the peripheral lymphatics are commonly irradiated following surgical removal of the primary tumour. The principal lymphatic drainage of the breast is to the axillary nodes lying between the second and third intercostal spaces. Additional drainage occurs to the supraclavicular nodes through the pectoralis major and to the internal mammary chain adjacent to the sternum.

PATHOLOGY
Epidemiology

Breast cancer is the commonest form of malignancy in Western countries and accounts for 12% of all cancers, 10% of all cancer deaths and 20–25% of all female cancer deaths. Worldwide there are 500 000–700 000 new cases annually. In the UK over 12 000 women die of the disease per year, and at least half a million worldwide. The risk of a woman developing the disease at some stage of her life is 1 in 12. The mortality from breast cancer has remained unchanged for the last 50 years. England, Wales, Scotland and Ireland have the highest mortality for breast cancer in the world. The majority of cases occur between the ages of 40 and 70 years. It is rare below the age of 30. Male breast cancer is rare (1% of all breast cancer).

Aetiology

The aetiology of breast cancer is unknown in most cases but a number of predisposing factors have been

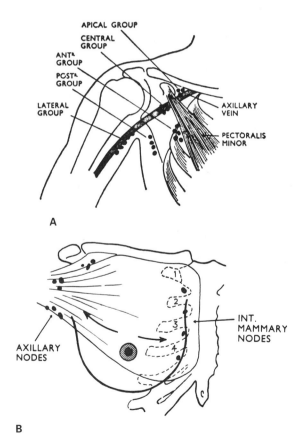

Fig. 23.1 **A** The lymph nodes of the axilla. **B** Diagram of the principal pathways of lymphatic drainage of the breast. These follow the venous drainage of the breast—to the axilla and to the internal mammary chain. (Reproduced with permission from Ellis, Clinical Anatomy, 5th edn, Blackwells, 1975.)

identified. Both genetic and acquired factors are thought to play a part.

Genetic

A family history of breast cancer is often elicited from women with breast cancer. The sisters and daughters of a woman with breast cancer have a threefold increased risk of developing the disease. The risk of breast cancer for a woman whose sister is affected is doubled. This rises to tenfold for women who have a mother and a sister affected. Women who have a first-degree relative with premenopausal or bilateral breast cancer are at particularly high risk.

Acquired

Benign breast disease. A number of benign conditions in the breast increase the risk of breast cancer, although the effect is small. The risk of breast cancer is raised twofold in women with breast hyperplasia and a family history of an affected first-degree relative.

Menstruation. Breast tissue is subject to repeated monthly cyclical changes under hormonal stimulation. The epithelium of the breast proliferates during ovulatory cycles. This may be due to the stimulus of either progesterone or oestrogen. This causes temporary growth of the milk-secreting glandular tissue, in preparation for possible pregnancy. The greater the number of years of menstruation, the higher the risk of breast cancer. If the menarche starts before the age of 12, the risk of breast cancer is nearly double that of women who begin to menstruate after the age of 13.

If menstruation continues above the age of 55, the risk of breast cancer is doubled compared with a normal menopause at 45 years. Furthermore, if a woman undergoes an artificial menopause (e.g. due to a hysterectomy and oophorectomy under the age of 40), there is a fourfold fall in the incidence of breast cancer.

The role of the ovarian oestrogens in the genesis of breast cancer is strongly suspected. Reductions in oestrogen levels may protect against breast cancer. Oral oestrogens, either as the contraceptive pill or as hormone replacement therapy, may accelerate the development of breast cancer.

Age at time of first pregnancy. The risk of breast cancer in a woman rises with her age at first pregnancy. It is three times higher in women who have their first baby over the age of 30, compared with those under the age of 18.

Lactation. Women who have breast fed their children are slightly less prone to breast cancer.

Age at first full-term pregnancy. Pregnancy itself seems to have a protective role. Women who first become pregnant before the age of 30 have a lower risk of breast cancer than women who first give birth after the age of 30. This effect only applies to completed pregnancies.

Diet. A diet high in animal fats may promote the development of breast cancer. It is possible that the link between fat and breast cancer may be that many of the carcinogens acting on the breast are absorbed in the diet and are soluble in fat.

There is some evidence that a high intake of alcohol is linked to breast cancer.

Weight. In obese postmenopausal women, the risk of breast cancer is increased. This might be due to increased quantities of oestrogens stimulating malignant transformation of the breast.

Radiation. Exposure to ionising radiation increases the risk of breast cancer. This is true of women who underwent low dose breast irradiation for benign mastitis. There is a linear relationship between dose and incidence of breast cancer, up to 4 Gy. Beyond this the incidence plateaus. Children irradiated by the atomic bombs dropped on Nagasaki and Hiroshima showed an increased risk of breast cancer with dose.

Oral contraceptive pill. Whether or not the use of the oral contraceptive pill, particularly those preparations high in progestogen, increases the risk of breast cancer remains uncertain despite intensive study.

Ductal and lobular carcinoma-in-situ

Premalignant in situ carcinoma may occur in the lobules (lobular carcinoma-in-situ (LCIS)) or ducts (ductal carcinoma-in-situ (DCIS)). With the advent of breast screening the diagnosis of DCIS has increased 3–4 times and now accounts for 15% of cases detected by mammography. Before screening DCIS was mostly associated with symptomatic breast disease. Its natural history among asymptomatic women selected for screening is unknown and may differ. At post mortem the incidence of DCIS is much commoner in women with breast cancer (40%) compared with those with normal breasts (5%). DCIS is associated with a substantial risk of progression to invasive carcinoma, with a mean delay of about 7 years.

LCIS is associated with an increased risk of tumour in both breasts, particularly infiltrating ductal carcinoma. The risk of developing breast cancer is estimated to be 1% per year for either breast, indicating that local measures to the breast where LCIS was found are not appropriate.

Malignant transformation from carcinoma-in-situ

When malignant cells are confined to the ductal–lobular system, they are termed *carcinoma-in-situ* (see later this chapter and p. 247). In situ carcinoma has the potential to become invasive cancer but it is not clear how often this transformation occurs.

Histology

A lump in the breast may be benign or malignant. Benign lesions include cysts, fibroadenomas and papillomas. Malignant tumours mainly arise from the glandular epithelium (adenocarcinomas).

The histological types of breast cancer are shown in Table 23.1.

Invasive cancers have traditionally been classified by their microscopic appearance and by histological grade. In general, microscopic appearance does not correlate well with prognosis. Exceptions are medullary and inflammatory carcinomas.

Inflammatory carcinomas are typified by an enlarged warm breast, associated with an ill-defined underlying mass. Histologically, there is infiltration of the subdermal lymphatics. Prognosis is poor. In contrast, medullary carcinoma is slow growing and has a much better prognosis.

Most malignant tumours (80–90%) are described as scirrhous adenocarcinomas because of the fibrous stromal reaction they elicit. This explains their hard and irregular outline on palpation and gritty texture on sectioning, similar to an unripe pear. Scirrhous carcinomas are commoner in elderly women.

Lobular invasive carcinomas are often bilateral (40%) and multicentric.

Table 23.1 WHO histological classification of breast cancer

A. Intraductal and intralobular non-infiltrating carcinoma
B. Infiltrating carcinoma
C. Special histological variants of carcinoma
   1. Medullary carcinoma
   2. Papillary carcinoma
   3. Cribriform carcinoma
   4. Mucous carcinoma
   5. Lobular carcinoma
   6. Squamous cell carcinoma
   7. Paget's disease of breast
   8. Carcinoma arising in cellular intracanalicular fibroadenoma

Paget's disease of the nipple is commonly associated with an underlying ductal adenocarcinoma.

Histological grading

Grading is of practical use in determining the need for postoperative radiotherapy (since it correlates with the likelihood of local recurrence) and prognosis. Five-year survival for grade 1 is 80% and falls to 25% for grade 3.

Lymphatic spread

Most tumours develop within the ducts and spread along the ducts and fascia into the mammary fat, the lymphatic channels of the breast and into the peripheral lymphatics. Invasive tumour may infiltrate the dermal lymphatics of the breast, causing oedema of the skin (*peau d'orange*). Tumours of the upper outer quadrant are more likely to have involved axillary nodes. The larger the tumour, the higher is the incidence of involvement of the axillary nodes. The higher the level of axillary involvement, the worse is the prognosis. Palpable supraclavicular nodes reflect advanced regional disease. In the presence of palpable axillary nodes there is a higher probability of involvement of the internal mammary nodes in tumours of the lower inner quadrant (72%), upper inner quadrant (45%) and central part of the breast (45%) compared with the lower outer quadrant (19%) and upper outer quadrant (22%).

Natural history

Tumours are commoner on the left side. Bilateral tumours are detected at the time of diagnosis (synchronous) in 1–2% of patients. A subsequent (metachronous) tumour in the opposite breast occurs in 7–8%.

Breast cancer shows a very wide range of behaviour, with great differences in rate of growth and tendency to metastasise. The majority of tumours (40%) originate in the upper outer quadrant of the breast. Thirty per cent occur in the central part of the breast, 15% in the upper inner quadrant, 10% in the lower outer quadrant and 5% in the lower inner quadrant. Although many tumours do progress locally and then regionally, blood-borne metastases do occur even when the primary is small or impalpable. A few, often premenopausal patients may die from rampant metastatic disease within a few weeks of the diagnosis. By contrast, particularly in the elderly, the disease may grow slowly and remain confined to the breast.

Course of untreated disease

The clinical course of untreated disease (usually in patients who have concealed their tumour for many years) is typically as follows. A lump becomes palpable in the breast of a middle-aged woman and is followed by the appearance of a node in the axilla. As the tumour increases in size, it becomes tethered to the skin, resulting in skin dimpling. Peau d'orange and nodules develop over the breast. In the extreme case confluent skin infiltration extends from the breast around to the back (cancer *en cuirasse*).

Symptoms of metastases may occur at any stage of the primary. They include back pain (vertebral deposits), cough and dyspnoea (pleural effusion, lung parenchymal deposits or lymphangitis carcinomatosa); anorexia, weight loss and jaundice (liver metastases); symptoms of raised intracranial pressure (p. 473) (cerebral deposits). The final phase of the disease is often that of cachexia and terminal bronchopneumonia.

Local recurrence

Local recurrence (Fig. 23.2) is most commonly seen following mastectomy. It generally presents as painless reddish nodules, usually less than 1 cm in diameter, over the skin flaps, or sometimes as a diffuse erythematous rash (Fig. 23.3). It may subsequently cross the midline to the opposite breast and extend to the ipsilateral axilla and skin of the back. Postoperative radiotherapy is given (see indications below) to reduce the likelihood of locoregional recurrence.

DIAGNOSIS

The patient may present with a lump she has found herself on routine or casual examination. Sometimes

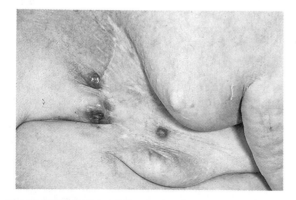

Fig. 23.2 Nodular local recurrence on the skin flaps of a mastectomy scar.

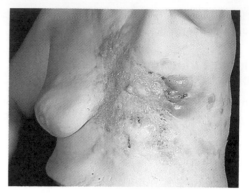

Fig. 23.3 Widespread nodular recurrence over left chest wall following mastectomy, extending to the other breast.

it is detected by her general practitioner or during admission to hospital for an unrelated condition.

Paget's disease of the nipple presents as a red, eczematous unilateral lesion. It may bleed and eventually destroys the nipple. An underlying carcinoma may be palpable.

Increasingly frequently early breast cancer is being detected through breast screening in asymptomatic women. Occasionally presentation is with features of metastatic disease (e.g. pathological fracture, pleural effusion or jaundice).

Obtaining a histological diagnosis

The patient should be referred urgently to a surgeon with a special interest in breast cancer. If the tumour is palpable (usually 1 cm or more in diameter), needle aspiration is performed with a 10 ml syringe and a 22 (green) gauge needle. Examination of the suitably-stained aspirate by a pathologist may show normal, equivocal or obviously malignant cells.

If the lump is not palpable but the mammogram shows an abnormal density or calcification (see p. 239 and Figs 13.7 and 13.8), needle biopsy under radiological control is carried out.

If the fine needle aspirate is negative or equivocal but the lump is considered to be malignant on clinical or radiological grounds, a biopsy under general anaesthesia is necessary to confirm the diagnosis before proceeding to conservative or more extensive surgery.

STAGING

Staging is most important in determining the choice of local treatment, hormonal or cytotoxic therapy. It is based upon clinical, radiological and laboratory examinations. The simplest staging scheme still in use

Table 23.2 Clinical staging of breast cancer

Stage	Clinical findings
I	Freely movable (on underlying muscle). No suspicious nodes
II	As stage I but mobile axillary node(s) on the same side
III	Primary more extensive than stage I, e.g. skin invaded wide of the primary mass or fixation to muscle. Axillary nodes, if present, are fixed; or supraclavicular nodes involved
IV	Extension beyond the ipsilateral chest wall area, e.g. opposite breast or axilla; or distant metastases

Table 23.3 TNM classification of breast cancer

Stage	Clinical findings
Primary tumour	
Tis	Carcinoma-in-situ
T0	No demonstrable tumour in the breast
T1	Tumour less than 2 cm in greatest dimension confined to the breast
T1a	Tumour 0.5 cm or less in maximum dimension
T1b	Tumour more than 0.5 cm but not more than 1 cm in greatest dimension
T1c	Tumour more than 1 cm but not more than 2 cm in greatest dimension
T2	Tumour > 2 cm but < 5 cm in greatest dimension
T3	Tumour more than 5 cm in its greatest dimension
T4	Tumour of any size with direct extension to chest wall or skin
T4a	Fixation to chest wall
T4b	Oedema, infiltration or ulceration of the skin of the breast
T4c	Both of above
Regional lymph nodes	
N0	No palpable nodes
NI	Mobile ipsilateral nodes
N2	Fixed ipsilateral nodes fixed to each other or to other structures
N3	Ipsilateral internal mammary nodes
Distant metastases	
M0	No distant metastases
M1	Distant metastases including skin involvement beyond the breast area

is shown in Table 23.2. However the TNM classification (Table 23.3) of the International Union Against Cancer (UICC) has gained wide acceptance.

The size and mobility of the tumour are noted and any involvement of the skin or underlying muscle. The regional lymph nodes (axillary and supraclavicular on both sides) and the other breast are examined. The chest is examined for signs of a pleural effusion. The abdomen is palpated for liver enlargement. The spine is percussed for bony tenderness, often associated with bone metastases.

Whether palpable nodes are histologically involved is difficult to assess. About 30% of axillary nodes clinically considered to contain tumour are histologically free of disease. However 30% of patients without clinically palpable nodes have histological evidence of nodal involvement.

The following investigations are performed:

— Full blood count
— Liver biochemistry
— Radiographs of chest, lumbar spine and pelvis
— Bone scan (in selected cases—see below)
— Liver ultrasound.

Radiographs of the chest, thoracolumbar spine and pelvis (Fig. 23.4) are recommended, since they are common sites of metastatic disease.

A bone scan is worthwhile (p. 185) if the patient has bone pain, the tumour is advanced (T3 or T4) or the regional nodes are involved.

An ultrasound examination of the liver should be performed to detect liver metastases.

Treatment of carcinoma-in-situ

The best treatment of ductal and lobular carcinoma-in-situ (DCIS and LCIS) is uncertain. Traditionally

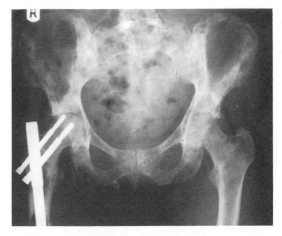

Fig. 23.4 Radiograph of the pelvis and upper femurs showing widespread mixed lytic and sclerotic metastases. The right hip has been pinned to stabilise a pathological fracture.

DCIS has been treated by total mastectomy. Axillary dissection is not routinely performed because of the low incidence of involved nodes (0–2%). However total mastectomy, while curative in nearly all patients, probably overtreats some patients, especially those with small lesions detected by screening. An alternative is wide local excision, provided that DCIS is not multifocal. However multicentricity is often underestimated by mammography. If wide excision shows that the margins are clear of DCIS, no further surgery is needed. However if the margins are not clear of DCIS, further excision is needed until the margins are clear. If DCIS is multifocal or extensive, mastectomy is necessary.

The value of adjuvant breast irradiation and of tamoxifen in DCIS detected by screening is being evaluated in national trials in the UK.

Lobular carcinoma-in-situ is not normally an indication for excision or mastectomy. Patients should be kept under close surveillance, with regular breast screening. It is not known whether tamoxifen inhibits the development of invasive cancer in the presence of LCIS.

TREATMENT OF EARLY BREAST CANCER

The treatment of breast cancer, particularly in its early stages, is one of the most controversial. By 'early' is meant operable disease (T1–3a, N0, N1, M0).

Historical perspective

For much of this century it was believed that lymphatic spread was the most important pathway of spread of breast cancer and that the regional lymphatics offered the main barrier to the blood-borne dissemination of the disease. The logical treatment was a radical mastectomy, an operation in which an 'en bloc' resection of the breast, local musculature and axillary dissection was performed. This was an extremely mutilating procedure.

Radiotherapy was first employed as an alternative to radical surgery in the 1920s. A limited excision of the tumour was carried out and radium needles implanted throughout the breast. The local control and survival using this conservative approach were comparable with the results of radical surgery. In patients where the tumour was confined to the breast the 5-year survival was about 70%. This conservative approach did not, however, fit in with the theory of the sequential spread of breast cancer from the breast to the draining nodes and thence to the bloodstream. Surgeons understandably did not adopt it.

In 1955 it was demonstrated that a less mutilating form of surgery, *simple mastectomy*, with postoperative radiotherapy to the chest wall and regional lymphatics could provide local control and survival comparable with more radical surgery. At the same time it was appreciated that breast tumours can disseminate by the bloodstream, even when the primary is apparently localised. This weakened the case for radical surgery. Experience over the last 15 years has shown that for selected early breast cancers more limited surgery and postoperative breast irradiation can provide comparable local control and survival compared with mastectomy. The main benefit to women has been the opportunity of retaining the breast with a high chance of local control and good cosmesis. Mastectomy remains an option for local recurrence.

Mastectomy or conservation therapy?

The decision as to whether a mastectomy or a more conservative approach of local excision and postoperative radiotherapy should be adopted depends on close liaison between surgeon and radiotherapist. A joint decision should ideally be taken after the patient has been seen by a radiotherapist following pathological confirmation of malignancy. The radiotherapist can decide whether locoregional radiotherapy is technically possible and assess the likely cosmetic result. In patients in whom local excision of the tumour would result in a substantial loss of breast tissue, mastectomy may be preferable.

The discussion of the options with the patient requires great sensitivity since she is usually distressed by the recent diagnosis of breast cancer. Such anxiety may impair her capacity to concentrate on the details of alternative treatment options. The assistance of a nurse counsellor during this period can be invaluable.

Conservation therapy (limited surgery and postoperative radiotherapy)

In patients with T1 and T2 tumours up to 4 cm in size some form of limited excision should be considered. This may be a lumpectomy, in which the tumour is removed with a 1–2 cm margin of normal tissue, or a more extensive excision such as a quadrantectomy, in which a quarter of the breast is excised.

Local excision is generally not advised in the following circumstances:

1. The likely cosmetic result will be poor (e.g. the removal of a 4 cm tumour from a small breast) due to loss of breast tissue.

2. Postoperative radiotherapy to the breast and regional lymphatics is not technically feasible (e.g. due to limited movement of the shoulder caused, for example, by arthritis.
3. Sufficiently frequent follow-up is unlikely.
4. The elderly.

In patients in whom a conservation approach is not feasible or acceptable to the patient, a simple mastectomy and axillary node sampling is recommended.

Management of the axilla

The main surgical options for the axilla are sampling of the lower axillary nodes, a lower axillary dissection or a complete axillary clearance. If a complete axillary clearance is carried out, postoperative irradiation of the axilla is unnecessary.

Radical radiotherapy

The role of postoperative radiotherapy is to sterilise any residual disease in the breast, chest wall and regional nodes and to reduce the probability of locoregional recurrence.

Postmastectomy

The indications are:

a. Pathological involvement or unknown histology of axillary nodes.
b. Adverse features of primary tumour:
   (i) Moderately (grade 2) or poorly differentiated (grade 3) histology
   (ii) Lymphatic invasion in the operative specimen
   (iii) Tumour at or close to the deep resection margin or involving the skin
   (iv) Tumours 4 cm or greater in size
   (v) Advanced local disease (stage III)
   (vi) Inner quadrant or central tumours.

Target volume and technique

The aim of postoperative radiotherapy is to deliver a homogeneous radical dose to the chest wall or breast and regional lymphatics. This is not an easy task because of the awkward shapes and curves of this area and the need to limit the dose to the underlying lung.

A variety of techniques is used. They are of two main types: en bloc and multifield.

En bloc. The chest wall/breast, axilla and supraclavicular nodes are encompassed in two large tangential fields with skin bolus. No computer plan is used. The ipsilateral arm is placed behind the head and the body rotated slightly to the opposite side.

This technique is suitable postmastectomy or for locally advanced breast cancer where a junction between shoulder and breast fields through the disease would be undesirable.

Theoretically this technique should be ideal—only two fields to set up and no junctions to worry about. But there are drawbacks. Dosage is likely to be too low, especially above the clavicle. The dosage to the supraclavicular fossa can be monitored by thermoluminescent dosimetry (TLD) while the patient is treated and the field adjusted if necessary to ensure adequate coverage. In an attempt to include both the parasternal and axillary nodes, the medial edge has to be beyond the midline and the lateral edge far enough back on the lateral chest wall to cover the apex of the axilla. There is the danger of including an excessive amount of lung tissue within the irradiated volume.

Multi-field. Separate fields are planned to cover (1) supraclavicular fossa, axilla and upper internal mammary chain (shoulder field) and (2) chest wall and lower internal mammary chain. The junction of the shoulder and chest wall fields are carefully matched to avoid overdosage or underdosage. A computer plan of the dose distribution on the chest wall field is commonly made.

Shoulder field. A direct anterior megavoltage field (Fig. 23.5) covers the supraclavicular fossa and axilla. The upper margin should be at the level of the thyrohyoid groove. The lateral margin should encompass the lateral border of the axilla. It is important that the length of the shoulder field does not exceed 10–11 cm since this risks irradiating a substantial amount

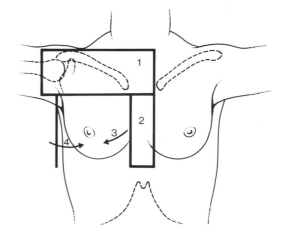

Fig. 23.5 Technique of megavoltage irradiation of the breast. Four fields are shown: 1, axillary–supraclavicular; 2, parasternal; 3 and 4, chest wall tangential (the breast may or may not be present). A posterior field is usually added. (Redrawn from Robinson's Surgery, Longmans.)

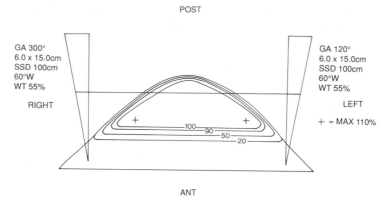

Fig. 23.6 The isodoses of a pair of wedged tangential chest wall fields of Figure 23.5 in cross-section. This technique minimises the amount of lung irradiated.

of lung and causing pneumonitis. The average size of the shoulder field is about 10 cm long and 20 cm wide.

The shoulder joint and the part of the larynx included in the field may be shielded with lead.

A direct *posterior axillary boost* may be necessary to supplement the dose to the axilla. It should encompass the nodes shown in Fig. 23.1A. The upper margin should be along the upper border of the clavicle. The medial limit should not incorporate more than 1–2 cm of lung. An average field size would be 10 cm in length by 8 cm in width.

If the axilla is to be cleared, the surgeon should be asked to place metallic clips at the medial extent of the dissection. Using the simulator, a field can be planned to treat the medial supraclavicular fossa, extending laterally as far as the clips.

Chest wall. The chest wall can be encompassed in a pair of wedged glancing fields (Figs 23.6 and 23.7). This should cover the scar of the local excision or mastectomy. It normally extends from the level of the suprasternal notch at the level of the second costal cartilage down to 2 cm below the submammary fold. The medial margin is at the midline or 1 cm to the contralateral side of it. The lateral margin should lie in the mid-axillary line. A typical dose distribution is shown on Figure 23.6. A breast jig may assist setting up parallel opposed glancing fields (Fig. 23.8).

As the separation between the medial and lateral chest wall limits increases, so too does the volume of lung irradiated by the tangential glancing fields. Where this separation exceeds 21 cm, the medial chest wall can be treated by a direct internal mammary field and

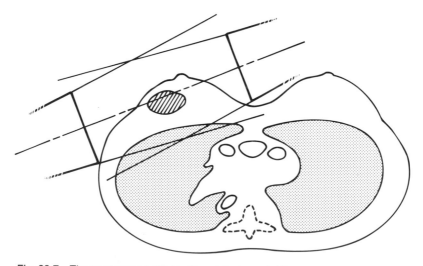

Fig. 23.7 The two tangential fields (3 and 4) shown in Figure 23.5.

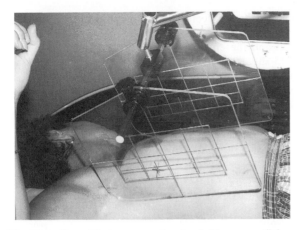

Fig. 23.8 Breast jig to ensure glancing fields are parallel opposed.

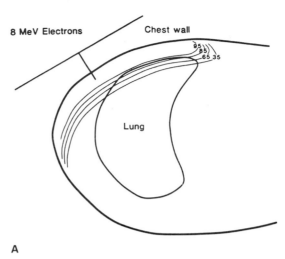

A

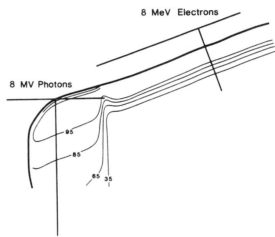

B

Fig. 23.9 **A** A typical dose distribution in the electron field. (8 MeV). **B** A typical dose distribution in the sagittal plane showing the junction between the 8 MV photon field irradiating the supraclavicular fossa (left of diagram) and the electron field irradiating the chest wall. (Reproduced with permission from Magee et al, Clinical Oncology, Springer-Verlag, 1991.)

the rest of the chest wall by medial and lateral glancing fields with a smaller separation encompassing less lung tissue.

The internal mammary nodes lie deep to the midline and 2–3 cm lateral to it. They may be included within the chest wall glancing fields or by a separate direct internal mammary field (Fig. 23.5). However unless the tumour is situated in the centre or inner quadrants of the breast and the axillary nodes are involved, the internal mammary nodes do not need to be treated routinely.

Alternative techniques

Megavoltage to shoulder field and electron beam to chest wall. The supraclavicular fossa and axilla can be treated with a direct single megavoltage field. The chest wall can be treated with 8–10 MeV electrons depending on the thickness of the chest wall (Fig. 23.9A). They have the advantage of sparing underlying lung because of their limited range (p. 391). Using a single electron field there is inevitably a fall-off in dose at the lateral end of the field as the chest wall curves posteriorly. The 80% isodose typically lies 22 cm from the midline, when measured over the skin surface.

To enable optimal matching of the photon and electron beams in the sagittal plane (Fig. 23.9B), the electron beam is applied at 30° to the vertical and 20° from the vertical in the sagittal plane. The nominal beam edges (i.e those of the light field) of the megavoltage and electron fields are matched. The matching of the isodoses at all depths is not perfect, with slight upward deviation of the isodoses towards the surface at the junction.

Electron energy for chest wall. The average thickness of the chest wall is 1.7 cm. The maximum thickness

is at the upper end of the anterior axillary line (3.1 cm) over the pectoralis major. However the latter area is included in the shoulder field. So for practical purposes 8–10 MeV electrons are adequate; 10 MeV electrons are used when the chest wall thickness exceeds 2 cm.

Dose and energy for en bloc and multifield techniques

Megavoltage rather than orthovoltage is chosen to limit the dose to the ribs. Unless the skin is involved by tumour clinically or in the operative specimen, it is not necessary to apply bolus material to the chest wall fields unless the bolus, as in the en bloc technique, is acting as a tissue compensator.

1. En bloc
   45 Gy in 20 daily fractions over 4 weeks (4–6 MV photons)

2. Multifield
   a. Shoulder field (supraclavicular and axillary nodes)
      45 Gy in 20 fractions over 4 weeks with the posterior axillary boost bringing the midaxillary dose to 45 Gy

   b. Chest wall fields
      45 Gy in 20 fractions over 4 weeks

Palpable chest wall disease or involved supraclavicular or axillary nodes can be boosted with electrons of suitable energy (9–12 MeV):
15 Gy in 5 daily fractions over 1 week

Conservation therapy

Most radiotherapists prefer to use a multifield technique for the intact breast following lumpectomy since it avoids the widespread telangiectasia which inevitably follows the en bloc technique with bolus.

Boost to the tumour. Some form of boost of irradiation to the primary tumour is desirable to bring the tumour dose to 60 Gy. This is either given by electrons or by an iridium-192 implant (Fig. 19.9). Either form of boost will give comparable local control. However the higher surface dose of electrons will cause telangiectasia on the treated skin. In implants telangiectasia is confined to the skin entry and exit points of the iridium wire and can be avoided if the sources lie just beneath the skin surface. In general the breast tissue tends to be thinner in the more medial and lateral parts of the breast. In these sites there may be inadequate tissue for an implant and electrons are preferable.

An iridium implant does enable a higher dose to be delivered than do electrons for a similar level of morbidity. However there is no compelling evidence that electrons are inferior to an implant in terms of local control in conservation therapy.

Electrons. The appropriate electron energy, usually 9–12 MeV, is chosen according to the depth of the breast tissue at the site of the tumour bearing area. This is usually judged clinically but is more accurately measured by ultrasound. In order to avoid unnecessary transmission of electrons to the underlying lung, Perspex of suitable thickness can be interposed between the skin and the end of the applicator. The length of the field should include the scar, or known tumour site if this does not correspond to the scar, with a 1–2 cm margin at each end to allow for the inward bowing of the isodose curves at depth.

Dose
15 Gy in 5 daily fractions over 1 week

Interstitial implant (Ch. 19)
20–25 Gy to 85% isodose

Boost to axillary or supraclavicular nodes. Palpable nodes can be boosted to the same dose as postmastectomy (see above).

Locoregional recurrence

If recurrence occurs on the chest wall or in the axillary, supraclavicular or, very rarely, in the internal mammary nodes, the chest wall and peripheral lymphatics should be irradiated after gross disease has been resected. Either en bloc or multifield technique may be used. Residual palpable disease is boosted with electrons. Dosage is the same as postmastectomy.

Practical points in setting up the patient

1. Ensure that the patient lies in a comfortable and relaxed position with a supporting pillow. If not she will tend to relax and sag during actual treatment. A glancing field may then miss the chest wall almost completely.
2. Take care to avoid overdosage and underdosage at field junctions.

Planning difficulties

The very mobile breast. In some patients in the treatment position a very mobile breast tends to fall beyond the midaxillary line. This has the effect of the lateral margin of the glancing field extending more posteriorly to encompass the breast. More lung is therefore included in the field. The position of the breast can sometimes be stabilised by applying a Netelast sling which the patient wears over the breast and is secured over the ipsilateral shoulder.

Inadequate coverage at the junction of the internal mammary and medial glancing field. As the light beam of the medial glancing field falls on the breast, the curvature of the chest wall tends to create inadequately covered areas at the upper and lower ends of the field. This can be overcome by rotating the gantry medially until these untreated areas are adequately covered. The area of overlap with the internal mammary field can be shielded by lead blocks on the shadow tray when the internal mammary field is treated.

General care

During treatment
— Avoid washing the treated area during treatment.
— Advise loose fitting clothes, omitting a bra since this tends to cause abrasion.
— Apply proprietary baby powder to the treated area to keep it dry.
— If the skin becomes uncomfortable during treatment, the application of cold air from an ordinary hairdrier is soothing.
— Shoulder exercises to keep the joint supple should be taught by a physiotherapist and practised daily by the patient during and after treatment.

After treatment
— Apply an emollient cream, such as Oilatum or hydrocortisone, to the areas of dry desquamation. A small amount should be rubbed into the treated area twice daily.
— Apply gentian violet or Flamazine to the areas of moist desquamation. These tend to occur in the axilla and the submammary fold.
— Where possible, the resolution of moist desquamation, particularly if extensive, is facilitated by keeping the treated areas uncovered.
— Continue shoulder exercises indefinitely.

Morbidity

Intact breast
1. Breast oedema is common. It is usually mild, often confined to the lower half of the breast and may last up to a year after treatment before resolving.
2. Subcutaneous fibrosis is usually mild throughout the breast but often marked in the area of the boost to the primary tumour.

Intact breast and postmastectomy
1. Skin—telangiectasia (Plate 16).
2. Lymphoedema of the arm. This is uncommon following axillary irradiation if the axilla has been sampled but not dissected. The risk is considerably increased if axillary clearance precedes axillary irradiation.
3. Rib fractures. These are rare. They tend to occur in the lateral 4th–7th ribs where the maximum dose

is delivered from the glancing chest wall fields (Fig. 23.7).
4. Pneumonitis and lung fibrosis. Virtually all patients will develop evidence of apical fibrosis on chest radiograph. About 9% of patients will have symptomatic radiation pneumonitis. This usually settles without long-term sequelae (p. 379).
5. Fibrosis of the shoulder joint can occur, restricting movement. The patient should be taught appropriate shoulder exercises by a physiotherapist to maintain a normal range of movement.
6. Cardiac morbidity. Patients, particularly with left-sided tumours, are at slightly increased risk of death from coronary artery disease. It is uncertain if this risk applies to megavoltage as well as to orthovoltage irradiation.
7. Radiation induced sarcoma. This is extremely rare. Mean latency between irradiation and diagnosis is 13 years. Prognosis is very poor. The mean survival is 15 months.
8. Hypothyroidism may occur due to inclusion of the thyroid gland in the radiation field.

Results of radical radiotherapy

Postmastectomy. Adjuvant postoperative radiotherapy reduces the local recurrence rate from 33% (without radiotherapy) to 13%. Typical locoregional recurrence rates following radiotherapy are 4% (stage I), 10% (stage II) and 20 % (stage III). In general postoperative radiotherapy does not improve survival, although a modest 3–5% reduction of mortality may occur in patients with involved axillary nodes.

Conservation therapy. The 5-year survival free of disease is 95% for T1 and 75% for T2. These results are similar to those of mastectomy and postopera-

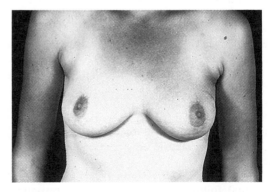

Fig. 23.10 Excellent cosmetic result of postoperative radiotherapy and iridium implant following lumpectomy for early carcinoma of the left breast. (Courtesy of Dr D Ash, Leeds.)

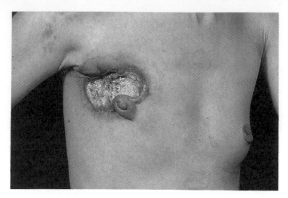

Fig. 23.11   Locally advanced and inoperable carcinoma of the right breast (T4).

tive radiotherapy. Cosmetic results are very good (Fig. 23.10) in T1 and T2 in 87% and 54% of cases respectively. The recurrence rate within the first 5 years following treatment is 8–10% for T1 and T2. Surgical salvage by mastectomy is successful for most local recurrences.

TREATMENT OF LOCALLY ADVANCED BREAST CANCER (T3B-T4, N2 OR N3M0)

For advanced inoperable disease (Fig. 23.11) a trial of 6–8 weeks of Tamoxifen (20 mg daily) is worthwhile if the pace of the local disease is not too aggressive. If there is no or only a partial response (e.g. reduced but persistent ulceration and discharge), toilet mastectomy (if there is adequate clearance of the tumour for the skin flaps) and postoperative radiotherapy to the breast and peripheral lymphatics should be considered.

The probability of local control with radical radio-therapy is much lower (10–30%), compared with early breast cancer. Palliative irradiation (see below) of the primary alone should be offered to frail patients uncontrolled by hormonal therapy.

Even if local control is maintained by radical therapy, distant relapse is common. Only 12–40% will remain relapse free at 5 years. Five-year survival rates are poor (25–50%).

Dose and energy
In the presence of macroscopic disease the dose needs to be higher than the 45 Gy prescribed for microscopic disease.

45 Gy in 20 daily fractions over 4 weeks (4–6 MV photons) followed by a boost to the tumour site by: (a) implant (20 Gy to 85% isodose)
or
(b) electrons 15 Gy in 5 daily fractions (9–12 MeV)

PALLIATIVE TREATMENT

In many patients radical treatment of any kind is inappropriate, either due to locally advanced disease, distant metastases, old age or poor general medical condition. The aim is to relieve symptoms. These aspects of palliative care are described in Chapter 33.

Palliative surgery

Surgery usually has little part to play in the local management of advanced breast cancer. Occasionally, however, if there is adequate skin uninvolved to allow skin flaps to be formed, a toilet mastectomy can provide rapid and effective local control of an ulcerated and odorous tumour.

Palliative radiotherapy

Palliative radiotherapy has a very useful role in the relief of a variety of distressing symptoms.

Primary tumour

External beam irradiation can reduce bleeding, discharge, ulceration and tumour bulk. Concurrent treatment with metronidazole may reduce infection and offensive odour caused by anaerobic bacteria.

Technique
This should be simple. A parallel opposed pair of tangential fields at megavoltage using a small jig and bolus or a direct orthovoltage (250–300 kv) or electron field will suffice.

Dose and energy
30–35 Gy in 10 daily fractions over 2 weeks (4–6 MV photons or 9–12 MeV electrons)

Bone metastases

Technique
Single or parallel opposed fields are used. Single fields suffice for the spine. It is worth simulating spinal fields since care needs to be taken not to overlap with previously treated fields. Overlap risks permanent spinal cord damage, particularly in patients surviving for many years with metastatic disease.

Dose and energy
8–10 Gy as a single fraction, or 20–22.5 Gy in 4–5 daily fractions over 1 week (4–6 MV photons, cobalt-60 or orthovoltage)

Cerebral metastases

Cerebral metastases are treated as described in Chapter 27 (p. 488).

ADJUVANT HORMONAL OR CYTOTOXIC CHEMOTHERAPY

Rationale

It is generally accepted that a substantial number of patients with operable breast cancer have micro-metastases which current techniques are unable to detect. This premise is supported by the fact that many of these patients develop distant metastases despite radical surgery to remove the primary tumour. It seems logical therefore to administer some form of hormonal or cytotoxic therapy at the time of primary surgery in an attempt to eradicate these micrometastases. This is what is meant by adjuvant therapy.

Who benefits?

A report of the Early Breast Cancer Trialists Group of 75 000 women with early breast cancer shows clearly that adjuvant therapy, whether it be hormonal (tamoxifen or oophorectomy) or with cytotoxic combination chemotherapy can increase 10-year survival. It seems reasonable to confine combination chemotherapy to patients with a very poor prognosis (e.g. premenopausal with more than 10 axillary nodes involved). Adjuvant ovarian ablation might be used for premenopausal women with less than 10 involved axillary nodes, and tamoxifen for node-negative premenopausal and all postmenopausal women irrespective of nodal status.

Adjuvant tamoxifen

Tamoxifen 20 mg given for at least 2 years reduces the risk of recurrence by 28% and mortality by 21%. Tamoxifen confers survival benefit in both pre- and postmenopausal women irrespective of oestrogen receptor status (p. 545). In women under the age of 50 the benefits of tamoxifen are less substantial.

Toxicity

The side-effects of tamoxifen are minimal. 'Hot flushes' occur in 15%, transient mild thrombocytopenia or leucopenia in 5–10% and vaginal bleeding in 5%. Hypercalcaemia very occasionally occurs on starting therapy. There is a small increase in the incidence of endometrial cancer.

Adjuvant oophorectomy

Until the report of the Early Breast Cancer Trialists Collaborative Group the value of adjuvant oophorectomy was not well supported because of small numbers in individual studies. However the overview of large numbers of patients treated with adjuvant ovarian ablation shows a highly significant increase in recurrence-free survival (26%) and in overall survival (25%) in premenopausal women under the age of 50.

For node-positive premenopausal women the gains in recurrence-free and overall survival at 15 years are 10.5% and 13% respectively. Much smaller but just as statistically significant benefits in both forms of survival are seen in premenopausal node-negative patients.

Adjuvant combination cytotoxic chemotherapy

The most influential of these trials was conducted in Milan. In this study women with histologically involved nodes with operable breast cancer were randomised to 12 cycles of cyclophosphamide, methotrexate and 5-fluorouracil (CMF) over 1 year or to no further therapy. At 10 years following treatment, the largest benefit accrued to premenopausal women, in whom there was a 40% reduction in risk of death. Improved survival was confined to premenopausal women with 1–3 axillary nodes involved by tumour. For those with 4–10 nodes involved, there was a significant improvement in relapse-free but not overall survival.

It is probable that some of the benefit of adjuvant chemotherapy is due to the endocrine effect of a chemical oophorectomy. However this is unlikely to be the only mechanism by which cytotoxic chemotherapy works since there is some, though smaller, benefit in postmenopausal women.

Duration of treatment

The optimal duration of adjuvant cytotoxic therapy is not known. Six cycles of chemotherapy are generally recommended.

Choice of drugs

Combination chemotherapy is more effective than single agent therapy. No particular combination is best. However CMF is amongst the most effective and widely used (Table 23.4).

Toxicity

Despite the evidence of a modest reduction in

Table 23.4 Adjuvant CMF cytotoxic chemotherapy in breast cancer

Cyclophosphamide	100 mg/m² orally	Days 1–14
Methotrexate	40 mg/m² i.v. bolus	Days 1 and 8
5-fluorouracil	600 mg/m² i.v. bolus	Days 1 and 8

Repeated every 28 days

mortality, enthusiasm for adjuvant cytotoxic therapy has been tempered by its toxicity.

Morbidity may be both physical and psychological. Of women undergoing adjuvant CMF, 30–40% become anxious or depressed. Even 6 months after the end of this combination, persistent psychiatric disturbance occurs in about 10% of patients.

Most patients treated with CMF will experience nausea and vomiting. Temporary alopecia is common, understandably a major concern to women. Hair normally starts regrowing about 2 months after the last cycle of treatment.

MEDICAL TREATMENT OF METASTATIC DISEASE

Although nearly 90% of patients will have operable disease at presentation, the majority will relapse. Treatment for metastatic disease is essentially palliative. This is important to bear in mind when selecting therapy. Maintaining good symptomatic control without undue toxicity is the aim. This is often not easy to achieve, since, in life-threatening disease (e.g. liver metastases), the most effective cytotoxic agents, such as Adriamycin, are inevitably accompanied by some unpleasant side-effects such as nausea, vomiting and alopecia. Some measure of quality of life of the patient (Ch. 34) needs to be monitored during treatment to assess whether therapy has really benefited the patient. If toxicity exceeds relief of symptoms, treatment should be stopped.

Selection of treatment

The choice of therapy must take into consideration age and general medical condition, menopausal and hormonal status, the sites and tempo of the disease, disease-free interval and the severity of symptoms. There are two main types of systemic treatment: hormonal and cytotoxic therapy. A general schema for selection of therapy is shown in Figure 23.12.

Age and general medical condition

The elderly and those who are in poor general medical

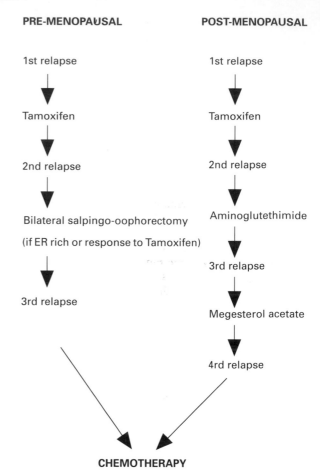

Fig. 23.12 Schema of systemic therapy for recurrent breast cancer.

condition tolerate cytotoxic therapy poorly. Hormonal therapy is preferable in such patients.

Anthracyclines such as Adriamycin or epirubicin should be avoided in patients with a history of ischaemic heart disease. Similarly, fluid retaining drugs such as megestrol acetate (p. 547) should be used with caution in patients with ischaemic heart disease since they may exacerbate angina and precipitate heart failure.

Menopausal and hormone receptor status

In general, hormonal therapy tends to be more successful in postmenopausal patients and in those with oestrogen receptor-rich tumours (p. 545). Premenopausal women can respond to hormonal therapy such as oophorectomy. However, rapidly progressive and life threatening disease is common in this group and requires cytotoxic chemotherapy.

Bilateral salpingo-oophorectomy should be considered in premenopausal patients who are known to be oestrogen receptor rich or have demonstrated a previous response to other hormonal therapy. An alternative means of inducing the menopause is the use of a luteinising hormone releasing hormone (LHRH) agonist, such as goserelin, which can be combined with tamoxifen.

Sites of metastases

Soft tissue (chest wall, breast, lymph nodes) and bone disease tend to respond to hormonal therapy, whereas visceral metastases (e.g. liver) respond less well or not at all. Liver and bone marrow metastases almost invariably need cytotoxic chemotherapy. The doses of myelosuppressive drugs often have to be reduced if there are bone marrow metastases.

Tempo of disease and disease-free interval

Both the site and the rapidity of the disease are important in determining the need for the early introduction of cytotoxic chemotherapy. Lung metastases may be indolent, without giving rise to symptoms, or rapidly progressive with severe dyspnoea. For disease with a slower tempo, a trial of hormone therapy (usually tamoxifen) is justifiable. Aggressive disease requires cytotoxic chemotherapy.

A more aggressive course of the disease can be expected in patients with a short disease-free interval (< 2 years) and involvement of multiple organs. In such patients primary cytotoxic therapy should be considered to halt the rapid and fatal progression of the disease.

By contrast, with a disease-free interval of 5 years or more, the tempo of the disease is often slower and the probability of response to hormonal therapy is higher. Tamoxifen 20 mg daily is recommended as initial therapy.

Hormonal therapy

The principles of hormonal therapy and the properties of commonly used agents in breast cancer are described in Chapter 32. The general scheme of hormonal therapy for recurrent or metastatic breast cancer is summarised in Figure 23.12.

Cytotoxic chemotherapy

Breast cancer is moderately sensitive to chemotherapy. Responses to single agents are 40% or more for Adriamycin and epirubicin, 35–40% for cyclophosphamide,

Table 23.5 CMFP and VAP combination chemotherapy for breast cancer

CMFP		
Cyclophosphamide	600 mg/m² i.v. bolus	Day 1
Methotrexate	40 mg/m² i.v. bolus	Day 1
5-fluorouracil	600 mg/m² i.v. bolus	Day 1
Prednisolone	40 mg daily orally	Days 1–5

Repeated every 21 days

VAP		
Vincristine	1.4 mg/m² (max 2 mg) i.v. bolus	Day 1
Adriamycin	40 mg/m² i.v. bolus	Day 1
Prednisolone	40 mg daily orally	Days 1–5

Repeated every 21 days

mitoxantrone, methotrexate and vincristine, and 25% for 5-fluorouracil. The objective response rates to combination chemotherapy are generally higher (60%) but with greater toxicity. Median duration of response is 10–12 months. Response to second line chemotherapy is much lower (20%).

Two commonly used regimes of combination chemotherapy (Table 23.5) are cyclophosphamide, methotrexate, 5-fluorouracil and prednisolone (CMFP) and vincristine, Adriamycin and prednisolone (VAP).

As a guideline, three courses (e.g. of CMFP) should be given initially, subject to patient tolerance. If there is evidence of a clinically useful response, a further three courses are given. If the disease continues to respond and the toxicity is acceptable to the patient, further courses are given. If there is no evidence of response and the patient is fit for alternative chemotherapy, an alternative regime (e.g. VAP) is given. In practice, nine courses are rarely exceeded.

Chemotherapy of patients with bone marrow metastases is complicated by low blood counts as a result of the disease and from the myelotoxic effects of drugs. The doses of chemotherapy have to be reduced accordingly.

Tamoxifen in the prevention of breast cancer

There are theoretical grounds for believing that tamoxifen might be able to prevent the development of breast cancer in women at high risk of the disease (e.g. a strong family history). Certainly the use of adjuvant tamoxifen following primary surgery was associated with a lower than expected incidence of contralateral breast tumours. Such evidence suggests that tamoxifen may be able to suppress the development of breast cancer in some women. Large randomised

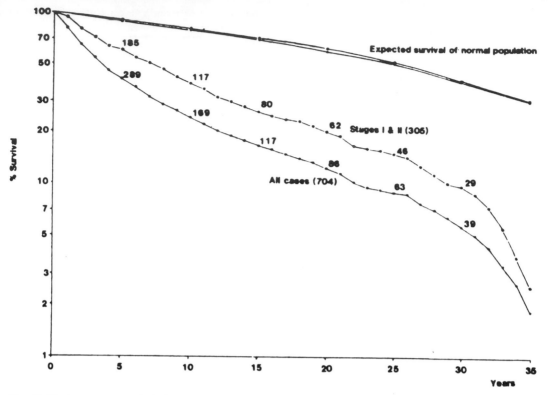

Fig. 23.13   Long-term survival of women with breast cancer. Survival curves for all patients and for stage I and II only. (Reproduced with permission from The Lancet, 1984.)

trials comparing the incidence of breast cancer among normal women taking tamoxifen and untreated controls are in progress to try to answer this very important question.

OVERALL SURVIVAL OF BREAST CANCER PATIENTS

As seen in Figure 23.13 the mortality from breast cancer exceeds that of the unaffected women, even up to 30 years or more after initial treatment.

Survival is influenced by a variety of prognostic factors, of which size of the primary tumour and axillary node involvement are the most important. At 10 years age-corrected survival is 92% (up to 1 cm), 70% (1–2 cm), 55% (2–3 cm) and 45% (over 3 cm) (Fig. 23.14).

Overall survival from time of diagnosis of metastatic disease is about 18 months. The tempo of metastatic disease varies considerably. It may be relatively indolent in bone. However the survival of patients with liver or cerebral metastases is often only a few months.

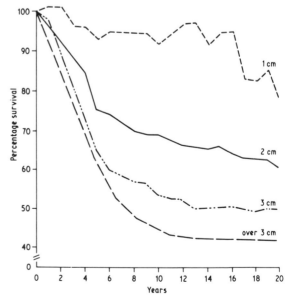

Fig. 23.14   Age-corrected survival rates by tumour size for patients treated for breast cancer apparently confined to the breast. (Reproduced with permission from Halnan, Treatment of Cancer, Ist edn, Chapman and Hall, 1982.)

FOLLOW-UP

Patients with breast cancer represent the largest group of patients followed up in most general oncology clinics. The main aim of follow-up is to detect local recurrence or a contralateral breast primary. Most locoregional recurrences tend to occur within the first 2 years. Routine investigations for the detection of metastatic disease (e.g. chest radiographs and bone scans) in the absence of symptoms are not recommended since there is no evidence that early introduction of treatment influences survival. Restaging investigations should be only be instituted if there is locoregional recurrence or symptoms suggestive of metastases.

For patients disease-free after treatment following mastectomy and postoperative radiotherapy, 3-monthly follow-up for the first 2 years and 6-monthly from 3 to 5 years is probably adequate. After 5 years a 2-yearly mammogram to detect a new tumour in the remaining breast and early access to the clinic if the patient notices any abnormality on the chest wall or in the opposite breast may suffice. No further follow-up is needed unless the mammogram is abnormal or the patient re-presents with symptomatic disease. Some oncologists prefer to keep patients on lifelong follow-up since they remain at long-term risk of relapse.

The duration of follow-up for patients treated with a conservation approach should be longer than following mastectomy: this is to detect recurrence within the breast sufficiently early for a salvage mastectomy to be carried out. Follow-up to 15 years is suggested. A yearly mammogram is suggested in the first 5 years and 2-yearly thereafter.

Breast cancer and pregnancy

Breast cancer diagnosed during pregnancy can present difficult problems. The interests of both mother and child must be considered, and they may at times conflict. Management will be influenced by the stage of pregnancy and of the disease.

In the first trimester, termination is followed by standard therapy. If a termination is not acceptable to the mother, simple mastectomy is advised. No adjuvant radiotherapy or chemotherapy (hormonal/cytotoxic) is given.

In the second trimester the choice is between simple mastectomy or termination of pregnancy followed by standard therapy.

In the third trimester of pregnancy the breast becomes more vascular. Close liaison is necessary between obstetrician and oncologist. For a tumour of 4 cm or smaller in size, wide local excision with postoperative radiotherapy delayed until after delivery is advised. For larger tumours, simple mastectomy with axillary node sample or clearance is recommended. Elective induction or caesarian section at 36 weeks is followed by postoperative irradiation of the peripheral lymphatics if the axillary sample contains a tumour.

During lactation tumours may grow more rapidly and carry a poor prognosis. Lactation should be suppressed by drugs and treatment carried out along conventional lines.

Breast cancer in males

Only about 1% of breast cancer occurs in males—about the same ratio as the amount of breast tissue. Most cases occur over the age of 60. The basic principles of staging, grading and treatment are similar to those in women. Since the distance to the underlying tissue of the chest wall is so much shorter, fixation often occurs before the mass is noticed. The stage is therefore liable to be more advanced, and the prognosis correspondingly worse, than in women.

Simple mastectomy is the normal surgical procedure. The paucity of breast tissue normally precludes wide local excision. Postoperative radiotherapy to the chest wall and peripheral lymphatics is advised if the axillary nodes are involved, the tumour is greater than 4 cm in diameter or there is residual disease at the resection margins. Primary radical radiotherapy is indicated for inoperable localised disease. The value of adjuvant tamoxifen is unproven because of the rarity of the tumour, but is a reasonable policy on the basis of its efficacy in women. Tamoxifen is useful in advanced and metastatic disease. The indications for cytotoxic therapy are as for female breast cancer.

24. Cervix, body of uterus, ovary, vagina, vulva, gestational trophoblastic tumours

CANCER OF THE CERVIX

Anatomy

The cervix (Figs. 24.1 and 24.2) projects into the vaginal vault. Adjacent are the anterior, posterior and lateral vaginal fornices. Anteriorly the cervix is related to the base of the bladder and posteriorly to the rectum and the pouch of Douglas. Laterally it is related to the ureters.

Lymphatic drainage (Fig. 24.3) is to the paracervical, obturator, presacral, external and internal iliac nodes and finally to the para-aortic nodes. The common iliac nodes extend up to the junction of the L4 and L5. Above this level lie the para-aortic nodes, which extend up to the junction of the T12 and L1.

Pathology

Epidemiology and aetiology

Cancer of the cervix is the second commonest gynaecological malignancy with an incidence of 13 per 100 000 in England and Wales. The average age at diagnosis is 50 years.

No immediate cause for cervical cancer is known. There is strong circumstantial evidence that it is a sexually transmitted disease. The disease is extremely rare in virgins. The incidence is higher in married than in single women and increases with the number of pregnancies. There is a fivefold higher incidence among prostitutes. It is commoner in women of lower socioeconomic groups. This is thought to be due to

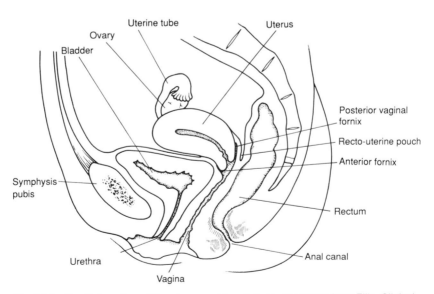

Fig. 24.1 Sagittal section of the uterus and its relations. (Redrawn from Ellis, Clinical Anatomy, 5th edn, Blackwells, 1975.)

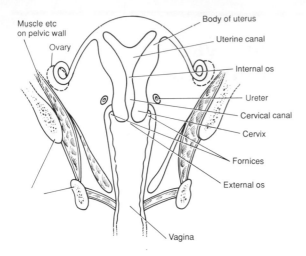

Fig. 24.2 Coronal section of the uterus and vagina. Note the important relationship of the ureter to the cervix.

the early age of first intercourse. There is evidence of an association with herpes simplex virus infection but no proof of its causative role. Male factors may play a part. There is a slight increase in the incidence of the disease in the second wife of a man whose first wife died of the disease.

PREINVASIVE CARCINOMA

Cervical intraepithelial neoplasia (CIN III)

Cervical intraepithelial neoplasia (CIN) has now combined and replaced the previously used terms of carcinoma-in-situ and cervical dysplasia. CIN is graded according to the degree of histological abnormality. The features examined are (a) the degree of differentiation, (b) mitotic activity, and (c) the appearance of the cell nucleus. CIN III is the most abnormal grade. It corresponds to carcinoma-in-situ and is most likely to progress to invasive cancer. Minor degrees of CIN (I and II) may regress or go on to invasion. Overall about 30–40% of CIN will, if untreated, progress to invasive cancer. In one study 18% of CIN III had progressed to invasive malignancy at 10 years and 36% at 20 years.

Microinvasive cancer

Microinvasive cancer is defined as non-confluent invasion less than 3 mm from the basement membrane of the epithelium into stroma. It requires an adequate biopsy (normally a cone biopsy, Fig. 24.4) for the diagnosis to be made.

Treatment

Cervical intraepithelial neoplasia is treated by laser therapy or cold coagulation (cryosurgery). Micro-

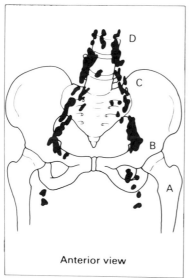
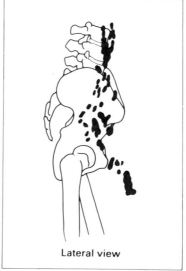

Fig. 24.3 Lymphatic drainage of the cervix: A, obturator; B, internal, external and common iliac; C, lateral sacral; and D, para-aortic. (Reproduced from Souhami and Tobias, Cancer and its Management, Blackwells, 1986.)

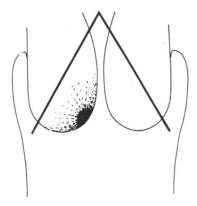

Fig. 24.4 To show the area of cervix removed by the operation of conisation. (Reproduced with permission from Jeffcoate, Principles of Gynaecology, Butterworths.)

invasive carcinoma is treated by conisation (Fig. 24.4) in young patients and by hysterectomy in those who do not plan to have children.

INVASIVE CARCINOMA

Invasive cervical cancer appears as a warty growth or ulcer on the cervix; 90–95% are due to squamous cell carcinoma and about 5% are due to adenocarcinomas. Sarcomas, lymphomas and melanomas are very rare.

Local spread is to the adjoining tissues (Fig. 24.5): vaginal vault, fornices, upward to the corpus, laterally to the parametria, anteriorly to the bladder and posteriorly to the rectum.

Clinical features

The cardinal symptom is vaginal bleeding or blood-stained discharge. This may occur irregularly between periods, after intercourse or after the menopause. Unfortunately, menstrual irregularities are common at the menopause and pathological bleeding may not be recognised, leading to delay in diagnosis. The growth may be obvious on clinical examination (inspection and palpation) but should be confirmed by biopsy. This will also establish the histological grade.

Pain is a late feature and indicates considerable spread beyond the cervix. Later invasion of the parametrial tissues and pelvic nerves causes lumbar aching, then pain radiating to the hip and thigh. In ulcerated lesions there will be associated infection, which will aggravate the symptoms.

Invasion of the base of the bladder will cause dysuria with urinary frequency and pain; destruction of the tissue between the base of the bladder and the vagina can cause a fistula allowing urine to leak from the bladder to the vagina (vesicovaginal fistula). The ureters pass through the parametria close to the cervix (Fig. 24.2). Compression of the ureters will lead to back pressure on the kidney and renal failure with uraemia. This is common in advanced or recurrent disease and is a common cause of death.

Staging and investigation

Clinical staging is carried out under general anaesthesia. Initially a colposcopy and curettage is performed by a gynaecologist. A cone biopsy is performed if the abnormal epithelium extends into the endocervical canal. The tumour is inspected and palpated. Bimanual examination of the size, shape and mobility of the cervix is carried out. The presence and degree of parametrial or posterior extension is assessed by rectovaginal examination. Cystoscopy is performed to exclude involvement of the bladder. Oedema of the base of the bladder is a common appearance associated with frank invasion.

Investigations

Essential investigations are a full blood count, serum urea, creatinine and electrolytes, chest radiograph and intravenous urogram (IVU). IVU may show hydro-ureter or hydronephrosis due to infiltration at the lower end of the ureters.

Lymphography is useful and reasonably reliable in demonstrating involvement of the pelvic and para-aortic nodes. The incidence of pelvic and para-aortic nodes rises with stage. For stages I–IV, pelvic nodes are involved in 15, 30, 45 and 55% and para-aortic nodes in about 5, 15, 35 and 40% respectively. However the results of lymphography may not necessarily influence treatment if the pelvic nodes are routinely irradiated with the primary tumour. Some radiotherapists irradiate the para-aortic nodes if the pelvic nodes are involved.

The contrast medium, an oily dye, is retained within the lymphatics for many months and may provide a useful guide to the response of nodes to treatment. Abnormalities within nodes can be followed for up to about a year after lymphography. There is a small risk of the dye embolising to the lungs.

CT scanning is less reliable than lymphography in demonstrating nodal involvement since metastases less than 1 cm cannot be diagnosed with confidence. Lymphography may show pathological filling defects in nodes smaller than 1 cm but CT scanning is less invasive and carries less morbidity.

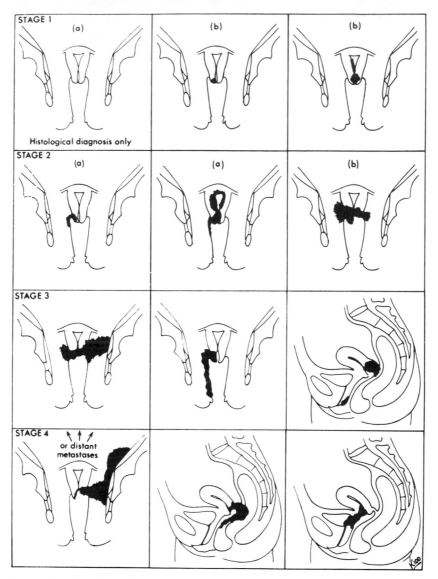

Fig. 24.5 Illustrations of the stages of cancer of the cervix. For details see Table 24.1. (Reproduced with permission from Jeffcoate, Principles of Gynaecology, Butterworths.)

The FIGO clinical staging system is the most widely used (Table 24.1 and Fig. 24.5).

Treatment

Surgery and radiotherapy alone or in combination are curative in cervical cancer. Factors which influence the choice of treatment will include the age and general condition of the patient, the stage of the tumour, and the patient's own preference. For patients symptomatic of pelvic disease but not fit for radical radiotherapy,

palliative intracavitary or external beam therapy should be considered. Dosage is as for endometrial cancer (p. 415).

1. Stage Ib

For young women with non-bulky tumours who have a negative lymphogram or CT scan of the pelvic and para-aortic nodes, a radical Wertheim's hysterectomy is the treatment of choice. The latter includes removal of the uterus, tubes, ovaries, parametria and upper

Table 24.1 FIGO staging of carcinoma of the cervix

Stage	Clinical findings
0	Carcinoma-in-situ*; also called preinvasive or intraepithelial carcinoma
I	Growth confined to the cervix. Upward spread to the corpus does not change the classification.
Ia	Microinvasive carcinoma
Ib	Clinically invasive carcinoma
IIa	Spread beyond the cervix to the upper two-thirds of the vagina
IIb	Spread to parametrium but not as far as the lateral pelvic wall
IIIa	Spread to the lower third of the vagina
IIIb	Spread to the pelvic side wall and/or hydronephrosis or non-functioning kidney due to ureteric compression by tumour
IVa	Spread to the bladder or rectum and/or extending beyond the true pelvis
IVb	Spread to distant sites outside the true pelvis

third of the vagina and a pelvic lymphadenectomy. This has the advantage that the ovaries can be preserved and avoids the narrowing of the vagina which pelvic irradiation induces. If at operation the para-aortic nodes are found to be involved, the operation is abandoned and treatment given by irradiation. Where many pelvic nodes are found to be infiltrated in the operative specimen, or the resection margins are very close to the tumour, postoperative pelvic irradiation should be given.

For patients who are older or have a positive lymphogram or are not fit for or refuse surgery, radical radiotherapy with intracavitary therapy with or without pelvic external beam irradiation should be given. External beam is not essential unless the tumour is poorly differentiated or the lymphogram is positive. Many radiotherapists, however, treat all stage I cases with pelvic external beam in addition to intracavitary therapy.

2. Stages Ib (bulky), IIa–IIIb

Radical radiotherapy

Radical radiotherapy is the treatment of choice for bulky stage Ib, IIa–IIIb. This normally requires a combination of uterine and vaginal intracavitary therapy and pelvic external beam irradiation.

In patients with stage III disease, uraemia may be advanced at presentation if there is bilateral ureteric obstruction. Where the patient is in renal failure, particularly if young, the insertion of temporary nephrostomies (tubes placed in the renal pelvis under ultrasound control to drain the urine) should be considered to relieve renal tract obstruction prior to

pelvic irradiation. Radical radiotherapy should only be started if renal function and general condition improve sufficiently. Since the prognosis with bilateral obstruction is very poor, it may be better to allow death painlessly from uraemia, particularly in those not too old and frail for radical radiotherapy.

General medical care. It is important to maintain patients in as good a medical condition as possible. Anaemia (Hb <10 g/dl) should be corrected by blood transfusion before treatment since the prognosis of the anaemic patient is less good.

Combined surgery and radiotherapy

A combination of surgery and radiotherapy, if carefully combined, can achieve equally satisfactory cure rates in patients with stage Ib, IIa and early IIb disease. A colpohysterectomy and external iliac lymphadenectomy is followed 2–6 weeks later by uterine and vaginal intracavitary therapy. In most cases this avoids the need for pelvic external beam irradiation and its associated morbidity in patients with no histological evidence of nodal involvement. Involved nodes or residual disease are indications for postoperative external beam irradiation.

3. Stage IVa

The outlook for this stage is grim and many patients are in poor medical condition. A vesicovaginal or rectovaginal fistula or both may be present, with or without renal tract obstruction. A preliminary colostomy or urinary diversion is desirable if radical radiotherapy is to be attempted. Intracavitary therapy may not be feasible because of fistula formation and treatment is limited to pelvic external beam irradiation alone.

Radical radiotherapy

Target volume
The aim is to treat the cervix, parametria and the pelvic nodes.

Because of the greater tolerance of the vagina to radiation it is possible to deliver a higher dose to it than to the rest of the pelvic tissues. The central disease is conventionally treated by uterine and vaginal intracavitary caesium. The sources provide a very high central dose. The isodoses from the uterine and vaginal sources are pear-shaped (Fig. 24.6) The dose falls off inversely with the square of the distance from the source (p. 60). External beam irradiation to a lower dose is used to treat the pelvic nodes and complement

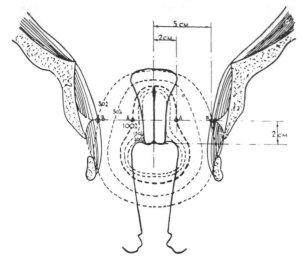

Fig. 24.6 Isodose curves in the pelvis for a typical radium distribution. The position of points A and B is shown. (Reproduced with permission from Tod, British Practice in Radiotherapy, Butterworths.)

the dose to the distal parametrium where the intra-cavitary dose falls off rapidly. A specially designed wedge is placed over the central part of the pelvic field during external beam irradiation. The wedge reduces the dose of external beam to the central pelvis, which is heavily irradiated by intracavitary therapy.

Intracavitary therapy. A variety of techniques are in use. Previously the live sources used to be placed directly by the operator into the uterine cavity and vagina (e.g. the Manchester and Sheffield systems) or manually afterloaded in the ward by the nursing staff. This radiation exposure to medical and nursing staff is now unnecessary with the development of 'remote afterloading' (p. 152). Remote afterloading has replaced manual insertion of live sources in most centres in the UK.

Remote afterloading

Cathetron. The first high-dose rate remote after-loading system using cobalt-60 was the Cathetron. The Cathetron has a number of advantages. Accuracy is high due to the rigidity of the applicator system (two vaginal ovoids and a central uterine tube). Treatment times (a few minutes) and duration of hospital stay are short, allowing more patients to be treated than with lower dose rate systems. Drawbacks are the number of treatments required (commonly five), each under a general anaesthetic with its attendant risks.

Selectron. The most popular type of remote after-loading medium dose rate system in the UK is currently the Selectron (Fig. 8.16B). The Selectron uses caesium-

137 sources for low and medium dose rate and cobalt-60 for high dose rate. The different dose rates are summarised in Table 8.5.

Many radiotherapists have adopted low dose rate remote afterloading machines to provide similar dose rates to the manually afterloaded systems with whose clinical effects they were familiar. Their aim has been to achieve similar pelvic dosimetry and cure rates without any increase in morbidity.

Intracavitary insertion. The insertion of the applicators is carried out in the operating theatre under general anaesthesia. The vagina, cervix and pelvis are assessed by inspection and bimanual examination. A cystoscopy should be carried out to exclude bladder invasion. A biopsy is taken for microscopy if not previously done. The cervical canal normally allows the passage of a very narrow 'sound' of about 3 mm diameter. To hold a uterine applicator the canal has to be widened. This is done gently and gradually, by passing a series of long narrow metal sounds of in-creasing size until it is wide enough to admit a uterine applicator. Occasionally a growth begins inside the canal (endocervical) and there may be nothing obvious at first, until the canal is widened enough to give the operator access. An average uterine canal (cervix and body) is about 6 cm long.

Sheffield technique. Although soon to be replaced by a remote afterloading system, the Sheffield manual intracavitary system illustrates the general principles of intracavitary therapy.

At the vault are kidney-shaped holders (Fig. 24.7)—

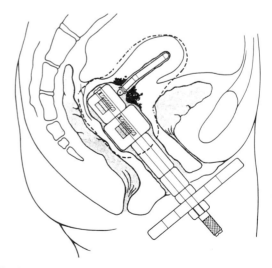

Fig. 24.7 The Sheffield uterovaginal applicator in position, with two caesium-holding 'kidneys' and uterine tube. (Courtesy of Dr F Neal, Sheffield)

Table 24.2 Dosimetry for typical intracavitary therapy for cervical cancer (Sheffield technique). Dose rates are drawn from tables based on standard insertions

Position	1st insertion		2nd insertion		Total dose: two insertions
	Dose rate (Gy/h)	Total dose (Gy)	Dose rate (Gy/h)	Total dose (Gy)	(Gy)
Cervix	1.640	60.50	1.562	61.70	122.2
Point A	0.810	29.97	0.760	30.03	60.00
Point B	0.228	8.44	0.200	7.90	16.34
Bladder	0.644	23.85	0.427	16.97	40.72
Rectum	0.401	14.80	0.362	14.30	29.10

1st insertion: treatment time to deliver 30 Gy to Point A = 30/0.81 = 37 hours
2nd insertion: treatment time to deliver 30 Gy to Point A = 30/0.76 = 39.5 hours

one or two according to the space available—made of transparent plastic, mounted by sliding on to a metal tube. They are made in three sizes, and the appropriate one can be chosen to suit the individual case. Tungsten inserts of 8 mm maximum thickness screen off about 50% of the gamma rays posteriorly, to reduce the rectal dose.

In a typical case, the uterine tube (total length 5.5 cm) contains 45 mg radium equivalent of caesium-137 (25 mg above, 20 mg below). The upper vaginal holder contains 2×20 mg and the lower 2×10 mg.

At the second insertion, a week after the first, the lower vaginal holder is usually omitted. No packing is needed, and the plastic is less irritant than gauze to the vagina. The apparatus is held in position by attachment to a belt strapped round the waist.

Dosimetry is based on tables drawn up for different combinations of uterine and vaginal sources. The tables assume ideal positioning of the sources. A calculation of a typical insertion is shown in Table 24.2.

Practical problems

Failure to identify the cervical os. If it is impossible to insert a uterine applicator because the cervical os cannot be confidently identified or because of local haemorrhage, a vaginal applicator alone may be inserted or the whole procedure deferred until more pelvic irradiation has been given to shrink the tumour and/or stop the haemorrhage. Intracavitary insertion may be possible once the tumour has shrunk (e.g. after 20 Gy in 10 daily fractions over 2 weeks (9–10 MV photons)).

Perforation of the uterus. Occasionally, in error, the uterus may be perforated by the applicator, particularly if the external os is difficult to identify because the tumour has distorted it. If perforation has occurred the applicator should be withdrawn and the patient started on antibiotics. A further attempt is made to carry out the insertion successfully a week later.

Verification of intracavitary insertion. After the

insertion of the uterovaginal applicator, lateral and anteroposterior radiographs of the pelvis are taken to show the exact position of the applicators. This is best done in theatre itself, with a portable X-ray machine. Occasionally their position is found to be unsatisfactory. The most serious mishap is that the central uterine tube may have slipped out and come to lie in the vagina alongside the vaginal applicators. This would mean an inevitable overdose to the rectum, leading to ulceration of the rectal wall and probable fistula. If positioning is seen to be poor, it can be corrected before the patient leaves the theatre.

The patient is returned to the ward and remains flat on her back for the period of insertion (typically about a day and half) to prevent displacement of the applicators.

Afterloading and care during intracavitary irradiation. Ideally a remote afterloading system is used to load the applicators from the source container (Fig. 8.16) in a specially protected ward. Essential nursing and medical procedures can be carried out by withdrawing the sources to their container for short periods of time.

In a manual afterloading system, the applicators are normally loaded by the nursing staff. A mobile lead screen 2.5 cm thick is placed at the bedside to reduce the dosage to staff and visitors. Nursing and medical procedures are minimised to avoid unnecessary radiation exposure.

For removal of the applicators at the appointed time, no anaesthetic is required. In a remotely afterloaded system the sources are hydraulically withdrawn into the source container before the uterovaginal applicator is withdrawn. Any vaginal packing is removed. Manually directly or afterloaded sources are placed at once in a lead box in a trolley which is then wheeled away to the isotope safe.

Dosimetry

Manchester points A and B. Most radiotherapists in

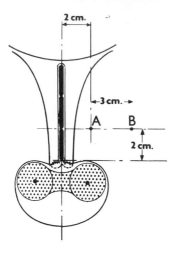

Fig. 24.8 Diagrammatic uterus and vagina, showing intrauterine tube, cross-sections of ovoids in lateral fornices, separated by spacer, and points A and B. (Reproduced with permission from Paterson, Treatment of Malignant Disease, Edward Arnold.)

the UK still prescribe intracavitary and external beam therapy to Manchester points A and B (Fig. 24.8). The position of point A is defined in relation to the midline but may vary according to whether the uterine cavity lies in the midline or is displaced to one side.

ICRU 38 recommendations. Many centres in Europe have adopted the ICRU 38 recommendations on dose prescription in gynaecological intracavitary therapy. These are summarised in Table 24.3.

The reference points for the measurement of doses to distal parametrium, bladder, rectum and to the pelvic and para-aortic nodes are shown in Figs 24.9 and 24.10.

The dosimetric points of the para-aortic and pelvic nodes are shaped like a trapezoid with the narrow end in the para-aortic region and the broad end at the level of the external iliac nodes. Computerised dosimetry based on radiographs taken with the unloaded uterovaginal applicator in situ allow the rapid calculation of the doses to these reference points.

The ICRU 38 reference points differ from the

Table 24.3   ICRU 38 recommendations for dose and volume specification for reporting intracavitary therapy in gynecology

1. The treatment technique must be completely described
2. The total reference kerma should be stated (p. 71)
3. The *reference volume* should be described in terms of the *height*, *width* and *thickness* of the volume enclosed in the 60 Gy isodose surface for low dose rate treatment of carcinoma of the cervix
4. The absorbed dose at reference points in organs at risk (*rectum, bladder*) should be determined (computed or measured) and expressed in well-codified ways to provide additional safety limits
5. The absorbed dose(s) at reference point(s) related to bony structures (*lymphatic trapezoid* and *pelvic wall* reference points should be reported)
6. The time–dose pattern should be completely specified

1. The **reference volume** is defined by three dimensions: (a) the height is the maximum dimension along the intrauterine source and is measured in the oblique frontal plane containing the uterine source; (b) the width is the maximum dimension perpendicular to the intrauterine source and is measured in the same oblique frontal plane; (c) the thickness is the maximum dimension perpendicular to the intrauterine source and is measured in the oblique sagittal plane containing the uterine source.
2. The **bladder reference point** (Fig. 24.10) is obtained by filling the balloon of a catheter in the bladder with 7 ml of radio-opaque fluid. The balloon is pulled down against the urethra. On the lateral radiograph the reference point is obtained on an anteroposterior line drawn through the centre of the balloon. The reference point is taken on this line on the posterior surface of the balloon. On the frontal radiograph the reference point is taken at the center of the balloon.
3. The **rectal reference point** (Fig. 24.10) is located on an anteroposterior line drawn on the lateral radiograph from the lower end of the uterine source (or from the middle of the intravaginal sources). The point is on this line 5 mm behind the posterior vaginal wall.
4. **Lymphatic trapezoid** (Fig. 24.9A). A line is drawn from the junction of S1–S2 to the top of the symphysis pubis. Then a line is drawn from the middle of that line to the middle of the anterior aspect of L4. A trapezoid is constructed in a plane passing through the transverse line in the pelvic brim plane and the midpoint of the anterior aspect of the body of L4. A point 6 cm lateral to the midline at the inferior end of this figure is used to give an estimate of the dose rate to the mid-external iliac nodes (R. EXT and L.EXT for the right and left external iliac, respectively).
   At the top of the trapezoid, points 2 cm lateral to the midline at the level of L4 are used to estimate the dose to the lower para-aortic area (labelled R.PARA and L.PARA). The midpoint of a line connecting these two points is used to estimate the dose to the low common (labelled R.COM and L. COM) iliac nodes.
5. The **pelvic wall reference point** is intended to be representative of the absorbed dose at the distal part of the parametrium and at the obturator nodes. On an AP radiograph the pelvic wall reference point is intersected by a horizontal line tangential to the highest point of the acetabulum and a vertical line tangential to the inner aspect of the acetabulum (Fig. 24.9B). On a lateral radiograph the highest points of the right and left acetabulum in the craniocaudal direction are joined and the lateral projection of the pelvic wall reference point is located midway between these points.

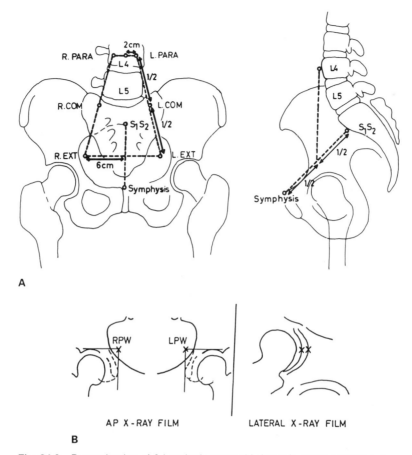

Fig. 24.9 Determination of **A** lymphatic trapezoid shown in anteroposterior view (left) and lateral view (right) and **B** the right (RPW) and left (LPW) pelvic side wall reference points. (Reproduced with permission from I.C.R.U. Report 38: Dose and Volume Specification for Reporting Intracavitary Therapy in Gynecology, I.C.R.U, 1985.)

Manchester system. They exclude points A and B because, though valid when the uterus is in the midline position, the dose to the parametrium and pelvic side wall may be underestimated if the uterus is deviated to one side and overestimated if it deviates to the opposite side. Instead the dose is prescribed to the 60 Gy isodose surrounding the uterine and vaginal sources (Fig. 24.11). This isodose has a more consistent position in the parametrium than point A since it is related to the actual position of the sources rather than to the midline. Whether or not these new reference points prove useful in setting dose limits to minimise rectal and bladder complications remains to be established.

Rectal probe. A further possible aid in avoiding rectal overdosage in directly loaded systems is a scintillation counter at the end of a narrow probe. This can be inserted at the end of the operation and the maximum dose rate at the rectal mucosa obtained by a series of readings at various distances along the rectal wall. If the dose is found to be excessive, the application must be adjusted.

Dosage. Cancericidal doses, e.g. 75 Gy at point A or to the 60 Gy isodose, from central sources can be safely delivered. This would give point B about one-fifth of the central dose (15 Gy), much too low to deal effectively with secondaries. To achieve adequate dosage to B, e.g. 50 Gy, from the same sources would take about 10 days and involve 250 Gy at A. This would result in acute necrosis, early fistulae of rectum and bladder, and probable death from sepsis.

It is obvious from Figure 24.6 that the dose at the surface of the cervix and immediately adjoining is 200%, i.e. about 150 Gy. This is a very high dose, but

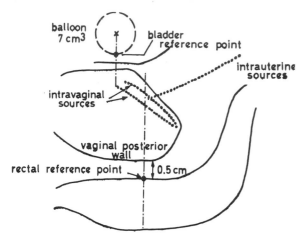

Fig. 24.10 Determination of the reference points for bladder and rectum. (Reproduced with permission from I.C.R.U Report 38: Dose and Volume Specification for Reporting Intracavitary Therapy in Gynecology, I.C.R.U, 1985.)

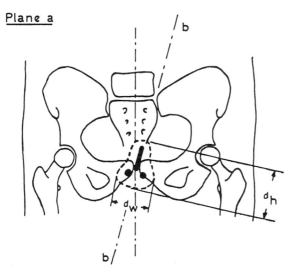

Fig. 24.11 Diagram showing the 60 Gy isodose and its dimensions in the frontal oblique plane surrounding the uterovaginal applicator. d_h, height; d_w, width). (Reproduced with permission from I.C.R.U Report 38: Dose and Volume Specification for Reporting Intracavitary Therapy in Gynecology, I.C.R.U, 1985.)

this region is, fortunately, unusually tolerant and so permits an effective dose as far out as point A. If this were not so treatment would be impracticable.

It is possible to make accurate dose calculations from the radiographs taken after the insertions, and some departments have done this routinely. Doing the calculations manually was very laborious and most clinicians preferred to rely on simple inspection of the films, in the light of experience, to assure themselves that the source layout was reasonable. With the availability of a modern planning computer and remote afterloading these calculations are much faster and more accurate. Dose distribution can be individualised and optimised to fit the tumour and minimise dose to bladder and rectum.

External beam pelvic irradiation. For genuine stage I disease, intracavitary caesium alone is adequate, and capable of achieving a cure rate of 90% or more. However nodal metastases can hardly ever be ruled out with confidence. Most radiotherapists therefore supplement intracavitary therapy with megavoltage irradiation delivered to the lateral parts of the pelvis to bring this dosage to a tumoricidal level.

External beam can precede or follow intracavitary therapy.

Target volume
This should include the whole of the pelvis (Fig. 24.12). It will encompass the primary and any local spread, and the common, internal and external iliac nodes. The upper border of the field is the junction of the fourth and fifth lumbar vertebrae. The lower border is the bottom of the obturator foramina of the pubic bones. It may need to extend a few centimetres more inferiorly

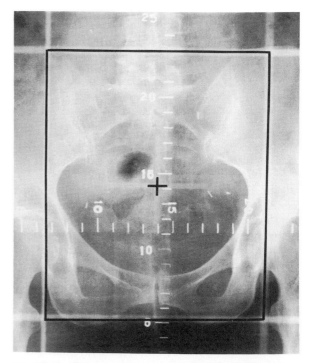

Fig. 24.12 Pelvic external beam field for carcinoma of the cervix and endometrium.

if there is involvement of the lower third of the vagina. The outer margin is 1 cm lateral to the pelvic brim.

Technique

A pair of anterior and posterior opposed fields is planned on the simulator. There is a central wedge filter (4–5 cm wide) to protect midline structures (cervix, bladder and rectum). A typical field size is 16 × 14 cm. Alternatively an anterior field is supplemented by two lateral wedged fields to reduce the dose to the rectum.

If the para-aortic nodes are involved, a separate single direct para-aortic field can be added at the end of pelvic irradiation. The width is normally about 8 cm. It extends from the T12/L1 junction to just above the upper border of the pelvic field. The length of the gap on the skin between the lower end of the para-aortic field and the upper end of the pelvic field is calculated so that no more than the 50% isodoses overlap at the depth of the spinal cord.

Energy and dose

Megavoltage therapy is advised. The aim is to give the desired dose at point B, additional to the dose already given from intracavitary therapy, while giving a much lower dose to A which is already heavily irradiated. There will be some photon dosage to A, if only from scattered irradiation. The dose to A can be varied while leaving the dose at B unchanged, by using different thicknesses of central filter, and changing them, if need be, during the course. In this way, the doses can be arranged to summate to the required levels. Table 24.2 summarises the intracavitary external beam

doses from a typical insertion using the Sheffield technique. In Table 24.4 are summarised the intra-cavitary and external beam doses for different stages of the disease.

Para-aortic nodes
45 Gy maximum dose in 20 daily fractions over 4 weeks (4–6 MV photons)

Acute reactions. The cervix and body of uterus are unusually tolerant of high dosage (see above). The more vulnerable organs that are potential sources of trouble are the rectum, bladder and any loops of bowel trapped or adherent in the pelvis.

Bowel. As we have noted, special precautions are taken for rectal protection—packing or heavy metal filter. A minor degree of rectal irritation, with perhaps slight diarrhoea, is usual after intracavitary caesium and settles rapidly.

During external irradiation diarrhoea is often troublesome, occasionally requiring treatment to be suspended for a few days. Treatment is with an antidiarrhoeal agent (e.g. loperamide), and a high fibre diet, avoiding fruit and vegetables. The reaction has normally settled 3–4 weeks after the end of treatment.

Bladder. Irritation of the bladder with dysuria and frequency is both less common and less troublesome. An anticholinergic (e.g. propantheline) often relieves the discomfort. The timescale for resolution is the same as for the bowel.

Skin. Reactions are minor if megavoltage is used. Washing the treated area is permitted.

Table 24.4   Treatment of carcinoma of the cervix

Stage	Treatment	Point	Cs (Gy)	Ext. beam (Gy)	Cs + Ext. beam (Gy)
0 I	Conisation/hysterectomy Hysterectomy (Wertheim's)/ Cs + ext. beam	— A B	— 60 15	— 15 35	— 75 50
IIa, b	Cs + ext. beam	Dosage as stage I			
IIIa, b	Cs + ext. beam or ext. beam alone	Dosage as stage I			
IVa	Defunctioning colostomy (rectovaginal fistula) or urinary diversion (vesicovaginal fistula). Then radical/palliative ext. beam	50 Gy in 25 daily fractions (whole pelvis) or 30 Gy in 10 daily fractions (whole pelvis)			
IVb	Palliative ext. beam +/- chemotherapy or palliative Cs.	30 Gy in 10 daily fractions (whole pelvis) 20 Gy to point A (one insertion)			

Cs, caesium; ext. beam, external beam.

Infection. Cervical tumours are often infected. Manipulations involved in treatment, including dilatation of the uterine canal, may spread infection; hence the need for examination under anaesthetic and intracavitary insertions to be carried under sterile conditions. Collections of pus in the uterine cavity behind a cervical tumour should be drained and antibiotics started.

Late reactions. The probability of developing late major pelvic complications following radical intracavitary and external beam therapy is about 5%. These mainly affect the bladder and bowel. Small bowel complications are predominantly related to external beam irradiation. Many factors play a part in the development of pelvic complications, including total dose, dose rate, treatment volume, and previous pelvic surgery or pathology.

Bowel. The bowel is most frequently involved because of the proximity of the rectum to the region of high dose from intracavitary therapy and the inclusion of small bowel in the pelvic radiation field. Normally the bowel is mobile. As a result the same segment of bowel may not consistently lie within the same part of the pelvic external beam field. However previous pelvic inflammatory disease or surgery increases the likelihood of loops of bowel being trapped in the pelvis and irradiated to higher doses than mobile segments.

Large bowel. Large bowel complications develop earlier than in the small bowel, usually within 2 years of treatment. The average latent period is 6–18 months. Haemorrhage, rectal ulceration and fistulae occur. Symptoms are of colicky abdominal pain, rectal urgency, tenesmus, constipation and diarrhoea. The site of the ulceration is usually on the anterior rectal wall behind the posterior vaginal fornix where the intracavitary dose is high and the blood supply is meagre. Fistulae are usually confined to patients who have had intracavitary therapy. Strictures are commonly seen on barium enema but only about 25% are symptomatic. The commonest radiological appearance is a long narrowed segment. Changes in the submucosa may give rise to a 'thumb-printing' pattern.

The treatment of troublesome proctocolitis is initially conservative, for example with Predsol enemas. If conservative measures fail, then surgery is required with either a temporary or permanent colostomy.

Small bowel. Symptoms of small bowel damage can occur within the first few months following radiation but are usually delayed on average until 1–5 years following treatment. Obstruction is the commonest complication, occasionally with perforation. Radiological examination of the small bowel with barium contrast (small bowel meal) may show straightening or narrowing of the bowel and filling defects or thumb-printing due to oedema and fibrosis.

Malabsorption is common and often accompanies other evidence of late pelvic morbidity. There may be no symptoms or there may be diarrhoea, weight loss and fatigue. If the ileum is extensively involved, the stools become fatty (steatorrhoea). If segments of the small bowel lose their contractility, its stagnant contents may encourage bacteria to proliferate (bacterial overgrowth), leading to malabsorption of vitamin B_{12}.

Bladder. The bladder is similarly vulnerable, lying just in front of the anterior vaginal wall. Up to 25% of patients may have severe symptoms of bladder dysfunction. This seems to be mainly due to damage to the detrusor muscle rather than to contraction of the bladder. Late effects tend to occur 1–10 years after treatment. Blood in the urine (haematuria) may result from telangiectasia at the bladder base. Cystoscopy is advisable, to exclude invasion of the bladder by tumour or an unrelated cause. Diathermy to the bleeding points is usually effective. The bladder may become contracted as a result of scarring and infection of the submucosal and muscle layers.

Vesicovaginal fistula is a major complication which results in continual leakage of urine from the vagina. The diagnosis can be confirmed by passing a blue dye (methylene blue) through a urinary catheter and observing the dye escaping through the vagina. Treatment is by transplanting the ureters into the ileum (ileal conduit). The fistula will then usually heal. Urinary diversion may also be required if the intolerable urinary frequency occurs as a result of a contracted bladder. Occasionally ureteric obstruction may occur due to a 'frozen' pelvis. However malignant disease is by far the commoner cause.

Results of treatment

The results of primary radical surgery or radiotherapy or a combination of preoperative caesium followed by surgery for stage Ib are excellent, with a 5-year survival of about 90%. Cure rates from radical radiotherapy decline with advancing stage: 80% (IIa), 65% (IIb), 45% (IIIa) and 35% (IIIb) and 15% (IV).

Follow-up

Most recurrences in the cervix or regional nodes tend to occur in the first 2 years after treatment. A suggested follow-up policy is 1 month after treatment and then 2-monthly for the first year, 3-monthly in the second year and 6-monthly from years 3 to 5. The likelihood of relapse beyond 5 years is small and routine follow-up is probably not essential. Early review for assessment of new symptoms can be arranged as required. Cervical cytology is not a reliable method of detecting recurrence since the cytological changes following radiotherapy are often difficult to distinguish from the presence of tumour.

Sexual rehabilitation

Sexual counselling should be given. Patients should be warned of vaginal dryness and stenosis. An oestrogen-containing cream, dinoestrol, may reduce the dryness. The regular use of dilators to maintain the patency of the vagina should be encouraged.

Treatment of recurrence after radiotherapy

Sadly, recurrent disease is often too advanced for salvage surgery. Examination of the vaginal vault at follow-up is often limited by radiation induced vaginal stenosis. Typical symptoms are of buttock pain, radiating down the back of the leg. There may be no palpable recurrence in the pelvis. An ultrasound may show enlarged pelvic nodes and/or a dilated ureter. MRI scanning can sometimes distinguish radiation fibrosis from pelvic recurrence. However for recurrence confined to the central pelvis, radical surgery with removal of vagina and bladder (anterior exenteration) or rectum (posterior exenteration) may be possible. Long-term survival for recurrent disease is poor since recurrence is often inoperable (due to extension to the pelvic side wall) or associated with distant metastases.

CANCER OF THE CERVICAL STUMP

Subtotal hysterectomy, i.e. removal of the uterus above the level of the cervix (e.g. for fibroids) was a common operative procedure in former times, but now rarely practised. Carcinoma may develop in the remaining stump. A distinction needs to be made between true stump carcinoma which has arisen on the cervical stump a year or more following surgery and coinciden-tal stump carcinoma which is detected within a year of hysterectomy. In the latter case the cancer can be assumed to have been present but not suspected at the time of surgery. Intracavitary treatment is difficult, as the length of the canal left, about 2 cm, is rarely enough to hold a uterine applicator. Vaginal applica-tions can be made, supplemented, or replaced entirely, by external irradiation.

The results of radical radiotherapy for true cervical stump carcinoma seem to match those where the uterus is intact. However the outlook for coincidental carcinoma is less favourable, probably because it re-presents cancer which has been inadequately treated by surgery.

CERVICAL CANCER IN PREGNANCY

Carcinoma of the cervix is fortunately rare in pregnancy, about 1% of cases. Management will depend upon the extent of the disease at the time of diagnosis, the stage of the pregnancy and the wishes of the patient. Most patients present with early disease (stages I and II).

In the first 3 months (trimester) of pregnancy, stage I disease is treated by a Wertheim's hysterectomy. In more advanced stages, a vaginal termination is followed by radical radiotherapy.

In the second trimester, for stage I the pregnancy is terminated by removal of the fetus from the uterus (hysterotomy) followed by a Wertheim's hysterectomy. For stage II or more advanced, the termination of the pregnancy is induced with prostaglandins, followed by radical radiotherapy. External beam is started first to allow time for the uterus to involute. Intracavitary therapy can then complete the treatment.

In the third trimester, with a viable fetus, a caesarean section is carried out at 34 weeks for stage I followed by a Wertheim's hysterectomy. For stage II or more advanced, radical radiotherapy is given fol-lowing caesarean section. Treatment is started by external beam 10 days after delivery and completed by intracavitary therapy.

Occasionally at 24 weeks, a decision has to be taken whether or not to postpone treatment a short time until the baby is viable. The parents need to be aware of the risks to mother and child of doing so.

The outcome of treatment of cervical cancer occurring during pregnancy is not, stage for stage, different from the results in women who are not pregnant.

CANCER OF THE BODY OF THE UTERUS (CARCINOMA CORPUS UTERI)
Pathology

Endometrial cancer represents 1.9% of all cancers and 0.9% of cancer deaths. The internal surface lining of the uterine cavity is called the endometrium. It is a glandular epithelium. Tumours arising from it are adenocarcinomas and account for over 80% of cancers of the corpus (body); 70% are well-differentiated endometrioid adenocarcinomas. Papillary adeno-carcinomas (5%) occur in an older age group and, like clear cell carcinoma (5%) have a less favourable prognosis. Adenoacanthoma has squamous metaplasia, and has identical prognosis to other endometrioid adenocarcinomas. True adenosquamous carcinoma of the corpus is very rare and is much more frequent in the cervix. Sarcomas are rare (5%), arising from the muscular walls of the uterus.

Aetiology

Endometrial cancer is associated with diabetes mellitus, hypertension, obesity and polycystic ovarian syndrome. What these conditions have in common is excessive stimulation by oestrogenic hormone uninfluenced by progestogens. This results in endometrial overgrowth and eventual malignancy. Oestrogen secreting ovarian tumours (p. 416) are a rare cause of the same phenomenon.

Oestrogens given as hormone replacement therapy at the menopause also cause endometrial hyperplasia and eventually endometrioid adenocarcinoma.

Spread

Spread of endometrial cancer may be downwards to the endocervix, and it may be impossible to say whether a growth arose in the cervix or the body. Such cases should be regarded as primary growths of the cervix. It may invade the uterine wall deeply and even penetrate into the parametrium. Secondary deposits in the ovaries are common, likewise in the vagina. The lower uterine segment and endocervical canal is involved in 5–10% of patients.

Lymph node metastases to pelvic and then to para-aortic nodes occur later and are less frequent than with cervical growths. The greater the depth of myometrial invasion and the less differentiated the tumour, the higher the incidence of nodal metastases and of vaginal recurrence. For example if the tumour is confined to the endometrium the incidence of pelvic node metastases is only 3%. It rises to 8% if there is superficial myometrial invasion and to 45% if there is deep invasion (to the outer third).

Myometrial invasion occurs in less than 5% of well-differentiated tumours and about 30% of poorly differentiated tumours. Blood spread to lungs, liver and bone is relatively common in later stages.

Clinical features

Irregular bleeding, especially after the menopause, is the cardinal symptom. It is occasionally detected as an incidental finding in the cervical screening programme.

Table 24.5 FIGO staging of endometrial cancer (T stages of TNM classification in parentheses)

Stage	Clinical findings
I	Carcinoma confined to the corpus (T1)
Ia	Uterine cavity 8 cm or less in length (T1a)
Ib	Uterine cavity >8 cm in length (T1b)
II	Extension to the cervix (T2)
III	Extension beyond the uterus but confined to the true pelvis (T3)
IV	Extension beyond the true pelvis or involvement of the bladder or rectum (T4)

Diagnosis and investigation

The diagnosis is established by dilatation and curettage (D and C) under general anaesthesia. The uterine canal is dilated and the cavity explored by a curette to remove fragments of the lining tissue. The diagnosis may be immediately obvious, or only when confirmed by microscopy.

Staging

Staging is by the FIGO classification (Table 24.5).

Treatment

The standard treatment is surgical, i.e. total hysterectomy (removal of uterus, ovaries and tubes) in early operable cases where there are no contraindications such as hypertension, diabetes and obesity. Inoperable cases, e.g. appreciable extension outside the uterus, or cases technically operable but unsuitable for surgery, are treated by radical radiotherapy, either intracavitary, external beam or a combination of both.

Radical radiotherapy

For a well-differentiated adenocarcinoma which is clinically stage I and penetrating less than a third of the myometrium, there is no need for supplementary pelvic irradiation.

The indications for postoperative radical radiotherapy are:

— Moderately or poorly differentiated histology
— Myometrial invasion greater than a third of its thickness
— Stage II or III disease
— Tumour at the surgical resection margins
— Invasion of vascular spaces.

Target volume
For stage 1 disease, some workers prefer to confine

the treatment volume to the vaginal vault using postoperative vaginal intracavitary caesium. This reduces the incidence of recurrence at the vaginal vault from about 10–15% to 2%. It seems more logical, however, to treat the whole of the pelvis by external beam since those at risk of recurrence at the vaginal vault are also at increased risk of pelvic nodal metastases.

The field margins for external beam irradiation of the pelvis are the same as for cervical cancer (p. 410).

Technique and dosage

Intracavitary therapy alone (postoperative). The principles are similar to those for the cervix, usually with a single insertion.

60 Gy to point A or to the reference isodose (Fig. 24.11)

Intracavitary combined with external beam (no surgery). Two intracavitary uterovaginal insertions are carried out. Dosage of intracavitary therapy and external beam is as for cervical cancer (p. 411)

The uterine cavity is usually on the large side, and will hold a longer applicator (e.g. 7.5 cm) than most cases of cervical cancer. In the Sheffield system a typical distribution would be 25 mg uterine and two 20 mg vaginal sources (total 65 mg).

Vaginal applicators are of various types, as for the cervix. Some workers apply vaginal caesium at only one of the two insertions. The Manchester and Sheffield techniques are also applicable to the corpus.

In the Stockholm method (Fig. 24.13), the uterine cavity is packed with as many small caesium sources as it will accommodate—Heyman capsules, holding 8–10 mg each. Each capsule has an attached numbered

thread, so that they can be removed in the correct sequence.

External beam alone (postoperative). A parallel opposed pair of fields is used.

45 Gy in 20 daily fractions over 4 weeks (9–10 MV photons)

External beam alone (no surgery). If the patient is unfit for a general anaesthetic or if there is any contra-indication to intracavitary insertion (p. 405), external pelvic irradiation alone is used.

A parallel opposed pair of fields is used.

50 Gy in 25 daily fractions over 5 weeks (9–10 MV photons)

Vaginal recurrence. If vaginal recurrence occurs in a patient who has not received previous pelvic irradiation, intracavitary therapy is the treatment of choice. The aim is to give 100 Gy to the vaginal surface in two intracavitary insertions. It is the dose to the vaginal epithelium and not to point A that is important.

Palliative radiotherapy

Palliative radiotherapy is indicated for troublesome vaginal bleeding in patients who are not fit for radical surgery or radical radiotherapy. If the patient is fit enough for a general anaesthetic a single uterine intracavitary insertion (20 Gy to point A or reference isodose) may be possible. If not, a simple parallel opposed pair of fields is used (field margins as above).

Energy and dose
30 Gy in 10 fractions over 2 weeks or 20 Gy in 5 daily fractions over a week (9–10 MV photons)

Hormone therapy

Well-differentiated locally advanced or metastatic endometrial adenocarcinoma may respond to progestogens in about 30% of cases. Treatment is with medroxyprogesterone acetate 100 mg orally t.d.s. At present it is uncertain whether progestogens have a useful role as an adjuvant following primary treatment.

Results of treatment

Cancer of the corpus is one of the more favourable cancers, as most are well differentiated, slowly growing and metastasise late. For stage I disease 5-year survival is up to 90%, for stage II it is reduced to 50%, and to 20% for stages III and IV. 5-year survival falls with increasing depth of myometrial invasion (80% if no invasion, 60% if greater than half of the myometrium

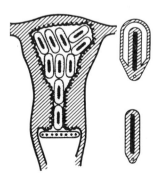

Fig. 24.13 Two types of Heyman applicators, and a uterine cavity packed with as many as it will hold. Note the flat box of caesium against the cervix, and the eyelets in the applicators for threads. (Reproduced with permission from Hulbert, Treatment of Cancer in Clinical Practice, Livingstone.)

invaded). Similarly increasing anaplasia impairs prognosis (5-year survival: 80% for well-differentiated, 75% for moderately differentiated and 50% for poorly differentiated).

UTERINE SARCOMAS

Uterine sarcomas are rare, representing less than 5% of uterine tumours. They may occur in young or in postmenopausal women. There are three principal histological types which, in order of frequency, are leiomyosarcoma, malignant mixed müllerian tumour and endometrial stromal sarcoma. Symptoms are of abnormal bleeding or of a pelvic mass. There is a high incidence of distant metastases, especially to lung. Treatment for stage I and II is a total hysterectomy and bilateral oophorectomy followed by postoperative pelvic external beam irradiation (50 Gy in 25 fractions over 5 weeks) for mixed müllerian and endometrial stromal sarcomas. For these two histological groups pelvic irradiation does reduce local recurrence and may improve survival. The exception is leiomyosarcoma which is highly radioresistant and postoperative irradiation is therefore not recommended. Chemotherapy with agents such as vincristine, DTIC and Adriamycin is palliative with only occasional responses. Overall 5-year survival is poor (20%).

CANCER OF THE OVARY

Anatomy

Each of the two ovaries is shaped like an almond and is attached to the back of the broad ligament on the side wall of the pelvis (Fig. 24.2). In front lie the external iliac vessels and, behind, the ureter and internal iliac vessels. Along one of its attachments pass the ovarian vessels and lymphatics. Lymphatic drainage is to the para-aortic nodes.

Cancer of the ovary accounts for 20% of gynaecological malignancy and for about 4000 new cases per year in the UK and for over 2000 deaths. Overall it represents 2.3% of all cancers and 4.2% of cancer deaths. The average yearly incidence is 15 per 100 000 women and is rising. The peak incidence is between 40 and 60 years. The aetiology is unknown, though oral contraceptive use seems to have a protective role.

Pathology

There is a wide variety of histological types.

1. Primary malignant tumours

a. Common epithelial tumours. Most ovarian tumours (90%) arise from the surface epithelium, or possibly its indentations, which produces the germ cells (ova, egg cells).

Of these epithelial tumours 10% are of 'borderline' malignancy (abnormal nuclei, increased mitotic activity, layers of tumour cells but no invasion). These borderline tumours may also be present as non-invasive implants on the omentum or on the pelvic side wall.

(i) Serous tumours (serous cystadenocarcinoma), often bilateral; so called because their fluid contents resemble serum in chemical composition. There are often papillary projections on the inner surface (papillary cystadenocarcinoma). This is the commonest type, amounting to about 42% of malignant tumours.

(ii) Mucinous tumours (12%). Mucin is the viscid secretion of intestinal and other glands, and is also produced by the epithelium of these tumours. They are typically multicystic.

(iii) Clear cell carcinoma (6%) (sometimes called mesonephroid).

(iv) Endometrioid carcinoma (15%). This resembles its uterine counterpart, and may sometimes arise in endometriosis.

(v) Undifferentiated carcinoma (17%).

b. From germ cells (6%). These resemble tumours of comparable origin in the testis.

(i) Dysgerminoma is a rare malignant tumour of children and young women. It is analogous to seminoma of the testis in males. It is highly sensitive to drugs and radiation.

(ii) Teratomas differentiate the various embryonic layers. Most are benign.

(iii) Choriocarcinoma.

(iv) Yolk sac tumour (endodermal sinus tumour = old term).

c. From specialised hormone-producing cells (2%).

(i) Granulosa cell tumours secrete oestrogenic hormones and so cause precocious puberty in children or excess feminisation in adults, with menorrhagia or postmenopausal endometrial hyperplasia and bleeding. Most occur in postmenopausal women. Their malignancy is difficult to predict and variable, though they generally run a very long course over many years.

(ii) Androblastomas are very rare and are usually benign. They may secrete androgenic hormones and so produce signs of virilism (hair growth and deepening of the voice).

2. Secondary tumours—uterus, breast, gastrointestinal tract. Krukenberg tumours are metastases from a gastric cancer simulating ovarian cancer.

Table 24.6 FIGO staging of ovarian cancer

Stage	Clinical findings
I	Tumour confined to the ovary
Ia	One ovary involved
Ib	Both ovaries involved
Ic	Tumour on the surface of one or both ovaries; capsular rupture; ascites containing malignant cells or positive peritoneal cytology
II	Tumour confined to the pelvis
IIa	Tumour extension to the adnexae
IIb	Tumour spread to other pelvic tissues
IIc	Tumour of IIa or IIb with tumour on the surface on one or both ovaries or capsular rupture; ascites containing malignant cells or positive peritoneal cytology
III	Tumour extending to the abdominal cavity, including peritoneal surfaces or the omentum
IV	Distant metastases

Staging is according to the FIGO staging system (Table 24.6).

Spread

Most tumours are cystic. Malignant change occurs within the cyst. As the tumour progresses, it spreads through to the outer peritoneal surface, or the cyst may rupture into the peritoneal cavity. Cells become attached to or invade adjacent structures—fallopian tubes, uterus, large and small bowel and bladder.

Seeding may deposit them far and wide on peritoneal surfaces, and multiple small nodules with some ascites are commonly found at operation. The main sites of spread are shown in Figure 24.14.

Spread to the para-aortic nodes occurs in 15% of stage I and II and 50% in stage III and IV disease. Blood-borne metastases occur late, typically to liver and lungs.

Natural history and clinical features

Ovarian tumours usually grow slowly and silently for some years and are usually advanced at the time of diagnosis; 60% have spread outside the pelvis at the time of presentation. In the uncommon hormone-secreting types the first signal may be from the effects described above. Benign tumours can attain enormous size, resembling advanced pregnancy. Eventually pressure symptoms from the enlarging mass occur: pain, swelling of the abdomen and lower limbs, dysuria from interference with the bladder. Anorexia and weight loss are common. Vaginal bleeding from uterine involvement or backache from para-aortic nodes may occur. Ascites and palpable pelvic masses, neck nodes or bowel obstruction may be present.

Staging and investigation

Current staging of ovarian cancer has become more

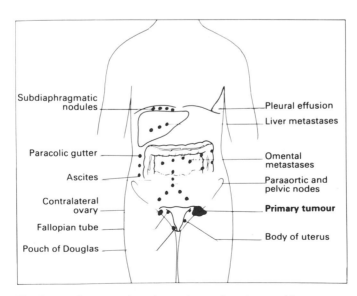

Fig. 24.14 Common sites of metastases of carcinoma of the ovary. (Reproduced with permission from Souhami & Tobias, Cancer and its Management, Blackwells, 1986.)

accurate. Many patients with apparently early disease were previously understaged. The main staging classification (Table 24.6) is clinical and has a profound effect on prognosis. A laparotomy is required to assess the intra-abdominal extent of the disease. The whole of the abdominal cavity is examined for evidence of spread, particularly the subdiaphragmatic areas and the paracolic gutters. Additional investigations include full blood count, liver function tests, serum urea, creatinine and electrolytes, chest radiograph, abdominopelvic ultrasound and CT scan of the abdomen.

Tumour markers

There are no tumour markers specific to ovarian cancer. CA-125 is the most helpful tumour marker and is raised in about 80% of patients with advanced disease.

Treatment

The management of ovarian cancer requires a multidisciplinary approach. Surgery, radiotherapy and chemotherapy all have a part to play, although, sadly, more intensive treatment of advanced disease has not produced much improvement in survival.

Surgery

Surgery is central to the treatment of stages I–III ovarian cancer. If possible a total abdominal hysterectomy and bilateral salpingo-oophorectomy is carried out. It is essential to remove the other ovary in most cases since 20% of tumours are bilateral or have metastasised to the other ovary. Following removal of the uterus and ovaries and in the absence of visible residual disease, any peritoneal fluid is sampled for evidence of malignant cells. If there is no peritoneal fluid, peritoneal washings are taken for cytology, which may reveal malignant cells.

In young women who are keen to maintain their fertility, removal of the affected ovary alone may be justified. Such conservative surgery is only justified if the following criteria are met:

1. Unilateral, well-differentiated mucinous, endometrioid or clear cell tumours (not serous).
2. Negative peritoneal washings.
3. Negative wedge biopsy of the other ovary and the omentum.
4. Close surveillance is possible.

For stages Ia and Ib, where the capsule of the ovary is intact, there is no need for postoperative adjuvant therapy.

For stages II–IV the aim is to remove as much tumour as possible since the greater the amount of residual disease following surgery, the worse the prognosis. This requires an experienced surgeon. The best results are achieved if the size of the largest residual mass is less than 1.5 cm. About 75% of patients will be amenable to this form of surgery. In the remaining 25% surgical debulking is not possible and only a biopsy is taken. A 'second-look' laparotomy has been used to assess the response to chemotherapy/radiotherapy following initial surgery and to remove any residual disease. However this is not recommended routinely since it has not increased survival.

Radiotherapy

The role of radical radiotherapy in epithelial ovarian cancer remains uncertain. The whole of the abdomen is at risk of spread. This probably explains why pelvic irradiation alone for stage I and II disease is ineffective. For stages I–III where there is minimal residual disease, whole abdominal irradiation is advised. Contraindications are multiple abdominal operations (increased risk of late gastrointestinal morbidity) or impaired pulmonary function (risk of late pulmonary fibrosis).

Target volume
The volume should include the whole abdominal cavity. The upper border should be 2 cm above the diaphragm (in full expiration). The lower margin is the bottom of the obturator foramen of the pubis. The lateral margin extends to the outer border of the abdomen.

Technique
Anterior and posterior fields are used, simulated in the supine and prone positions. The kidneys are identified by an intravenous urogram (IVU) during planning and shielded from the front and the back by customised MCP blocks to limit the dose to each kidney to 20 Gy. A boost is given to the pelvis by parallel opposed fields. The field margins are as for cervical cancer (p. 410).

Dose and energy
22.5 Gy is given in 20 daily fractions over 4 weeks to the whole abdomen (9–10 MV photons). The boost to the pelvis is 22.5 Gy in 10 daily fractions over 2 weeks at the same energy.

Monitoring of whole abdominal irradiation. Full blood count is monitored twice weekly since marrow impairment is normal after such wide field irradiation. Liver function tests become abnormal since the liver is irradiated. Full pulmonary function tests should be carried out before treatment since part of the lower lobes are included in the volume.

Acute reactions. Nausea, anorexia, vomiting and diarrhoea are normal during treatment but resolve usually within three weeks of the end of treatment. Antiemetics (e.g. metoclopramide), low residue diet and anti-diarrhoeal therapy (e.g. lopcramide) are usually needed. Tiredness may last several months. White blood count and platelets fall and may require temporary suspension ·of treatment if they fall below certain thresholds (white count $< 2 \times 10^9/l$ or platelets $< 60 \times 10^9/l$). Liver function tests become abnormal but resolve following treatment.

Late reactions. Late complications are usually related to gastrointestinal toxicity (9%), particularly to small bowel. Stenosis and haemorrhage are the main risks, particularly if more than one abdominal operation has been carried out.

It is not recommended that radioactive isotopes (e.g. gold-198 or phosphorus-32) are introduced into the abdominal cavity to deal with residual disease. Dose distribution is uneven and loculation risks serious bowel damage.

Chemotherapy

Ovarian cancer is moderately sensitive to chemotherapy. Cures are extremely rare. Treatment is therefore essentially palliative. The most active drugs are cisplatin, its analogue carboplatin and the alkylating agents (e.g. chlorambucil and cyclophosphamide). Care should be taken to balance toxicity of chemotherapy against the probability of symptomatic benefit. The response rates of combination chemotherapy are greater than single agents, although overall survival is no different. Since the toxicity of combination therapy tends to be more substantial, single agent therapy is preferable.

Chlorambucil has the advantages of oral administration on an outpatient basis and minimal toxicity (mainly leucopenia). A suitable dosage is 10 mg daily for 2 weeks out of every month, subject to satisfactory blood count. About 50% of patients respond. Similar response rates are achieved by oral cyclophosphamide. There is, however, an increased risk of leukaemia (usually acute myeloid) being induced by therapy with alkylating agents. Melphalan carries the highest risk. The cumulative incidence after 2 years of therapy with alkylating agents is of the order of 5%.

Cisplatin ($80–120$ mg/m^2 3-weekly) has a response rate of 40–60% but is toxic, causing severe nausea and vomiting, renal impairment and deafness. Renal function and hearing should be carefully monitored. Carboplatin (400 mg/m^2 monthly) is preferred since it is much less emetic and causes no renal toxicity. Its limiting toxicity is to the bone marrow (leucopenia and thrombocytopenia). Both carboplatin and cisplatin are given intravenously.

Results of treatment

Ovarian cancer has a poor prognosis, largely due to its advanced state at the time of diagnosis. The overall survival rate is 50%. In patients who have had adequate surgery 5-year survival is 95% in stage I, 70% in stage II, 20% in stage III and 0–5% in stage IV. Where surgery has been inadequate, the survival for stages I–III is poorer (70, 60 and 10% respectively).

DYSGERMINOMA

This tumour occurs in a younger age group than do epithelial tumours. Average age is 20 years. Presentation is often with abdominal pain and a pelvic mass. Precocious puberty and abnormal menstruation may occur. Dysgerminoma does not normally produce tumour markers unless there are teratomatous elements (secreting beta human chorionic gonadotrophin and alpha-fetoprotein). A pregnancy test may be positive.

Staging

Staging investigations should include a chest X-ray and CT scan. If the CT scan is normal, a lymphangiogram is recommended. Most (75%) are stage I.

Treatment

Treatment for stage I is removal of the affected ovary alone (oophorectomy). For stage II or III disease, pelvic and para-aortic irradiation ('dog leg') as in testicular abdominal node irrradiation (Fig. 25.12) or whole abdominal node irradiation is very effective, achieving a 5-year survival of 85%. However this is also a very chemosensitive tumour and combination chemotherapy is progressively replacing radiotherapy for stages II and III. Chemotherapy is the treatment of choice for stage IV. A commonly used combination is vincristine, actinomycin D and cyclophosphamide.

GRANULOSA CELL TUMOURS OF THE OVARY

These tumours are rare. The majority occur in

postmenopausal women although they may occur in girls before puberty. They often secrete hormones such as oestrogens, progestogens and androgens. Oestrogens are mainly derived from the cells of the theca and give rise to symptoms of menorrhagia, postmenopausal bleeding and breast tenderness. Precocious puberty occurs in young girls. Ninety per cent are stage I and are curable by abdominal hysterectomy and bilateral oophorectomy. The role of chemotherapy is uncertain. Responses in recurrent disease may occur with alkylating agents.

Results of treatment

Prognosis is good: 5-year survival is 80%.

CANCER OF THE VAGINA

Most cancers in the vagina are secondary deposits from uterus, rectum or ovary. Primary tumours of the vagina are rare with an incidence of less than 1 in 100 000 women. It usually occurs over the age of 60 years. The aetiology in most cases is unknown. However there was an outbreak of adenocarcinoma of the upper third of the vagina in teenage children whose mothers had been treated with very high doses of diethylstilboestrol for threatened abortion. Most tumours occur in the upper vagina. Lymphatic drainage of the upper two-thirds is to the pelvic nodes, and of the lower third to the inguinal and pelvic nodes. Blood-borne metastases are rare. Over 90% are squamous cell carcinomas. Symptoms are of vaginal bleeding.

FIGO staging is shown in Table 24.7. To distinguish primary vaginal cancer from cervical cancer, the tumour must be sited in the vagina, not involve the cervix and not be a secondary deposit from a primary elswhere. A biopsy is necessary to confirm the diagnosis. Staging investigations are as for cervical cancer.

Stage I and IIa squamous cell carcinomas in the lower third can be treated by interstitial implantation using iridium-192. For stages I–III in the upper third and stages IIb and III in the lower third vaginal intracavitary and external beam are used (45 Gy in 20 daily fractions over 4 weeks; 9–10 MV photons) using an anterior and two posterior oblique fields. This is followed by vaginal intracavitary therapy delivering a further 25–30 Gy to the vaginal mucosa.

For stage IVa external beam alone is given (50 Gy in 20 daily fractions over 4 weeks; 9–10 MV photons).

Results of treatment

Prognosis is less favourable than for cervical cancer: 5-year survival following radical radiotherapy is about 75% for stage I, 60% for stage II and 20% for stage III.

CANCER OF THE VULVA

Cancer of the vulva is rare, one-fifth of the frequency of cervical cancer. It mainly occurs in elderly women.

Pathology

Aetiology

The aetiology is unknown. An association with viral infection (herpes simplex virus type 2, human papilloma virus) is suggested (but unproven), and vulval intra-epithelial neoplasia (VIN) has been postulated. Viral vulval condylomata are also associated with vulval cancer. However these condylomata rarely contain human papilloma virus (HPV) type 16, identified in invasive vulval cancer.

Macroscopic and microscopic appearance

Tumours may be exophytic or ulcerative. There is often associated leucoplakia.

Virtually all are squamous cell carcinomas. Adenocarcinoma is rare.

Spread

Local spread is to the surrounding skin, perineum, vagina and urethra. Lymphatic spread commonly occurs to the inguinal and femoral nodes and may be bilateral. Subsequent spread is to the external iliac nodes. Blood-borne spread is late.

Clinical features

Vulval itching is common (70%), often with a vulval mass or ulcer. Discharge and bleeding are less common. There is frequently a long delay between the development of symptoms and referral to a gynaecologist,

Table 24.7 Modified FIGO staging of vaginal cancer

Stage	Clinical findings
I	Tumour confined to vaginal mucosa
IIa	Infiltration beneath the vaginal mucosa but not infiltrating the parametrium
IIb	Parametrial invasion but not to the pelvic side wall
III	Parametrial extension to the pelvic side wall
IVa	Spread to rectum or bladder
IVb	Distant metastases

often because the significance of the changes on the vulva has not been appreciated by other doctors.

Diagnosis and staging

The vulva, vagina and cervix should be carefully examined since multicentric lesions may be found elsewhere in the genital tract. A pelvic examination should be carried out under anaesthesia, noting the site, size and extent of the tumour. A biopsy is taken. A chest radiograph is necessary to detect lung metastases.

Treatment

Surgery

Surgery is the treatment of choice. Referral to a specialist gynaecological oncologist is advised since inadequate initial surgery may result in unsalvageable local and groin node recurrence.

In the few cases where invasion is less than 1 mm, a wide local excision may be adequate without groin node dissection. For all other cases of localised disease, a radical resection of the vulva and groin node dissection is recommended.

Radiotherapy

The role for radiotherapy is in the postoperative radical treatment of the pelvis for involved groin nodes and the palliation of local symptoms of advanced disease.

Involved groin nodes

Target volume
The groin and pelvic nodes bilaterally.

Technique
Parallel opposed anterior and posterior fields.

Dose and energy
45–50 Gy midplane dose in 20 daily fractions over 4 weeks (9–10 MV photons)

Inoperable local disease

Target volume
The field should cover the tumour with a generous margin.

Technique
Direct field with bolus.

Dose and energy
30 Gy in 10 daily fractions over 2 weeks (9 MeV electrons)

Radiation reaction. The perineum is relatively intolerant of radiation due to natural moisture and friction. Painful moist desquamation is inevitable. Analgesics and good nursing care are required.

Chemotherapy

There is no established role for chemotherapy in vulval cancer.

Results of treatment

If the groin nodes are free of disease the 5-year survival is reasonable (70–80%). If the nodes are involved, survival falls to 20–50%. Involved pelvic nodes carry a very poor prognosis (20% 5-year survival).

GESTATIONAL TROPHOBLASTIC TUMOURS

Gestational trophoblastic tumours (GTTs) include hydatidiform mole, choriocarcinoma and its rare variant the placental site trophoblastic tumour. They affect women during and after their reproductive period. The unique feature of these tumours is that they are derived from the trophoblast of the placenta rather than from the patient's own tissues. Trophoblastic tumours retain the property of normal trophoblast to invade the muscular wall of the uterus (myometrium), and its vessels.

Hydatidiform mole is the simplest form of GTT. Histologically it is characterised by hyperplasia of the trophoblast and hydropic change in the placental villi. A mole is an abnormal embryo. In the complete form there is no embryo since the conceptus has been abnormal from its beginning, containing only paternal genes. In the partial form there is an abnormal conceptus associated with an embryo. The latter dies early and the only residual evidence of the embryo is the presence of fetal red cells in the mole. Over 90% of moles degenerate spontaneously once the uterus has been evacuated. A further 8% do not settle and continue as persistent trophoblastic disease (such as an invasive mole), but are readily cured. A very small percentage transform to the highly malignant choriocarcinoma.

The remainder of gestational choriocarcinomas arise following about 1 in 50 000 pregnancies. They can develop from both normal and abnormal pregnancies (normal full-term pregnancy, an ectopic pregnancy, abortion or stillbirth). They contain both syncytiotrophoblast and cytotrophoblast. They are haemorrhagic tumours with a strong tendency to blood-borne spread, especially to the lungs.

Diagnosis

Clinical presentation of GTT is usually with a hydatidiform mole. Typically there is vaginal bleeding at the end of the first trimester. The uterus may be unduly large for the stage of pregnancy. The cystic trophoblastic villi give rise to multiple echoes on ultrasound. No fetus is present. Occasionally there is no immediate antecedent history and a woman may present several years following pregnancy. The diagnosis of choriocarcinoma should be borne in mind in any woman of reproductive age with disseminated cancer of unknown origin.

GTTs all secrete human chorionic gonadotrophin (HCG). This tumour marker is of great use in both establishing the diagnosis and monitoring the response to treatment. Current immunological assays can detect very small amounts of HCG in blood and urine (down to 2 iu/l). It is also detectable in the CSF in association with brain metastases. A baseline chest radiograph is taken to detect lung metastases.

Treatment

As soon as the diagnosis is suspected the patient should be referred to a specialist centre for management. In the UK these centres are in Dundee, Sheffield and London.

The initial treatment of a GTT should be suction evacuation of the uterus. Serial blood HCG levels are measured before and after evacuation. In most uncomplicated hydatidiform moles, HCG levels fall to normal as the mole degenerates. Most GTTs are exquisitely chemosensitive, particularly to methotrexate. The following are indications for chemotherapy:

— Blood HCG levels over 20 000 iu/l for more than a month after evacuation of the uterus
— Rising levels of HCG
— Histological evidence of choriocarcinoma
— Presence of lung metastases greater than 2 cm in diameter or metastases in brain, liver or bowel
— Persisting uterine bleeding
— HCG detectable in body fluids 4–6 months post evacuation.

The choice of drugs depends on a variety of prognostic factors (e.g. age, sites and number of metastases, level of HCG). On this basis patients can be divided into low, medium and high risk groups.

Low risk patients are treated with low dose methotrexate and folinic acid; medium risk with a combination of etoposide, methotrexate with folinic acid, 6-mercaptopurine and actinomycin D, and high risk with actinomycin D, etoposide, high dose methotrexate, vincristine and cyclophosphamide.

Patients with brain metastases should additionally receive intrathecal methotrexate. Isolated brain metastases should be excised if possible since chemotherapy may precipitate intracranial bleeding.

Results of treatment

Virtually all low and medium risk patients with GTT are cured. Even in the high risk group, cure rates are about 90% in the best centres.

25. Kidney, bladder, prostate, testis, urethra, penis

KIDNEY

Anatomy

The kidneys lie retroperitoneally on the posterior abdominal wall. They are approximately 11 cm long and 6 cm wide in adults. The left kidney is 1 cm higher than the right. The right kidney is related in front to the liver, the second part of the duodenum and the ascending colon. In front of the left kidney are the stomach, the pancreas, descending colon and the

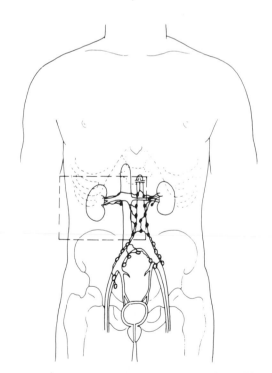

Fig. 25.1 Anatomical relationships of the kidney with lymphatic drainage pathways and typical treatment volume when irradiating the renal bed. (Reproduced with permission from Souhami & Tobias, Cancer and its Management, Blackwells, 1986.)

spleen. On the top of each kidney lies an adrenal gland. Behind the kidneys lie the diaphragm and the 12th rib. On the medial side of the kidney there is an opening, the hilum, through which pass the renal artery and vein, and the ureter. The renal vein drains into the inferior vena cava. The lymphatic drainage is to the para-aortic nodes. The anatomical relationships relevant to the oncologist are shown in Figure 25.1.

Pathology

The three principal malignant tumours of the kidney are Wilms' tumour (nephroblastoma) in children (described in Ch. 29), renal cell adenocarcinoma (also called clear cell carcinoma, hypernephroma and Grawitz's tumour) and transitional cell carcinoma of the renal pelvis.

The term, hypernephroma, means 'above the kidney', in the same sense as suprarenal or adrenal. The name was given because the tumour cells resemble adrenal cells microscopically and most tumours do in fact arise at the upper pole of the kidney, near the adrenal gland. It is a misnomer and should be dropped. (Grawitz believed the tumour arose from misplaced 'ectopic' adrenal tissue.)

Renal cancer is uncommon, accounting for 1.4% of all cancers and 1.5% of cancer deaths. Adenocarcinoma arising from the renal tubules accounts for 80% of tumours. It is approximately twice as common in men and occurs mainly in the 5th–7th decades of life. The aetiology of renal cell carcinoma is unknown, though smoking is a risk factor.

Macroscopically the tumour appears as a yellowish vascular mass. Microscopically the tumour cells are large with a foamy or clear appearance to the cytoplasm. The nucleus is small, central and densely staining.

Spread

There is direct spread through the renal substance

and into the perinephric fat of the renal bed. The characteristic mode of spread is permeation along the renal vein and into the inferior vena cava. Tumour may rarely extend up to the right side of the heart, completely blocking the inferior vena cava. Lung, bone and brain metastases are common. The tempo of metastatic disease may be slow and survival with metastases over several years is not uncommon. Occasionally metastases may be solitary (particularly in bone). Removal of the primary and the metastasis may be followed by prolonged survival. Rarely spontaneous regression of a metastasis may occur.

Clinical features

Presentation is usually with local symptoms. Of these, painless haematuria is the commonest. However colicky pain may be produced by clots of blood. Other symptoms are aching or a mass in the loin which may be noticed by the patient. A distant metastasis may be the first presentation—pathological bone fracture, haemoptysis from pulmonary metastases or symptoms of raised intracranial pressure from cerebral deposits. Systemic features such as anaemia, loss of weight and unexplained fever may occur. The kidney may be palpably enlarged.

Investigation and staging

The urine may contain frank or microscopic evidence of blood. Urine cytology may show malignant cells. The most important investigation is an intravenous urogram (IVU), which may show distortion of the calyces (the channels that drain urine to the renal pelvis and are outlined by the contrast medium) by the tu-

mour. Calcification within the tumour may be visible on plain radiographs. Ultrasound and CT scanning (Fig. 25.2) are helpful in distinguishing between solid and cystic renal masses. Ultrasound may show extension of tumour into the renal vein or inferior vena cava. CT scanning is now preferred to angiography and venography in most cases and may show direct tumour spread, venous and lymph node involvement and liver metastases. Angiography has the disadvantage of being an invasive procedure. It may show widening of the renal artery and new vessel formation within the tumour. It is used when the kidney is to be embolised (i.e. material introduced into the renal arterial supply to cut off its blood supply and cause death of part or the whole of the kidney).

Bone metastases are typically osteolytic (Fig. 25.3)

No staging system for renal cell cancer has universal acceptance. The TNM classification is shown in Table 25.1.

Treatment

Surgery is the main treatment for localised renal cell cancer. Radiotherapy and embolisation have more limited roles. Chemotherapy is of unproven value. Immunotherapy is currently being evaluated.

Surgery

Nephrectomy is indicated for tumours confined to the kidney and/or regional nodes. Extension into the inferior vena cava is not necessarily a contraindication

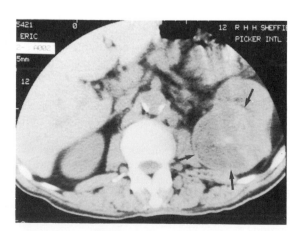

Fig. 25.2 CT scan showing renal cell carcinoma (arrowed). (Courtesy of Dr R Nakielny, Sheffield.)

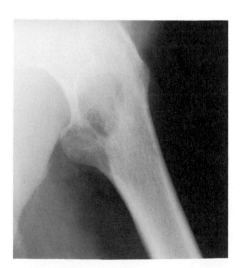

Fig. 25.3 Radiograph showing osteolytic metastasis of the femoral neck from renal cell carcinoma.

Table 25.1 TNM staging of primary renal tumours

Stage	Clinical findings
Tumour	
T0	No tumour
T1	Small tumour, no enlargement of the kidney. IVU shows minimal calyceal abnormality
T2	Kidney enlarged or distorted and involvement of the calyces or renal pelvis
T3a	Invasion of perinephric tissues
T3b	Invasion of the renal vein
T3c	Invasion of the inferior vena cava
Nodes	
N0	No regional nodes involved
N1	Single ipsilateral regional node
N2	Contralateral, bilateral or multiple regional nodes
N3	Fixed regional nodes
N4	Juxtaregional nodes involved
Metastases	
M0	No distant metastases
M1	Distant metastases

to surgery. Palliative removal of the kidney may be required to control pain or haemorrhage or if a painful syndrome following embolisation occurs. If presentation is with solitary lung or brain metastases, nephrectomy and resection of the metastasis may be associated with surprisingly long survival (30–50% 5-year survival).

Embolisation

Embolisation of the kidney via a catheter inserted into the renal artery is useful in both operable and inoperable cases. In operable cases embolisation is indicated where there is concern about blood loss at nephrectomy, e.g. in patients who refuse blood transfusion on religious grounds. In inoperable cases it is effective in controlling renal pain and haematuria. Embolisation may be complicated by a postembolisation syndrome with pain, ileus, and infection.

Radiotherapy

Renal cell carcinoma is relatively resistant to radiation. Pre- or postoperative radiotherapy does not reduce local recurrence where the tumour has spread locally outside the kidney. Its role is palliative to relieve symptoms from the primary tumour or from distant metastases.

Kidney

Target volume
The whole of the kidney and the regional nodes should be included (Fig. 25.1).

Technique
A parallel opposed anterior and posterior pair of fields is used.

Dose and energy
30 Gy in 10 daily fractions over 2 weeks (4–6 MV photons)

Distant metastases

Brain and bone metastases are treated by palliative radiotherapy, as described on page 488 and page 512 respectively.

Chemotherapy

Chemotherapy has little value in renal cancer. Oral progestogens have been claimed to benefit 20% of patients but the evidence for their benefit is scanty. Cytotoxic therapy has not proved of value.

Immunotherapy

The role of immunotherapy with interferon and interleukin 2, which stimulate the body's immunological attack on tumours, is under assessment but cannot be recommended for routine use. Since some metastases from renal cell carcinoma may undergo spontaneous regression, the true impact of immunotherapy on the evolution of metastatic disease is difficult to demonstrate.

Results of treatment

The outlook depends on the stage at diagnosis. Extra-renal local invasion and blood-borne metastases confer a poor prognosis. For tumours confined to the kidney 5-year survival varies from 50 to 80%. If there are lymph node metastases or the renal vein is invaded, survival falls to 50% or less. Nearly 75% of patients presenting with metastases are dead within a year.

BLADDER
Anatomy

The bladder is related anteriorly to the pubic symphysis, superiorly to the small intestine and sigmoid colon, laterally to the levator ani muscle, inferiorly to the prostate gland and posteriorly to the rectum, vas deferens and seminal vesicles (Fig. 25.7) in the male and to the vagina and cervix in the female.

At cystoscopy the bladder mucosa and ureteric orifices can be inspected.

Lymphatic drainage is to the iliac and para-aortic nodes.

Pathology

The bladder, ureters and renal pelvis are lined by transitional cell epithelium (urothelium). The same type of tumours may arise anywhere along the urinary tract but cancers in the renal pelvis and ureter are rare compared with those in the bladder. The bladder is also sometimes secondarily involved by prostatic adenocarcinoma and other pelvic tumours.

Aetiology

In the majority of cases of bladder cancer, the aetiology is unknown. However, as discussed in Chapter 14, occupational exposure to certain carcinogens has accounted for some cases. The production of aniline dyes and processing of rubber are associated with 2-naphthylamine, now recognised as a procarcinogen. Workers in these industries are now offered regular cytological examination of urine to detect abnormalities or tumours at an early stage. Bladder cancer sometimes shows a point mutation in the *ras* oncogene, illustrating the issue of gene alterations in the process of tumour development.

Smoking also predisposes to bladder cancer. Bladder cancer is up to six times commoner in smokers than non-smokers and increases in frequency with the number of cigarettes smoked.

Phenacetin, formerly used as an analgesic drug, and, in low doses, the cytotoxic alkylating agent cyclophosphamide may give rise to urothelial tumours.

Some foodstuffs such as coffee and artificial sweeteners have been incriminated in the development of bladder cancer in experimental animals but not in man.

Squamous carcinoma tends to complicate chronic irritation of the bladder including a parasitic disease, schistosomiasis (formerly known as bilharziasis), which is common in Egypt and Central Africa. Adenocarcinoma occurs on the dome of the bladder in relation to embryological remnants of the urachus, and also from the trigone at the bladder base.

Epidemiology

Bladder cancer is common and accounts for 4.4% of all cancers and 3.4% of cancer deaths. The male to female ratio is 3.8:1 and it has a peak incidence at the age of 65. It is twice as common in Caucasians as in Blacks. Over 90% are transitional cell carcinomas.

Macroscopic appearance

The chief types on inspection of the bladder are (1) papillary and (2) solid. Multiple growths are common.

Papillary carcinoma has a base with surface fronds. The tumours tend to be multiple and to appear in crops. Confined at first to the mucosa and submucosa, they eventually invade the submucosa, muscle coat and then outside the bladder.

Solid carcinoma is nodular, often ulcerated, grows more rapidly and infiltrates early.

From the point of prognosis a division can be made between superficial (papillary) and invasive (solid) bladder cancer. Superficial bladder tumours are the commonest (80%) and become malignant in less than 15% of cases. By contrast, invasive cancer, untreated, carries a very poor prognosis. The degree of invasion correlates with the risk of metastatic disease. Invasion of the lamina propria (the layer of tissue between the epithelium and the muscle layer of the bladder), superficial and deep muscle is associated with 20%, 30% and 60% incidence of lymphatic invasion.

Microscopic appearance

Benign tumours of the bladder are very uncommon. However low grade transitional cell malignant tumours are often erroneously referred to as papillomas.

Malignant tumours of the bladder include:

— Transitional cell carcinoma; papillary and solid variants
— Adenocarcinoma (uncommon)
— Squamous carcinoma (rare in the UK)
— Sarcomas (all very rare).

Transitional carcinoma accounts for 90% of bladder cancer and is classified histologically into well, moderately and poorly differentiated tumours. The degree of differentiation is important. Anaplastic tumours grow faster and infiltrate sooner.

After muscle has been invaded, lymphatic spread is to the pelvic and then para-aortic nodes.

Clinical features

The presenting symptom is usually painless haematuria. Occasionally clots of blood are passed and are even more suggestive of the diagnosis. Papillomatous types grow slowly and may cause no other symptoms for a long time. When anaplastic growths invade muscle, there may be urinary frequency, dysuria and pain, especially when there is extravesical (i.e. outside the bladder) spread into the pelvic soft tissues. Bacterial cystitis may be associated with the tumour and may aggravate symptoms.

Obstruction of one or both ureters can occur at any time, with no symptoms at first. Later there may be upper urinary tract infection, pain in the flank(s) and eventual renal failure from back pressure.

In localised bladder disease clinical examination is usually unremarkable.

Investigation and staging

Urine. The urine should be examined for red cells, pus cells and bacteria as well as undergoing cytology for malignant cells. Urine cytology is a valuable screening method for industrial workers at risk. Malignant cells are present in the urine of 60% of cases of bladder cancer, particularly the more anaplastic tumours. However negative cytology does not exclude malignancy since it is negative in 30% of patients with bladder cancer.

Biochemistry. Serum urea, creatinine and electrolytes are measured for evidence of renal impairment.

Radiology. Radiology is important in the diagnosis and staging of bladder cancer. An intravenous urogram is essential to determine the site of the tumour in the bladder and to exclude a lesion higher up in the renal tract. Obstruction at the lower end of the ureter(s) will be shown by dilatation of the ureter and renal pelvis (hydroureter and hydronephrosis). Filling defects in the bladder can also be shown.

Cystourethroscopy. This is the most important investigation of all. Under general anaesthesia the urethra and the whole of the bladder are inspected. The number, site, size and character of the tumours are noted and a biopsy taken. While the patient is relaxed under the anaesthetic, a bimanual examination of the pelvis is made, with a finger in the rectum and the other hand on the lower abdomen. In this way the tumour may be palpated and any extravesical spread assessed.

Clinical staging of bladder cancer is according to the TNM classification (Fig. 25.4 and Table 25.2).

Treatment

Treatment will depend on the staging, histology, size and multiplicity of tumours and the age and general medical condition of the patient.

Superficial Ta and T1 tumours

Superficial tumours are biopsied and removed by transurethral resection (TUR) or diathermy. Superficial

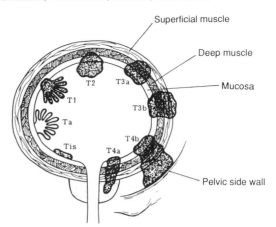

Fig. 25.4   T staging of bladder cancer—UICC classification. (Modified from Wallace et al, British Journal of Urology, 1975.)

Table 25.2   TNM staging of bladder cancer

Stage	Clinical findings
Tumour	
Tis	Carcinoma-in-situ
Ta	Papillary non-invasive carcinoma
T1	Invasion of submucosa but not beyond the lamina propria
T2	Invasion of superficial muscle
T3a	Invasion of deep muscle
T3b	Invasion of perivesical fat
T4	Invasion of adjacent structures, progressing to fixation to pelvic side wall
Nodes	
N0	No evidence of nodal involvement
N1	Single ipsilateral nodal involvement <2 cm diameter
N2	Single nodal metastasis 2–5 cm diameter or multiple nodes none exceeding >5 cm
N3	Node >5 cm
Metastases	
M0	No metastases
M1	Distant metastases

tumours do respond completely to radical radiotherapy in over 75% of cases but there is recurrence in more than 50%. For this reason radical radiotherapy is rarely used in T1 lesions. It may have a limited role in poorly differentiated T1 tumours, where 50% 5-year survival has been obtained.

The instruments are passed by an operating cystoscope. Random biopsies of the bladder are carried out to exclude carcinoma-in-situ. In the majority of patients these tumours tend to recur rather than invade. For this reason cystoscopic follow-up needs to be lifelong.

If recurrences are multiple or high grade, intravesical chemotherapy or BCG should be used.

Carcinoma-in-situ is treated by intravesical chemotherapy or intravesical BCG. Cystectomy is indicated if these measures fail.

Invasive bladder cancer (T2 and T3)

Surgery and radiotherapy are the standard treatments for invasive bladder cancer.

T2 tumours. These may be controlled by endoscopic treatment. However if the tumour is shown on histology not to have been completely resected or is poorly differentiated (and therefore more likely to invade the deep muscle and pelvic nodes) radical radiotherapy is indicated.

T3 tumours. These have invaded too deeply for removal by endoscopic means. There is no firm agreement on the best treatment for T3 tumours. Some oncologists favour preoperative radiotherapy and primary cystourethrectomy (removal of the bladder and prostate with diversion of the ureters on to the abdominal wall). Most British surgeons and oncologists (including the author) prefer a policy of primary radical radiotherapy with cystectomy for salvage of locally persistent or recurrent tumour. This policy has the advantage that the patient has a better chance of tumour control with the bladder intact. If radiotherapy fails there is a 30% chance of successful salvage by cystectomy. By contrast, if primary cystectomy fails, radical radiotherapy is rarely successful for recurrent disease. Each policy carries a similar 5-year survival of about 40%. The use of adjuvant cytotoxic chemotherapy, to reduce tumour bulk and deal with microscopic lymph node metastases, followed by radical radiotherapy is being evaluated. At present adjuvant chemotherapy cannot be routinely recommended for T3 tumours.

T4 tumours. A distinction must be made between T4a and T4b tumours. T4a means tumour penetration into the prostate or vagina. T4a includes both aggressive deeply invasive tumours infiltrating the prostate and less aggressive superficial tumours extending into the prostatic urethra and/or ducts. The latter has a much better prognosis than the former. T4a tumours should be treated radically. T4b tumours are fixed to neighbouring structures, are inoperable and should be treated with palliative radiotherapy.

Adenocarcinoma and squamous carcinoma of the bladder

Neither of these is very radiosensitive and they are better treated by cystectomy.

Radical radiotherapy

The following are criteria for accepting patients for radical radiotherapy:

— Age <80 years
— Adequate general medical condition
— Transitional cell carcinoma/squamous carcinoma
— Tumour <10 cm maximum diameter
— Stage T1–T4a
— No metastases

Target volume

The treatment volume is 1–2 cm around the tumour, judged by bimanual examination and CT scanning. The bladder is emptied before CT planning and before each treatment.

Radiation planning technique

The tumour is localised by intravesical contrast medium (cystogram) on a simulator (Fig. 25.5) or by a CT planning scan.

With localisation by cystogram a radio-opaque solution is introduced into the bladder via a catheter. The rectum is identified by the introduction of a small volume of a barium solution through a rectal tube. Simulation is carried out in the prone position with the toes together, heels apart and the head resting on the hands. Anteroposterior and lateral radiographs are taken. An open anterior and two posterior oblique wedged fields are used, treating isocentrically (Fig. 25.6).

The posterior oblique fields should include 1 cm of

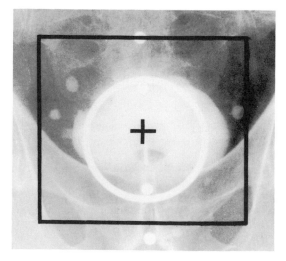

Fig. 25.5 Simulator radiograph showing anterior treatment volume for radical radiotherapy of a T3 carcinoma of the right bladder wall. (Courtesy of Dr J Bolger, Sheffield.)

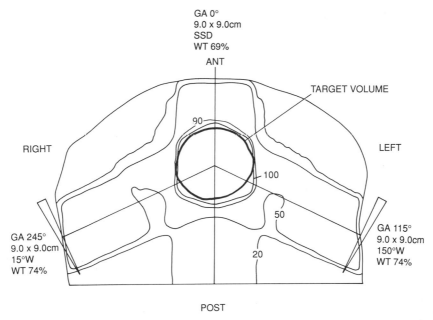

Fig. 25.6 Isodose distribution for radical radiotherapy of the bladder using anterior and two posterior oblique fields. (Courtesy of Dr J Bolger, Sheffield.)

the anterior wall of the rectum. An external contour of the body surface through the centre of the treatment volume is taken, as described on page 107. The position of the rectum, just in front of the sacrum, is marked. The rectum is the critical organ of tolerance where the dose should be kept as low as possible. It cannot be completely avoided but the posterior fields are angled so as to give a favourable distribution with rapid fall-off towards the rectum.

If CT planning is available, the patient is planned in the same position on the CT scanner as on the simulator and treatment couches. The levels 1 cm above and below the upper and lower limits of the bladder are determined and marked on a 'scout' film of the pelvis marked with transverse lines at 1 cm intervals. On the planning computer the width of the field to encompass the tumour with a 1–2 cm margin is chosen. In our experience the treatment volume using CT planning tends to be larger than that using a cystogram.

Dose and energy
55 Gy in 20 daily fractions over 4 weeks (9–10 MV photons)

Radiation reaction. Before radiation begins, attention is paid to the patient's general condition and nutrition. The patient's haemoglobin level should be maintained over 12 g/dl, by blood transfusion if necessary, since anaemia will reduce the amount of oxygen available to the tumour. It is known that reduced oxygenation in parts of the tumour contributes to resistance to radiation. Urinary infection should be treated with antibiotics. The urine should be made sterile if possible before radiation begins, since inflammation has adverse effects on radiation response. However with an ulcerated mass this may not be possible until the tumour has shrunk in response to radiation.

Acute reactions
1. Frequency and urgency, from radiation cystitis during and after the course, are common but not usually serious unless bacterial infection is gross. Painful spasm may require an antispasmodic drug. Fluid intake must be strongly encouraged. The patient should be warned that he or she may pass fragments in the urine (blood clot and tumour) and a little fresh blood.
2. Bowel reactions are also to be expected in almost every case—usually mild diarrhoea and tenesmus. If they are severe treatment may have to be suspended or dosage reduced.

Late reactions
1. Fibrosis of the bladder. The bladder wall may be so contracted by fibrosis and the bladder volume so reduced that uncontrollable frequency may make life intolerable. Ureteric diversion may be required.

2. Telangiectasia on the bladder lining may develop, with repeated bleeding. It may be possible to seal them off with the diathermy point at cystoscopy. If they are uncontrolled by this means, cystectomy may be required.

3. Late bowel reactions are similar to those after the irradiation of cancer of the cervix (p. 412), though less common. Loops of bowel trapped in the pelvis by adhesions after previous surgery or inflammatory disease are especially at risk. There may be bleeding from telangiectasia on the bladder mucosa, ulceration, even necrosis and perforation. If conservative measures, e.g. steroid enemas, fail, a defunctioning colostomy may be required.

Palliative radiotherapy

Palliative radiotherapy should be considered in the following circumstances: age (>80 years) or poor general condition with either significant local symptoms (e.g. haematuria) or symptomatic metastases, e.g. bone and skin.

Technique
A four field 'box' technique of an anterior and posterior opposed pair of fields and a pair of lateral opposed fields is used. A cystogram is recommended for bladder localisation.

Dose and energy
30 Gy in 10 daily fractions over 2 weeks (9–10 MV or with cobalt-60)

Results of treatment

The 5-year survival for radical radiotherapy is 30–40% for T2 and 5–20% for T3 and T4 tumours.

PROSTATE
Anatomy

The prostate gland lies just below the base of the bladder and in front of the rectum (Fig. 25.7). It resembles a chestnut in size and shape. Through it passes the prostatic urethra. Into the urethra empty the ejaculatory ducts which carry sperm from the seminal vesicles which lie behind and to each side of the prostate gland. The prostate is divided into two lobes by a median groove. It is surrounded by a thin layer of fibrous tissue (true capsule) and a layer of fascia continuous with that surrounding the bladder (false capsule). Between these two layers lies the

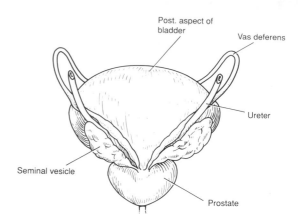

Fig. 25.7   Prostate, seminal vesicles and vas deferens in a posterior view of the bladder. (Redrawn from Ellis, Clinical Anatomy, 5th edn, Blackwells, 1975.)

prostatic venous plexus. Part of the venous drainage is to a plexus of veins lying in front of the vertebral bodies. This may account for the tendency of prostate cancer to spread to the vertebrae.

Pathology

Cancer of the prostate gland is the third commonest malignancy in men in the UK. It represents 3.8% of all cancers and 4.2% of cancer deaths. There are about 5700 new cases per year in the UK. It is commonest in the seventh and eighth decades and rare under the age of 40.

The aetiology of prostatic cancer is unknown. The increased incidence of the disease in patients with a family history of the disease and the wide variation in incidence between countries suggest the role of genetic factors. Possible environmental factors include exposure to radiation, heavy metals and chemical fertilisers.

Over 95% are adenocarcinomas arising from the peripheral part of the gland. The tumour is commonly well differentiated, though the differentiation may vary from one part of the tumour to another. In 75% of cases the tumour has spread beyond the gland at the time of presentation, and 50% will have distant metastases. Direct spread is to the bladder, seminal vesicles and rectum. Lymphatic spread is to the obturator, presacral, internal and external iliac nodes. Further spread is to the common iliac and para-aortic nodes. It readily invades the pelvic veins and thence the pelvic bones and vertebrae. Bone secondaries are typically of sclerotic type, showing as an increased density on the radiograph because they induce new bone formation.

The natural history of the disease is very variable. It may be indolent in the elderly patient with a well-differentiated tumour and an incidental finding at post mortem. The disease tends to run a more aggressive course in men under the age of 40, particularly with poorly differentiated tumours.

Hormonal sensitivity

The prostate has analogies with the breast and is under hormonal control. Removal of male hormones by orchidectomy, or administration of female hormones (oestrogens), causes shrinkage of the normal gland, and of 80% of tumours.

The normal and malignant prostate gland secretes an enzyme, *acid phosphatase*, measurable in the blood. It is raised in 80% of patients with metastases. Similarly, *prostate specific antigen* may serve as a marker of this disease. Both these substances are of value in the histological recognition of prostatic adenocarcinoma when metastatic.

Clinical features

The prostate often undergoes benign enlargement, and the early symptoms of cancer may be similar, i.e. increased frequency and difficulty of micturition. Clinical evidence of disease is rare under the age of 45.

Nearly 50% present with urinary outflow obstruction, 25% in acute urinary retention, 5% with haematuria and 7% with bone pain. Pathological fracture may be the first symptom. Back pressure on the kidneys may cause renal impairment. Sacral, sciatic or perineal pain may occur from infiltration of nerves in the pelvis.

Diagnosis and staging

The presence of a hard irregular gland on rectal examination suggests the diagnosis. This should be confirmed by a biopsy of the prostate. Ultrasound of the prostate carried out with the probe in the rectum is useful in identifying small peripheral tumours and guiding the surgeon to the appropriate site for biopsy.

Serum acid phosphatase is increased in 80% of patients with metastases compared with 11% where the disease is confined to the prostate. In patients with a negative bone scan and an elevated alkaline phosphatase, the incidence of pelvic nodal involvement is 60% compared with 25% in those with normal levels.

Prostatic carcinoma is staged using the TNM classification (Table 25.3). The local stage of the disease is mainly based on rectal examination. This may be supplemented by ultrasound or CT scanning. CT

Table 25.3 TNM staging of prostate cancer

Stage	Clinical findings
Tumour	
T1a	No tumour palpable (focal disease)
T1b	No tumour palpable (diffuse disease)
T2	Palpable tumour confined to the gland
T3	Tumour extending beyond the capsule and/or into the seminal vesicles
T4	Tumour fixed or invading adjacent structures
Nodes	
N0	No nodes involved
NI	Single node metastasis <2 cm in diameter
N2	Single node metastasis 2–5 cm in diameter or multiple nodes, none >5 cm
N3	Node >5 cm
Metastases	
M0	No distant metastases
M1	Distant metastases

scanning is helpful in showing enlarged pelvic nodes and local invasion of the bladder, seminal vesicles and rectal wall. However none of these imaging techniques is entirely reliable. Surgical dissection of the pelvic nodes is the only reliable means of assessing pelvic node involvement but has not gained wide acceptance in the UK since it does not improve survival. Plain radiographs of painful bones should be obtained. A bone scan is recommended in view of the high incidence of bone metastases. Serum acid phosphatase should be measured before digital rectal examination since palpation of the gland may increase blood levels.

Treatment

1. Clinically localised disease

Untreated, the disease will progress locally in about 85% of patients. However there is no consensus on the treatment of clinically localised disease. Radical surgery (total prostatectomy) and radical radiotherapy can be curative in patients where the tumour is confined to the prostate (T1–3). The lack of agreement is due in part to the unpredictable course of the untreated disease, and the absence of good information on the comparative benefits on local control and survival of radical surgery and radiotherapy.

Factors which should influence the choice are the age and general condition of the patient, the likelihood of progression to symptomatic disease and the morbidity of treatment, particularly on sexual function. The higher the T stage and degree of anaplasia, the higher the chance of local progression and metastatic spread.

There is some evidence that, at least for T1 tumours,

radical radiotherapy can be curative. The likelihood of local control is less with more advanced disease (T2 and T3) but none the less probably better than with hormonal therapy deferred until local symptoms progress.

Radical surgery is only suitable for medically fit patients. Its main complication until recently was impotence, but the operation can now be carried out sparing the parasympathetic nerves involved in erection of the penis.

Radical radiotherapy

Target volume

If the tumour is T1–T3 and CT scan shows that the tumour is confined to the prostate and there is no obvious involvement of the pelvic nodes, the target volume is confined to the tumour and any local extension (e.g. seminal vesicles), with a 1 cm margin of normal tissue around it. If there is pelvic nodal involvement, the author sees no value in trying to include the pelvic nodes in the treatment volume for two reasons. First, the likelihood of curing pelvic disease is negligible, and secondly, pelvic morbidity is substantially increased.

Technique

A three field technique is used with an anterior and two posterior oblique fields at 120° to each other. The patient lies prone. Localisation is ideally done with a

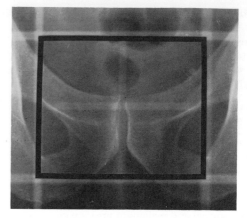

Fig. 25.8 Simulator radiograph showing anterior treatment volume for radical radiotherapy of carcinoma of the prostate. (Courtesy of Dr J Bolger, Sheffield.)

CT planning scan. The bladder should be full to displace the dome of the bladder and small bowel out of the field. If CT planning is not available, a cystogram is performed for planning. The urinary catheter is drawn down on to the bladder base. The anterior field is defined. This is normally about 8 × 8 cm with the centre of the volume 1 cm below the top of the pubic symphysis in the midline. An anteroposterior film is taken for verification (Fig. 25.8). A small amount of barium is introduced into the rectum through a soft plastic tube and the lateral field is defined. The posterior border should include no more than 1 cm thickness

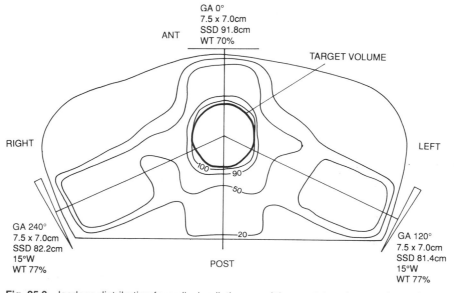

Fig. 25.9 Isodose distribution for radical radiotherapy of the prostate using anterior and two posterior oblique fields. (Courtesy of Dr J Bolger, Sheffield)

of the rectum. The oblique fields are viewed to ensure adequate coverage. A typical isodose distribution is shown in Figure 25.9.

Dose and energy
55 Gy in 20 daily fractions over 4 weeks (9–10 MV photons)

Acute reactions. About half way through a radical 4-week course, urinary frequency and occasionally dysuria occur. These can often be relieved by mist. pot. cit. or an anticholinergic (e.g. propantheline) and normally settle within 3 weeks of the end of treatment. Diarrhoea and tenesmus from acute proctitis have a similar time course.

Late reactions. The main late urinary effects are chronic cystitis, urethral stricture or incontinence. Loss of sexual potency also occurs. Bowel morbidity includes rectal ulceration or stricture and small bowel obstruction. Symptoms are tenesmus, rectal bleeding or incontinence. Proctitis may respond to steroid (Predsol) enemas but ultimately a defunctioning colostomy is required in 2% of cases.

Results of radical radiotherapy. The 5-year survival for T1 and T2 is 78% and for T3 59%.

2. Metastatic disease

Hormonal therapy

Most prostatic tumours contain elements sensitive to the androgenic hormone testosterone. Hormonal treatment is designed to reduce levels of testosterone circulating in the blood. This may be achieved in a number of different ways: (1) removal of the testes, which secrete testosterone (orchidectomy); (2) oral oestrogens, e.g. stilboestrol; (3) chemical compounds, similar to luteinising hormone releasing hormone (LHRH), which diminish the pituitary production of luteinising hormone (LH) and thus reduce testosterone production—these are administered as snuff, subcutaneously or by monthly depot intramuscular injection; (4) oral agents which block the cellular action of androgens (e.g. cyproterone acetate).

About 80% of patients will respond to hormonal therapy. Whether hormonal treatment should be instituted as soon as metastases are demonstrated or should be delayed until symptoms occur remains controversial. It is probable that starting hormonal treatment early does delay the onset of symptoms but does not improve overall survival. About 70% of patients with bone metastases die within 2 years of diagnosis.

Palliative radiotherapy

Radiotherapy has a useful role in relieving pain from bone metastases. It can also shrink advanced local disease causing symptoms of outflow obstruction and pelvic nodes causing lymphoedema and nerve compression.

Technique
Parallel opposed field or single fields.

Dose and energy

1. Prostate
30 Gy in 10 daily fractions over 2 weeks (9–10 MV photons)

2. Bone metastases

Confined to a limited area e.g. lumbar spine
Single fraction of 8 Gy or 20 Gy in 4 daily fractions (4–6 MV photons or cobalt-60)

Widespread
Hemibody irradiation. Where there are widespread painful bony metastases, hemibody irradiation may be considered to encompass all the painful areas. Improvement in pain control tends to be prompt and may last the few months until death. Treatment of the lower half of the body is better tolerated because the side-effects are minimal. Upper hemibody irradiation is not recommended on the basis that palliative treatments should induce little toxicity.

Preparation. The patient is given intravenous fluids and fasted before treatment. Regular antiemetics are given before and after treatment.

Treatment volume
For the lower half, the field usually extends from the top of the iliac crests to the knees and for the upper half from the top of the head to the lower abdomen. Overlap with the lower field is avoided.

Acute reaction. Nausea and vomiting occur at the end of treatment and last for up to 6 hours. Lethargy is common. If the upper half is treated, hair loss starts at about 10 days. The mouth becomes dry and taste sensation is altered. The blood count reaches its low point at 10–14 days. Haemoglobin, white blood cell and platelet counts are all reduced (pancytopenia) and remain so for up to 8 weeks. Cough and shortness of breath occurring at 6 weeks are usually indicative of radiation pneumonitis. If both halves of the body are treated, an interval of at least 6 weeks is left after the first hemibody irradiation to allow the systemic effects to settle and the blood count to recover.

Technique

The patient is treated supine. Parallel opposed anterior and posterior fields are used at extended FSD (140 cm).

Dose and energy

Lower half of body

8 Gy midplane dose in a single fraction (9–10 MV photons)

Upper half

6.5 Gy midplane dose in a single fraction (9–10 MV photons)

Strontium-89. Strontium-89 is a pure beta emitter with a half-life of 50 days. It is selectively taken up by bone metastases. Doses of 74–740 MBq have resulted in relief of bone pain in 60–70% of patients, with little haematological toxicity.

Cytotoxic chemotherapy

Cytotoxic chemotherapy has no useful role to play in prostatic cancer to date.

TESTIS

Anatomy

Each testis (the diminutive form 'testicle' is also in common use, with its adjective testicular) lies within a fibrous capsule (tunica albuginea) within the scrotum (Fig. 25.10). In the embryo, the testes arise on the posterior abdominal wall and migrate downwards through the inguinal canal to the scrotum.

The testis is divided into 200–300 lobules. Each of these contains 1–3 seminiferous tubules. These drain into the epididymis which lies on the posterior border of the testis. The lymphatic drainage of the testis is to the para-aortic nodes. It is important to note that the skin of the scrotum drains to the inguinal nodes. To avoid surgical contamination of the scrotal skin, the testis is surgically removed through an inguinal incision.

Pathology

Aetiology

The main factor predisposing to the development of germ cell tumours of the testis is an undescended testis. This accounts for 10% of cases. The risk is increased fivefold if one testis is maldescended and twelvefold if both are maldescended. However, even if one testis is maldescended, there is an increased risk of testicular

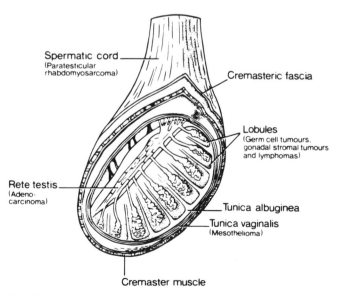

Fig. 25.10 Diagram of testis and spermatic cord indicating sites of tumour origin. Paratesticular rhabdomyosarcoma may arise from connective tissue of the cord or of adjacent structures. (Reproduced with permission from Williams, Krikorian & Green, Textbook of Common Cancers, John Wiley, 1988.)

cancer in the normally descended testis on the other side. Intratubular germ cell neoplasia or carcinoma-in-situ is a premalignant condition which gives rise to malignancy in 50% of patients within 5 years.

Testicular cancer is the commonest form of malignancy in men between the ages of 20 and 40. The incidence is rising and currently there are about 900 new cases per year in England and Wales. It accounts for 0.1% of deaths from cancer. The types of common (germ cell tumours) and rarer tumours and their sites of origin in the testis are illustrated in Fig 25.10.

Germ cell tumours

There are two main tumour types which arise from the germ cells: seminoma and teratoma. Teratoma occurs mainly between the ages of 20 and 35, and seminoma between 25 and 40 years. Over the age of 50 tumours are more likely to be non-germ cell tumours. These are non-Hodgkin lymphomas and tumours arising from other structures of the testis (Sertoli and Leydig cell tumours). Paratesticular rhabdomyosarcoma (Fig. 25.10) occurs in infancy and in young adult life.

1. Seminoma. Seminoma is the commonest type (60%). It arises from the cells of the seminiferous tubules. It is solid with a pale cut surface like a potato. There are two principal types: *classical* and *spermatocytic*. The characteristic histological feature of classical seminoma is its uniform appearance. The cells are rounded with a central nucleus and clear cytoplasm. The tumour is divided into lobules by a fibrous stroma, associated with a variable infiltration of lymphocytes.

Spread of seminoma may be local to the epididymis and to the spermatic cord, but lymphatic spread is more important. The first group of nodes to be invaded is the upper para-aortic, at the level of the renal hilum. Further lymphatic spread may be upwards to the mediastinum and even the supraclavicular nodes through the thoracic duct, or downwards to the lower para-aortic and pelvic nodes. If extratesticular tissues of the scrotum are invaded, including the scrotal skin, their draining inguinal lymph nodes may be invaded. Blood-borne spread is much less common.

Spermatocytic seminoma is uncommon and generally seen in older men. The tumour cells show differentiation to spermatocytes, and their behaviour is benign. Metastases are extremely rare.

2. Teratoma. Teratoma accounts for the remainder of germ cell tumours. Strictly speaking, a teratoma shows differentiation towards all three embryological germ cell layers of ectoderm (e.g. skin, neural tissue),

endoderm (e.g. gut, bronchi) and mesoderm (e.g. fat, cartilage). In practice, the British classification applies the term more widely (while American terminology refers to this group as non-seminomatous germ cell tumours). Teratomas are subtyped according to their cell constituents as:

— Teratoma differentiated
— Malignant teratoma intermediate
— Malignant teratoma undifferentiated
— Malignant teratoma trophoblastic.

Teratoma differentiated (TD) shows cysts lined by various mature-looking epithelium surrounded by smooth muscle, with islands of cartilage and neural tissue. In infants its behaviour is benign, but in adults it is rare and can give rise to metastases. *Malignant teratoma undifferentiated* (MTU), by contrast, has no recognisable differentiated structures, but has undifferentiated rather than carcinomatous tissue. It often has tissue resembling yolk sac (YST), and there are frequently syncytiotrophoblast giant cells. These account for secretion of alpha-fetoprotein (AFP) and human chorionic gonadotrophin (HCG) respectively, which can be measured in the blood and are invaluable as markers of tumour load. It has an aggressive clinical behaviour with early metastasis via lymphatics to para-aortic lymph nodes, and blood-borne spread to the lungs. *Malignant teratoma intermediate* (MTI) has a mixture of differentiated and undifferentiated tissues. *Malignant teratoma trophoblastic* (MTT) has tissue resembling gestational choriocarcinoma (i.e. syncytiotrophoblast and cytotrophoblast), either throughout or in combination with features of other teratomas. Large amounts of HCG are secreted and the clinical course is very aggressive with widespread blood-borne metastases.

Tumour markers

The two tumour markers AFP and HCG are helpful in the diagnosis, staging and monitoring of response to treatment (Fig. 25.11). AFP has a half-life of about 5 days. It is produced by yolk sac elements but is not specific to teratoma. Elevated levels occur in the presence of liver damage. HCG is mainly a marker of trophoblastic neoplasms; it can, however, occur in seminoma. The half-life of HCG is 24 hours and of the beta subunit 45 minutes. Markers for the presence of seminoma are much less reliable. Serum placental alkaline phosphatase (PLAP) is often raised in the presence of seminoma, particularly if there is bulky disease. However false-positive and false-negative results for PLAP are common.

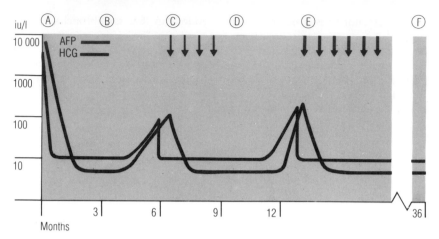

Fig. 25.11　Tumour markers in the management of testicular cancer. **A**. Both HCG and AFP are elevated before orchidectomy but fall following operation (HCG more rapidly because of its short half-life). **B**. No evidence of recurrence, followed by a rise in marker levels. **C**. Combination chemotherapy for recurrence is followed by a fall in levels to normal (**D**). **E**. A further rise in marker levels is treated more intensively and the patient is disease free at 3 years **F**. (Reproduced with permission from Souhami & Moxham, Textbook of Medicine, Churchill Livingstone, 1990.)

Clinical features

The usual presentation is a gradually enlarging painless testicular swelling. The tumour feels hard. In 10–20% of patients there is associated pain in the testis or the lower abdomen. The first symptoms and signs may be of metastatic spread (haemoptysis from lung metastases, back pain from para-aortic metastases, loin pain from ureteric obstruction or neck lymphadenopathy). Malignant teratoma trophoblastic (choriocarcinoma) may produce gynaecomastia (breast enlargement).

Table 25.4　The Royal Marsden Hospital staging classification of testicular tumours

Stage	Clinical findings
I	No evidence of metastases
Mk+	Rising serum markers with no other evidence of metastases
II	Abdominal node involvement
a	<2 cm diameter
b	2–5 cm diameter
c	>5 cm diameter
III	Nodal involvement above the diaphragm
IV	Extralymphatic metastases
L1	Lung metastases three or less in number
L2	Lung metastases more than three in number (all 2 cm or less in diameter)
L3	Lung metastases more than three in number (more than 2 cm in diameter)

Diagnosis and staging

The diagnosis is made by surgical removal of the testis through an inguinal incision (inguinal orchidectomy) and histological examination. Immunocytochemical stains of the tumour for the presence of AFP and HCG may be positive. Blood levels of AFP and HCG are measured pre- and postoperatively. A chest radiograph is required (for overt lung metastases), together with a CT scan of the thorax (for small volume lung and mediastinal metastases) and of the abdomen (abdominal nodal and liver metastases). If the CT scan is equivocal about the presence of small volume (<1 cm) abdominal nodes, a lymphangiogram may help clarify whether or not the nodes are involved.

The Royal Marsden staging classification (Table 25.4), based on the extent of spread and the bulk of disease, is widely used for determining management.

Treatment

1. Seminoma

Stage I. Postoperative abdominal node irradiation should be given routinely.

Target volume
Postoperative radiotherapy to the ipsilateral pelvic and para-aortic nodes is recommended (Fig. 25.12). The field should include the inguinal scar. The upper margin of the para-aortic field is at the level of the junction of

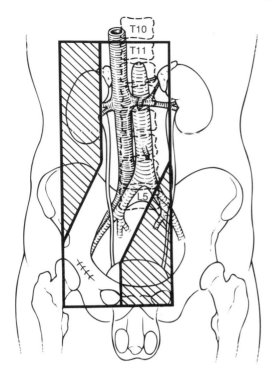

Fig. 25.12 Treatment volume for ipsilateral pelvic and para-aortic ('dog leg') irradiation for testicular seminoma.

Table 25.5   BEP chemotherapy regime

Bleomycin	30 mg i.v. bolus	Days	2,9,16
Etoposide	120 mg/m^2 i.v. infusion	Days	1,3,5
Cisplatin	20 mg/m^2 i.v. infusion	Days	1,2,3,4,5

Repeated every 21 days for 4 cycles

urogram (IVU) during simulation is essential to verify the position of the kidneys.

Stage IIa and IIb. For this stage the pelvic nodes are treated on both sides in addition to the para-aortic nodes. The field shape is that of an inverted Y. Planning is as for an 'inverted Y' used for the lymphomas (p. 448).

Dose and energy
Seminoma is one of the most radiosensitive of all cancers and can be cured with relatively modest doses. **30 Gy in 20 daily fractions over 4 weeks (9–10 MV photons)**

Acute reaction. About 50% of patients will experience nausea lasting for 2–3 hours following treatment.

Late reactions. Late side-effects are rare. Dyspepsia occurs in 5%, occasionally with evidence of peptic ulceration. Using the radiation technique and dosage described the dose to the contralateral testis is very low (less than 0.5 Gy). None the less this dose is sufficient to cause a moderate reduction in sperm count for 2–3 years, but it is not associated with permanent infertility.

Stage IIc, III and IV. In stage IIc where there are bulky abdominal nodes it is difficult to avoid irradiating more than one-third of the renal substance on both sides. Combination chemotherapy with bleomycin, etoposide and cisplatin (BEP) (Table 25.5) is recommended for these stages. Some radiotherapists still irradiate the abdominal nodes (inverted Y) following chemotherapy but this is probably not essential. It may be difficult to deliver the planned dose due to bone marrow suppression from chemotherapy.

Mediastinal relapse. Mediastinal relapse of seminoma can be controlled by mediastinal irradiation.

Target volume
This includes the mediastinal nodes and the supraclavicular fossae.

Technique
Parallel opposed anterior and posterior fields are used (Fig. 25.13).

Dose and energy
30 Gy in 20 daily fractions over 4 weeks (9–10 MV photons)

the 10th and 11th thoracic vertebrae. The lower limit is the lower border of the obturator foramen. This 'dog leg' shaped field is vertical in the para-aortic region and diverges at the level of the junction of the fourth and fifth lumbar vertebrae.

It is not necessary to include the scrotum and inguinal nodes on the affected side except under the following circumstances:

1. Surgical removal of the tumour through a scrotal incision.
2. Previous surgical transposition of an undescended testis into the scrotum (orchidopexy).
3. Previous repair of a scrotal hernia (herniorrhaphy).
4. Direct tumour infiltration of the scrotal skin.

Technique
An anterior and posterior pair of fields is used. The patient is simulated supine for the anterior field and prone for the posterior field. Extended FSD is required (about 140 cm). Ideally customised MCP blocks should be made to protect tissue outside the treatment volume. Care should be taken not to include more than one-third of the renal substance within the para-aortic fields on either side. The width of the para-aortic field is normally 8–10 cm. An intravenous

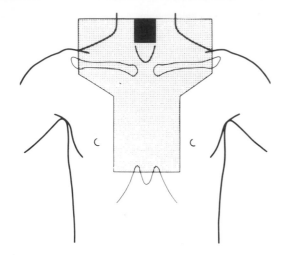

Fig. 25.13 Treatment volume for irradiation of the mediastinum and supraclavicular fossae. (Reproduced with permission from Easson & Pointon, The Radiotherapy of Malignant Disease, Ist edn, Springer-Verlag, 1985.)

Results of treatment

The results of treatment in early stage seminoma are excellent, reflecting its radiosensitivity: 5-year survival rates are 95% for stage I and 90% for stage IIa and IIb. For more advanced stages cure rates have improved with the availability of effective combination chemotherapy: 5-year survival for stages IIc and III is 75% and for stage IV 65%.

2. Teratoma

Stage I. Teratoma is less radiosensitive than seminoma and has a higher incidence of extralymphatic spread. About 25% of patients with stage I disease will have subclinical metastases and will relapse. For this reason a policy of close surveillance only is recommended for selected patients with stage I disease. In the presence of extralymphatic metastases, irradiating the para-aortic nodes prophylactically may compromise the ability to deliver subsequent combination chemotherapy at desired dosage and frequency.

A number of histological features of the primary tumour increase the risk of relapse in stage I disease. These are:

— Lymphatic invasion
— Vascular invasion
— Presence of undifferentiated cells (MTU)
— Absence of yolk sac elements.

If the patient has three or more of these risk factors, the risk of recurrence is 60%. Such patients are best treated by adjuvant combination chemotherapy rather than surveillance.

Surveillance. For patients for whom a surveillance policy is adopted, tumour markers are measured monthly in the first year with 2-monthly outpatient clinical examination and 3-monthly CT scans of chest and abdomen. In the absence of evidence of disease, outpatient examination, measurement of tumour markers and CT scan should be 3-monthly in the second year, 4-monthly in the third year, 6-monthly in the fourth year and annually from the fifth year. If the original tumour markers were negative, CT scans in the second year can be delayed until 24 months.

Stages II–IV. These stages should be managed by combination chemotherapy (see below).

Cytotoxic chemotherapy. The development of curative combination chemotherapy for advanced testicular cancer in the 1980s has been one of the most important advances in oncology.

The combinations of drugs used for treating seminoma are the same for teratoma. The most effective regimes contain cisplatin. Cisplatin was successfully combined with vinblastine and bleomycin (PVB). Now vinblastine is commonly replaced by etoposide, which is less myelotoxic, without loss of efficacy. This regime is known as BEP (Table 25.5). Carboplatin is much less toxic than cisplatin and appears to be as effective. It is not toxic to the kidney or the auditory or peripheral nerves and is less antiemetic. Carboplatin is likely to progressively replace cisplatin.

Before each course of chemotherapy a number of investigations are carried out to assess fitness to treat and, if necessary, to modify dosage due to the toxicity of the agents. A full blood count is required because of the myelotoxicity of vinblastine and etoposide.

Cisplatin is toxic to the kidney and to hearing. Renal function tests (serum urea, electrolytes and creatinine, 24-hour urine creatinine clearance) and hearing (audiometry) should be measured before, during and after treatment.

Bleomycin can be toxic to the lung (see below). Full lung function tests (including gas transfer factor) are carried out before treatment and repeated if toxicity is suspected.

Sperm storage, if available, is desirable for men wishing to father children following chemotherapy since sterility is commonly induced. Normally an initial sample is examined tc count the number and motility of the sperm. If satisfactory, two additional samples are taken for sperm banking. However chemotherapy, if urgently required, should not be delayed to await this procedure.

Dosage and scheduling. Normally a minimum of four

and a maximum of six courses of BEP are given at 3-weekly intervals. This usually represents two courses beyond clinical, radiological and tumour marker evidence of complete remission.

Monitoring response to treatment. Clinical examination, chest radiograph, tumour markers, full blood count, renal function tests and audiometry are repeated before each cycle of treatment to monitor the response to and toxicity of treatment.

Following surgery a fall in tumour marker levels in line with their half-lives usually indicates that there is no residual disease. A slower fall or rising levels suggest residual disease.

It may be necessary to delay the next cycle of chemotherapy or modify its dosage if blood count, renal function or hearing deteriorate below certain thresholds. Chemotherapy should not be given if the white blood cell count is below $2.0 \times 10^9/l$. CT scan of chest and abdomen is repeated after three cycles to confirm that the disease is responding. Rapid resolution of disease is usual after the first course. Residual 2–4 cm masses may however persist for several years.

Management of residual abdominal masses. Resection of residual abdominal masses following chemotherapy shows that most of them (44%) are due to differentiated (mature) teratoma or to fibrosis and necrosis (34%). Residual tumour is found in 22%. If recurrence occurs, as it does in 10–20% of patients, it is most likely to develop at a site of initial involvement. If surgical expertise is available, resection of residual masses is desirable. It serves both as a diagnostic and therapeutic procedure. Further chemotherapy is indicated if residual disease is found, but the outlook is poor, with less than 50% of such patients remaining free of disease.

An alternative, where such surgery is not undertaken and in absence of disease elsewhere, is to irradiate these residual abdominal masses.

Target volume

This should cover the residual mass with a margin of 1–2 cm of normal tissue.

Technique

As for seminoma (see above). Individualised MCP blocks are not required.

Dose and energy

35 Gy in 20 daily fractions over 4 weeks (9–10 MV photons)

Toxicity. In addition to renal damage and ototoxicity (impaired hearing), cisplatin causes severe nausea and

vomiting and peripheral neuropathy. Nausea and vomiting can be reduced by the anti-5HT antagonists (ondansetron and granisetron). Regular sedation (e.g. lorazepam) is given during chemotherapy. Intravenous hydration is required 24 hours before cisplatin is given and for 24 hours afterwards to reduce the risk of renal damage. None the less the majority of patients will experience renal damage. A 20–25% reduction in glomerular filtration rate is usual.

Etoposide causes alopecia and myelosuppression. The incidence of septicaemia with etoposide is less than with vinblastine since it is less myelosuppressive.

Bleomycin may cause pneumonitis. Presentation is with progressive dyspnoea. This complication may occur after relatively modest doses (e.g. 200 mg). It can be progressive, is irreversible and carries a 1% mortality. Other side-effects are fever, skin rashes, pigmentation and Raynaud's phenomenon.

Results of treatment

Ninety per cent of patients with small volume disease are cured following chemotherapy. For large volume disease in extralymphatic sites, the probability of survival is reduced to 50–70%.

The 5-year survival is 90% for stages I and IIa, 70% for stages IIb and III, and 50–60% for stage IV.

TESTICULAR LYMPHOMA

Testicular lymphomas are rare (4% of testicular tumours). They are mainly non-Hodgkin lymphomas. Clinical features that help to differentiate them from germ cell tumours are bilaterality (20% at presentation or subsequently), older age group (over 50 years), different pattern of metastases, absence of maldescent and of gynaecomastia. They are usually of high grade (poorly differentiated lymphocytic or histiocytic). Stages I and IIa should be treated by radical orchidectomy and postoperative combination chemotherapy followed by para-aortic and pelvic irradiation. If the patient is fit enough, CHOP (Table 26.8) is an appropriate chemotherapy regime (Ch. 26). Treatment technique is as for seminoma. For stages III and IV, chemotherapy is the treatment of choice. For the lymphoblastic type, prophylactic CNS irradiation should be considered.

Dose and energy

35 Gy in 20 daily fractions over 4 weeks (9–10 MV photons)

Results of treatment

The prognosis is poor. Overall 5-year survival is 20%.

For stage I and IIa it is 40%. Average survival with stage IV disease is about 8 months.

URETHRA

Tumours of the urethra are rare and are usually transitional carcinomas. Predisposing factors are as for bladder cancer (p. 426). Presenting symptoms and signs are pain and haematuria.

Female urethra

The tumour is twice as common in women as in men. In the proximal third transitional carcinoma predominates and in the distal two-thirds squamous carcinoma predominates. The distal urethra drains to the inguinal nodes and the proximal urethra to the iliac nodes. Presenting features are offensive discharge, bleeding or a mass.

Treatment

For superficial squamous carcinoma of the urethral orifice, a permanent gold grain (gold-198) implant delivering 55 Gy at 0.5 cm is used. For more proximal lesions radical external beam irradiation using an anterior and two lateral wedged fields is used. A dose of 55 Gy is given in 20 daily fractions over 4 weeks at megavoltage.

Results of treatment

The cure rates with surgery and radiotherapy are similar at about 50%.

PENIS

Cancer of the penis is a rare tumour responsible for 0.4% of all cancers and 0.1% of cancer deaths. It occurs in older men, typically between 50 and 70 years old. The disease is commoner in South-east Asia, China and Africa.

Pathology

Aetiology

The disease rarely occurs among peoples who practise circumcision (for example Jews and Muhammadans). There is a high incidence in Hindus, who are never circumcised. Phimosis is present in up to 50% of cases. Poor penile hygiene is thought to be an important predisposing factor. No infective agent has been conclusively demonstrated, although there is an association with human papilloma virus infections. There are several premalignant conditions, including viral warts (condyloma acuminata) and erythroplasia of Queyrat. The primary tumours are squamous carcinomas, usually well differentiated. Secondary deposits are rare but can occur from prostate and bladder cancer.

Clinical features

These tumours occur as warty growths or, more commonly, as indurated ulcers on the glans or the sulcus at the base of the glans. Symptoms have often been present for a year or more before presentation. The first sign may be an infected or bloody discharge from beneath the prepuce. Growth is superficial at first, then by invasion of the penile shaft. If the lesion is visible the diagnosis is usually obvious. If phimosis hides it, the glans must be exposed by incising and peeling back the prepuce (dorsal slit) or by complete circumcision, under anaesthesia. A biopsy is taken at the same time.

Lymphatic spread occurs early to the inguinal nodes, though enlargement here may simply reflect infection. The nodes may eventually ulcerate. Blood-borne metastases are rare and late.

Staging

Both TNM and Jackson staging systems are in use (Table 25.6). If inguinal nodes are enlarged, needle aspiration to distinguish tumour from infection should be carried out. A CT scan of the pelvis may show the extent of abdominal lymphadenopathy.

Table 25.6 TNM and Jackson staging systems for penile cancer

Stage	Clinical findings
Tumour	
T1	Superficial tumour <1 cm
T2	Superficial tumour >1 cm
T3	Invasion of underlying tissues
T4	Invasion of local structures: corpora cavernosa, urethra, perineum or prostate
Nodes	
N0	No regional nodes
N1	Unilateral regional nodes
N2	Multiple unilateral nodes or bilateral nodes
N3	Deep inguinal or pelvic nodes
Metastases	
M0	No distant metastases
M1	Distant metastases present
Jackson classification	
I	Tumour confined to the glans or prepuce
II	Tumour extending on to the shaft of the penis
III	Tumour with operable inguinal nodes
IV	Tumour with inoperable metastases

Treatment

Surgery and radiotherapy are the main treatments for penile cancer. Factors which influence the choice of treatment are the age and general condition of the patient, the extent of the disease, the desire to retain sexual function and the capacity to pass urine in the standing position for young males.

Surgery

Surgery involves amputation of part or the whole of the penis. Although curative in 70% if the inguinal nodes are not involved, the procedure is obviously objectionable, especially for young males.

Radiotherapy

Radical radiotherapy is the treatment of choice for early penile cancer since it permits the organ to be conserved. However if there is deep invasion of the shaft, the chances of control by radiation are poor and surgery is preferable. Invasion of the urethra also favours surgery, since postradiation fibrotic stricture is very liable to occur.

Treatment techniques and dosage

The choice of technique and energy will depend on the extent and site of the disease. For tumours confined to the glans or the prepuce, superficial, orthovoltage, electron beam or implant are possibilities. For infiltrating tumours or where the inguinal nodes are involved, megavoltage irradiation is required.

Implantation. A single or double plane implant with iridium-192 should include within the target volume a 2 cm margin around the tumour. Tumours greater than 4 cm in any dimension or invading the corpora cavernosa should not be implanted.

The implant (Fig. 19.6) is carried out under a general anaesthetic and following catheterisation. The penis is held upright and away from the testicles and thighs by foam padding secured by adhesive tape to the thighs. The dose to the testis is usually up to 3 Gy. This can be reduced by interposing 2–3 mm of lead shielding, if fertility needs to be conserved. The dose to the reference isodose using the Paris system should be 60–65 Gy. Duration of treatment is normally 6–7 days.

Superficial or orthovoltage therapy. For very small (T1) superficial tumours 100 kV or 250 kV X-ray therapy may suffice. A 0.5 cm margin of normal surrounding tissue is included in the treated volume. A dose of 50 Gy is given in 15 fractions over 3 weeks. Alternatively low energy (6 MeV) electrons can be used using an appropriate thickness of Perspex over the lesion to bring up the surface dose to 100%.

Megavoltage

Treatment volume

If there is evidence of spread on to the shaft of the penis, the whole of the penis should be treated.

Technique

A rectangular wax block with a central cylindrical cavity is made to encompass the penis and ensure homogeneous irradiation of the whole volume. The penis is treated en bloc by a parallel opposed pair of lateral fields.

Dose and energy

50–55 Gy in 20 daily fractions over 4 weeks at megavoltage (4–6 MV photons)

Acute reactions. These are like skin reactions elsewhere but more marked, and moist desquamation is commoner. The urethral reaction causes discomfort and dysuria. If very severe it may result in acute retention requiring catheterisation.

Late reactions. These include telangiectasia, skin atrophy, urethral stricture and necrosis. Urethral dilatation is required for stricture. Necrosis occurs in less than 10% of cases.

Management of regional nodes

If inguinal nodes are found to be histologically involved at presentation, a block dissection of the groin should be carried out, followed by radical radiotherapy to the primary. There is no value in giving prophylactic groin node irradiation. The only role for radiotherapy in the treatment of groin nodes is for palliation.

Palliative radiotherapy

Technique

A simple parallel opposed pair of fields to the affected groin.

Dose and energy

30 Gy in 10 daily fractions over 2 weeks at megavoltage or cobalt-60

Results of treatment

Early superficial tumours have a high cure rate: 5-year survival for stage I disease is about 90%. This falls to 60% in stage II and 30–40% in stage III.

26. Lymphoreticular tissues and bone marrow

MALIGNANT LYMPHOMAS

The term 'lymphoma' covers all the primary malignancies of lymph nodes. The two main types of lymphoma are Hodgkin's disease and non-Hodgkin lymphoma. The histological classification of Hodgkin's disease, known as the Rye classification, is widely accepted. In contrast, the classification of the non-Hodgkin lymphomas is more complex. This is due to the variety of cytological appearances and the capacity to identify different cell surface markers using immunohistochemical techniques. As a result there are several different classifications in use.

HODGKIN'S DISEASE

Pathology

Epidemiology

Hodgkin's disease is uncommon. It accounts for 0.7% of all cancers and 0.4% of cancer deaths. In the UK the incidence per 100 000 population per year is 2.65 for men and 1.81 for women. It has two age peaks. The first is between 25 and 34 years in males and the second in old age. The disease is commoner in Jews in the UK , USA and Israel. The incidence is substantially lower in the Japanese and black Americans. The reasons for these ethnic variations are unclear.

Hodgkin's disease is commoner among the higher social classes. One hypothesis is that the disease is a rare sequel of a common infection in children (for nodular sclerosing but not other histological subtypes). Children in higher social classes who tend to be educated in a protected environment may be exposed to the infection later than children of lower social class. This may explain the later age of onset in children of higher social class.

Considerable differences in incidence occur between regions of the UK. No satisfactory explanation for these differences is available. There is no evidence that they are related to pollution from industrial plants.

Aetiology

The aetiological agent(s) responsible for Hodgkin's disease have not been identified. It seems likely that a number of factors may have to interact in order for the disease to develop. These include genetic susceptibility, infection and altered immunity.

The higher incidence in males and the slight excess of the disease in Jews suggest that genetic factors may be important. A genetic basis is also supported by the higher incidence in certain families. In Yorkshire 6% of all cases had one or more additional lymphoma or leukaemia sufferers among blood relatives; 50% of these were due to Hodgkin's disease.

Some time ago it was suggested that the disease had a different aetiology for each age peak. The peak in early adulthood (<35 years) was postulated to be due to infection. Common viral infections were thought to be responsible. Part of the Epstein–Barr virus (EBV) was particularly commonly isolated in Hodgkin's disease. The link between EBV and Hodgkin's disease was thought to be similar to that between EBV and both nasopharyngeal carcinoma (p. 327) and Burkitt's lymphoma. The link between EBV and Hodgkin's disease is not a strong one. It may be that other agents, as yet unknown, are operating.

In addition, Hodgkin's disease has been associated with certain dusty (particularly wood dust) occupations thought to induce allergic reactions.

Microscopic features

Hodgkin's disease is characterised by the replacement of normal lymphoid tissue by atypical mononuclear cells, multinucleate Reed–Sternberg cells and a variable number of chronic inflammatory cells. Oddly for a neoplasm, malignant cells are in the minority. The majority are made up of cells such as lymphocytes, histiocytes, plasma cells, granulocytes and fibroblasts.

Reed-Sternberg cells are large. They have eosinophilic cytoplasm and often a perinuclear halo. The presence of Reed-Sternberg cells in an appropriate context is essential for the diagnosis of Hodgkin's disease.

Histological classification (Rye). There are four main types of Hodgkin's disease.

1. Lymphocyte predominant (LP) <10%. This is uncommon. Reed–Sternberg cells are very scarce, and the tumour is dominated by lymphocytes and sometimes histiocytes.

2. Nodular sclerosing (NS) 60%. This is characterised by the division of the node into nodules. The nodules of tumour contain Reed–Sternberg (RS) cells; these often lie in little spaces or lacunae. Nodular sclerosing disease has been further subdivided into grades 1 (low grade) and 2 (high grade). Grade 2 shows depletion of lymphocytes or numerous Hodgkin's cells. All other cases are assigned to grade 1. These two grades have different prognoses (see later in this chapter).

Nodular sclerosing Hodgkin's disease has an equal sex distribution. It tends to affect the mediastinum and to occur in the young adult.

3. Mixed cellularity (MC) 15%. As the term implies, a variety of cells are present. These include Reed–Sternberg cells and non-neoplastic cells such as plasma cells, eosinophils, neutrophils and lymphocytes.

4. Lymphocyte depleted (LD) 5%. This is characterised by very atypical RS cells and few lymphocytes. Diffuse fibrosis is present.

Before accurate staging and curative chemotherapy was available, each histological subtype had prognostic significance. Prognosis was best for lymphocyte predominant and worst for lymphocyte depleted. Now the only histological type with definite prognostic significance is lymphocyte depleted. This carries a poor 5-year survival of 20%. All other subtypes have a similar survival. Grade 1 tends to have a better prognosis than grade 2.

Clinical features

The first symptom is usually painless enlargement of a group of nodes, most commonly in the neck (60%) (Fig. 26.1), but occasionally in the axilla (20%) or in the inguinal/femoral region (15%). The left side of the neck is slightly more commonly involved than the right. The size of the nodes may wax and wane. The spleen (10%) or liver (7%) may be palpably enlarged.

In 25–30% of patients systemic or B symptoms are the presenting features. There are three B symptoms: fever (>38°C), night sweats and weight loss (>10% of body weight in previous 6 months). General malaise also occurs.

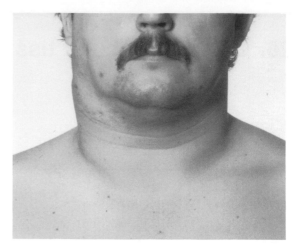

Fig. 26.1 Typical cervical lymphadenopathy in early Hodgkin's disease.

There may be a characteristic fever (Pel–Ebstein) in waves lasting a week or two separated by afebrile intervals. Itching (pruritus) occurs in 12% but is not a B symptom. Patients without systemic symptoms are designated as A (i.e. absence of systemic symptoms). The designation of 'A' or 'B' is always added as part of the Ann Arbor staging classification (see under Investigations).

A peculiar symptom of unknown cause is severe pain in lymph nodes after taking even very small quantities of alcohol.

Investigations

The first step is usually lymph node biopsy to establish the diagnosis and the histological type. It is essential

Table 26.1 Ann Arbor staging classification of Hodgkin's disease

Stage	Clinical findings
I	Involvement of a single lymph node region (I) or of a single extralymphatic organ or site (IE)
II	Involvement of two or more lymph node regions on the same side of the diaphragm (II) or localised involvement of an extralymphatic organ or site and one or more lymph node regions on the same side of the diaphragm (IIE)
III	Involvement of lymph node regions on both sides of the diaphragm (III) which may be accompanied by localised involvement of an extralymphatic organ or site (IIIE) or by involvement of the spleen (IIIS) or both (IIISE)
IV	Disseminated involvement of one or more extralymphatic organs or tissues with or without associated lymph node involvement

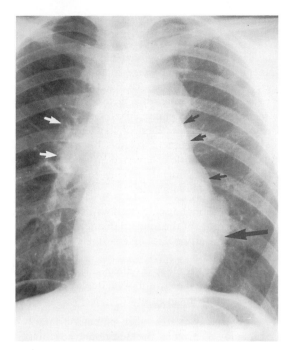

Fig. 26.2 Chest radiograph showing enlarged mediastinal nodes (small arrows) and pericardial nodes (large arrow) due to Hodgkin's disease. (Courtesy of Dr R Nakielny, Sheffield.)

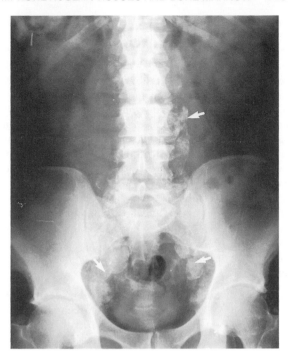

Fig. 26.3 Lymphangiogram showing typical enlarged 'foamy' pelvic and para-aortic nodes (arrowed) due to Hodgkin's disease. (Courtesy of Dr R Nakielny, Sheffield.)

to establish the extent of the disease (staging) since this will influence the choice of treatment. The Ann Arbor staging classification is the most commonly used and is applicable both to Hodgkin's disease and non-Hodgkin lymphoma. It describes the anatomical distribution of lymph node involvement as well as of extranodal disease (Table 26.1)

The following basic tests should be carried out:

1. Full blood count and ESR (erythrocyte sedimentation rate)
2. Serum urea and electrolytes, calcium
3. Liver function tests
4. Chest X-ray (Fig. 26.2)
5. CT of chest and abdomen.

Radiological detection of intra-abdominal disease

At presentation about 35% of patients will have disease below the diaphragm. Of these only 8% will have clinically detectable nodes. It is therefore of considerable importance to know whether the nodes are involved or not. CT scanning has largely replaced bipedal lymphangiography (Fig. 26.3) as the principal radiological investigation. Lymphangiography is useful if the CT scan is normal or equivocal and there is a strong suspicion that the nodes are involved.

CT scanning can detect significant enlargement of nodes (>1 cm) but cannot detect evidence of Hodgkin's disease in normal sized nodes (≤1 cm).

Clinical and pathological staging

There are two types of staging, *clinical* and *pathological*. Clinical staging is based upon the history, physical examination, blood chemistry, biopsy and radiological investigations. Pathological staging includes, in addition to the above, a staging laparotomy to establish the extent of intra-abdominal disease.

A staging laparotomy involves the careful inspection of the abdominal contents, a splenectomy and liver biopsy. In addition, the lymph nodes in the porta hepatis, coeliac axis and in the mesentery (none of which are demonstrable by lymphography), as well as the upper para-aortic, iliac and mesenteric nodes are biopsied. Any suspicious nodes on lymphography or CT scanning can also be sampled.

This operation has provided a great deal of information about the intra-abdominal extent of the disease. However it is now no longer carried out as a routine procedure for a number of reasons.

1. Combination chemotherapy is able to cure a substantial proportion of patients who relapse after

radiotherapy. Hence, knowing whether there is intra-abdominal disease at presentation is not essential.

2. A variety of prognostic factors (e.g. ESR, pathological grade and age) are able to predict with reasonable accuracy the probability of intra-abdominal involvement in an individual patient.

3. The morbidity and mortality even in skilled hands are not insubstantial. There is a major complication rate of about 8%, of which half are fatal. Serious infections (particularly pneumococcal) occur in 3% of patients. There is a minor complication rate of about 30% (e.g. wound infection).

4. The survival of patients who have not undergone staging laparotomy is similar to comparable patients who have.

Prognostic factors and their influence on the need for laparotomy

A variety of prognostic factors have been identified in stage I and IIa Hodgkin's disease which appear to predict the outcome of therapy. The British National Lymphoma Investigation (BNLI) analysis shows the following to be adverse prognostic factors:

— Age over 60
— High ESR
— Male sex
— High grade histology
— Multiple nodal sites
— Bulky disease
— Reduced lymphocyte count
— Low serum albumin
— Extranodal extension.

Treatment of Hodgkin's disease

In general radical radiotherapy is the treatment of choice for early Hodgkin's disease and chemotherapy for those with advanced disease (III and IV), systemic 'B' symptoms or poor prognostic factors. Treatment by stage is summarised in Table 26.2.

Table 26.2 Treatment of Hodgkin's disease by stage

Stage	Treatment
Ia IIa	Radiotherapy
IIa (bulky mediastinum)	Chemotherapy + radiotherapy
Ib IIb IIIa IIIb IVa IVb	Chemotherapy

Treatment of early Hodgkin's disease in adults (Stages I and IIa)

In the early 1980s locoregional radiotherapy was the treatment of choice for stage I and IIa Hodgkin's disease. This approach has changed for two reasons: the recognition of prognostic factors for relapse and treatment-induced second malignancy.

Prognostic factors. First, it has been shown that some of these patients if treated by extended field irradiation (e.g. mantle or inverted Y) run a higher risk of relapse. They frequently require to be salvaged by chemotherapy. These include:

— Bulky mediastinal disease (tumour mass occupying a third or more of the internal diameter of the thoracic cage at the level of T5–6)
— ESR >50 mm/hr
— Unfavourable histology (nodular sclerosing grade 2, mixed cellularity, or lymphocyte depleted histology)
— Three or more involved sites.

It seems logical to treat such patients primarily by chemotherapy. This has the additional advantage of avoiding the myelosuppressive effects of extended field irradiation which may limit the patient's capacity to tolerate subsequent chemotherapy in full dosage.

Choice of target volume. The terms 'involved' and 'extended' fields are commonly used in relation to the radiotherapy of Hodgkin's disease. 'Involved' field means one confined to the involved area of disease plus a small margin of surrounding normal tissue. 'Extended' field means encompassing the involved nodes plus all the other nodal areas above the diaphragm (mantle) or below the diaphragm (inverted Y). Both mantle and involved field radiation are in common use.

Radiation technique. Hodgkin's disease in lymph nodes tends to spread in continuity to adjacent lymph nodes. The inclusion of both involved and adjacent uninvolved nodes (extended field irradiation) within the irradiated volume increased the cure rate compared to irradiating the involved nodes alone. 'Mantle' (Fig. 26.4) and 'inverted Y' (Fig. 26.5) radiotherapy are the techniques of extended field irradiation for disease above and below the diaphragm respectively.

Mantle technique. The term derives from the similarity of the treatment fields to a cloak.

Target volume
The nodes of the neck, axilla, infraclavicular, para-tracheal, hilar and anterior mediastinal regions are included (Fig. 26.4).

Technique
The patient lies supine. The chin is extended to exclude

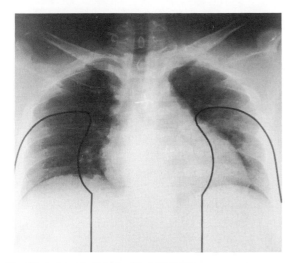

Fig. 26.4 Mantle field for Hodgkin's disease.

as much of the oral cavity as possible. The arms are slightly abducted with the hands on the hips. Anterior and posterior fields are used at extended SSD (120–140 cm).

The upper limit of the field is on a line joining the chin to the external occipital protuberance. This line passes through the mastoid process. The occipital, submental and submaxillary nodes are included in the volume. However Waldeyer's ring, the preauricular and parotid nodes are excluded. If Waldeyer's ring is involved, the field should extend up to the base of the skull.

The lower limit is the junction of the 10th and 11th thoracic vertebrae. The lateral border runs along the lateral margin of the axilla through the acromioclavicular joint.

The width of the mediastinal field is usually 8–10 cm, depending on the size of the nodes. It can be shaped to encompass any nodal masses. These can be measured most accurately from a CT scan of the thorax. It is helpful to outline palpable lymph node masses with lead wire prior to simulation to ensure adequate coverage.

Shielding

1. The lung is shielded lateral to the mediastinum, a curved line running along the lower border of the fourth rib posteriorly (Fig. 26.4).

2. The larynx may be shielded for half of the treatment by lead on the anterior field. However this should be avoided if there is adjacent lymphadenopathy, in case underdosage occurs.

3. Some clinicians also shield the cervical part of the spinal cord by a narrow 2 cm strip on the posterior

field to limit the spinal cord dose to 30 Gy. However, so doing results in a small area of underdosage in the middle of the mediastinum. Although the incidence of transient Lhermitte's sign is probably commoner if the cervical cord is not shielded, there is no evidence that the incidence of chronic radiation myelopathy is increased.

Spinal shielding should be avoided particularly where the cervical nodes or mediastinum are involved.

It is important not to shield the axilla and the infraclavicular areas since these may be sites of recurrence.

Three points are tattooed on the front and back of the chest: (1) the centre of the field, (2) a point 10 cm below the centre of the field, and (3) a third point is made midway between the first two points and 5 cm lateral to the midline (to ensure there is no rotation of the thorax). Lead markers are placed on all three points and a radiograph taken. The same procedure is repeated with the patient lying prone. The clinician draws on the simulator films the outline of the lung blocks (Fig. 26.4). Lung blocks are then prepared (p. 51). A verification film is taken on the linear accelerator and compared with the simulator film. The medial ends of the clavicles and the spinous processes of the vertebrae usually provide useful bony landmarks on the portal film.

Dose distribution. The neck and the axilla are the thinnest structures in the anteroposterior plane. The midplane dose to the axillae and neck would receive 10–15% and 15–20% more dose respectively, compared with the mediastinum, if no attempt was made to compensate for these variations in thickness. This can be overcome by applying Lincolnshire bolus bags in the axillae and over the upper chest for anterior and posterior fields. The superior level of the bolus should be at the topmost point of the chest wall. The effect of the bolus is to convert an irregular volume into a box-shaped volume of uniform thickness.

Dose and energy
35 Gy midplane dose in 20 daily fractions over 4 weeks at megavoltage (6–10 MV photons)

Boost to involved sites given on successive days after mantle treatment completed:
5 Gy in 3 daily fractions (orthovoltage or 6–10 MV photons)

Bulky mediastinal disease. In the presence of Ia or IIa bulky mediastinal disease, the risk of pneumonitis is increased because of the greater volume of lung included in mantle fields. Initial treatment with three cycles of combination chemotherapy is advised. This usually shrinks the mediastinal nodes sufficiently for them to be encompassed with a conventional 8–10 cm wide field. If chemotherapy is not possible for any reason, a 'shrinking field' technique can be adopted. An initial 10 Gy in five daily fractions is given to mantle fields encompassing all the mediastinal disease. A week is then allowed without treatment to allow disease regression. New lung blocks are then made for a smaller mantle field and treatment continued over the remaining 3 weeks, giving a further 25 Gy. The same boost of 5 Gy in three daily fractions is given after 35 Gy in 5 weeks.

Side-effects

Acute. The main acute side-effects of mantle radiotherapy are anorexia, nausea, vomiting, sore throat, dry mouth, dysphagia, impaired taste and hair loss in the occipital region. Apart from altered taste and dry mouth, the other side-effects have normally settled by a month after treatment. Mucaine 10 ml p.r.n. and before meals usually diminishes dysphagia.

Dry mouth and altered taste. Inclusion of the sublingual, submaxillary and part of the parotid gland results in reducing the output of saliva and making it more viscous. Taste is impaired but usually returns within a period of 3 months. Artificial saliva may help. Regular mouth washes are encouraged. A dental assessment before treatment is essential. Caries should be dealt with. Regular dental assessment is necessary following treatment since caries are more likely to occur once the protective effect of normal saliva is diminished.

Skin reaction. In the latter half of treatment skin erythema develops. This is followed by desquamation, dry in most areas but often moist in the axilla. Exposure to the sun should be avoided during treatment and until the acute reaction has settled. Simple analgesia may be necessary. An emollient cream such as Oilatum is applied to areas of dry desquamation and gentian violet to moist desquamation once treatment is completed.

Alopecia occurs over the occiput, and beard growth is inhibited. The hair in both areas normally regrows by 3 months after treatment. Dry shaving is recommended during treatment to protect the skin.

Inverted Y technique

Target volume
This includes the paraortic, pelvic, iliac and femoral nodes (Fig. 26.5).

Technique
The patient is simulated supine for the anterior field

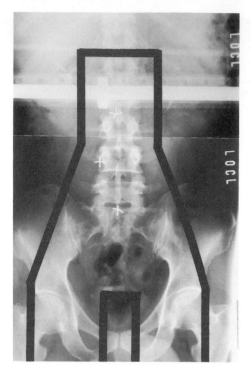

Fig. 26.5   Inverted Y fields for Hodgkin's and non-Hodgkin lymphoma.

and then prone for the posterior field. The patient lies straight with the legs together and hands straight at the side of couch. Anterior and posterior fields are used at extended SSD.

The upper margin of the field is the junction of the 10th and 11th thoracic vertebrae or inferior to the gap calculated to allow overlap of the 50% isodose at the level of the spinal cord if a mantle field has been previously treated. This gap is usually about 2 cm on the skin. The lower border is the inferior margin of the obturator foramen. The width of the field is guided by the size of the nodes on lymphography and on CT scanning. It is normally 8–10 cm wide.

The abdominal cavity lateral to the nodal areas outlined above is shielded with individualised MCP blocks.

Kidney. The medial 1–2 cm of each kidney are necessarily included in the field. In the absence of pre-existing renal damage, up to a third of each kidney can be irradiated without compromising renal function. The position of the kidneys is verified by an IVU carried out at the start of simulation

Ovaries. In young women the ovaries can be protected by transposing them at the time of surgery centrally to the inferior part of the body of the uterus (oophoropexy) and marking their position with clips. Lead blocks can then be placed over the new site of the ovaries. The only radiation that the ovaries then receive is from scattered radiation. This operation makes it possible for women to become pregnant while still receiving radical doses of radiation. Children born to such mothers do not show any evidence of impaired development.

Bladder and genitalia. A central rectangular block placed in the midline protects the ovaries (if transposed), the bladder and genitalia. Care should be taken not to shield involved nodes adjacent to the block. The block should be omitted if there is a risk of underdosage to these nodes.

The dose to the testis can be reduced by applying 1 cm thick lead cups around the testis. These can reduce the dose to the testis to 0.6 Gy out of a total dose of 40 Gy.

Acute reaction. Anorexia, nausea, vomiting, colicky abdominal pain and diarrhoea occur but should settle by 3 weeks after treatment. They can be reduced by avoidance of a low residue diet, particularly avoiding fruit and green vegetables.

Low blood counts are an inevitable consequence of wide field irradiation. The full blood count should be checked twice weekly on treatment. If the white cell count falls below $2 \times 10^9/l$ or platelets to less than $60 \times 10^9/l$, treatment should be suspended for a few days untill the blood count has risen above these levels. The blood count may need to be monitored more frequently thereafter.

Late effects. Late effects of radiation occur months or years after radiotherapy and tend to be permanent. These tend to be more marked in children because irradiation interferes with bone growth. Chemotherapy does not have this effect. It is therefore chosen in preference to wide field irradiation. Radiotherapy, if given, is restricted to the site of involvement.

Most late effects occur after mantle rather than inverted Y irradiation. The organs mainly affected are the thyroid, lung and heart.

Thyroid. Abnormally low thyroid function (biochemically) develops in 40% of patients. Less than 10%, however, are clinically hypothyroid. This complication usually develops insidiously several years after radiotherapy. Low serum thyroxine levels are often associated with elevated TSH (thyroid stimulating hormone). If the TSH level remains above normal, there is an increased risk of malignant transformation of the thyroid gland. Thyroxine should be given to suppress TSH. Thyroid function should be monitored intermittently.

Neurological. The most common syndrome is of numbness, tingling (paraesthesia) or an 'electric shock'-like sensation in the arms or legs following mantle or neck irradiation. It is often precipitated by flexion of the neck (Lhermitte's syndrome). It is thought to be due to transient demyelination of the spinal cord within the irradiated volume due to damage to oligodendrocytes. It occurs 2–4 months after treatment. It is important to stress that it does not lead on to permanent spinal cord damage (transverse myelitis) but it may last up to 6 months.

Transverse myelitis should not occur if the above dose and fractionation schedule is observed. It may however occur if there is mismatching of supra- and infradiaphragmatic fields or retreatment of a previously treated area.

Lung. Radiation pneumonitis is an uncommon complication unless substantial volumes of lung are included in the mantle field. This is more likely to occur where the mediastinal disease is bulky. Lung function is minimally impaired in about a third of patients undergoing mantle therapy. Symptoms are of nonproductive cough and dyspnoea, with or without fever. Chest radiography may show hazy shadowing in the central part of the lung fields. Treatment is with steroids (prednisolone 40–60mg /day). Provided that sufficient normal lung lies outside the treated area, the symptoms usually settle.

Lung fibrosis usually develops within the irradiated areas of lung in the mantle field over 4–18 months. Most patients have no respiratory symptoms.

Cardiac. Radiation induced cardiac disease occurs in less than 5% of patients. The incidence is higher in patients treated by a single anterior field rather than the conventional equally weighted parallel opposed pair of mantle therapy. It usually presents with features of acute pericarditis (fever, chest pain, pericardial friction rub), asymptomatic pericardial effusion noted on chest radiograph or rarely (<5%) with constrictive pericarditis and tamponade. Acute pericarditis usually settles with conservative management. Asymptomatic pericardial effusion usually resolves over several months. Constrictive pericarditis is more serious and may require surgery.

Bone. Avascular necrosis of the femoral head occurs in 2% of patients treated for Hodgkins's disease (Fig. 26.6). This is particularly likely following chemotherapy and intermittent steroid treatment. Inverted Y irradiation is also a contributory factor. Often, but not invariably, the patient has had the affected hip irradiated. Symptoms of hip pain develop on average about 2 years following the start of chemotherapy. If the condition progresses, total hip replacement may be necessary. Changes are not confined to the hips. The humeral head, for example, may also be affected.

Ovary and testis. Although the ovaries of younger women are more resistant to radiation, a dose of

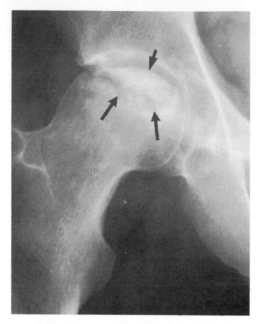

Fig. 26.6 Radiograph showing avascular necrosis of the femoral head in a patient treated with chemotherapy for Hodgkin's disease. (Courtesy of Professor B Hancock, Sheffield.)

1.2 Gy results in a high incidence of amenorrhoea, irrespective of pubertal status. Loss of ovarian function is rare if the dose to the ovary is 0.15 Gy or less. Transposition of the ovaries (see oophoropexy under Inverted Y) can achieve this.

The dose to the testes is determined by their relative depth and proximity to the edge of the beam during abdominopelvic irradiation. Little can be done to adjust the beam edge if pelvic nodes are to be adequately treated. With cobalt-60 the testicular dose may be up to 10% of the tumour dose (i.e. 3.5 Gy). This dose is sufficient to induce prolonged or permanent azoospermia and sterility. The dose can be reduced by 75% to 2.5% of the tumour dose (<1 Gy) by a lead protective shield surrounding the testis.

Growth. Growth retardation with reduction in both standing and sitting height is common in children who have received mantle radiotherapy. Thinning of the neck muscles and shortening of the clavicles may occur. The appreciation of these complications has resulted in the avoidance of mantle irradiation in children where possible, and treatment by primary chemotherapy and/or limited field irradiation (see below).

Chemotherapy

Combination chemotherapy has been outstandingly

Table 26.3 Chemotherapy regimes for Hodgkin's disease

MOPP

Nitrogen mustard 6 mg/m² i.v.	Days 1 and 8
Vincristine 1.4 mg/m² (max. 2 mg) i.v.	Days 1 and 8
Procarbazine 100 mg/m² orally	Days 1–14
Prednisolone 40 mg/m² orally	Days 1–14

Repeated every 6 weeks for 8 courses

LOPP

Chlorambucil (Leukeran) 10 mg orally	Days 1–10
Vincristine (Oncovin) 1.4 mg/m² (max. 2 mg) i.v. bolus	Days 1 and 8
Procarbazine 100 mg/m² (max. 200 mg) orally	Days 1–10
Prednisolone 25 mg/m² (max. 60 mg) orally	Days 1–14

Repeated every 28 days for 8 courses

ChlVPP

Chlorambucil 6 mg/m² (max. 10 mg) orally	Days 1–14
Vinblastine 6 mg/m² (max. 10 mg) i.v.	Days 1 and 8
Procarbazine 100 mg/m² orally	Days 1–14
Prednisolone 40 mg orally	Days 1–14

Repeated every 28 days

LOPP/EVAP
LOPP (as above) alternating with EVAP as below (minimum 4 courses)

EVAP

Etoposide 150 mg/m² (max. 200 mg) orally	Days 1–3
Vinblastine 6 mg/m² (max. 10 mg) i.v. bolus	Days 1 and 8
Adriamycin 25 mg/m² i.v. bolus	Days 1 and 8
Prednisolone 25 mg/m² (max. 60 mg) orally	Days 1–14

Repeated every 28 days

ABVD

Adriamycin 25 mg/m² i.v.	Days 1 and 15
Bleomycin 10 mg/m² i.v.	Days 1 and 15
Vinblastine 6 mg/m² i.v.	Days 1 and 15
DTIC 375 mg/m² i.v.	Days 1 and 15

Repeated every 28 days

successful in obtaining complete and prolonged remissions. It is the treatment of choice for stages Ib, IIb, IIIa, IIIb, IVa and IVb. It is also indicated in bulky mediastinal Hodgkin's disease to reduce the volume of disease before mantle radiotherapy (see above). Commonly used regimes are shown in Table 26.3.

Initially most chemotherapy was with MOPP. The nitrogen mustard component is highly emetic and has largely been replaced by chlorambucil (as in LOPP) because it is not emetic. LOPP has been found to be as effective and less toxic than MOPP. EVAP is one example of a non cross-resistant regime (i.e patients resistant to LOPP may respond to EVAP). LOPP/ EVAP is a hybrid regime under evaluation in which alternating courses of LOPP and EVAP are given. If a patient does not respond to LOPP or ChlVPP or responds and then relapses, EVAP or ABVD are possible salvage regimes. ABVD has a lower incidence of second malignancies than MOPP but has unpleasant side-effects. Two of its components, DTIC and bleomycin, are only moderately active against Hodgkin's disease. Adriamycin and etoposide in EVAP are more effective. EVAP is also generally better tolerated than ABVD. Responses are seen with these second line combinations but cure is rare.

Second malignancy. An increased incidence of both leukaemia (usually acute myeloid) and solid tumours has been observed in patients treated by radiotherapy, chemotherapy or both. For example the risk of patients developing acute myelogenous leukaemia is about 3–5% at 5 years in unselected cases of Hodgkin's disease followed for more than 5 years. The highest risk (10%) is in patients treated by a combination of chemotherapy (MOPP) and radiotherapy. The risk of leukaemia in patients treated with radiotherapy alone is thought to be small. It appears to be the chemotherapy, especially in regimes containing alkylating agents such as procarbazine, rather than radiotherapy that is mainly carcinogenic.

The risk of developing a solid tumour is more modest, at 4%, and is not associated with any particular form of treatment. A variety of tumours are seen. As a consequence, the current practice is to use either primary radiotherapy or chemotherapy but, if possible, to avoid combining them. An exception is bulky mediastinal disease. In this case initial chemotherapy is given (often three cycles) followed, if there has been adequate shrinkage, by mantle radiotherapy, and further chemotherapy (three cycles). The average number of cycles to achieve a complete response is three. Most patients require 6–8 courses. Maintenance chemotherapy beyond eight courses has not improved survival.

Response and survival. Both MOPP and LOPP can achieve complete response rates of 60–80% in advanced disease. Over half of those who achieve a complete response remain disease free at 5 years.

Toxicity. MOPP has considerable toxicity. It causes hair loss, nausea, severe vomiting and peripheral neuropathy. It renders virtually all males and a substantial number of females sterile.

ABVD causes more severe nausea and vomiting but moderate myelosuppression. There is an increased risk of late cardiac and pulmonary damage. However the risk of infertility and of second malignancies is reduced.

Results of treatment

The prognosis of Hodgkin's disease has improved with the advent of effective combination chemotherapy and more accurate staging. The overall 5-year survival is 70–80%. The results of treatment by stage and grade of histology are summarised in Table 26.4.

Relapsed Hodgkin's disease

Forty per cent or more of patients treated with MOPP or LOPP will relapse. Failure to achieve a complete response is more likely in the following groups of patients:

Table 26.4 Results of treatment of Hodgkins' disease

Stage	Symptoms	% Total	Histological grade	CR rate (%)	5-year survival (%)
I	A	20	1	99	92
			2	98	83
	B	v.rare	—	—	—
II	A	21	1	96	94
			2	90	77
	B	7	1	74	78
			2	55	70
III	A	17	1	85	80
			2	70	71
	B	13	1	69	77
			2	60	55
IV	A	6	1	62	74
			2	44	56
	B	14	1	61	64
			2	43	46

(Reproduced with permission from Souhami R L and Moxham J 1990 Textbook of Medicine, Churchill Livingstone, Edinburgh.)
CR = Complete Response

— Prior chemotherapy
— Stage IV
— Multiple extranodal sites
— Systemic symptoms
— Age >40 years
— Nodular sclerosis (unfavourable types)
— Bone marrow involvement
— Bulky disease.

Most relapses occur at the original site of disease, especially in nodes, and usually in the first 3 years after treatment. Relapse occurring within a year of the end of treatment has a particularly poor prognosis. Only a third of patients who relapse within a year of the end of treatment and who are retreated with the same drugs achieve a complete remission. They are rarely cured. If relapse is confined to the neck, axilla, mediastinum or to the para-aortic or pelvic nodes, mantle or inverted Y radiotherapy is recommended. If there is disease outside these sites, second line chemotherapy is needed.

Second line chemotherapy with EVAP or ABVD can achieve complete remissions in 30% of patients and partial remissions in a further 30%.

Absence of systemic symptoms in relapsed patients has the closest correlation with response (59% with symptoms compared with 35% without). Overall survival at 7 years is 27%. Average duration of remission varies between 17 and 38 months.

Hodgkin's disease in children

Although the same histological subtypes occur in children, lymphocyte-depleted Hodgkin's disease is even less common than in adults. Lymphadenopathy is the presenting feature in 90%, of which 60% is cervical or supraclavicular.

CT scanning has the advantage of being non-invasive but may require sedation in young children. Lymphangiography is possible but should be avoided if there is mediastinal disease or a history of asthma.

Staging laparotomy used to be carried out if primary radiotherapy was the sole proposed treatment. The stage of the disease is altered in 30% of children undergoing laparotomy. However severe life-threatening pneumococcal infection is a particular problem in up to 15% of children following splenectomy, with 2–5% mortality. It is now felt that the prognosis of childhood Hodgkin's disease is so good that the risks of staging laparotomy outweigh the benefits.

In view of the growth retardation, pneumonitis, pericarditis and hypothyroidism following mantle irradiation, limited involved field irradiation with lower doses than in adults is recommended in children for pathologically-staged I–IIa disease, e.g. unilateral isolated cervical or inguinal lymphadenopathy. Doses of 25 Gy to the vertebral column result in much less truncal shortening than doses of 35 Gy.

Chemotherapy and radiotherapy can be combined and tailored to the severity of the disease as shown in Table 26.2.

Combination chemotherapy with MOPP or ChlVPP results in complete remissions in 80%. Two-thirds of these children will have prolonged disease-free remissions.

Relapse following chemotherapy carries a bad prognosis. Second line chemotherapy, as in adult disease, is rarely successful.

Management of Hodgkin's disease in pregnancy

Most patients who develop Hodgkin's disease during pregnancy have localised disease. Patients with advanced symptomatic disease often have impaired ovulation and therefore are less likely to become pregnant.

One is concerned with the health of both the mother and the fetus. However there is little evidence that pregnancy worsens the prognosis of Hodgkin's disease or that the disease adversely affects the fetus.

The management of Hodgkin's disease in pregnancy will depend upon the stage of the disease and of the pregnancy and the mother's wishes.

Radiotherapy is potentially teratogenic during the first trimester. Above a dose of 0.1 Gy to the fetus there is a risk of inducing a fetal abnormality.

It seems probable that chemotherapy is also potentially teratogenic. It is unknown if chemotherapy is carcinogenic to the fetus. There is no evidence that either radiotherapy or chemotherapy is teratogenic during the third trimester.

The staging of Hodgkin's disease in pregnancy should minimise exposure to ionising radiation. Thus initial investigations should include only a chest radiograph, full blood count, ESR and liver function tests.

In the first trimester or early weeks of the second trimester, if radiotherapy would deliver more than 0.1 Gy to the fetus or chemotherapy was indicated, therapeutic abortion should be considered. If the diagnosis is made later in the second trimester or in the third trimester, it may be possible to postpone treatment until after the child has been delivered by induced labour between 32 and 34 weeks. If urgent treatment has to be given because of advanced disease or therapeutic abortion is declined by the patient or is not feasible, combination chemotherapy is the treatment of choice. ABVD is recommended because of its probable low risk of carcinogenicity and lower risk of reduced fertility in the child. Localised radiotherapy above the diaphragm can be safely given.

Patients who have been successfully treated for Hodgkin's disease should be advised to avoid pregnancy for 2 years after the end of treatment. This is because it is within this period that relapse is most likely. Beyond it the risk of relapse falls markedly. Patients can be reassured that subsequent pregnancy does not increase the risk of relapse of the disease.

NON-HODGKIN LYMPHOMAS

This group of tumours includes a very wide spectrum of malignancy, from almost benign to highly aggressive disease.

Pathology

Epidemiology

Non-Hodgkin lymphomas (NHL) are responsible for 1.4% of all cancers and 0.4% of cancer deaths. The peak incidence is in the fifth and sixth decades. Children in developed countries are rarely affected. The incidence among children in developing countries is higher, particularly of high grade Burkitt's lymphoma. Males are slightly more commonly affected than females. The sex ratio is 1.7:1.

Aetiology

The cause of most NHL is unknown. The risk of developing NHL is increased in certain inherited genetic syndromes such as combined immunodeficiency syndromes and ataxia telangiectasia. Chromosomal defects have been identified in some types of NHL (14:18 translocation in follicular lymphoma and 8:14 translocation in Burkitt's lymphoma). However, these are acquired as part of tumour development, not inherited abnormalities.

Some NHL are associated with, though not necessarily caused by, viral infection. For example endemic Burkitt's lymphoma, originally described in East African children, is associated with infection by the Epstein–Barr virus (EBV). These children have evidence of antibodies to the viral antigen. EBV is unlikely, however, to be the sole causative agent of Burkitt's lymphoma since the virus is distributed world-wide, whereas the tumour is limited to areas where malaria is endemic. Malaria has therefore been suggested as a possible cofactor. Some NHL are caused by infection with the human T lymphocytic virus (HTLV-1).

Conditions in which the body's immune system is impaired predispose to the development of NHL, particularly immunoblastic. Examples are rheumatoid arthritis, coeliac disease, hypogammaglobulinaemia and AIDS. There is a 60-fold excess of these tumours in patients who have undergone immunosuppressive drug therapy following renal transplantation.

Microscopic features

NHL are typified by the monoclonal proliferation, in order of frequency, of B lymphocytes or T lymphocytes.

The wide variation in histological appearance of NHL, and the difficulty in classifying many of them with certainty has led to a confusing variety of systems of pathological classification. The availability of modern immunohistochemical techniques to identify different cell types has contributed to the complexity. However the basis of classification is to recognise the malignant cell, and name it according to its normal counterparts.

In the UK the British National Lymphoma Investigation (BNLI) group and the Kiel (Table 26.5) classifications are the most commonly used. The Working Formulation of the US National Cancer Institute is also popular. Much expertise is required to classify the NHL. High grade NHL may be confused with a poorly differentiated carcinoma by the unwary. The management and prognosis of these two conditions is different. *Referral of all cases to a specialist pathologist for review before taking a decision on management is recommended.*

BNLI classification. The BNLI classification is based on morphological appearances. Its attraction to the clinician is the division into grade 1 and grade 2 disease which provides a comprehensible and practical guide to decision making. The BNLI classification has the advantage of wide usage in the UK. The BNLI offers an excellent centralised service for review of pathology to centres participating in its studies.

Table 26.5   Kiel classification of non-Hodgkin lymphoma (simplified abstract)

B cell	T cell
Low grade	
Lymphocytic	Lymphocytic
Lymphoplasmacytoid	
Centroblastic-centrocytic	Pleomorphic small cell
High grade	
Centroblastic	Pleomorphic medium and large cell
Immunoblastic	Immunoblastic
Large cell anaplastic	Large cell anaplastic
Lymphoblastic	Lymphoblastic

Kiel classification. The Kiel classification (Table 26.5) is based on scientific principles and microscopic appearances. It also divides lymphomas into low or high grade malignancy. Both the Kiel and another classification (Luke–Collins) take account of the T or B cell origin of the tumour.

Low grade tumours tend to behave in a less aggressive manner than high grade tumours. However this applies more to B cell than to T cell lymphomas. In general, low grade tumours tend to have smaller cells with a closer resemblance to normal lymphoid cells. High grade tumours usually have larger cells, often multinucleate with prominent nucleoli. Some tumours contain a mixture of cells, which can make them difficult to classify.

Clinical features

NHL differ in several respects from Hodgkin's disease. These differences are summarised in Table 26.6. In contrast to Hodgkin's disease, very few patients (10%) at presentation have localised disease. Systemic B symptoms (p. 444) are common. A further difference is the frequency of presentation (15%) with involvement of extranodal sites. The most common of these are in the head and neck, particularly in the lymphoid tissue of the tonsil, nasopharynx and base of tongue (Waldeyer's ring). Second in frequency is the gastrointestinal tract (stomach > small bowel > large bowel). Less common sites are the thyroid, skin, CNS, bone, and testis. Epitrochlear and mesenteric nodes and the bone marrow are rarely involved by Hodgkin's disease but not infrequently by NHL.

Table 26.6 Comparison of clinical features of Hodgkin's disease and non-Hodgkin lymphoma

Feature	Hodgkin's disease	Non-Hodgkin lymphoma
Localised	+++	+
Nodal spread		
Contiguous	+++	+
Non-contiguous	+	+++
Bone marrow infiltration	+/−	++
CNS involvement	+	++

Investigations

The staging investigations for NHL are similar to those for Hodgkin's disease. An adequate biopsy is essential for proper histological examination and cell surface marker studies. There are, however, the following differences:

1. Surface markers. A number of monoclonal antibodies to cell surface proteins made by these tumours are useful in determining whether they are of B or T cell origin. Most (about 85%) lymphomas are of B cell origin. Staining with antibodies against epithelial cell components (e.g. cytokeratins) usually identifies undifferentiated carcinomas, separating them from lymphomas.

2. CT scanning. Since NHL tend to be more generalised than Hodgkin's disease, CT scanning of the thorax and the abdomen is preferred to lymphangiography. In those unfit for CT scanning of chest and abdomen because of advanced age or poor general medical condition, a chest radiograph and abdominal ultrasound provide simpler alternatives.

3. Bone marrow examination. A bone marrow aspirate and a small core of bone (trephine) should be examined for tumour infiltration. The trephine may be positive when the aspirate is negative. Marrow involvement is much commoner in low grade (80%) than high grade (10–15%) NHL.

4. Staging laparotomy. This is not recommended since so few patients have localised disease. Many patients are elderly and unfit for surgery on medical grounds.

The following staging investigations are recommended:

1. Haematology
   a. Full blood count
   b. Bone marrow aspirate and trephine.
2. Biochemistry
   a. Liver function tests
   b. Serum immunoglobulins
   c. Serum urea, creatinine and electrolytes.
3. Radiology
   a. Chest radiograph
   b. CT scan of thorax and abdomen.

Principles of management

The management of NHL depends upon the age and general condition of the patient, the histology, the extent of the disease and whether the tumour is nodal or extranodal. NHL are generally very sensitive to radiation and to chemotherapy.

In general widespread low grade (BNLI grade 1) tumours are treated with 'gentle' chemotherapy (chlorambucil with or without steroids) or slightly more aggressive combination chemotherapy (chlorambucil, vincristine (Oncovin) and prednisolone (CV(O)P); Table 26.7). Radiotherapy at modest doses is used for localised disease.

High grade (BNLI grade 2) tumours usually require

Table 26.7 CV(O)P regime for low grade non-Hodgkin lymphomas

Vincristine (Oncovin)	1.4 mg/m² (max. 2 mg) i.v.	Day 1
Cyclophosphamide	400 mg/m² orally	Days 2–5
Prednisolone	25 mg b.d. orally	Days 2–5

Repeated every 21 days

more aggressive combination chemotherapy, e.g. with cyclophosphamide, Adriamycin, vincristine (Oncovin) and prednisolone [CHOP] (Table 26.8). Radiotherapy at higher dosage than for low grade tumours is required for truly localised (stage Ia) disease or for masses failing to resolve completely on chemotherapy.

1. Localised disease (stages I and II)

Low grade (grade 1)

For patients with localised stage I or II disease of low grade histology local radiotherapy is generally recommended.

High grade (grade 2)

Local radiotherapy is recommended for non-bulky (<2.5 cm) stage Ia disease of high grade histology. In view of the frequent failure of radiotherapy to control bulky stage I and stage II disease, cytotoxic chemotherapy is advised, often followed by radiotherapy to the initial site of involvement. Combination chemotherapy is most commonly with the CHOP regime (Table 26.8) to a total of six courses, subject to response and patient tolerance.

Results of treatment. For low grade stage I and II local control is about 80% at 5 years. For high grade local control of stage I disease is 65% at 5 years. Radiotherapy is less effective for high grade bulky (>2.5 cm) stage I or stage II (local control only 27% at 5 years).

2. Widespread disease (stages III–IV)

Low grade

There is little evidence that treatment influences the natural history of stage III–IV disease of low-grade histology. Despite treatment, 75% of patients will relapse within 5 years. Since cure is unrealistic with current radiotherapy or chemotherapy, it is important to minimise the toxicity of treatment.

In general, in the absence of life-threatening disease (e.g. liver metastases, bone marrow failure, renal or cerebral involvement), asymptomatic patients should be kept under regular surveillance on an outpatient basis. Treatment is only instituted with local radiotherapy or with chemotherapy if there is symptomatic progression or vital organs (e.g. kidneys) are threatened.

Chemotherapy. For symptomatic non-life-threatening disease, chlorambucil (0.2 mg/kg daily in divided doses (max. 10 mg)) and/or prednisolone (10–40 mg daily) can provide good control. To reduce the risk of leukaemogenesis and preserve adequate bone marrow tolerance to subsequent chemotherapy, if needed, treatment with chlorambucil should usually be stopped 3 months after a complete response has been achieved. Total duration of treatment should not exceed 6 months.

If disease progresses despite chlorambucil and/or steroids, more aggressive treatment is necessary. Combination chemotherapy such as cyclophosphamide, vincristine and prednisolone (CV(O)P) is advised (Table 26.7) to a total of six courses if a useful clinical response is obtained.

High grade

Chemotherapy has been more successful in the control of high grade than low grade lymphoma. Combination chemotherapy is the treatment of choice. Of the available regimes, CHOP (Table 26.8) is the most widely used. Six courses are given, subject to response and patient tolerance. The most aggressive forms of high grade disease (e.g. lymphoblastic) are often treated additionally, if the disease is responding to chemotherapy, with prophylactic CNS irradiation because of the high incidence of CNS involvement.

Results of chemotherapy for high grade disease. Complete response rates of the order of 60% are achievable. Overall cure rate is about 40%.

Relapse

High dose chemotherapy with or without autologous bone marrow transplantation should be considered for patients failing to respond or relapsing after CHOP chemotherapy. However the probability of cure is low.

Table 26.8 CHOP regime for high grade non-Hodgkin lymphomas

Cyclophosphamide	750 mg/m²	Days 1 and 8
Hydroxydaunorubicin	25 mg/m²	Days 1 and 8
Oncovin	1.4 mg/m²	Days 1 and 8
Prednisolone	50 mg/m²	Days 1 and 8

Repeated every 28 days from day 1

Radiotherapy

Localised disease (low grade)

Target volume

Since NHL do not necessarily spread to contiguous nodes, local radiotherapy should be confined to the affected nodes, with a generous (e.g. 5 cm) margin. This is in contrast to regional (e.g. mantle radiotherapy) in Hodgkin's disease where the cervical, mediastinal and axillary nodes are treated even if only one of these sites is involved.

Technique

For the treatment of neck nodes, if orthovoltage is used, the patient lies supine with the neck turned away from the affected side. A suitably sized applicator is used with bolus applied to the highest point of the field to fill the air gaps due to variation in the contour of the neck.

For deeper or more extensive nodes in the neck or groin and other nodal sites megavoltage or cobalt-60 X-ray therapy is advised. The patient lies supine with the head straight and the neck extended. A direct anterior field is simulated. Unless the nodal mass extends across the midline, the medial border of the field can usually be placed lateral to the spinal cord.

Where both the pelvic and para-aortic nodes are involved, an inverted Y technique is used (as in Hodgkin's disease, p. 448).

For involved mediastinal nodes, it is not necessary to include the cervical, infraclavicular or axillary nodes as in the mantle technique.

Dose and energy

The energy chosen will vary according to the site of involvement. For superficial nodes in the neck or the groin, orthovoltage (250–300 kV) is often adequate. For bulky nodes megavoltage is advised.

35 Gy (250–300 kV) or midplane dose (4–6 MV photons) in 20 daily fractions over 4 weeks

Localised disease (high grade)

Technique

This is similar to low grade disease. Care should be taken to avoid delivering more than 40 Gy in 20 daily fractions to the spinal cord, either by excluding it from the field or shielding the cord with a central lead block placed over the spine.

Dose and energy

A higher dose is required than for low grade disease.
40 Gy applied (250–300 kV) or midplane dose (4–6 MV photons) in 20 daily fractions over 4 weeks

Extranodal non-Hodgkin lymphomas

1. Gastrointestinal

Pathology. The stomach is the most common site (50%), followed by small bowel (30%). The large bowel is less commonly affected (10%). The majority are of B cell origin of high grade histological type.

Clinical features. Clinical presentation is usually with abdominal pain, weight loss and anorexia, often associated, in small bowel tumours, with acute intestinal obstruction.

Diagnosis. A biopsy is needed. The diagnosis of gastric NHL is often a surprise finding made either at endoscopic biopsy of what was thought to be a benign gastric ulcer or at laparotomy for what appeared on naked-eye examination to be a gastric carcinoma. Small and large bowel tumours are often only discovered by laparotomy.

Management. The management of gastrointestinal extranodal NHL differs from nodal lymphomas in a number of ways. First, surgery has a major role in the resection of localised disease. Secondly, the gastrointestinal tract is a mobile structure which makes localisation for radiotherapy planning more difficult. Thirdly, the dose that can be delivered to large volumes of the abdomen is limited. Finally, there is a significant risk of intestinal haemorrhage or perforation following a response to chemotherapy or radiotherapy.

a. Localised disease (stages IEA and IIEA). Wide excision of the tumour yields much better results than biopsy alone or subtotal resection.

The macroscopic appearance of a gastric NHL at laparotomy may be similar to that of a carcinoma. Unless the diagnosis of NHL is considered, inadequate resection or a palliative bypass procedure may be all that is attempted. Commonly the diagnosis is only made on the surgical specimen after surgery. If the patient's general condition allows and less than optimal resection or bypass has been carried out at the initial laparotomy, a second elective laparotomy should be considered to attempt a complete resection.

Staging. The same staging procedures should be carried out as for nodal NHL.

Postoperative management. Owing to the rarity of these tumours and the lack of prospective randomised studies, the role of postoperative radiotherapy and chemotherapy remains controversial.

For localised disease, there is probably no need for postoperative radiotherapy or chemotherapy if the following criteria are fulfilled:

1. Only one site of bowel is involved.
2. Surgical resection margins are clear of tumour.

3. Serosa is not penetrated.
4. Tumour is less than 10 cm in diameter.
5. There is no other evidence of intra-abdominal disease.

Postoperative chemotherapy. If there is high grade residual tumour or the initial tumour was >10 cm in diameter, postoperative chemotherapy is advisable. Doses may have to be reduced or cycles delayed because of poor general medical condition.

Postoperative radiotherapy. Radiotherapy is less frequently used as an adjuvant because of the difficulties in accurate tumour localisation and intolerance of the doses needed to eradicate disease (40 Gy) by normal tissues and the spinal cord.

Wide field abdominal irradiation may be offered for low grade residual disease where the necessary tumoricidal dose (35 Gy) can be delivered with acceptable morbidity while remaining within spinal cord tolerance.

Target volume
Localisation of the tumour bearing area or operative site with barium is helpful. A generous margin should be allowed around the tumour bearing areas to allow for the variability in the position of the bowel within the abdomen. In practice most of the abdomen is irradiated.

Technique
A parallel opposed pair of anterior and posterior fields is used.

Dose and energy
It is rarely possible to deliver more than 30–40 Gy over 4–5 weeks to large areas of the abdomen because of gastrointestinal toxicity.

30–40 Gy midplane dose in 20–25 daily fractions over 4–5 weeks (9–10 MV photons)

Critical organs. The kidneys should be identified during simulation by intravenous urogram. Anterior and posterior MCP blocks should limit the dose to the whole kidney to 20 Gy. The dose to the spinal cord should not exceed 40 Gy in 4 weeks.

b. Advanced disease (stages III, IV or B symptoms). This should be treated by chemotherapy appropriate to the type of tumour and provided that the patient's general condition will allow this.

2. Head and neck, bone, testis, brain and breast

Clinical features. Extranodal tumours in the head and neck commonly present in Waldeyer's ring, the thyroid gland and occasionally in the salivary glands, paranasal sinuses or in the orbit. In the tonsil they appear as smooth often vascular masses. Thyroid lymphoma typically presents as a rapidly growing painful thyroid mass and stridor from tracheal compression, sometimes with a previous history of Hashimoto's thyroiditis. In the orbit pink fleshy conjunctival deposits (Plate 17) are seen. The lacrimal glands and retrobulbar area may also be affected. Bilateral involvement is common.

Primary NHL of bone is very rare. It mainly affects long bones, especially the humerus and femur.

Primary testicular NHL tends to occur in the elderly, typically between 60 and 80 years of age. Bilateral involvement occurs in 20% at some stage.

Primary NHL of the CNS usually involves the brain. The spinal cord is rarely affected.

NHL of the breast usually presents with a breast mass clinically indistinguishable from carcinoma.

Management. In general, stages IEA (grades 1 and 2) and IIEA (grade 1) are treated by local radiotherapy. Stage IIEA (high grade), more extensive stages (grade 1 or 2) and those with B symptoms require chemotherapy. The choice of drugs will depend on the grade of the tumour, as for nodal lymphomas. Following chemotherapy radiotherapy may be required for residual masses.

Local radiotherapy as primary treatment is indicated for thyroid lymphoma (sometimes as an emergency for tracheal obstruction) and cerebral NHL. Intrathecal* methotrexate is needed if there is evidence of spread to the cerebrospinal fluid.

Primary NHL of the testis often has an aggressive course. It should be treated initially by orchidectomy followed by radiotherapy to the regional lymphatics (inverted Y, p. 448) and chemotherapy.

a. Waldeyer's ring

Target volume
For NHL of Waldeyer's ring the treatment volume should extend from the base of the skull to the clavicles, including the cervical lymph node chains on both sides of the neck.

Technique
Parallel opposed lateral fields are used.

b. Thyroid

Target volume
The thyroid gland and the cervical lymph node chains on both sides.

Technique
A parallel opposed pair of anterior and posterior fields is used.

c. Orbit (p. 495)

d. Bone

Target volume
The whole of the affected bone should be included in the initial volume. If possible the field should then be coned down to the site of involvement.

Technique
A parallel opposed pair of fields is used.

e. Brain

Target volume
The whole brain should be treated.

Technique
A pair of lateral opposed fields is used (Fig. 27.5A).

f. Breast

Target volume
The breast, axillary and supraclavicular nodes should be included.

Technique
(1) A pair of medial and lateral glancing fields (en bloc technique) is used to cover the whole of the treatment volume or (2) a direct anterior field to cover the supraclavicular fossa and axilla and a glancing pair of fields to the breast are used (Fig. 23.6).

Dose and energy

Waldeyer's ring, thyroid, breast, brain
40 Gy in 20 daily fractions over 4 weeks (4–6 MV photons)

Bone
Whole bone: 40 Gy in 20 daily fractions over 4 weeks (4–6 MV photons)
Tumour volume: 15 Gy in 10 daily fractions over 2 weeks (4–6 MV photons)

Testis

Target volume
Following orchidectomy, the para-aortic and pelvic nodes are irradiated.

Technique
Inverted Y (Fig. 26.5)

Dose and energy
35 Gy in 20 daily fractions over 4 weeks (9–10 MV photons)

Mycosis fungoides

Mycosis fungoides is a malignant skin tumour derived from T lymphocytes. It may develop a leukaemic form (Sézary syndrome). In its localised form groups of neoplastic cells aggregate in the epidermis. The average age of onset is in the fifth decade. It runs a long course, evolving typically over 10 years but occasionally up to 30 years.

There are three main stages: pre-mycotic (erythematous), plaque (infiltrative) and finally tumour formation. Typically erythematous patches (Plate 18) start on the buttocks, upper thighs or breasts. Rarely the whole skin becomes involved and red (erythroderma or 'homme rouge' (literally, red man)). The latter is often associated with blood-borne spread (Sézary syndrome). Erythematous patches become thickened to form plaque, and finally fungating tumours, often likened to tomatoes. Local and systemic infection, depression (sometimes resulting in suicide) are common in advanced disease. Terminally, there is systemic spread with visceral involvement (e.g. liver and spleen).

Treatment

Treatment of mycosis fungoides is palliative. Care should be taken to avoid aggressive treatment in the early phases of the disease because of its long natural history. Death often occurs from an unrelated illness.

In the premycotic stage topical steroid or cytotoxic therapy (nitrogen mustard), photochemotherapy using long-wave ultraviolet light with psoralens (PUVA) or radiotherapy may control the disease. PUVA tends to be used first but is only appropriate for very superficial lesions. Systemic chemotherapy is indicated for visceral spread.

Nitrogen mustard is applied by the patient, wearing protective gloves. Often treatment has to be stopped due to sensitisation to the drug.

Photochemotherapy involves exposing the patient to ultraviolet light (UVA) after administering a photosensitising agent, psoralen, orally.

Radiotherapy may be to local areas or to the whole body surface by low energy electrons (3 MeV) from linear accelerators or beta irradiation from a strontium-90 source (betatron).

1. Local

Dose and energy

10 Gy in 5 daily fractions (80–100 kV for superficial lesions, 250–300 kV or electrons of appropriate energy for plaque or tumour stage)

2. Whole body electron therapy. Four fields of approximately 45 cm in length can be used to cover the whole body at extended SSD (120 cm). Lead shielding is applied to protect the eyes and the finger nails. If the eyelids are involved by disease, a lead internal eye shield is used. If 5 or 8 MeV electrons are used, Perspex is needed to reduce the depth of penetration.

Dose

30 Gy in 6 fractions (once weekly) for 6 weeks

Side-effects. Temporary alopecia and loss of nails are followed by permanent skin atrophy, oedema and radiodermatis.

3. Chemotherapy. Combination chemotherapy with agents such as CHOP (Table 26.8) is indicated for systemic disease. Complete response rates are low (20–25%) with high rates of relapse.

Results of treatment

Five-year survival is 50%, with an average 15-year survival of 8.8 years.

Overall results of treatment of non-Hodgkin lymphomas

The 10-year relapse-free survival is 50% for stages I and II low grade NHL, and 30% for stages III and IV and those with patients with B symptoms. Cure is rarely achieved and relapse is common in all stages.

For high grade stage Ia or I$_E$ NHL radiotherapy is curative, with 70% 10-year relapse-free survival. For advanced disease a complete response is obtained in about 60% of cases, with long-term control in 30–40%.

MULTIPLE MYELOMA

Multiple myeloma is a relatively common haematological malignancy, accounting for 0.9% of all cancers and 1.3% of cancer deaths. Its incidence is 3 per 100 000 per year. It tends to occur in late middle age. The median age at diagnosis is 62 years. The male to female sex ratio is 1.5:1 The aetiology is unknown. Genetic factors may play a significant role since in the USA the incidence of the disease in Blacks is twice that of Whites. Exposure to alpha particles may be a risk factor since myeloma developed in higher than the expected proportion of the survivors of the atomic bombs dropped on Japan in 1945.

Pathology

Myeloma is a plasma cell tumour of B lymphocyte lineage, usually originating in the bone marrow. Plasma cells are immunoglobulin producing cells. Each immunoglobulin (Fig. 26.8) is composed of heavy and light chains. The neoplastic proliferation of plasma cells is thought to arise from a single cell (monoclonal). It leads to marrow destruction and failure and also to local destruction of bone. For this reason it is often classified with bone tumours.

There are four main types of myeloma:

1. Multiple myeloma (the commonest)
2. Solitary myeloma of bone (plasmacytoma)
3. Extramedullary myeloma
4. Plasma cell leukaemia.

Multiple myeloma is a generalised disease affecting many bones in its course. Rarely myeloma may be confined to one or two bones only (plasmacytoma). Extramedullary myeloma is even rarer and most often occurs in the upper respiratory tract, followed in decreasing order of frequency by the lymph nodes and spleen, skin and gastrointestinal tract.

Paraprotein production

Myeloma cells produce abnormal immunoglobulins (paraproteins) in 95% of cases. They are usually detectable in the blood as a monoclonal band on protein electrophoresis (Fig. 26.7). When light chains are produced in excess they are found in the urine as Bence-Jones protein. These are parts of or whole immunoglobulin molecules (Fig. 26.8).

The incidence of the different types of these pathological immunoglobulins (Ig) is similar to that in the healthy subject (IgG 50–60%, IgA 20–25%, light chain only 20%, IgD 2%, IgE and IgM <1%). The paraprotein production can be quantified and changes measured in response to treatment.

In 5% of cases no paraprotein is detectable. This is the *non-secretory* type. In the rare cases in which there is abnormal production of immunoglobulins D and E, they may fail to be detected by conventional techniques.

Natural history

This is very variable. The first abnormality detected

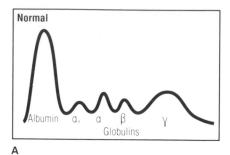

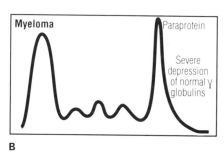

Fig. 26.7   Serum protein electrophoresis from **A** a normal individual and **B** patient with myeloma. (Reproduced with permission from Souhami and Moxham, Textbook of Medicine, Churchill Livingstone, 1990.)

may be the presence of a monoclonal band on protein electrophoresis (Fig. 26.7) many years before any clinical or radiological abnormality. This may remain static or rise slowly over many years or rapidly over a 1–3 year period.

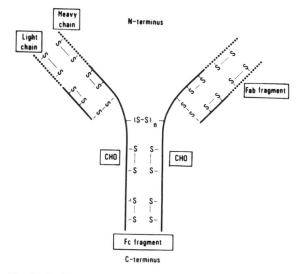

Fig. 26.8   Immunoglobulin molecule. (Reproduced with permission from Halnan, Treatment of Cancer, 1st edn, Chapman and Hall, 1982.)

In some patients the disease may have an indolent course, remaining localised for many years to a single bone (solitary plasmacytoma). It may subsequently disseminate in about 50% of cases. In others the disease has a much more aggressive course with death within a year. High levels of paraprotein production result in plugging of the renal tubules and, if unresponsive to treatment, death within a few months from kidney failure.

Clinical features

The commonest presenting feature is bone pain (70%), usually from a rib or a vertebra. The destruction of cortical bone leads to pathological fractures in about 25% and hypercalcaemia in 30%. Fewer patients (12%) present with infection and with bleeding (7%). Spinal cord compression is occasionally the presenting feature. Most patients are anaemic. A third have evidence of myelosuppression with reduced white count and/or platelets.

If the paraprotein level is high enough a *hyperviscosity syndrome* develops. This is characterised by visual impairment, lethargy and coma.

Soft tissue lesions (lymph nodes, spleen or liver) are uncommon at presentation.

Diagnosis

Two or more of the following features must be present to fulfil the diagnosis:

— Serum or urine paraprotein
— Plasma cell infiltration of the bone marrow (>20%)
— Typical radiological lesions (osteolytic deposits in the axial skeleton and ribs).

Occasionally the diagnosis is not clear-cut. For example the patient may have a modest level of paraprotein, a small increase in plasma cells in the bone marrow (<5%) and no radiological lesions. In such cases close observation is necessary to detect the development of other diagnostic features. Not all paraproteinaemias are malignant. The incidence of paraproteinaemia rises with age. It is 1% over 25 years, 3% over the age of 70 years and 25% over 90 years. For the most part they have a benign course. However about 20–25% of cases of paraproteinaemia diagnosed in hospital will develop multiple myeloma if followed up for 10 years, and 40% at 15 years. Paraproteinaemia is not an uncommon feature of lymphoma.

Other investigations are designed to detect common sites of metastatic spread:

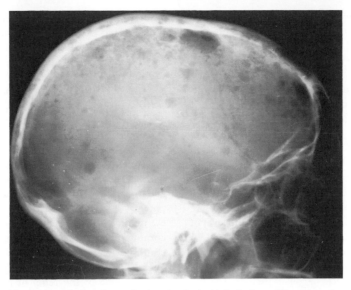

Fig. 26.9   Skull radiograph showing typical lytic lesions. (Courtesy of Dr M Greaves, Sheffield.)

1. Full blood count (anaemia, leucopenia, thrombocytopenia from marrow infiltration)
2. Blood urea, creatinine and electrolytes (renal impairment from myelomatous infiltration, nephrotic syndrome, hypercalcaemia, amyloid
3. Blood calcium (hypercalcaemia)
4. Serum electrophoresis (monoclonal paraprotein band) often accompanied by a reduction of immunoglobulins (immune paresis)
5. Bone marrow examination (excess plasma cells)
6. Skeletal survey (lytic lesions, especially skull (Fig. 26.9), ribs and vertebrae, or diffuse osteoporosis).

Prognostic factors

Certain factors confer a poor prognosis in myeloma. These are:
1. Presenting haemoglobin <8.5 g/dl
2. Hypercalcaemia (>3 mmol/l)
3. Blood urea >12 mmol/l (after correction of dehydration)
4. Poor performance status.

Treatment

Multiple myeloma

There is at present no curative therapy for multiple myeloma. Treatment is aimed at alleviating symptoms, controlling the advance of the disease and preventing complications. The main forms of treatment are cytotoxic therapy and palliative radiotherapy. Bone marrow transplantation is only appropriate for a minority of patients. Treatment with interferon is at an early stage of evaluation.

Cytotoxic therapy. Cytotoxic therapy is the only form of therapy known to prolong survival in multiple myeloma. One of the commonest initial regimes for multiple myeloma is:

Oral melphalan 7 mg/m^2 and prednisolone (1 mg/ kg) daily for 4 days every 3 weeks

The addition of prednisolone to melphalan increases the response rate but survival is not improved. This combination of drugs results in approximately 50–75% reduction in the level of paraprotein in about half the patients treated. Average survival is 2–3 years.

Whether more aggressive combinations of chemotherapy prolong survival more than melphalan and prednisolone is debatable. Comparison of different combinations has been limited by different criteria of response. The Medical Research Council in its fifth myeloma trial showed that a combination (ABCM) of a 6-weekly regime of: Adriamycin, BCNU, cyclophosphamide and melphalan had a significant survival advantage over intermittent melphalan alone. Two-year survival on ABCM is about 60%. The complete response rate is 7%; 20% of the complete responders will subsequently relapse. However other studies have not shown unequivocal benefit of combination alkylating agent therapy over melphalan alone.

Higher doses of intravenous melphalan can achieve higher response rates (up to nearly 80%) but with greater treatment-related mortality and morbidity. Such treatment should only be undertaken in specialised units by experienced staff.

Supportive measures. Pain control is important. Opiates are usually required. Palliative radiotherapy, either localised or hemibody irradiation, is effective (see below).

Hypercalcaemia is treated by intravenous hydration and bisphosphonates.

Hyperviscosity, if causing significant symptoms and signs, is treated by plasmapheresis. In this process some of the patient's plasma is replaced by an appropriate colloid solution (usually albumin) to reduce the level of paraprotein.

Renal failure may require dialysis.

Infection due to neutropenia and immune paresis should be vigorously treated.

Criteria of response. The following criteria of a response are widely accepted. All should be fulfilled:

1. A reduction in paraprotein level to 50% or less.
2. If urinary paraprotein >1 g/24 h, a reduction to 50% or less; if 0.5–1 g/24 h, a fall to less than 0.1 g/24 h.
3. Healing of radiological lesions.
4. More than 50% reduction of the plasmacytoma radiologically or by clinical measurement in the product of the two largest dimensions.

A complete response is defined as the absence of detectable paraprotein or urinary light chains and normalisation of the bone marrow with <5% plasma cells.

Most patients reach a plateau of response. Maintenance therapy after a plateau phase of 6 months is unnecessary. Further response after 6–12 courses of melphalan and prednisolone is uncommon. Complete response with disappearance of paraprotein is rare. Most patients improve symptomatically with chemotherapy, although lytic bone lesions do not usually heal. Of the 7% of patients who achieve a complete response to chemotherapy, 20% will relapse.

Relapse. If the disease does relapse after an initial period of a detectable but stable paraprotein level (plateau phase), a response may be obtained with further courses of melphalan. The paraprotein level may be stabilised again, but at a higher level. However the duration of subsequent plateau phases tends to be short-lived. High dose melphalan is less successful in relapsed disease than in untreated patients. Complete response rates of the order of 20% are obtainable but at the cost of considerable myelosuppression and gastrointestinal toxicity.

Bone marrow transplantation. The value and ideal timing of allogeneic transplantation in myeloma has yet to be established. Its applicability is limited by donor availability and the intolerance of the elderly of the morbidity of treatment. It is most effective when the tumour burden is small, for example when the first plateau phase has been reached. In future it may have a role at an early stage of the disease in selected patients with poor prognostic factors.

High dose chemotherapy and autologous bone marrow rescue may have a future role.

Interferon. Alpha-interferon appears to have some activity against myeloma, particularly in untreated patients. However its efficacy is inferior to conventional cytotoxic therapy. Preliminary encouraging results of its combination with conventional chemotherapy require confirmation. Lethargy is a common side-effect.

Palliative radiotherapy. Palliative radiotherapy has a useful role in the relief of pain from bony deposits, pathological fractures and spinal cord compression.

Bone deposits and pathological fractures. Patients may develop many painful bony deposits over the course of their illness. Pain often flits from one site to another, making the assessment of which sites to irradiate difficult. A new site of pain often emerges shortly after the last one has been irradiated. In addition, movement on and off the treatment couch may be limited by pain. For this reason prolonged fractionation should, if possible, be avoided. Single fractions using a single orthovoltage field or, for deeper seated lesions, megavoltage is used. Longer fractionation is desirable in some circumstances, for example to the lower dorsal spine to avoid duodenal upset or for spinal cord compression.

Spinal cord compression. This may occur at any stage of the disease. It is usually due to extradural disease rather than a collapsed vertebra. If the diagnosis of myeloma has been previously established surgical decompression is unnecessary since it is very radiosensitive. When, however, cord compression is the presenting feature of the disease, emergency laminectomy and biopsy are required to establish a histological diagnosis.

The management of spinal cord compression is as described in Chapter 27.

Dose and energy

Multiple myeloma
**Rib deposits: 7 Gy single fraction at orthovoltage
Lower dorsal and cervical spine and pathological fractures: 20 Gy in 5 daily fractions over a week (250–300 kV or 4–6 MV photons)**

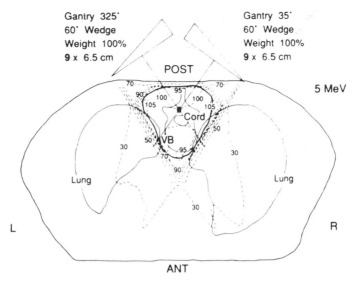

Fig. 26.10 Posterior oblique wedged pair of fields to treat tumour of vertebral body (VB). (Reproduced with permission from Dobbs et al 1992.)

Spinal cord compression: 20–25 Gy at the depth of the cord in 5 daily fractions over a week (4–6 MV photons)

Solitary plasmacytoma

For solitary myeloma, radical radiotherapy should be delivered to eliminate the local malignant plasma cell population. If the paraproteinaemia persists, chemotherapy should follow.

Target volume

Spine: the target volume should include the affected vertebral body and one normal vertebral body above and below. The scar from a laminectomy should be included.

Technique

This will vary with the site. For the spine a direct megavoltage field in the lumbar region (avoiding the kidneys) or a posterior oblique wedged pair (Fig. 26.10) in the cervical and thoracic region is usually adequate. Where there are multiple painful deposits in one or both halves of the body, hemibody irradiation may provide good palliation. The toxicity of treating the upper half of the body is greater, due to radiation pneumonitis.

Dose and energy

35 Gy in 15 daily fractions over 3 weeks (4–6 MV photons)

Hemibody irradiation. Patients with progressive myeloma frequently develop widespread painful bony deposits, too numerous to encompass with single fields and often difficult to localise. In these circumstances, either the upper or lower half of the body can be encompassed in a single megavoltage field (9–10 MV photons) at extended SSD (e.g. 140 cm). This should be carried out on an inpatient basis.

Treatment of the other half of the body is carried out 4–6 weeks later, depending on general condition, response to treatment of the first hemibody irradiation and a satisfactory blood count (white cell count $\geq 2.0 \times 10^9/l$, platelets $\geq 60 \times 10^9/l$).

Preparation. To reduce radiation induced nausea and vomiting, 100 mg of hydrocortisone is given i.v. in 500 ml of normal saline over an hour, 1 hour before treatment.

Target volume

1. Lower half. The field for the lower half extends from just below the 12th rib to just above the knee joints. The upper limit of the field should be tattooed to avoid overlap if the upper half is to be treated.

2. Upper half. The field extends from the vertex of the skull or the clavicles (if the eyes are to be avoided) to the level of the 12th rib in the midclavicular line. Because of the risk of pneumonitis, the dose to the upper half is less than to the lower half. If the skull is included the mouth should be shielded to avoid oral mucositis.

Dose and energy

Lower half: 8.5 Gy in a single fraction (9–10 MV photons)

Upper half: 6.5 Gy in a single fraction (9–10 MV photons)

Side-effects. About 30% of patients develop nausea and vomiting within a few hours of treatment. Regular antiemetics are necessary. When the lower half is treated, diarrhoea occurs in a third of patients, 3–5 days after radiotherapy. This is controllable with anti-diarrhoeal agents. Anaemia, leucopenia and thrombocytopenia are common. Blood transfusion may be required. The white count normally recovers by 6 weeks. The platelet count takes on average 10 days longer than the white count to recover.

Response. Prompt pain relief is achieved in most patients.

Overall survival

About 50% of patients will survive 2 years. For patients with poor prognostic factors, 2-year survival is 10%, and, with a good prognosis, 75%.

LEUKAEMIA

Leukaemia encompasses a group of diseases characterised by the uncontrolled accumulation of malignant leukopoetic tissue in the bone marrow and peripheral blood. It accounts for 2.1% of all cancers and 2.6% of cancer deaths. The sex ratio is 1.5:1 in favour of males.

Pathology

Classification

Leukaemia is divided into two main subgroups, acute and chronic:

1. Acute
   a. Lymphoblastic (ALL)
   b. Myeloblastic (AML)
2. Chronic
   a. Lymphocytic (CLL)
   b. Myeloid (granulocytic) (CML)

Aetiology

In most cases the cause of leukaemia is not known; however there are both acquired and genetic causes.

Acquired. With the exception of CLL, the other types of leukaemia can be induced by relatively high doses of ionising radiation. Typically this occurs 3–10 years following exposure. Evidence for this is:

1. Survivors of the atom bomb explosions at Hiroshima and Nagasaki showed a 20-fold increase as compared with the unirradiated population.
2. Patients irradiated for ankylosing spondylitis have a tenfold increase in incidence.

One form of acute T cell leukaemia which occurs predominantly in the West Indies and in southern Japan is caused by the human T cell leukaemia virus (HTLV-1).

Some industrial chemicals, of which benzene is the main culprit, induce acute leukaemia (mainly AML).

Cytotoxic drugs, especially the alkylating agents, can induce leukaemia, particularly when given in conjunction with radiation. The risk at 10 years of developing leukaemia (mainly AML) in patients who receive MOPP chemotherapy for Hodgkin's disease varies from 3 to 13%. Current evidence suggests that there is no synergistic effect between chemotherapy and radiation in increasing the risk of leukaemia, except when the radiation fields are large.

Major chromosomal abnormalities in the form of deletions or translocations are seen in many cases of leukaemia.

Genetic. Children with Down's syndrome account for the majority of genetic cases. The increase in leukaemia is 20-fold. Much rarer causes, such as ataxia telangiectasia predispose to ALL and Fanconi's anaemia to AML.

White blood cells are either of lymphoid or myeloid origin. Any of them may undergo malignant change. Virtually all leukaemias are derived from a single clone of cells. In acute leukaemia primitive cells, blasts, are found in the bone marrow and in the peripheral blood. In the chronic forms more differentiated but still abnormal lymphoid and myeloid cells are seen.

The normal process of transformation from primitive stem cells into mature adult cells is somehow disturbed and arrested, so that immature cells accumulate in the marrow and enter the circulation in large numbers, to give the typical peripheral blood picture. The marrow becomes filled with leukaemic cells which displace other components—red cells (causing anaemia) and platelets (causing bleeding tendency).

Resistance to infection is lowered because of the immaturity of the white cells. Death is usually due to infection in association with bone marrow failure.

ACUTE LEUKAEMIA

Acute leukaemia may be of lymphoid, myeloid or other type, but the clinical picture is similar in all. ALL constitutes 80% of childhood cases and AML 80% of adult cases. AML may occur at any age but mainly in middle age and in the elderly. The clinical features of ALL and AML are comparable. They are described in Chapter 29.

Acute monocytic leukaemia

Acute monocytic leukaemia is a subgroup of acute myeloid leukaemia. It accounts for 10% of leukaemia. It is commonest over the age of 30. Swollen painful gums are more common in this form of leukaemia than in other types. Treatment is on the same lines as acute myeloid leukaemia.

Treatment of AML

Most current regimes consist of combinations of daunorubicin, cytosine, thioguanine and etoposide. Remission is achieved in approximately 80% of patients under the age of 40 and 50–60% over that age. Once a remission has been achieved, several further courses are given as *consolidation* therapy. *Maintenance* therapy is not considered to be of value.

Bone marrow transplantation

If the patient is below the age of 45 and has a histocompatibility antigen (HLA)-matched sibling as a bone marrow donor, bone marrow transplantation is an option. Unfortunately only 1 in 4 patients have such a match.

The rationale for bone marrow transplantation is as follows. It allows higher doses of chemotherapy and radiotherapy than the bone marrow would tolerate if unsupported. The bone marrow depression induced by chemoradiotherapy is compensated for by the infusion of donor bone marrow.

Bone marrow grafts are of two types. The first and commonest is *allogeneic* transplantation in which bone marrow is taken from an immunologically compatible (HLA-matched) sibling. Allogeneic transplantation is the treatment of choice for patients with AML and an HLA compatible donor.

The second is *autologous* marrow transplantation. In this case some of the patient's marrow is removed and stored before chemotherapy is started. It is then reinfused after chemoradiotherapy to sustain the marrow. The advantage of autologous transplantation is that there is no immunological rejection of the marrow since it belongs to the patient. There is, however, the potential hazard of reinfusing leukaemic cells that may repopulate the bone marrow.

Procedure. In the first phase bone marrow (500–1000 ml) is aspirated from the donor's iliac crests under general anaesthesia. The patient then receives high dose chemotherapy (cyclophosphamide 100 mg/kg over 2 days) with total body irradiation (10 Gy) (see below) to eliminate residual tumour. The stored bone marrow is freshly infused via a Hickman central venous line into the recipient. Following chemoradiotherapy, the white cell and platelet counts drop within 10 days. They recover 3–6 weeks after the marrow transplant. Over this period supportive antibiotics, red cell and platelet transfusions are given. Blood products are irradiated to kill T lymphocytes which may precipitate graft-versus-host disease (GVHD). Immunodeficiency due to defects of T cell and B cell functions occurs during the first 6 months and for longer in the presence of GVHD. Viral, bacterial and fungal infections may be fatal.

The main problem of allogeneic transplantation is the immunological reaction that the the donor marrow elicits in the host. This is known as *graft-versus-host disease*. It may be acute or chronic. The acute effects take place in the first 8 weeks following the graft. The features of acute and chronic GVHD are as follows:

Acute
— Cholestatic jaundice
— Skin rashes
— Diarrhoea and weight loss

Chronic
— Arthritis
— Hepatitis and chronic liver disease
— Malabsorption and weight loss
— Oral mucositis and sicca syndrome
— Restrictive and obstructive lung disease
— Pericardial and pleural effusions
— Scleroderma
— Skin rashes

Prevention of GVHD. Since GVHD has a high mortality, its prevention is important. Cyclosporin, usually in combination with methotrexate, is very effective.

Total body irradiation (TBI)

Technique
A variety of techniques are in use. Some centres have dedicated machines for wide field irradiation. Others, as in Sheffield, use linear accelerators at extended SSD (about 4 metres) with the patient in a semi-sitting position. In Sheffield adults are treated seated and children supine on a specially designed mobile couch (Fig. 26.11). Extended SSD is necessary to enable the

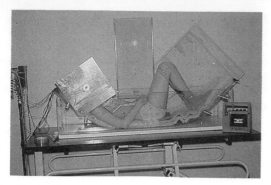

Fig. 26.11 Total body irradiation. Note tissue compensators over head and neck and below knee. (Courtesy of Dr K Dunn, Sheffield.)

whole patient to be encompassed within the photon beam directed at 90° to the long axis of the patient. Typical field sizes are 40 × 40 cm. After half the treatment the patient is turned through 180° and the other side is treated.

Careful dosimetry is needed using thermoluminescent dosimeters (TLD) positioned at regular intervals along each side and the midline of the body. The positions of the TLD probes and typical TLD values are shown in Figure 26.12. In general, doses to the thinner structures, the neck, lungs and the lower legs tend to be higher. To obtain a more even dose distribution (i.e. less than 10% variation), compensators are placed lateral to the head and neck, thorax and lower leg. Typically, 8 mm, 1 mm and 6 mm brass compensators are placed over the head, neck and thorax respectively. Sheets of Perspex (3–10 mm) are placed lateral to the legs from the knees downward.

Dose and energy
14.4 Gy midplane dose in twice daily fractions over 4 days (6 MV photons)

Side-effects
   1. *Pneumonitis.* Since pneumonitis commonly occurs following bone marrow transplantation in the absence

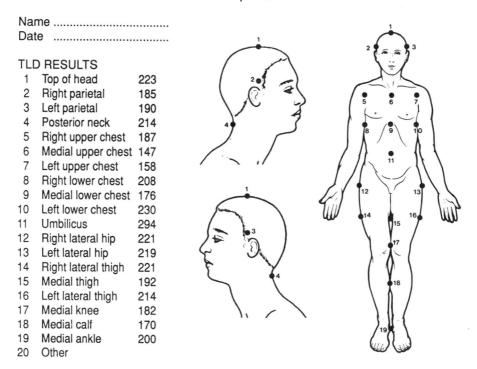

Fig. 26.12 Position for thermoluminescent dosimetry (TLD) measurements and typical doses for total body irradiation. (Courtesy of Dr J Conway, Sheffield.)

of radiation, the role of TBI in its causation is difficult to assess. In about half the cases there is an infectious cause. It is known however that lung damage is related both to total dose and to dose rate. Total doses above 8–9 Gy and dose rates above 0.05 Gy/min substantially increase the risk of lung damage. The incidence of pneumonitis is 50% for a total single TBI dose of 12 Gy given at low dose rate. This incidence is higher than might be predicted for the same dose given at higher dose rates. The explanation is probably that chemotherapy given at the same time reduces lung tolerance to irradiation.

2. Cataract. The incidence of cataract varies with both dose and dose rate. At a dose rate of 0.02 Gy/min the incidence is about 20% between 3 and 6 years for single fraction irradiation. The incidence is similar for fractionated TBI. At 0.05–0.08 Gy/min for single fraction TBI the incidence of cataract is 75% within 5 years. About 50% of patients with cataract need surgical treatment at some stage.

3. Hepatic veno-occlusive disease. Histologically confirmed veno-occlusive disease of the liver occurs in up to 25% of patients. In most patients symptoms are mild. However the mortality of established disease is high (30%).

4. Fertility. In females the retention of ovarian function and fertility is related to age at the time of TBI and chemotherapy. Under the age of 25, periods are likely to return within 6 months of treatment. Over the age of 25, permanent sterility is likely.

In males puberty is delayed in two-thirds and most patients are rendered azoospermic. Sperm production is unlikely to recover. Sperm storage should be considered in all patients who are sexually mature.

5. Hypothyroidism. Hypothyroidism, of varying severity, occurs in up to 30% of patients. The commonest finding is compensated hypothyroidism (i.e. raised TSH and normal T4). Thyroid hormone replacement may be required.

6. Growth delay. Growth hormone secretion may be impaired, especially if previous cranial irradiation has been given.

7. Second malignancy. This may very rarely occur (0.2%).

Radiotherapy

Local radiotherapy is useful for relieving the pain of skin, bony or retro-orbital deposits.

Technique

Single fields are used for skin, retro-orbital (p. 499) and most bone deposits. Parallel opposed lateral fields are used for gums and some bone deposits.

Dose and energy

Megavoltage or cobalt-60 (eye, bone, gums); superficial (skin) or orthovoltage (skin, bone).
5 Gy in single fraction to bone and skin deposits and in two daily fractions to eye or gums

Results of treatment

About 25% of patients with AML who achieve a complete remission and undergo further intensive chemotherapy are cured. If relapse occurs during chemotherapy, the probability of achieving a second remission is small. However if relapse occurs more than 6 months after treatment, a second remission can be induced in more than 50% of such patients.

CHRONIC MYELOID (GRANULOCYTIC) LEUKAEMIA

Chronic myeloid (granulocytic) leukaemia (abbreviated to CGL or CML) occurs mainly in the fifth and sixth decades. The incidence in the UK is 1 in 100 000. There is a slight male predominance (1.4:1).

A diagnostic feature is the presence of an abnormal chromosome 22, the *Philadelphia chromosome*. The long arm of chromosome 22 is translocated usually to chromosome 9 but occasionally to other chromosomes. It is present in over 90% of cases.

The typical picture is the insidious onset of progressive tiredness due to anaemia, with gross splenomegaly. The latter may cause a dragging sensation in the abdomen or acute pain if splenic infarction has occurred. The spleen may reach a huge size, filling the whole of the abdomen. Lymph nodes are not usually enlarged. Skin infiltration occurs rarely. The blood count shows a total white cell count typically between 100 and 500 × 10^9/l, of which 20–25% are myelocytes. Anaemia is often mild. The platelet count is normal or raised. The bone marrow is hypercellular.

The course of most of the illness is indolent (*chronic phase*). However eventually it transforms, on average after 3.5 years, to an *accelerated phase* and death. The accelerated phase is characterised by the presence of immature blast cells in the marrow. In most cases these are of myeloid type but in 20% they are lymphoid.

Treatment

1. Chronic phase

The aim of treatment is palliative in most patients. No treatment is needed if the patient's general condition is satisfactory and haemoglobin and white cell count are at reasonable levels. Indications for treatment are:

— Anaemia
— High platelet count
— High white cell count
— Uncomfortable splenomegaly.

Allopurinol (300 mg daily orally) should be given to prevent gout, particularly if the serum urate is raised.

Chemotherapy with alkylating agents (e.g. busulphan) in low dosage is given to improve the blood count and reduce the size of the spleen. It is aimed to keep the white count at $10–15 \times 10^9/l$. Hydroxyurea is an alternative to busulphan. The advantage of hydroxyurea is that its effects are reversible.

Dose: Busulphan oral 2–6 mg daily; hydroxyurea oral 1–2 g daily.

Care must be taken not to overtreat, reducing the white count to dangerous levels where infection may be life-threatening. This is a particular risk with busulphan due to its prolonged action (the nadir of the white count occurring at 4 weeks). For this reason busulphan is usually stopped when the white count reaches $20 \times 10^9/l$.

If clinical features of the hyperviscosity syndrome (p. 460) develop, leucopheresis is advised until chemotherapy has reduced the production of white cells.

Alpha-interferon has been shown to be effective in the control of a high white count and splenomegaly but whether it prolongs the chronic phase is as yet unproven.

Bone marrow transplantation. Allogeneic bone marrow transplantation should be considered for patients under the age of 45 with a compatible sibling donor.

2. Accelerated phase

The results of treatment of the accelerated phase in which myeloblasts appear is so poor that the clinician may decide not to offer chemotherapy. Hydroxyurea or 6-thioguanine may keep the blast cell numbers in check. For lymphoid transformation, the chances of obtaining a further remission with re-establishment of a second chronic phase are better. The drugs used are the same as for acute lymphocytic leukaemia (Ch. 29). If a remission is induced, craniospinal prophylaxis with intrathecal methotrexate and cranial irradiation are given.

Radiotherapy

CML is a very radiosensitive disease. In the past radioactive phosphorus-32 was used but has been replaced by chemotherapy. Irradiation still has a useful role for: (1) Uncomfortable splenomegaly uncontrolled

by chemotherapy, (2) myeloblastomas (local tumours composed of acute myeloblastic leukaemic cells), and (3) prophylactic cranial irradiation (in lymphoblastic transformation).

Spleen

Treatment volume
Irradiation of the whole of the spleen is not necessary to achieve shrinkage and symptomatic benefit. Splenic irradiation can be repeated if necessary, but eventually resistance develops.

Technique
Direct anterior or lateral fields (e.g. 15×10 cm) are used.

Dose and energy
0.25 Gy per day, increasing by 0.25 Gy per day up to 1.5–2 Gy daily to a total dose of 3 Gy (cobalt-60 or 4–6 MV photons)

Myeloblastomas. Single fractions of 5 Gy or 10 Gy by single or parallel opposed fields depending on site.

Prophylactic cranial irradiation. For patients who develop lymphoid transformation in the accelerated phase and achieve a second remission, prophylactic cranial irradiation is given. Technique and dosage are as described for ALL (Ch. 29).

Results of treatment

Average survival is about 3–4 years. With bone marrow transplantation in chronic phase, 50% are disease free at 4 years. This figure falls to 12% for patients transplanted in the accelerated phase.

CHRONIC LYMPHATIC (LYMPHOCYTIC) LEUKAEMIA

This disease is grouped both with the leukaemias and with low grade non-Hodgkin lymphomas (Ch. 26). Its incidence in the UK is 2 per 100 000. The male to female sex ratio is 2:1. It is usually seen in middle age.

The onset is insidious with tiredness from anaemia. Rapid onset of anaemia often indicates the development of an autoimmune haemolytic anaemia. Enlargement of lymph nodes of the neck and other peripheral sites (including the epitrochlear nodes at the elbow), spleen and liver is common. The spleen does not reach the large size of the chronic myeloid variety. Infiltration of the skin rarely occurs. Sometimes the entire skin is reddened and thickened (generalised leukaemic erythrodermia).

The white cell count is raised usually between 30–300 × 10⁹/l; 5–99% are small lymphocytes. In about 25% the diagnosis is made as an incidental finding on a blood count done for other reasons. As the disease advances, CLL may undergo prolymphocytoid immunoblastic change. 'Smudge' cells, which are cells that have been ruptured when making the blood film, are commonly seen. The platelet count is only markedly reduced in the terminal phase of the illness. The bone marrow is hypercellular with 30–90% of the cells being of the lymphoid series. Biopsy of enlarged nodes shows infiltration with lymphocytes (which differ from the lymphocytes of low grade diffuse lymphocytic lymphoma).

The course of the disease is usually slowly progressive.

Treatment

Treatment is only indicated if the patient has symptoms or if critical organs are involved by the disease (e.g. renal tract obstruction from enlarged para-aortic nodes).

Chemotherapy

Chemotherapy with chlorambucil is normally the initial treatment.

Dose: 2–10 mg per day orally. It is not necessary to achieve a complete response and treatment may be discontinued after a few months.

Steroids are helpful if the patient is thrombocytopenic or has an autoimmune haemolytic anaemia. The dose is gradually reduced if there is a response and eventually discontinued.

Dose: Prednisolone oral (5–40 mg daily).

Radiotherapy

If there is no response to chemotherapy, local radiotherapy to bulky tumour is indicated.

Technique
This will vary with site. An anterior and posterior parallel opposed pair of fields is suitable for axillary nodes. For the neck and groin, depending on the depth of the nodes, a single orthovoltage field may suffice.

Dose and energy
20 Gy in 4 daily fractions (250–300 kV, cobalt-60 or 4–6 MV photons)

Results of treatment

Five-year survival of CLL is about 50% but patients presenting with advanced disease may live for less than a year.

POLYCYTHAEMIA RUBRA VERA, PRIMARY POLYCYTHAEMIA

Polycythaemia rubra vera (PCRV) is an uncommon disease of the bone marrow, occurring mainly between the ages of 50 and 65 years. It is slightly more common in men than women. There is hyperplasia of all of the marrow constituents—erythroblastic, leucoblastic and megakaryocytic—i.e the precursors of red and white cells and platelets, which are all increased in the peripheral blood. The aetiology is unknown.

Clinical features

The clinical picture is dominated by the greatly increased number of red cells in the peripheral circulation (hence the name), but there may eventually be complete marrow exhaustion (aplastic anaemia), or the erythroblastic tissue may be exhausted first and the leucoblastic proliferation continue, leading to leukaemia.

The patient complains of headache, dizziness and tiredness, and has a cyanosed plethoric appearance. Pruritus occurs, particularly on exposure to heat or cold.

The spleen is palpable in 75% of patients at presentation. The increase in red cell volume increases the viscosity leading to thromboses (especially in brain, heart and limbs) and to haemorrhages. Other complications include peptic ulceration (10%), myelofibrosis, hyperuricaemia (30%) and gout (10%). Late leukaemic transformation develops rarely, either as a feature of the disease or due to treatment with radioactive phosphorus (see below).

Diagnosis

Typically the red cell count is raised (over 5.5×10^{12}/l in men and 5.0×10^{12}/l in women). The haemoglobin concentration is usually above 18 g/dl in men and 17 g/dl in women. The packed cell volume is normally in excess of 0.55 in men and 0.52 in women.

Other causes of polycythaemia must be excluded before making the diagnosis. Secondary polycythaemia can occur from the stimulus of hypoxia at high altitudes, in congenital heart disease and certain lung diseases (e.g. chronic obstructive airways disease and pulmonary fibrosis). It may also occur in association with renal lesions, especially renal adenocarcinoma.

True polycythaemia should be distinguished from spurious or stress polycythaemia in which raised haematocrit is due to a depleted plasma compartment. The mechanism is unknown, but it commonly occurs in overweight males who smoke and drink heavily.

Treatment

The aim is to produce prolonged reduction in the red cell volume to a fairly normal level. This may be achieved by (a) venesection (b) chemotherapy and (c) radiation.

Venesection

Venesection reduces the blood volume rapidly. Five hundred ml of blood may be removed initially and this affords quick symptomatic relief. A further 500 ml can be withdrawn 24 hours later and then every 48 hours until the packed cell volume reaches less than 0.50. The effect of venesection is temporary since it does not correct the defect in the bone marrow. It may be useful, e.g before an operation, to reduce the risk of thrombosis. When the plasma viscosity has been controlled by venesection, treatment with chemotherapy (usually with busulphan) or radioactive phosphorus is needed.

Cytotoxic therapy

Cytotoxic therapy can be given in short courses. Busulphan in a dose of 4–6 mg daily for 4–6 weeks is recommended. Busulphan has a very prolonged action. Care is necessary to ensure that the drug is stopped if the platelet count falls below $120 \times 10^9/l$. Chlorambucil (4–10 mg daily) and melphalan (2–4 mg daily) are alternatives. However, they carry a higher risk of inducing leukaemia than busulphan or radioactive phosphorus. More recently, hydroxyurea has been used extensively. This requires continuous oral therapy but may carry a lesser leukaemogenic risk.

Radioactive phosphorus (phosphorus-32)

Radioactive phosphorus (phosphorus-32) has the advantage that it is simple to administer and requires less frequent monitoring by blood counts than chemotherapy. It is given as an intravenous injection, usually as a phosphate salt. It is a beta emitter with a maximum energy of 1.7 MeV. Its physical half life is 14.3 days and its biological half life approximately 11 days.

Phosphorus is an essential constituent of all cells, especially of nuclei, and is therefore taken up to a greater extent in rapidly dividing than in slowly dividing cells.

It should be reserved for patients who are elderly or relatively immobile since the risk of leukaemogenesis is smaller and the likelihood of death from other causes greater in old age.

Phosphorus-32 is drawn up behind a perspex protective screen (to absorb the beta rays). Protective goggles and gloves are worn. Absorbent paper lines the tray on which the phosphorus-32 is dispensed to minimise contamination from accidental spillage. The syringe used to draw up the phosphorus-32 is also protected by an additional outer covering of perspex.

Dose
111–185 MBq as a single injection according to weight and the severity of the condition

A total dose of more than 1100 MBq is avoided to reduce the risk of inducing leukaemia.

Haematological effects

The maximum effect on the white cells and platelets occurs 3 weeks later. The red cell count falls at 6–8 weeks. The dose can be repeated if necessary at 3-monthly intervals depending on clinical and haematological findings. About 85% of patients go into remission, mostly after a single injection. A remission once achieved may last several years.

The risk of inducing acute non lymphocytic leukaemia is 3–4% and rises with the total dose of phosphorus-32.

Results of treatment

Without treatment the average survival is about 5 years. With treatment this is doubled. The end comes with marrow failure, leukaemia, thrombosis, haemorrhage or heart failure.

27. Central nervous system, eye and orbit

TUMOURS OF THE CENTRAL NERVOUS SYSTEM

Anatomy

A knowledge of normal neuroanatomy (Fig. 27.1) is important in appreciating the site of origin of different tumours of the central nervous system (CNS) (Fig. 27.2).

Tumours of the CNS are uncommon, accounting for 1.7% of all cancers and 1.8% of cancer deaths. They occur in both adults and children. The male: female ratio is 1.4:1. Benign tumours can be as important as malignant tumours, because, as space occupying masses within the rigid skull, they can cause pressure symptoms and may be fatal if vital brain centres are compressed.

Eighty per cent of CNS tumours are primary and 20% are secondary deposits from primary tumours elsewhere. Lung cancer accounts for 60% of metastases, followed by breast (15%) and then a variety of tumours including urogenital (particularly kidney), colon, ovary, leukaemia and lymphoma. Metastases are usually multiple but occasionally solitary.

Pathology

Table 27.1 gives details of the chief histological types. It is noteworthy that none are tumours of actual nerve

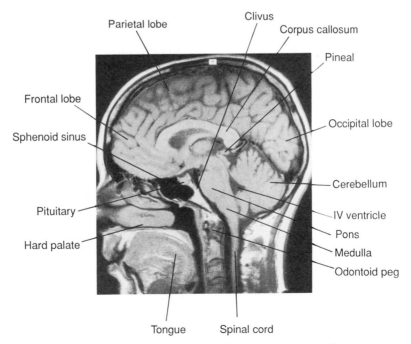

Fig. 27.1 Normal anatomy of the central nervous system shown. MRI midline sagittal section. (Courtesy of Dr L Turnbull, MRI Unit, Sheffield.)

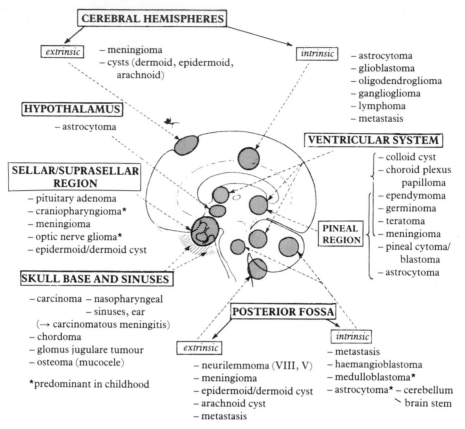

CEREBRAL HEMISPHERES

extrinsic
– meningioma
– cysts (dermoid, epidermoid, arachnoid)

intrinsic
– astrocytoma
– glioblastoma
– oligodendroglioma
– ganglioglioma
– lymphoma
– metastasis

HYPOTHALAMUS
– astrocytoma

VENTRICULAR SYSTEM
– colloid cyst
– choroid plexus papilloma
– ependymoma
– germinoma
– teratoma
– meningioma
– pineal cytoma/ blastoma
– astrocytoma

SELLAR/SUPRASELLAR REGION
– pituitary adenoma
– craniopharyngioma★
– meningioma
– optic nerve glioma★
– epidermoid/dermoid cyst

PINEAL REGION

SKULL BASE AND SINUSES
– carcinoma – nasopharyngeal
– sinuses, ear
(→ carcinomatous meningitis)
– chordoma
– glomus jugulare tumour
– osteoma (mucocele)

★predominant in childhood

POSTERIOR FOSSA

extrinsic
– neurilemmoma (VIII, V)
– meningioma
– epidermoid/dermoid cyst
– arachnoid cyst
– metastasis

intrinsic
– metastasis
– haemangioblastoma
– medulloblastoma★
– astrocytoma★ – cerebellum
         ↘ brain stem

Fig. 27.2 Classification of intracranial tumours according to site. (Reproduced with permission from Lindsay et al, Neurology, Neurosurgery, Churchill Livingstone, 1991.)

Table 27.1 Tumours of the central nervous system

Tissue of origin	Histological type	Typical site and degree of malignancy	Incidence (%)
	Glioma		
Neuroglia (connective tissue of CNS)	Astrocytoma	Commonest glioma. Ranges from benign to highly malignant. Adult: cerebral cortex. Child: cerebellum	
	Oligodendroglioma	Adult: cerebral cortex	50
	Ependymoma	Children: ventricles, esp. 4th. Wide range of malignancy. Seeds via CSF	
	Medulloblastoma	Child: cerebellum. Anaplastic, highly malignant. Seeds via CSF	
Meninges	Meningioma	Adults: benign. Malignancy rare	30
Pituitary gland	Chromophobe adenoma	Benign	12
	Eosinophil (acidophil) adenoma		
	Basophil adenoma		
Acoustic nerve	Acoustic neuroma	Benign, slowly growing	8
Pineal gland	Pinealoma	Mostly malignant, especially children. Seeds via CSF	<5
Blood vessels	Haemangioblastoma	Adults: malignant. Cerebellum	
Developmental anomaly	Craniopharyngioma	Benign (but can be fatal by pressure)	<1

cells, but only of supporting tissues and glands. The CNS is composed of *neurones* and their processes, surrounded by *glial cells*, consisting of *microglia*, *oligodendrocytes* and *astrocytes*. Tumours arising from nerve cells are extremely rare. In excess of 45% of intracranial tumours are *gliomas* (of glial origin). Microglial tumours are rare. *Astrocytomas* (75% of gliomas) have a wide-spectrum of malignancy. The Kernohan grading system is commonly used. This ranges from relatively well-differentiated (grades 1 and 2) to anaplastic tumours (grades 3 and 4). The most malignant is *glioblastoma multiforme* (grade 4). Tumours can rarely occur in the choroid plexus as papillomas in the lateral ventricles in children and in the posterior fossa in adults. *Gliomas* may occasionally develop in the optic nerve, more commonly in children.

Oligodendrogliomas are less common (5% of gliomas) than astrocytomas. They occur almost exclusively in adults. Growth is usually slow but they may transform to a more aggressive tumour after many years. Calcification within the tumour is common. The frontal lobes are a common site.

Medulloblastoma is a highly malignant tumour in children. It is rare in adults. It arises in the midline of the cerebellum from the floor of the fourth ventricle. The age of peak incidence is 4–10 years. The male to female ratio is about 2:1. It may block the cerebrospinal fluid (CSF) pathway and cause hydrocephalus. It spreads to the cerebrospinal fluid and spinal cord. It is the only intracranial tumour that gives rise to distant metastases, particularly to bone.

Ependymomas are tumours arising from the lining cells of the ventricles, central canal of the spinal cord and the filum terminale; 50% are of low grade malignancy; 60% of intracranial ependymomas are infratentorial. Tumours in the posterior fossa and high grade tumours are more likely to spread to the CSF than low grade and supratentorial tumours. The most malignant ependymomas develop in children.

Meningiomas are tumours, nearly always benign, arising from the arachnoid. They are attached to the meninges. Common sites are the parasagittal region, sphenoidal ridge and the olfactory groove.

Neurinomas are tumours arising from peripheral nerves. The commonest is the *acoustic neuroma* from the eighth or acoustic nerve. The main symptom is deafness.

There are some congenital tumours such as *craniopharyngiomas* and *chordomas*.

Craniopharyngiomas are histologically benign tumours developing from embryological remnants (Rathke's pouch) in the area above the sella turcica (suprasellar), the recess enclosing the pituitary gland. They usually present in adolescence with endocrine dysfunction (diabetes insipidus, hypogonadism and visual failure). They commonly contain viscous fluid containing cholesterol.

Chordomas arise from the primitive notochord, usually at the upper or lower ends of the neuraxis in the clivus or in the sacrum. Although they look benign histologically, they invade local structures but do not metastasise.

Tumours of the pineal region include malignant tumours such as *dysgerminoma* and *pineoblastoma*. Both have a tendency to spread to the CSF.

Spread of cerebral tumours

Spread is by local invasion; metastasis outside the CNS is rare. The absence of lymphatic vessels helps to account for this.

Metastatic spread outside the CNS is more likely if ventriculoperitoneal shunting has been carried out to relieve hydrocephalus. Local spread can occur by seeding of cells via the CSF, giving rise to multiple deposits on the surface of the brain and spinal cord. This is characteristic of medulloblastoma, ependymoma and pineoblastoma.

Clinical features

Though the tumours listed are very diverse in nature and have individual life histories, symptoms and signs arise in two distinct ways: (1) general effects from increased intracranial pressure, and (2) local effects which can arise from local pressure and damage to adjacent nervous tissue. These can arise from any space-occupying lesion, whether neoplastic, inflammatory or traumatic.

1. There is a classical triad of headache, vomiting and papilloedema (oedema of the optic disc, the white patch on the retina where the optic nerve emerges). It is important to recognise clinically that raised intracranial pressure can be present in an individual without each component of the triad being present. Headache, often worse in the morning, is of a throbbing kind and gradually becomes worse if the intracranial pressure is not relieved. Papilloedema can be seen on direct inspection through the pupil of the eye with an ophthalmoscope, even before the patient notices any disturbance of vision. Drowsiness, mental deterioration and personality changes may occur; with a slowly growing tumour, the behavioural disturbance may be considered to be psychiatric in origin. The patient may initially be admitted to a psychiatric ward.

2. Localising symptoms and signs depend very much

on the site of the tumour. Some typical examples are as follows:

Cerebellum : loss of coordination of movement
Frontal lobe : intellectual impairment and personality change
Temporal lobe : epilepsy, speech disturbance and visual field defects
Parietal lobe : sensory or visual inattention
Occipital lobe : visual field defects
Brainstem : cranial nerve defects, involvement of motor and sensory tracts

Epileptic attacks are common with tumours of the cerebral hemispheres, especially slow-growing oligodendrogliomas.

Diagnosis and investigation

A full history is taken. Information from the patient's family may indicate a change in personality or behaviour of which the patient may be unaware. The history and neurological examination may suggest the site of the tumour within the brain. However the diagnosis is most frequently made on the basis of a CT scan.

Plain radiographs of the skull may show calcification in a tumour (craniopharyngioma and some oligodendrogliomas), separation of cranial sutures (between bones) from raised intracranial pressure in a child and erosion of the sella in an adult, enlargement of the sella in pituitary tumours and erosion of the skull by meningioma.

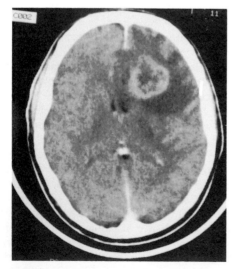

Fig. 27.3   CT scan showing grade 4 astrocytoma of the frontal lobe with surrounding oedema. (Courtesy of Dr T. Powell, Sheffield.)

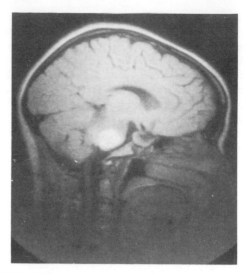

Fig. 27.4   MRI scan, sagittal section, showing brainstem glioma.

Isotope brain scanning is still useful in diagnosing brain tumours, although it has largely been replaced by CT scanning. It will show about 80% of tumours.

CT scanning is the most useful investigation in the diagnosis of brain tumours. It can show both the tumour and associated oedema or hydrocephalus. Figure 27.3 shows the typical appearance of a high grade astrocytoma.

Uptake of intravenous contrast (enhancement) occurs in the same conditions in which radioactive isotopes are taken up and is commonly seen with malignant tumours. Some areas of the brain are not well seen on CT because of the artefacts caused by bone, particularly in the posterior fossa and the spine. For these sites magnetic resonance imaging (MRI) is preferred. MRI shows tumours of the brainstem particularly well (Fig. 27.4).

Angiography—a radio-opaque medium is injected into the carotid or vertebral arterial circulation and may indicate the nature of the pathology. Angiography may help the planning of surgery. Displacement of the normal position of the vessels may help localise the lesion, or an area of abnormally profuse vascularity may be shown (e.g. meningioma).

Electroencephalography (EEG) may assist in showing abnormal waves, consistent with tumours in the hemispheres or with hydrocephalus.

Principles of treatment

Surgery

Biopsy. Radiological investigations should be followed by a biopsy, to confirm the suspected diagnosis. A tissue diagnosis is important since, despite the accuracy of modern neuroradiology, a mistaken diagnosis may be made on the basis of radiology alone in 5% of potentially salvageable cases. Biopsy may be performed under local or general anaesthetic. For small tumours, particularly in the posterior fossa and brainstem, biopsy should be carried out using a stereotactic system to ensure accuracy. A stereotactic frame is fixed to the skull and the coordinates of the tumour are measured in three planes from a CT scan performed with the frame in place. Knowing the coordinates the neurosurgeon can introduce the biopsy needle with the appropriate angulation to the required depth to minimise damage to critical structures. Sometimes, as in the brainstem, biopsy may be considered too hazardous because of the risk of damage to cranial nerve nuclei and motor and sensory tracts.

One disadvantage of any form of biopsy is that the specimen may represent only one part of the tumour. This may be the least malignant part. It is common for astrocytomas to contain a range of elements from benign to highly malignant. The biopsy therefore needs to be assessed in the context of the clinical and radiological features. If the history and CT scan suggest a highly aggressive tumour and the biopsy a low grade tumour, the biopsy result should be regarded with caution and not as a definitive guide to treatment. Repeating the biopsy may be necessary if the clinical behaviour is of a more malignant tumour. Alternatively, treatment is chosen on the presumption of higher grade malignancy being present.

Craniotomy. Surgical exploration by opening the skull (craniotomy) should always be considered, but the particular type and location of the tumour will determine what is done. Malignant intracranial tumours commonly infiltrate the surrounding tissues. It is therefore usually impossible to remove malignant tumours in their entirety. For example tumours in the brainstem are rarely surgically removable because of the proximity of cranial nerve nuclei and motor and sensory tracts. More complete removal with a margin of apparently normal tissue can be achieved in areas of the brain (frontal and occipital lobes) which are not concerned with speech (non-eloquent). Unfortunately, even apparently complete excision is almost invariably followed by recurrence in time, possibly because of a field change.

Subtotal excision with postoperative radiotherapy may be preferable to radical total removal in moderately radiosensitive tumours such as pituitary adenomas. Radical excision may risk damage to the optic chiasm and increase the possibility of the development of diabetes insipidus with electrolyte disturbance. Partial removal may be appropriate to prevent neurological complications, for example decompressing the optic nerves from a pituitary tumour.

Tumours in the region of the corpus callosum are unsuitable for even palliative surgery because of associated morbidity.

Palliative surgery. Palliative surgical procedures include relieving hydrocephalus by creating a drainage pathway for CSF between the atria of the heart or the peritoneum and the cerebral ventricles (ventriculoatrial or ventriculoperitoneal shunts). Aspiration of fluid within cystic tumours may relieve symptoms of raised intracranial pressure. Where fluid is likely to reaccumulate an Omaya reservoir inserted subcutaneously under the scalp may facilitate intermittent drainage under local anaesthesia.

Steroid therapy

Relief of raised intracranial pressure is assisted in the short term by treatment with corticosteroids. Dexamethasone in an initial dose of 16 mg/day often relieves symptoms in tumours with surrounding oedema, such as gliomas and metastases. The dose should be reduced to a level that controls symptoms and, if possible, withdrawn completely. Unwanted side-effects of corticosteroid therapy include obesity, diabetes mellitus, electrolyte disturbance and in the long term osteoporosis.

Radiotherapy

Radiotherapy may be radical or palliative in intent. In tumours such as medulloblastoma and pineal germinoma cure is achievable. For high grade astrocytomas, only short-term palliation is achievable even with radical doses.

Megavoltage external beam is the main form of irradiation used for treating brain tumours, both in adults and children. It is usually given postoperatively following biopsy or debulking of the primary tumour. Intracavitary therapy with yttrium-90 (for craniopharyngioma) or interstitial implantation with iridium-192 (to boost high grade gliomas or to treat recurrent disease after external beam) are occasionally indicated.

The volume of the CNS irradiated will vary with the local extent and pattern of actual and likely spread of the tumour. There are three broad groups: (1) tumours treated by small volume brain irradiation because they tend to remain localised, e.g. brain stem gliomas; (2) tumours treated by wide field brain irradiation because of their tendency to infiltrate within the cerebral hemispheres, e.g. high grade astrocytomas; and (3) tumours treated by whole CNS (craniospinal) irradiation, e.g. medulloblastoma, ependymoma and pineoblastoma, where seeding of tumour to spinal cord via the CSF may occur.

Radiation tolerance of the central nervous system

It is important to have an appreciation of the radiation tolerance of the CNS since it influences the volume that can be safely irradiated.

The radiation tolerance of the CNS (brain and spinal cord) is of basic importance, in addition to the sensitivity of the actual tumour cells. Nerve cells are among the most resistant in the body. This is due to the fact that mature nerve cells never go into mitosis. Once destroyed they are never replaced. They are vulnerable to damage to their supporting tissues (neuroglia), and especially the small blood vessels on which they depend for oxygen and other nutrients. Obliterative endarteritis induced by radiation is the limiting factor in the tissue tolerance of the nervous system. The supporting glial cells can be renewed, albeit slowly. During the acute reaction to radiation there is direct damage to nerve cells, blood vessels and the glial cells. Damage to normal tissue arises from: (1) impairment of renewal of glial cells, and (2) narrowing of the small vessels of the arterial system leading to death of the tissues supplied. Typical late effects of brain irradiation are fibrosis, loss of cerebral white matter (demyelination), vascular damage and cell death (necrosis). The mechanisms are similar to those seen in other organs but the effects are more serious because of the irreplaceability of nerve cells.

The parts of the CNS most sensitive to radiation are the spinal cord (particularly the cervical part), the hypothalamus and the brainstem. The frontal, temporal and occipital lobes will tolerate higher doses.

Dose per fraction is an important factor in CNS tolerance. The tolerance to high doses per fraction is reduced. For this reason doses are conventionally kept to 2 Gy per fraction or less for radical treatment.

If the whole brain is irradiated, total dosage should generally not exceed 35 Gy in 10 daily fractions, 45 Gy in 20 daily fractions, 50 Gy in 25 daily fractions or 54 Gy in 30 daily fractions. For the brainstem, 45 Gy in 20 daily fractions or 55 Gy in 30 fractions should not be exceeded.

Radiosensitivity of brain tumours

The radiosensitivity of brain tumours varies con-siderably. At one end of the spectrum are low grade astrocytomas and meningiomas which are relatively radioresistant. At the other end are pineal germinomas which are highly radiosensitive.

Treatment of cerebral gliomas

The treatment of both low grade and high grade gliomas is controversial.

Low grade tumours (1 or 2)

In general, low grade astrocytomas should be treated by total or macroscopic excision. Whether postoperative radiotherapy should be given is uncertain. Non-randomised studies suggest some prolongation of 5- and 10-year survival. Many radiotherapists do not routinely offer postoperative radiotherapy to low grade gliomas. Occasionally a tumour behaves more ag-gressively than is suggested by the low grade histology. This sometimes reflects sampling from better dif-ferentiated areas of a glioma which contains more malignant grade 3 or 4 elements. In this circumstance it is reasonable to give postoperative irradiation on the presumption of high grade tumour.

High grade astrocytomas (3 or 4)

Surgery. Surgical debulking should be carried out if possible since it reduces the need for steroids and facilitates the delivery of postoperative radiotherapy. Where no debulking is carried out, postoperative radio-therapy may be accompanied by clinical deterioration due to radiation induced oedema. Where a tumour lies in an eloquent area, e.g. the left parietal lobe, biopsy alone is often preferred to avoid damaging the speech area.

Radiotherapy

Postoperative radiotherapy. Opinions differ on the indications for postoperative radiotherapy. High grade astrocytomas are relatively radioresistant. Cure is ex-ceptional and local persistence or recurrence of tu-mour the rule, even with radical doses. Treatment is therefore palliative, prolonging survival by only a few months compared with surgical debulking alone. Sadly the quality of life of many of these patients is poor as a result of both the disease and its treatment. With such limited benefits from postoperative radiotherapy, careful selection of patients most likely to benefit is particularly important. A discussion with the patient and the family on the likely additional survival and anticipated side-effects of radiotherapy may help the patient to decide whether or not to accept postoperative radiotherapy.

It is important not to irradiate patients who have a particularly poor prognosis. These include the elderly, those in poor general medical condition or patients who have a major neurological deficit (e.g. a hemiparesis) which fails to improve with steroids or surgery.

Target volume

Since high grade cerebral gliomas infiltrate widely, often well beyond the macroscopic limits of the tumour, the target volume should include a generous margin of normal tissue. On this basis many clinicians treat the whole brain. However in order to minimise late sequelae, it is reasonable to allow a 3 cm margin around the limits of the tumour if well defined on CT scan.

Technique

For extensive, diffusely infiltrating and all bilateral tumours a parallel opposed pair of lateral fields is used covering the whole brain (Fig. 27.5A).

For well-defined tumours a right-angled wedged pair (Fig. 27.6) is appropriate. A third unwedged field between the wedged fields may be necessary to bring up the dose to the posteromedial part of the target volume.

Since local relapse is most common at the primary site, there has been increasing interest in boosting the tumour, if well defined on CT scan, with an iridium-192 implant following external beam. Longer survival compared with external beam alone has been reported with this approach. These preliminary findings need to be confirmed in randomised prospective studies comparing external beam plus implant with external beam alone. In general, increasing the dose to large volumes of brain increases the risk of radionecrosis without increasing local control. However the tolerance of the brain to very focal irradiation may prove to be better.

Dose and energy

45 Gy in 20 daily fractions over 4 weeks (4–6 MV photons or cobalt-60)

Side-effects. Acute side-effects are hair loss within

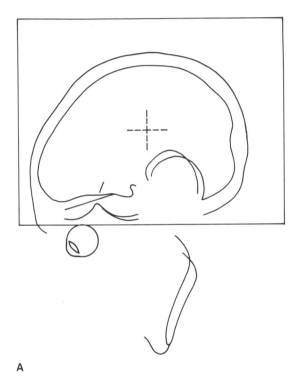

A

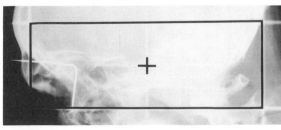

B

Fig. 27.5   A Field for whole brain irradiation. (Reproduced with permission from Perez & Brady 1987.) **B** Field for palliative irradiation of the base of skull. (Courtesy of Dr J Bolger, Sheffield.)

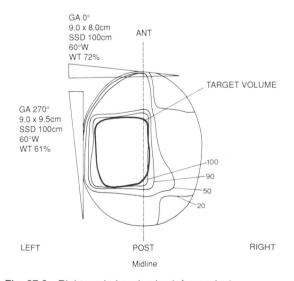

Fig. 27.6   Right-angled wedged pair for grade 4 astrocytoma of the frontal lobe.

the irradiated area, skin erythema, impaired hearing (if the ear is included in the treated volume) and somnolence. The most important late side-effect is radionecrosis.

Chemotherapy. Where there is recurrence or persistent disease after surgery and radiotherapy, palliative chemotherapy may result in temporary growth restraint. CCNU, BCNU and procarbazine are used since they cross the blood–brain barrier. Response rates are poor. **e.g. CCNU 120–130 mg/m² orally or 40 mg/m² orally daily for 3 days, repeated 6–8-weekly.**

The dose limiting factor for CCNU is bone marrow suppression.

Results of treatment of astrocytomas

Five-year survival is: grade 1: 60%, grade 2: 40%, grade 3: 10% and grade 4: 2%.

Treatment of ependymomas

Low grade supratentorial ependymomas should be treated by cranial irradiation alone. High grade ependymomas and all infratentorial ependymomas should be treated by craniospinal irradiation.

Radical radiotherapy

Technique, volume (Figs 27.7–27.11) and dose are as for medulloblastoma (below).

Macroscopic disease identified on MRI or myelography is boosted by an additional 10 Gy in 5 daily fractions.

Results of treatment

Overall 5-year survival of intracranial ependymomas is 40–60%. Survival is better for low grade tumours (80%).

MEDULLOBLASTOMA

Children with medulloblastoma of the cerebellum usually present with features of raised intracranial pressure and of cerebellar dysfunction (unsteady gait and lack of coordination). CT scan shows the primary tumour, often accompanied by hydrocephalus. Some children are in extremis at presentation and die without prompt neurosurgical intervention. Treatment is initially aimed at macroscopic removal of the tumour. A ventriculoperitoneal shunt is often needed to relieve hydrocephalus.

Adjuvant cytotoxic therapy with vincristine and CCNU has been shown to be beneficial in certain high risk groups (e.g. age <2 years, partial or subtotal removal or with brainstem involvement).

Postoperative craniospinal irradiation is given as described below.

Radical radiotherapy

Target volume

The aim is to irradiate the entire craniospinal axis at the same time. This should encompass any malignant cells in the neuraxis.

Technique

Separate megavoltage fields are used for the skull and the spine. A shell which encompasses the head and shoulders is constructed in the prone position (Figs 27.7–27.9).

In the few cases where the child is too restless, general anaesthesia may be necessary for each treatment.

Cranial and upper spinal field. Irradiation of the brain is carried out in three phases to progressively smaller volumes.

The initial volume is the whole brain and upper cervical cord extending to the lower margin of the second cervical vertebra. The anterior face is protected with lead shielding. The head of the gantry is twisted (usually 8–10°) so that the lower margin of the cranial field is matched to the divergence of the posterior spinal field.

In the second phase the volume is reduced to include the posterior fossa, the third ventricle, the hypothalamus and the pituitary. The anterior margin of

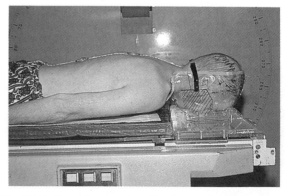

Fig. 27.7 Prone treatment position for craniospinal irradiation. Hatched area on mould indicates shielding of the eye and anterior face. Midline strip of ball bearings on the back identifies the skin surface for measuring depth of spinal cord along the treatment volume.

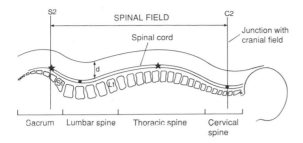

A

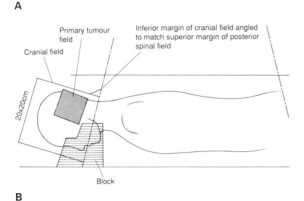

B

Fig. 27.8 A Diagram showing patient in the prone treatment position for craniospinal irradiation. d, Depth from skin surface to posterior margin of the spinal cord. Points of maximum (★) and minimum (●) spinal cord dose are shown. (Modified from Dobbs et al 1992.) **B** Diagram showing matching of the upper junction of the spinal field with the lower border of the cranial field.

this second phase is the anterior clinoid process of the pituitary fossa.

In the third phase, the field is reduced to cover the posterior fossa alone. The anterior margin of this field is the posterior clinoid process of the pituitary fossa.

Spinal field(s). The spinal field(s) extends down from C2 to cover the whole of the spinal cord and dural sheath to the lower border of the second sacral piece (Figs 27.8 and 27.9). In children the whole of the spine can often be encompassed in one field. In adults two fields are usually needed, separated by an optical gap on the skin. The latter is calculated to match the 50% isodoses at the posterior margin of the spinal cord.

The width of the spinal field(s) covers the dural sleeves and spinal ganglia. The outer limit of the field is 1 cm lateral to the pedicles on each side (Fig. 27.10). In children the spinal field is not widened to cover the upper sacral nerves in order to minimise the dose to the gonads. The width of the spinal field is normally 4 cm in children and 6 cm in adults.

Radio-opaque markers are placed on the skin in the midline over the spine. Lateral radiographs are taken.

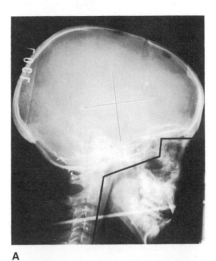

A

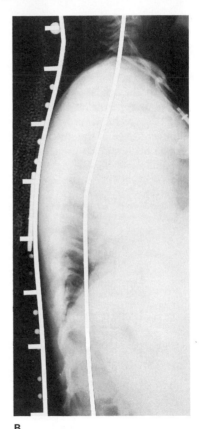

B

Fig. 27.9 A Planning radiograph showing field for irradiation of whole brain and upper spinal cord (phase 1). **B** Lateral simulator radiograph showing points on skin surface from which depth of spinal cord is measured. (Courtesy of Dr M J Whipp, Sheffield.)

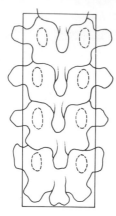

Fig. 27.10   In the posterior spinal field the lateral border should be 1 cm lateral to the pedicles on each side to cover dural sleeves and spinal ganglia. (Reproduced with permission from Perez & Brady 1987.)

This enables the depth from the skin surface, at 5 cm intervals, to the posterior margin of the spinal cord to be calculated (Fig. 27.9B). If the maximum dose exceeds ± 5%, wax compensators are used to obtain a more even dose distribution along the spinal axis. The maximum dose to the spinal axis tends to occur in the midthoracic and upper sacral region (Fig. 27.8).

'Feathering' the field junctions. A further measure to avoid overdosage at the junctions between (1) cranial and spinal fields and (2) upper and lower spinal fields is the technique of 'feathering'. This is achieved

by shifting the junctions of (1) and (2) 1 cm upwards or downwards on a daily basis while maintaining the same optical gap between the fields (Fig. 27.11).

Dose and energy
Phase 1: 30 Gy in 20 daily fractions over 4 weeks (4–6 MV photons)
Phase 2: 10 Gy dose in 6 daily fractions (4–6 MV photons)
Phase 3: 10–15 Gy in 6–8 daily fractions (4–6 MV photons)

Primary tumour. In children under the age of 3 years the total dose should be 40–45 Gy in 6–7 weeks. Over the age of 3, the dose is 50–55 Gy in 6–8 weeks. Doses to the lens should be measured using thermoluminescent dosimetry and should generally not exceed 10% of the tumour dose.

Spinal field(s)
Mean tumour dose of 30 Gy in 25 daily fractions over 5 weeks

Radiation reaction. With proper shielding, constitutional reactions should be mild.

1. Acute reaction
Bone marrow suppression. The blood count will fall during treatment due to the large volume of bone marrow irradiated. Treatment should be suspended if the white blood count falls below $2 \times 10^9/l$ or platelets

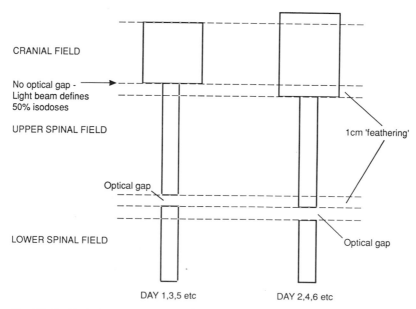

Fig. 27.11   Technique of 'feathering' of field junctions in craniospinal irradiation.

below $60 \times 10^9/l$. The blood count normally recovers after a few days' rest, allowing treatment to be resumed. Delays in radiotherapy due to marrow suppression are more frequent if adjuvant cytotoxic chemotherapy is given (e.g. in medulloblastoma).

Skin and oesophageal reaction. Acute effects include total epilation of the scalp, erythema and dysphagia (from the exit dose passing through the pharynx and oesophagus).

2. Late effects. Late effects include impairment of vertebral growth either as a direct effect or due to irradiation of the hypothalamo-pituitary axis causing a reduction of growth hormone.

Hypothyroidism may result from irradiation of the thyroid gland from the exit dose. Thyroid function should be regularly monitored.

Mental impairment may occur in long-term survivors. This is often multifactorial. The effects of the tumour, surgery and radiotherapy probably all contribute.

Results of treatment

The overall 5-year survival of medulloblastoma in the UK is 18%. This relatively low figure reflects the inclusion of children who die as a result of surgery or who do not complete a course of radiotherapy. Major centres with substantial experience of treating the disease report much better results (40–50% 5-year survival). This difference argues for such children to be treated in specialised centres.

PINEAL AND THIRD VENTRICULAR TUMOURS

Clinical features of tumours of the pineal and posterior end of the third ventricle are mainly due to CSF obstruction causing symptoms and signs of raised intracranial pressure. Upward gaze may be impaired (Parinaud's syndrome) due to compression of the midbrain. The cerebellum may also be compressed, giving rise to unsteady gait. Diabetes insipidus with absent or delayed secondary sexual development in a teenager is typical of dysgerminoma.

Tumours of the anterior end of the third ventricle cause impaired vision and hypopituitarism.

Diagnosis and treatment

Management depends on the site, clinical features and likely histology. A stereotactic biopsy should be obtained from tumours of the pineal or the posterior end of the third ventricle. If dysgerminoma is suspected on clinical grounds, ventriculoatrial shunting should

be avoided if possible to reduce the risk of disseminating tumour cells throughout the CSF pathways.

Often it is considered too hazardous to carry out a biopsy in deep-seated pineal tumours. In this circumstance the need for craniospinal irradiation is determined by the response to local irradiation. If after 20 Gy a repeat CT scan shows marked regression, the presence of germinoma or pineoblastoma is virtually certain. So radiosensitive are these tumours that 20–30 Gy often shrinks the tumour sufficiently to relieve hydrocephalus without the need for shunting.

For tumours of the anterior part of the third ventricle an open craniotomy is required. Tumour markers, alpha-fetoprotein and human chorionic gonadotrophin (HCG), may be detectable in blood and CSF in teratomas. Serial tumour markers and CT scanning should be carried out to assess the response to treatment.

Because of the cumulative risk of CSF dissemination (10% for pineal tumours overall and 50% for dysgerminomas) craniospinal irradiation is advised for all biopsy proven dysgerminomas and for tumours which are locally invasive or involve both the pineal and the hypothalamus.

Radical radiotherapy

Target volume
Phases 1 and 2: (as medulloblastoma).
Phase 3: the boost volume is confined to the pineal tumour with a margin of normal tissue.

Technique
Craniospinal irradiation (as medulloblastoma) except that one proceeds directly to boost the pineal after the initial 4 weeks of whole brain irradiation.

Dose and energy: as medulloblastoma.

Brain and upper cervical cord (4–6 MV photons)
Phase 1 (whole brain): 30 Gy in 20 daily fractions over 4 weeks
Phase 2 (primary tumour): 20 Gy in 10 daily fractions over 2 weeks

Spinal field (4–6 MV photons)
30–35 Gy mean dose in 25 daily fractions over 5 weeks

Chemotherapy

In the presence of tumour it does not appear that the blood–brain barrier prevents systemic cytotoxic agents entering the CNS. Chemotherapy using the same regime as for testicular teratoma (Table 25.5) can cure intracranial germ cell tumours. In future, chemotherapy may reduce the dose of radiation necessary for local control.

Results of treatment

Overall 5-year survival is about 60% for pineal tumours and higher for germinomas. Follow-up of growth, endocrine function and intellectual development is particularly important in children. Endocrine function should be monitored in adults.

BRAINSTEM TUMOURS

Tumours of the brainstem are inoperable and, because of their site and vascularity, even biopsy is hazardous. A diagnosis has usually to be made on the clinical and radiological findings. Astrocytoma is the commonest histological type. Occasionally secondary tumours occur (e.g. from breast cancer). MRI gives good definition of the tumour (Fig. 27.4). Treatment is by radical radiotherapy.

Radical radiotherapy

Target volume
The tumour and the whole of the brainstem and a 1–2 cm margin of normal tissue should be included. The lower border of the field is the inferior margin of the second cervical vertebra.

Technique
A parallel opposed pair of fields or a three field technique with wedges is used.

Dose and energy
45 Gy in 20 daily fractions over 4 weeks (4–6 MV photons)

Results of treatment

The results of treatment are poor. Five-year survival is 15–20%.

PRIMARY CNS LYMPHOMA

Primary extranodal lymphoma of the CNS is much less common than secondary intracerebral involvement. The incidence is increased in patients whose immune system has been suppressed, for example after renal transplantation or in acquired immunodeficiency syndrome (AIDS). The disease is normally confined to the brain. The histology is usually a high grade histiocytic lymphoma. It invades locally and may seed to the CSF. Symptoms and signs are as for other primary brain tumours.

Diagnosis and investigation

A biopsy should be obtained. Debulking of the tumour is not carried out since it is very sensitive to radiation. Lumbar puncture and cytology of the CSF should be performed to look for malignant cells.

Treatment

If the CSF shows no evidence of spread, the whole of the brain is treated by external radiotherapy. If there is spread to the CSF craniospinal irradiation and intermittent intrathecal methotrexate are indicated.

Radical radiotherapy

Technique
Whole brain (Fig. 27.5A or craniospinal irradiation (Fig. 27.8) is used.

Dose and energy
Brain: 45 Gy in 20 daily fractions over 4 weeks to whole brain (4–6 MV photons)
Spinal cord: 30–35 Gy mean dose in 25 daily treatments over 5 weeks (4–6 MV photons)

Results of treatment

The prognosis is poor with 5-year survival of less than 20%.

MENINGIOMA

Meningiomas usually grow very slowly. Surgical removal is the principal treatment. If complete, no further treatment is required. The response to radiotherapy is therefore difficult to assess. There is some evidence that external beam irradiation reduces local recurrence where surgical removal is subtotal. Radiotherapy technique will depend on site.

Radical radiotherapy

Target volume
This includes the tumour and a small margin of normal tissue.

Technique
A two or three field technique with wedges is used.

Since this is a benign tumour, a CT planning scan is helpful to minimise the volume of normal brain irradiated.

Dose and energy
45 Gy in 20 daily fractions over 4 weeks (4–6 MV photons)

Results of treatment

The value of radiotherapy is difficult to measure since the natural history of the tumour itself is often very slow. Postoperative radiotherapy probably reduces the recurrence rate but this requires confirmation in randomised studies of surgery with and without post-operative radiotherapy.

OPTIC NERVE GLIOMA

This rare tumour is normally slowly growing and of low grade malignancy. Treatment is by biopsy and radical radiotherapy or surveillance alone.

Radical radiotherapy

Target volume
This includes the tumour with a 1 cm margin of normal tissue.

Technique
The patient lies supine. An open anterior field and two lateral wedged fields are used. A shell is required.

Dose and energy
45 Gy in 20 daily fractions over 4 weeks (4–6 MV photons)

Results of treatment

Following radical radiotherapy, vision can be preserved or improved in the majority of patients.

PITUITARY TUMOURS

Anatomy

The pituitary gland (Fig. 27.12) lies in the sella turcica, a recess in the base of the skull. The sella has a floor and front and back walls bounded by anterior and posterior clinoid processes. It is composed of anterior and posterior lobes. It is connected structurally and functionally to the hypothalamus above. Above the pituitary gland lies the optic chiasm, where

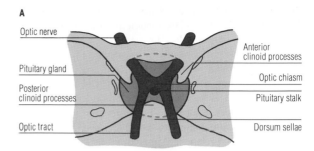

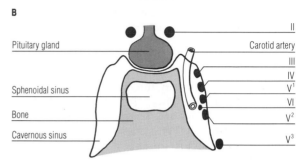

Fig. 27.12 Gross anatomy and relations of the pituitary gland. (Reproduced with permission from Souhami & Moxham, Textbook of Medicine, Churchill Livingstone, 1990)

the visual pathways cross. To each side lie the cavernous sinuses through which pass the 3rd, 4th and first and second divisions of the 5th cranial nerve, the 6th cranial nerve and the carotid artery. Below lies the sphenoid sinus.

The pituitary gland exerts control, through the hormones that it secretes, on the gonads, thyroid and adrenal glands and upon growth. The anterior lobe, under the influence of releasing factors from the hypothalamus, secretes the following hormones: prolactin, thyroid stimulating hormone (TSH), adrenocorticotrophic hormone (ACTH), follicle stimulating hormone (FSH), luteinising hormone (LH) and growth hormone (GH). The posterior lobe secretes antidiuretic hormone (ADH) and oxytocin.

Pathology

Tumours of the pituitary are relatively common, accounting for about 12% of tumours of the CNS. Virtually all arise from the anterior lobe of the gland. Histologically primary pituitary tumours are all benign. Their danger is due to the proximity of vital structures such as the optic nerves, compression of which can lead to partial or complete blindness. In addition to this local pressure, clinical syndromes due to underproduction or overproduction of hormones develop.

Secondary tumours, of which breast cancer is the commonest, are rare. The principal clinical syndromes are described below.

It is the type and amount of hormone secreted rather than the staining characteristics (e.g. eosinophilic or basophilic) that correlate best with clinical features and behaviour of the tumour. A functional classification is therefore adopted. Tumours are classified as secretors or non-secretors and subclassified by the hormone they produce. Approximately 30% of large pituitary tumours (macroadenomas, i.e. >1 cm in size) are non-secretory or functionless. The latter are normally chromophobe adenomas.

Hormone secretion

The commonest secretory tumours are prolactinomas, producing prolactin. They are usually eosinophilic. Occasionally tumours may secrete both prolactin and growth hormone. ACTH is most commonly secreted by basophilic tumours causing Cushing's syndrome. Tumours which secrete TSH, FSH or LH are rare.

Clinical features

1. Local effects of pituitary and suprasellar tumours
a. Pressure on the optic chiasm—visual field defects (blindness). Typically the upper visual fields are affected initially. A bitemporal hemianopia, in which the outer half of both visual fields is lost, may subsequently develop.
b. Headache, often persistent.
c. Extension into the cavernous sinus is rarely symptomatic unless extensive. If so, the 3rd, 4th, 5th and 6th cranial nerves and first and second divisions of the 5th nerve can cause pain in the eye, diplopia (double vision), closure of the eye (ptosis), sensory loss over the part of the same side of the nose and loss of the corneal reflex.
d. Increased appetite and thirst.
e. Pressure on the floor of the third ventricle (loss of recent memory).
2. Clinical syndromes
a. Panhypopituitarism
   (i) Children—failure of growth and of pubertal development.
   (ii) Adults—non-specific malaise, pale 'waxen doll' skin complexion, cold intolerance (features of hypothyroidism are rarely gross), amenorrhoea (women), loss of sex drive and potency, loss of secondary sexual hair, hypopituitary crisis (acute abdominal pain) and low blood sugar.
b. Acromegaly, Cushing's syndrome (p. 549)

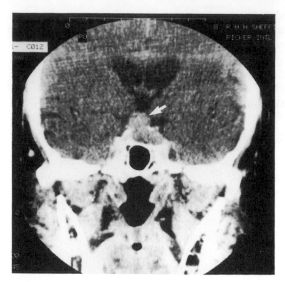

Fig. 27.13   Coronal CT scan showing pituitary tumour with suprasellar extension (arrowed). (Courtesy of Mr R Battersby, Sheffield)

Diagnosis and investigation of pituitary tumours

CT and MRI scanning are the investigations of choice. However the initial diagnosis may be suspected from enlargement of the pituitary fossa on lateral skull radiograph. CT scanning shows local extension, e.g. above the pituitary (suprasellar, Fig. 27.13) and into the cavernous sinus. Basal levels of the anterior pituitary hormones should be measured. Dynamic tests of pituitary function are performed in which the ability of the pituitary to secrete particular hormones in response to hypothalamic releasing factors is assessed.

Treatment of pituitary tumours

Surgery, radiotherapy and medical therapy are the treatments available for pituitary tumours. Close liaison is required between surgeon, radiotherapist and endocrinologist in choosing the appropriate combination of treatments.

Surgery

The surgical approach to the pituitary gland (Fig. 27.14) is most commonly through the nose (trans-sphenoidal) and less commonly through a craniotomy incision (transfrontal). Trans-sphenoidal surgery is used for small or medium sized pituitary tumours with or without symmetrical extension above the sella (suprasellar). This approach allows small tumours (microadenomas)

Operative approach

From BELOW:

1. Trans-sphenoidal
Through an incision in the upper gum the nasal mucosa is stripped from the septum and the pituitary fossa approached through the sphenoid sinus.

2. Transethmoidal
An incision is made on the medial orbital wall and the pituitary fossa approached through the ethmoid and sphenoid sinuses.

With the transethmoidal and trans-sphenoidal routes the pituitary gland can be directly visualised and explored for microadenoma. Even large tumours with suprasellar extensions may be removed from below, avoiding the need for craniotomy.

From ABOVE

3. Transfrontal
Through a craniotomy flap the frontal lobe is retracted to provide direct access to the pituitary tumour. This approach is usually reserved for tumours with large frontal or lateral extensions.

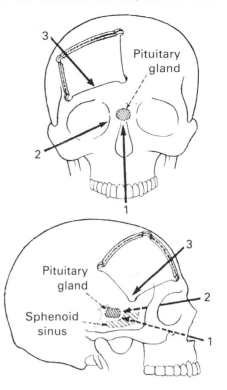

Fig. 27.14 Surgical approaches to the pituitary gland. 1, Trans-sphenoidal. 2, Transethmoidal. 3, Transfrontal. (Reproduced with permission from Lindsay et al, Neurosurgery, Neurology, Churchill Livingstone, 1991.)

to be removed while leaving adjacent normal pituitary tissue intact. The morbidity of trans-sphenoidal surgery is low.

Transfrontal surgery is appropriate either to relieve compression of the optic nerves or to remove tumours which are (1) large, (2) have asymmetrical suprasellar extension, or (3) have spread laterally into the cavernous sinus. Removal of the tumour is subtotal and post-operative radiotherapy is required. The morbidity of transfrontal surgery is higher than trans-sphenoidal surgery and carries an operative mortality of 1% or less.

Hypopituitarism may occur, depending on how discrete the adenoma is and how radical the surgery needs to be. Hormone replacement is required (see below).

Radical radiotherapy

There are a variety of ways of irradiating the pituitary gland. These are photons, yttrium implantation and proton beam therapy. Of these, photontherapy remains the most effective and, with appropriate dosage and fractionation, the safest. Yttrium-90 and gold-198 have been used to implant tumours confined to the sella.

Although they can deliver a high dose to the pituitary gland, with more rapid effects than external beam, complications such as damage to the optic nerve and meningitis discourage use.

Target volume

This should include the pituitary tumour with a 1–2 cm margin. Postoperative field sizes normally range between 4 × 4 cm and 5 × 5 cm.

Technique

A head mould is required. The patient is treated with the chin flexed to allow the anterior field to enter above the eyes. A three field technique is commonly used (Fig. 27.15B). An alternative is a parallel opposed pair of fields. A theoretical disadvantage of the latter is that the maximum dose is delivered to the temporal lobes. However there is no clinical evidence of temporal lobe damage after conventional central tumour doses of 40 Gy over 4 weeks.

Dose and energy
40 Gy in 20 daily fractions over 4 weeks (4–6 MV photons)

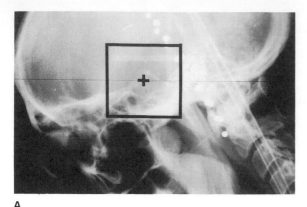

A

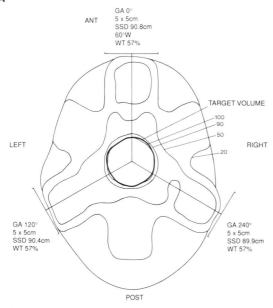

ANT

GA 0°
5 x 5cm
SSD 90.8cm
60°W
WT 57%

TARGET VOLUME

100
90

50

20

LEFT

RIGHT

GA 120°
5 x 5cm
SSD 90.4cm
WT 57%

GA 240°
5 x 5cm
SSD 89.9cm
WT 57%

POST

B

Fig. 27.15 A Lateral simulator radiograph showing treatment volume for pituitary tumour. **B** Isodose distribution from anterior and two posterior obique fields for a pituitary tumour (6 MV photons).

Radiation reaction. Acute reactions are minimal. Erythema and hair loss occur. The commonest late effect is hypopituitarism, which is nearly universal. Hormonal replacement therapy is with thyroxine, hydrocortisone and the sex hormones (oestradiol + progesterone as the oral contraceptive for women and testosterone for men). Using the doses and fractionation stated above, chiasmal damage should not occur.

Treatment of specific tumours

1. Prolactinomas

Large prolactinomas (macroprolactinomas) are greater than 1 cm in size. They behave differently from small prolactinomas (microprolactinomas, less than 1 cm). Large prolactinomas expand the pituitary fossa and compress the chiasm and require prompt treatment.

Macroprolactinomas. Bromocriptine is the initial treatment of choice for macroprolactinomas and can shrink very rapidly even large tumours compressing the optic chiasm. If bromocriptine fails to relieve chiasmal compression completely, surgical decompression is required. Postoperative external beam irradiation is advised to sterilise the tumour. If, however, a macroprolactinoma is untreated, there is a small risk that it may expand during pregnancy. For this reason normalisation of the serum prolactin with surgery or bromocriptine is advised before conception occurs. If bromocriptine is not tolerated, trans-sphenoidal surgical removal of the tumour should be carried out.

Microprolactinomas. Not all patients with an elevated serum prolactin have a prolactin secreting tumour. In some patients there is no obvious cause. However if the serum prolactin is in excess of 1000 mu/l, a microprolactinoma is likely to be present. The natural history of these tumours is more benign than that of macroprolactinomas. Treatment is not necessarily essential. Surgery is the only treatment which can effectively cure the disease. Bromocriptine may achieve temporary growth control.

Indications for treatment are: amenorrhoea, low oestrogen levels (which favour the development of osteoporosis), impaired sexual desire and function.

The risks of tumour expansion during pregnancy are smaller than for macroprolactinomas. Pregnancy may proceed with regular clinical assessment for signs of chiasmal compression.

Postoperative radiotherapy is only required if the serum prolactin is markedly raised preoperatively, fails to fall following surgery or the tumour is locally invasive.

2. Functionless tumours

These account for about a third of large pituitary tumours. Compression of the optic chiasm is common. Treatment is surgical, by trans-sphenoidal surgery if possible. Postoperative radiotherapy is given to reduce the rate of local recurrence. Medical treatment with bromocriptine is of little value.

3. Acromegaly and gigantism

Aetiology. Excessive secretion of growth hormone causes gigantism in a child who is still growing and acromegaly in an adult in whom skeletal growth is complete.

Clinical features. The effects of excess growth hormone in acromegaly are enlargement of the hands and feet and of the skeleton in general, coarsening of the facial features, prominence of the jaw, sweating, arthropathy, amenorrhoea and impotence. Impaired vision and headache are local effects of tumour extension. Nerve entrapment occurs due to overgrowth of the soft tissues, e.g. compressing the median nerve at the wrist (carpal tunnel syndrome). Arterial hypertension and diabetes mellitus are common. Untreated, the disease may be fatal, usually due to cardiovascular damage.

Diagnosis and investigation. The most useful test to make the diagnosis of acromegaly is to give an oral glucose load. In normal individuals this suppresses growth hormone levels to < 2 mu/l. In acromegaly, however, growth hormone levels are not suppressed.

Treatment. Treatment is required for virtually all patients with acromegaly. Cure of acromegaly is rare but control can commonly be achieved. Trans-sphenoidal removal of the adenoma is normally the first line of treatment and is urgent if vision is impaired. This is followed by postoperative radiotherapy (see radiation technique and dosage below) since it is often difficult for the surgeon to be confident that all the tumour has been removed.

Bromocriptine is the main medical therapy for acromegaly. It lowers growth hormone secretion from the pituitary in about 70% of patients but substantial falls in growth hormone levels are only achieved in 15–20% of patients. It is particularly effective in shrinking tumours that secrete both growth hormone and prolactin. It is used after surgery if growth hormone levels do not return to normal postoperatively or if the patient is unfit for or refuses surgery. Maintenance doses are normally 10–30 mg per day. Side-effects such as gastrointestinal intolerance may limit its use. A more recent drug, octreotide, derived from the hormone somatostatin, can considerably reduce growth hormone levels. Its role in the treatment of acromegaly is yet to be established.

Results of treatment. Cure of acromegaly, defined as a serum growth hormone level of less than 1 mu/l, is rare. The effects of radiotherapy on growth hormone levels are very slow. The average time to reach the normal range of growth hormone is about 7 years.

Cushing's disease. Cushing's disease (pituitary-dependent Cushing's syndrome) is treated by trans-sphenoidal surgical removal of the tumour. Metyrapone is used to block adrenal steroid production. Pituitary irradiation is employed for persistent or recurrent disease.

CRANIOPHARYNGIOMA

This is a congenital benign tumour arising from Rathke's pouch. Remnants of this may persist and form cystic tumours which may compress the pituitary.

Presentation is usually in early adulthood with endocrine dysfunction, with failure of growth and of sexual maturation, and diabetes insipidus. Visual impairment and signs of raised intracranial pressure are common.

Diagnosis and investigation

The presence of calcification above the pituitary fossa on skull radiograph may suggest the diagnosis. CT scanning demonstrates both solid and cystic components.

Treatment

Surgical removal is the treatment of choice. This is often complete, especially in children, and no further treatment may be needed. Sometimes it is impossible to remove the whole tumour due to its intimate relations with vital structures such as the optic chiasm or to the large size of the cyst. If the residual disease is predominantly cystic, the cyst can be drained under stereotactic CT guidance and a solution of radioactive yttrium-90 instilled. This reduces the likelihood of recurrence. If the disease is mainly solid, postoperative external beam is preferable. It is better not to delay irradiation until recurrence since the local control rate falls to 25%.

Radical radiotherapy

Target volume
This includes the tumour and a 1–2 cm margin of normal tissue.

Technique
A parallel opposed pair of lateral fields or a three field technique (as for the pituitary gland, see above) is used with a shell.

Dose and energy
45 Gy in 20 daily fractions over 4 weeks (4–6 MV photons)

Results of treatment

The prognosis is better in children than in adults. Five-year survival is nearly 100% for children and 95% for adults. Following external beam just over 50% of patients are free of disease at 5 years.

INTRACRANIAL METASTASES

Intracranial metastases may occur in the meninges, brain or the skull; 80% of brain metastases occur in the cerebral hemispheres and 16% in the cerebellum. Rarely deposits may occur in the basal ganglia, brainstem, pituitary gland and the choroid plexus. Metastases to the meninges may be isolated or part of carcinomatous meningitis where malignant cells are widespread in the CSF. Occasionally the source of the primary is not clinically evident. Two-thirds of metastases are multiple.

Clinical features

Presentation may be with raised intracranial pressure, epilepsy, or with a stroke. Frequently they develop in the context of advanced disease elsewhere and are often a terminal event. Lower cranial nerve palsies may indicate base of skull metastases.

Treatment

The treatment of brain metastases is virtually always palliative. Surgery, radiotherapy, chemotherapy and steroids are the treatments available. The choice is determined by the age, general condition, the number of metastases and the presence of disease elsewhere. If the patient is terminally ill, relief of intracranial pressure by steroids alone (dexamethasone 4 mg orally q.d.s.) may be all that is appropriate.

For those in better general condition the number of metastases is important. Isolated metastases may be amenable to surgical removal followed by postoperative radiotherapy. For multiple metastases surgery is inappropriate. Very occasionally it may be justified for two metastases if they are radioresistant and lie within the same operative field.

Palliative radiotherapy is helpful in relieving headache; 80% of patients obtain some symptomatic improvement and in about 50% relief is complete. Between 70 and 75% will have motor deficit improved, with complete resolution in 30–35%. The control of epilepsy requires anticonvulsant therapy. Phenytoin 300 mg nocte is the initial treatment of choice in adults.

Chemotherapy is of little value in treating most cerebral metastases. Intrathecal methotrexate may be of benefit to patients with cerebral lymphoma, leukaemia or choriocarcinoma.

Palliative radiotherapy

Target volume
This includes the whole brain if there are supratentorial metastases. If the metastases are confined to the cerebellum, the infratentorial region of the brain need only be treated.

Technique
For whole brain irradiation a simple parallel opposed pair of lateral fields is adequate, e.g. 15×12 cm using cobalt beam or megavoltage (Fig. 27.5A). The same technique for base of skull metastases is shown in Figure 27.5B.

Simulation is not essential and anatomical landmarks of the base of skull (a line from the outer canthus to the external auditory meatus) can be used.

Dose and energy
30 Gy in 10 daily fractions (4–6 MV photons or cobalt-60)

Results of treatment

The results of treatment of cerebral deposits are poor. With steroids alone average survival is 2 months. With palliative radiotherapy, it is between 3 and 5 months. In patients with isolated metastases treated by surgery and postoperative radiotherapy, median survival is about 6 months. Patients with an interval of more than a year between the diagnosis of the primary and that of cerebral metastases tend to have a longer survival.

Carcinomatous meningitis

Carcinomatous meningitis is an uncommon complication of a variety of tumours (e.g. lung and breast). Presentation is with headache which becomes progressively severe. Photophobia, neck stiffness and cranial nerve palsies are common. Treatment is palliative. Patients are rarely fit for more than palliative irradiation to the base of the skull by parallel opposed fields (Fig. 27.5B).

Palliative radiotherapy

Target volume
The base of skull is included. Typical fields sizes are 15×6 cm.

Technique
A parallel opposed pair of fields is used.

Dose and energy
30 Gy in 10 daily fractions over 2 weeks (4–6 MV photons or cobalt-60)

TUMOURS OF THE SPINAL CORD

Classification

Approximately 15% of tumours of the CNS develop in the spinal cord. They are classified according to whether they lie inside (intradural) or outside (extradural) the dura. Intradural tumours may lie within the cord (intramedullary) or outside it (extramedullary).

1. Extradural
   a. Primary
      (i) Chordoma
      (ii) Sarcoma
      (iii) Lymphoma
      (iv) Myeloma
   b. Secondary (e.g breast and lung cancer)
2. Intradural
   a. Extramedullary
      (i) Meningioma
      (ii) Neurofibroma
   b. Intramedullary (gliomas)
      (i) Ependymoma
      (ii) Astrocytoma.

The majority of intramedullary tumours in the cervical cord are astrocytomas. In the thoracic cord, astrocytomas and ependymomas are equally common. In the lumbosacral region, ependymomas predominate. In the cauda equina virtually all are ependymomas. Astrocytomas account for a third of primary spinal cord tumours. They are mostly well differentiated. Ependymomas represent the other two-thirds; 90% are well differentiated and rarely seed to the CSF.

Chordoma is a rare tumour arising from remnants of the notochord; 50% occur in the sacrococcygeal region, 35% in the base of the skull (e.g. clinoid process) and 15% at various levels of the vertebral column. It invades locally into the nasopharynx, pelvis, buttocks or retroperitoneal tissues. Metastases to lymph nodes, lung and liver occur in less than 10%.

Clinical features

Pain due to involvement of the nerve roots or vertebral body may precede signs of spinal cord compression (see below). Neurological function is lost at the level of and below the lesion. The loss may be motor and/or sensory. Upper motor neurone signs occur below the level of cord involved. Intramedullary tumours positioned laterally in the cord may give rise to hemisection of the cord (Brown-Séquard syndrome). In this syndrome there is loss of pain and temperature sensation on the opposite side of the body below the lesion, from compression of the lateral spinothalamic tracts which enter and cross the spinal cord from the opposite side, and loss of motor function and vibration and joint position sense on the affected side, from damage to the pyramidal tracts and posterior columns respectively.

Chordomas may present as an intracranial space occupying lesion with headache, cranial nerve palsies, spinal cord compression or pain, e.g. from destruction of the sacrum.

Treatment

Astrocytomas should be treated by surgical excision or maximal debulking. Ependymomas in the cauda equina cannot be treated by radical surgery because of the damage that would be done to nerve roots. In both tumours surgery should be followed by postoperative radiotherapy to reduce the incidence of local recurrence.

Chordomas are best treated by surgical debulking followed by postoperative radiotherapy. Because of their site in the base of the skull or sacrum, complete surgical excision is usually impossible. Chordomas are relatively radioresistant. However radiotherapy may relieve pressure symptoms.

Radical radiotherapy

Target volume
This should include the known extent of the tumour with a margin of 5 cm of normal tissue above and below the tumour.

Technique
   Ependymomas and astrocytomas. The patient is treated prone in a shell immobilising the trunk. In the cervical and thoracic cord two posterior oblique wedged fields are used. In the lumbar region a direct field is used instead of posterior oblique fields to avoid overdosage of the kidneys.

Chordomas
Base of skull: a parallel opposed pair of lateral fields.
Pelvis: anterior and posterior pair of fields.

Dose and energy
45 Gy in 20 daily fractions over 4 weeks (4–6 MV photons)

Results of treatment

Ninety per cent of well-differentiated ependymomas

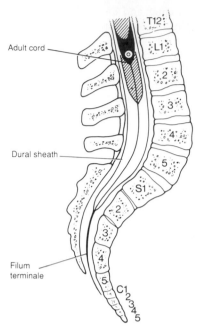

Fig. 27.16   Range of variation in the termination of the spinal cord. (Redrawn from Ellis, Clinical Anatomy, 5th edn, Blackwells, 1975.)

of the cauda equina are disease free at 5 years. For low grade gliomas 5-year survival is about 50%. High grade tumours respond poorly to treatment with a survival similar to cerebral gliomas of the same grade.

Malignant spinal cord compression

Anatomy

The spinal cord runs behind the posterior margin of the vertebral bodies from the upper border of the atlas (C1) to the lower body of L1. It is important to know that the lower level may vary from the lower border of T12 to the upper border of L3 (Fig. 27.16). The spinal cord ends in a group of nerve roots, the cauda equina. The cauda equina is not part of the spinal cord but it is convenient to consider its management in conjunction with spinal cord compression because of their anatomical proximity.

The levels of the spinal cord segments are not at the same level as the correspondingly numbered vertebral bodies. In the adult the spinal segment is about two segments above the corresponding vertebral level. For example the sixth thoracic segment is opposite the 4th thoracic vertebra and the first sacral segment is opposite the 12th thoracic vertebra.

Aetiology and pathology

Spinal cord compression is a common complication occuring in 5% of patients with malignant disease. It may be extradural or intradural (see above).

The majority (70%) of extradural bony deposits causing cord compression arise in the thoracic spine, 30% are in the lumbar spine and 10% in the cervical spine. Multiple levels of cord compression occur in approximately 20% of patients.

Clinical features

Spinal cord compression may develop acutely or insidiously. The common sequence is increasingly severe back pain followed by weakness, sensory disturbance and then sphincter dysfunction (urinary retention and bowel incontinence).

Early symptoms of involvement of the bladder sphincter are hesitancy and urgency of urination. These often precede urinary retention and overflow incontinence. Constipation with spurious diarrhoea are symptoms of interference with rectal continence. If the level of compression is at the level of or above the fifth cervical segment, all four limbs will be affected and may be completely paralysed (quadriplegia). If the lesion is below the first thoracic segment, the arms are spared but the legs may both be paralysed (paraplegia).

Diagnosis and investigation

Early diagnosis is essential since the smaller the neurological deficit, the better the prospect of recovery. Investigation is therefore urgent.

Plain radiographs of the whole spine are essential since there may be evidence of vertebral collapse or destruction of the pedicles corresponding to the clinical level of compression.

A myelogram is advised if its result is likely to influence subsequent management, e.g. suitability for surgery or choice of radiation fields. Myelography may show partial or complete (Fig. 27.17) obstruction of the flow of contrast up the spinal canal. If there is a complete block, the upper limit of the block cannot be assessed. A myelogram introducing contrast from above, through the cervical spine, or CT scanning (see below) should be performed if this information is required. CT scanning may show the upper level of the block, whether extradural deposits lie in front or behind the cord and whether there is any associated soft tissue mass.

MRI is extremely helpful in determining the site(s) of compression (Fig. 27.18). It has the advantage of being non-invasive and is likely progressively to replace myelography.

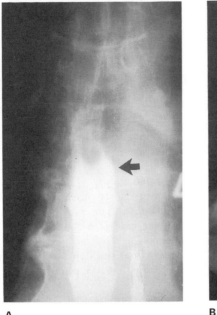

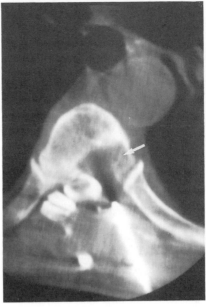

A   **B**

Fig. 27.17 **A** Myelogram showing complete block at T6 due to extradural compression from non-small cell lung cancer. **B** CT guided biopsy of T6. Note destruction of the right side of the vertebral body (arrows). (Courtesy of Dr T Powell, Sheffield.)

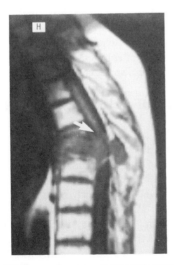

Fig. 27.18   MRI scan showing spinal cord compression (arrow) due to collapse of the 7th thoracic vertebra due to metastatic breast cancer (Courtesy of Dr L Turnbull, MRI Unit, Sheffield).

Management

Prevention. Spinal cord compression commonly occurs as a complication in patients with known metastases in the vertebral column. They should be advised to avoid movements which may precipitate vertebral collapse and cord compression (e.g. bending, twisting and lifting).

Treatment

Urgent treatment should follow the diagnosis. The aim of treatment is to improve or at least conserve neurological function and relieve pain by decompressing the spinal cord. Surgery, radiotherapy and steroids are the treatments available, individually or in combination. The choice between them is influenced by a number of factors: age and general medical condition, histology, degree of neurological deficit, site of compression and stability of the spine.

1. Surgical decompression

There has been an increasing trend among neuro-surgeons in the UK to avoid surgery if possible. This is due to experience in finding that a higher proportion of patients deteriorate neurologically after laminectomy than after radiotherapy alone. In addition, there is the major operative morbidity (wound infection, spinal instability) and mortality in up to 20% of cases.

Surgery is generally preferred in the following circumstances:

— Rapid onset
— Complete myelographic block
— Radioresistant tumours (melanoma, sarcoma, renal cell carcinoma)
— High cervical cord compression with the risk of respiratory failure
— Isolated site of compression.

Contraindications to surgery are:

— Old age and poor general medical condition
— Multiple levels of cord compression or vertebral collapse
— Histology (lung cancer).

Patients must be in good general medical condition. Multiple levels of involvement are usually a contra-indication because of the extent of the operation which would be required. Radioresistant tumours such as melanoma, sarcomas and renal cell carcinomas are better treated by surgery. Neurosurgeons are not keen on operating on patients with lung cancer because of the very poor prognosis.

Surgical decompression offers a means of quickly relieving cord compression. Laminectomy is the commonest operation for doing so. This involves the removal of the lamina, the bony shelf forming the back or the arch of the spinal canal. Removal will normally be necessary over several adjacent verterbrae. This operation allows inspection of the extent of the tumour, a biopsy to be obtained and sufficient tumour to be removed to relieve the compression.

For tumours compressing the front of the cord, anterior decompression and stabilisation is indicated in selected cases.

2. Radiotherapy

The vast majority of radiotherapy for malignant spinal cord compression is palliative. Patients are either treated postoperatively following laminectomy or biopsy or as a primary procedure in cases of a known malignancy. Occasionally solitary plasmacytoma of a vertebral body presents with spinal cord compression and should be treated radically.

Indications. Palliative radiotherapy is indicated postoperatively following surgical decompression. It is of little value in patients who are not in pain, have no motor or sensory function or have a radioresistant tumour. For the terminally ill the discomfort of transfer to and from the treatment couch is best avoided.

Target volume
This is based on the clinical, operative and radiological findings. In general a generous margin of two vertebral bodies should be taken above and below the site of compression.

Technique
A single direct posterior field is used. If the patient is unable to lie prone, he or she is simulated supine and an anterior skin mark is used for setting up. The patient is treated with the gantry underneath the couch. If this is not feasible the lateral decubitus position may be possible.

Dose and energy
Megavoltage is preferred to achieve an adequate depth dose. The average depth of the cervical and thoracic cord is 4–5 cm, and is 7 cm in the lumbar region.
20–25 Gy at the depth of the spinal cord in 5 daily fractions (4–6 MV photons)

Results of treatment

Pain is relieved in most patients. The degree of improvement in neurological function is related to the radiosensitivity of the tumour and the pretreatment neurological deficit. Radiosensitive tumours such as myeloma and lymphoma respond best. Patients with moderately radiosensitive tumours such as breast and prostate can be improved if they have reasonable limb power. Those who have no motor or sensory function and loss of sphincter function rarely improve, irrespective of the histology.

TUMOURS OF THE EYE AND ORBIT
Anatomy

The bony margins of the orbit contain the eyeball, the optic nerve and the recti and oblique muscles which move the eye. The optic nerve leaves the back of the globe and travels posteriorly, leaving the orbit via the optic canal. The eyeball is made up of three layers. The outer layer, the sclera, is fibrous. The middle layer, the uveal tract, is vascular and is composed of the choroid, the ciliary body and the iris. The choroid lines the inner surface of the sclera. The inner layer, the retina, is neural. The lens lies towards the front of the eyeball approximately 0.5 cm from the surface of the eye.

There are four rectus and two oblique muscles. The lateral rectus muscle moves the eyeball laterally and is supplied by the sixth cranial nerve. The other recti elevate, and the inferior oblique depresses, and move the eyeball inward. These three muscles are supplied by the third cranial nerve. The superior oblique moves the eye downward and outward and is supplied by the fourth cranial nerve.

The conjunctiva is a membrane lining the inner surface of the eyelids and is reflected over the anterior surface of the globe, terminating at the corneoscleral junction. The lacrimal gland lies in the upper lateral part of the orbit. Tears secreted by the gland drain into the nose through the nasolacrimal duct.

Pathology

Classification

Malignant tumours are best classified as orbital or intraocular. Orbital tumours may be primary or secondary. The principal sites of these tumours are shown in Fig. 27.19.

1. Orbital tumours
   a. Primary
      (i) Lymphoma
      (ii) Rhabdomyosarcoma
      (iii) Lacrimal gland carcinoma
   b. Secondary
      Metastases (e.g. breast cancer, neuroblastoma)

2. Intraocular
   a. Primary
      (i) Retinoblastoma
      (ii) Malignant melanoma

   b. Metastases
      (i) Choroidal deposits (e.g. breast and lung cancer).

Frequency

In childhood retinoblastomas are the commonest neoplasms. They arise from the retina and may be bilateral. Uveal melanomas are the commonest primary neoplasms in adults. Most adult intraocular tumours occur in the choroid. Secondary tumour spread may occur by invasion of the orbit from tumours of the paranasal sinuses, nasopharynx and eyelids or as metastases from a primary tumour elsewhere. Of the latter in order of frequency in adults are breast, lung, bowel and thyroid cancer. In childhood, neuroblastoma is the commonest tumour metastasising to the orbit, often bilaterally.

Radiation tolerance of the eye

The tolerance of different structures in the eye varies enormously. The most sensitive structure is the lens.

Lens

The probability of developing a cataract depends on the dose, the energy of radiation and the amount of

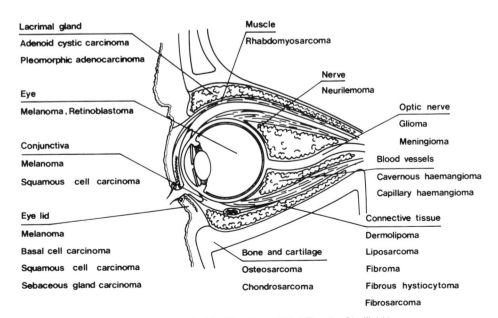

Fig. 27.19 Tumours of the eye and orbit. (Courtesy of Mr I Rennie, Sheffield.)

the lens that has been irradiated. Cataracts may occur over a wide range of doses. Cataracts have been observed at doses as low as 2 Gy. However normally doses of 5 Gy or more are required to cause clinically significant cataract. The tolerance of the lens to continuous low dose rate irradiation from an iridium-192 implant is greater and doses of less than 20 Gy may not result in the formation of cataract. If cataracts are radiation induced, the period from treatment to the development of cataract is usually 2–3 years. Surgical removal of the cataract is usually possible.

Cornea and lacrimal gland

The acute effects of radiation on the cornea are normally temporary with pinhead size erosions (punctate keratitis). Symptoms are local irritation and lacrimation. This normally occurs with doses of 30–50 Gy in 4–5 weeks and settles within a few weeks or months of irradiation. Topical steroids and antibiotics may alleviate the discomfort.

Megavoltage irradiation, because of its sparing of the superficial tissues, is less likely to cause acute keratitis than superficial and orthovoltage radiation.

The late effects are more serious. The lacrimal gland atrophies and tear production is impaired, if it has been irradiated to between 50 and 60 Gy. The result is a dry eye. At these dose levels, and those used for treating basal cell tumours at the inner canthus (e.g. 45 Gy in 10 daily fractions at 90–120 kV), the puncta and canaliculi of the lacrimal drainage apparatus may be occluded. As a result the eye may weep continuously (epiphora). In most cases epiphora following irradiation of basal cell carcinomas at the inner canthus is mild. However surgical reconstruction of the duct may need to be considered if it is troublesome in a younger patient.

Most patients treated to doses of 30–40 Gy to the whole orbit do not develop marked symptoms of a dry eye.

The sensitivity of the cornea to painful stimuli is reduced. The absence of corneal pain may delay the diagnosis of corneal damage. The tolerance dose of the cornea is 50 Gy over 5 weeks. With doses in excess of 60 Gy corneal ulceration occurs, usually following punctate keratitis and oedema, eventually healing with scarring and impairment of vision. Infection complicating the corneal radiation reaction increases the likelihood of corneal damage and should be treated with topical antibiotics.

Keratinisation of the cornea is a late complication. It tends to occur with doses in excess of 50 Gy. If the cornea is exposed to high doses of beta irradia-tion (e.g. 200–300 Gy from a strontium-90 applicator), secondary vascularisation and fatty infiltration may develop, causing blindness several years later.

Sclera

The sclera is rarely affected since it is avascular. Necrosis of the sclera is uncommon and doses of 100 Gy are needed to induce it. This may occur following irradiation with ruthenium-106 plaques for ocular melanoma.

Anterior chamber

Complications in the anterior chamber are rare. Rubeosis of the eye due to new vessel formation may follow cobalt-60 plaque therapy for retinoblastoma. Secondary glaucoma may follow.

Retina

No acute effects are experienced with conventionally fractionated external beam irradiation. Late effects are seen at doses in excess of 50 Gy. These changes are vascular. There are haemorrhages, exudates and degenerative changes. Optic atrophy may follow doses of 50–80 Gy over 4–8 weeks.

Principles of irradiation

It is difficult to irradiate the orbit uniformly while shielding the cornea and lens. A compromise is often necessary to enable adequate dosage to the tumour while limiting the dose to vulnerable structures, particularly the lens. It should be remembered that radiation induced cataract can usually be removed surgically. Inadequate tumour dosage, however, may prove fatal. In these circumstances a higher risk of radiation damage may have to be accepted, if tumour cure is to be achieved. Ultimately the radiation damaged eye may have to be surgically removed (enucleation).

Technique

For superficial tumours, for example lymphomas of the conjunctiva, a single anterior superficial (120 kV) or orthovoltage (250 kV) field may suffice. Treatment of basal and squamous cell tumours of the eyelids and inner canthus are described on page 296.

For deeper tumours (e.g. lacrimal gland carcinomas or rhabdomyosarcoma) an anterior and lateral wedged fields are used (Fig. 27.20). The front margin of the lateral field should lie at the outer canthus behind

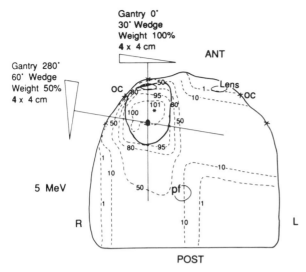

Fig. 27.20 Dose distribution for treatment of the orbit from an anterior and lateral field wedged pair of fields weighted 2:1. (Reproduced with permission from Dobbs et al 1992.)

the cornea and lens. The lateral field is angled 5–10° posteriorly to avoid the lens of the opposite eye.

If there is forward displacement of the eye or involvement of the posterior or anteromedial part of the orbit, superior and inferior oblique fields give a better distribution of dose (Fig. 27.21).

RHABDOMYOSARCOMA

Pathology

The tumour is usually of embryonal type (see Ch. 28 on soft tissue sarcomas).

Clinical features

Rhabdomyosarcoma is a malignant tumour arising from the soft tissues. It is the commonest primary orbital tumour in childhood. The majority present under the age of 10 years, usually with rapidly progressive protrusion of the eye (exophthalmos). It may spread locally to the nasopharynx or ethmoid air sinuses. It metastasises to the cervical lymph nodes, lungs and occasionally bone.

Diagnosis and investigation

A biopsy should be carried out. Staging includes a plain skull and chest radiographs, bone scan, orbital CT scan and bone marrow examination. Most patients are found to have localised disease.

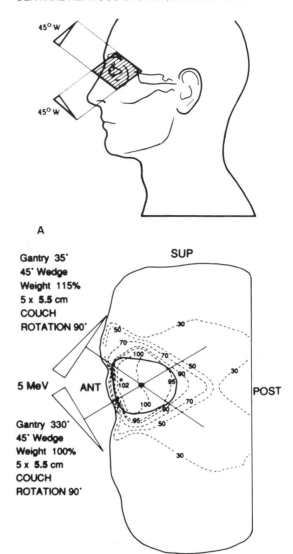

Fig. 27.21 **A** Superior and inferior oblique wedged fields for tumours displacing the globe. **B** Dose distribution from **A**. (Reproduced with permission from Dobbs et al 1992.)

Treatment

Treatment should be undertaken in a specialist centre. Initial cytotoxic chemotherapy is given to shrink the tumour (vincristine, actinomycin D and cyclophosphamide (VAC)). This is followed by external beam irradiation to the whole orbit. Vincristine and cyclophosphamide are given during the period of radiotherapy. After radiotherapy combination chemotherapy is continued for a further year.

Radical radiotherapy

Technique

An anterior and lateral wedged pair of megavoltage fields is used for posteriorly placed tumours. The eye is treated open to take advantage of the skin sparing effect and reduce the severity of keratoconjunctivitis.

For more anterior lesions an anterior electron field will suffice.

Dose and energy

40 Gy in 20 daily fractions over 4 weeks (4–6 MV photons or 16–20 MeV electrons)

Morbidity. The main acute reaction is painful keratoconjunctivitis. Cataract, impairment of bony growth of the orbit, and dry eye (xerophthalmia) are common late complications.

Results of treatment

The results of treatment are excellent, with over 90% of patients disease free at 5 years. Most relapses occur within the first 2 years. Careful follow-up by clinical and CT examination is essential.

OCULAR MELANOMA

Melanoma is the commonest primary intraocular tumour. In adults it most frequently affects the uveal tract, especially the choroid.

Clinical features and investigation

If the tumour arises on the iris, the patient or a relative may notice a pigmented spot. Melanomas more posterior in the eye are more difficult to diagnose and present with visual loss or symptoms of retinal detachment. Indirect ophthalmoscopy after dilating the pupil will reveal most tumours. Ultrasound is helpful in confirming the clinical diagnosis of choroidal melanoma (Plate 19). Fluoroscein angiography is used to demonstrate tumour vascularity. MRI is superior to CT scanning in demonstrating involvement of the optic nerve or extraocular spread.

Natural history

Metastases are rarely present at the time of diagnosis but develop up to 15 years later in about 50% of patients, mainly in the liver, and are the main cause of tumour related death.

Treatment

Iris melanomas

Melanomas of the iris are usually slow growing and can be kept under observation unless there is evidence that the tumour is growing, there is marked new vessel formation, impairment of vision or complications such as glaucoma. Small lesions can be locally excised. Removal of the eye (enucleation) is only very rarely indicated.

Choroid and ciliary body

The management of melanoma of the choroid and ciliary body is controversial. One of the main areas of disagreement is whether removal of the eye disseminates metastases. The aim of treatment is to preserve vision and to prolong survival.

For small melanomas of the choroid and ciliary body, the risks of a policy of observation alone are low. Laser therapy is suitable for very small tumours of the posterior choroid.

For medium-sized tumours (10–15 mm in diameter and 2–5 mm in height), the risks of observation alone are higher. The choice of treatment remains controversial. There is some evidence that the mortality of the disease is higher following enucleation. Radiotherapy does have a role in selected cases. Although melanoma is normally relatively radioresistant, brachytherapy to high doses with cobalt-60, ruthenium-106 or iodine-125 plaques and external irradiation with charged particles (protons and helium ions) have proved beneficial. It may be that radiation exerts its damaging effect on the tumour vasculature rather than by directly damaging tumour cells. Medium-sized tumours may also be locally resected.

The physical properties of protons are described on page 206. Doses of 47–67 Gy in 5 fractions over 8–9 days have been well tolerated. Cobalt-60 or ruthenium-106 plaques are sutured to the sclera. Doses of 50–100 Gy are delivered to the apex of the tumour. Ruthenium-106 has the advantage of emitting predominantly beta radiation. The more limited penetration of ruthenium-106 is better suited to the depth of the tumour and requires less radiation protection than cobalt-60, which emits more penetrating gamma rays.

For large melanomas greater than 15 mm in diameter and 5 mm in height, local resection or enucleation are recommended.

Results of treatment

Iris melanomas metastasise in <5% of cases and have a very good prognosis.

The prognosis of melanoma of the ciliary body and choroid is much poorer. Metastases usually occur within 5 years of diagnosis, typically first to the liver (60–70%). Most patients die within 6 months of the detection of metastases. Bad prognostic factors include large size, extrascleral extension, tumours arising in the ciliary body and old age. Fifty per cent of patients with large tumours die from melanoma. For small tumours of the choroid, the eye can be conserved, with useful vision in 75% of patients following proton irradiation.

RETINOBLASTOMA

Pathology

Retinoblastoma is a congenital tumour which develops from primitive cells in the retina. It is very rare (0.5% of CNS tumours). Both inherited and sporadic (spontaneously arising) forms occur. The abnormal gene that is responsible for the inherited form lies on chromosome 13. However only in about 10% of cases is a positive family history found, suggesting that spontaneous mutations account for the majority of cases. In the inherited form both eyes are affected (30% of cases).

Clinical features

Most (75%) of tumours present under 3 years of age and are sporadic. The presenting clinical features include an opaque light reflex (cat's eye reflex) in the normally dark pupil, or a squint. More advanced cases have raised intraocular pressure. Eventually there may be perforation of the globe. Local extension occurs within the orbit, often from tumour growth along the optic nerve. Metastases may occur to the central nervous system and the bone marrow.

Diagnosis and investigation

The management of children with retinoblastoma should be in specialised centres (e.g. St Bartholomew's Hospital, London in the UK) in view of the rarity of the tumour and the good prospects of cure in the hands of an experienced ophthalmic surgeon and radiotherapist.

The diagnosis is made by indirect binocular ophthalmoscopy of both eyes under a general anaesthetic. The tumour is identified and staged according to a clinical classification (Table 27.2). It should be remembered that this classification relates to the prospect of retaining vision (falling with increasing

Table 27.2 St Bartholomew's Hospital modification of Reese staging of retinoblastoma

Stage	Clinical findings
I	Single or multiple tumours less than 4 disc diameters at or behind the equator (1 disc diameter = 1.5 mm)
IIa	Solitary lesion 4–10 disc diameters at or behind the equator
IIb	Solitary lesion larger than 10 disc diameters at or behind the equator
III	Lesions anterior to the equator
IVa	Multiple tumours, some larger than 10 disc diameters
IVb	Any lesion extending anteriorly beyond the limit of ophthalmoscopy
Va	Massive neoplasms
Vb	Vitreous seedlings
VI	Residual orbital disease or optic nerve infiltration

stage) and not to survival. The diagnosis is clinical. Histological confirmation is not normally obtained unless the eye is removed. Additional staging investigations include a bone marrow biopsy, CSF examination and a bone scan to identify metastases.

Treatment

For small tumours every effort is made to conserve the eye and useful vision. Most unilateral non-inherited tumours present late and require enucleation. For advanced tumours or relapse following non-surgical treatment, enucleation is required.

1. Tumours up to 4 mm

Laser therapy is suitable for posteriorly placed tumours up to 4 mm in diameter. This form of treatment is not used for tumours just lateral to the optic disc because of the risk of damaging the macula. Cryotherapy (a method of freezing the tumour) is used for tumours lying more towards the front of the eye.

2. Tumours 4–13 mm in diameter

Tumours of 4–13 mm in diameter are treated with a radioactive plaque. Traditionally this was gamma ray emitting cobalt-60 or iodine-125. The external surface of the eyeball is exposed surgically and a specially prepared disc holding radioactive cobalt is sutured in position, overlying the tumour mass. The exact position of the growth must be determined by previous ophthalmoscopy. The disc is removed in a surgical operation a week later. A range of discs with diameters varying from 5 to 15 mm are available, each plaque forming part of a sphere which has an internal radius of 11 mm, corresponding to the radius of the eye.

Dose

A dose of 40 Gy is delivered to the apex of the tumour. The maximum dose at the surface of the eyeball is about 200 Gy.

3. Larger tumours

External beam irradiation is indicated for:
— Tumours in excess of 13 mm in diameter
— Two or more tumours which cannot be covered by a single plaque
— Vitreous seedlings
— Tumours close to the macula or optic disc.

Target volume

The whole of the eye should be treated.

Technique

Previously a direct anterior field was treated with cobalt-60 irradiation, shielding if possible the lacrimal gland and the nasolacrimal duct (Fig. 27.22). This ensured that the whole of the eye was treated to cover any vitreous seedling or second primary. The eyelid is taped to keep the eye open to spare the anterior part of the eye.

The technique using a lateral field illustrated in Figure 27.23 is recommended for single tumours lying at the back of the eye without vitreous seedlings. The child is sedated. A contact lens is placed over the cornea. The contact lens serves as a fixed point from

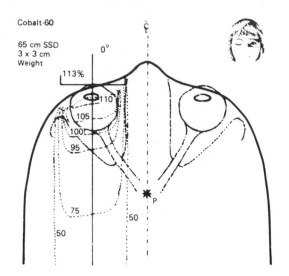

Fig. 27.22   A direct anterior megavoltage for treatment of the whole eye in retinoblastoma. The lacrimal gland and nasolacrimal duct may be shielded (see inset). (Reproduced with permission from Hope-Stone 1986.)

which measurements can be made. The beam from a linear accelerator is split to reduce divergence so that the front of the beam edge is sharply defined. The depth of the back of the lens can be measured by ultrasound. The front of the lateral beam can then be positioned at this point. It is angled back to avoid the lens of the opposite eye.

Dose and energy

40 Gy in 20 daily fractions over 4 weeks (4–6 MV photons)

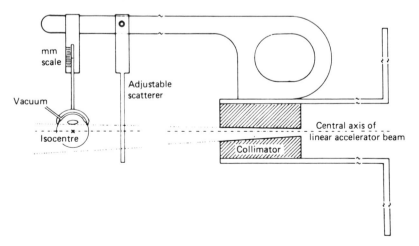

Fig. 27.23   Technique for megavoltage irradiation of nearly the whole retina with sparing of the lens and anterior chamber. (Reproduced with permission from Hope-Stone 1986.)

Morbidity. If the whole eye is irradiated cataract will develop, usually 2 years after treatment. This may be removed surgically. Xerophthalmia (dry eye) and retardation of the growth of the orbit are common.

Chemotherapy

Chemotherapy is reserved for palliation and is of limited efficacy. Agents such as vincristine, cyclophosphamide and derivatives of platinum have been used.

Results of treatment

Many tumours present late with no prospect of useful vision. The eye is therefore removed.

Most posterior tumours can be controlled by radiation, with useful vision in up to 90%. This falls to 30% for multiple growths or those in the anterior part of the eye. About 50% of patients with extensive involvement of the optic nerve or residual disease in the orbit will die from metastatic disease.

CHOROIDAL DEPOSITS

Blood-borne metastases to the eye tend to lodge in the choroid, resulting in retinal detachment. Choroidal deposits generally present with sudden or rapidly progressive visual loss, usually in a patient with known breast or lung cancer. In 50% of cases, both eyes are affected. The typical 'honeycomb' appearance of the fundus is shown in Plate 20. Choroidal metastases usually infer a poor prognosis, with most patients dying within 1 year of the appearance.

Urgent radiotherapy is required to preserve vision.

Palliative radiotherapy

Target volume
The whole of the eye is included.

Technique
Choroidal deposits can be treated by a single anterior megavoltage photon or cobalt field or a lateral field angled 5–10° posteriorly. If an anterior field is used, the eye is taped open to take advantage of the skin sparing effect of megavoltage to reduce the dose to the cornea and lens.

Dose and energy
30 Gy in 10 daily fractions over 2 weeks (4–6 MV photons or cobalt-60)

Results of treatment

Choroidal metastases are well worth treating, with improvement or at least conservation of vision in most patients.

28. Soft tissues and bone

SOFT TISSUE SARCOMAS

Soft tissue sarcomas (Fig. 28.1) are malignant tumours arising from supporting connective tissues anywhere in the body. These structures (fibrous tissue, fat, blood vessels, smooth and skeletal muscle, tendons, cartilage and synovial tissue) are derived embryologically from the mesoderm. Sarcomas of bone also occur and are discussed in this chapter under bone tumours. Tumours of peripheral nerves are generally included.

Despite arising from a wide variety of tissues, they have many similarities in pathology, clinical findings and behaviour.

Pathology

Soft tissue sarcomas are rare, representing 0.4% of all cancers and 0.3% of cancer deaths. The incidence is about 0.6 per 100 000 population per year. However they constitute 6% of tumours in children under the age of 15. Most occur in the 40–70 age group. The sex ratio is virtually the same.

Their aetiology is largely unknown. In a minority of cases genetic factors are involved. There is, for example, an increased incidence of the tumour in association with certain genetically transmitted diseases, e.g. Gardner's Syndrome, tuberous sclerosis, Von Recklinghausen's disease. Rarely soft tissue sarcomas may occur in the children of mothers with breast cancer of early onset.

Some sarcomas are radiation induced and occur within previously irradiated areas (especially for benign angiomas). The incidence of sarcomas among young people who have been treated with both chemotherapy and radiotherapy for Ewing's sarcoma may reach 18%.

Oncogenes may well have a role in malignant transformation, although the mechanism is as yet unknown. The *ras* gene has, for example, been identified in rhabdomyosarcoma, and there are chromosome 12 abnormalities in tumours of fat.

Rhabdomyosarcoma and soft tissue Ewing's sarcoma, although included in some lists of histological subtypes of soft tissue sarcomas, are quite different from the rest of the group, both in natural history and in being in general more chemo- and radiosensitive. Thus the principles of treatment outlined below, do not apply to these two histological types.

The World Health Organization (WHO) classification is the most frequently used (Table 28.1). In some tumours it is not possible to be certain of the cells from which they originate (malignant fibrous histiocytoma for example). Many others defy classification because they lack an obvious pattern of differentiation. From the point of view of management and prognosis the histological subtype is generally less important than the histological grading and the size of the tumour. However grading is imprecise and itself depends in part on the tumour subtype. Low grade tumours have a recognisable pattern of differentiation, relatively few mitoses, and no necrosis. High grade tumours include all examples and certain subtypes (e.g. synovial sarcoma), tumours with little or no apparent differentiation, and those with necrosis and a high mitotic rate. The tumour size is also important, and those over 5 cm are much more likely to recur locally or give rise to distant metastases.

Table 28.1 WHO histological classification of soft tissue sarcomas

Tumour	Tissue of origin	Incidence (%)
Rhabdomyosarcoma	Skeletal muscle	20
Fibrosarcoma	Fibrous tissue	19
Liposarcoma	Fat	18
Malignant fibrous histiocytoma	Fibrous tissue	10
Synovial sarcoma	Joints	10
Leiomyosarcoma	Smooth muscle	6
Neurogenic sarcoma	Nerves	5
Angiosarcoma	Blood vessels	3
Others	Miscellaneous	2

Initial spread from the primary site is into adjacent tissue and along tissue planes between structures such as muscle bundles. Soft tissue sarcomas do not possess a true capsule but are often surrounded by a pseudocapsule of compressed surrounding tissues. This apparent encapsulation may tempt the surgeon to try and 'shell out' the tumour. Local recurrence from residual tumour at the periphery is then very likely (up to 90% within 2 years). Lymph node spread is infrequent, while blood-borne spread is common, giving rise to distant metastases, predominantly in the lungs.

Clinical features

Approximately 40% of soft tissue sarcomas occur in the upper and lower limbs. Of these about 75% occur at or above the knee. Ten per cent of sarcomas arise in the upper half of the body. Of the sarcomas of the trunk, 10% occur in the retroperitoneum and 20% in the chest or abdominal wall.

The history is usually of a painless lump developing over a few weeks or months and occasionally over years. Pain may occur from pressure on local structures, e.g. nerves and joints. Occasionally non-metastatic effects are seen (e.g. hypoglycaemia in malignant fibrous histiocytoma).

Diagnosis and staging

A biopsy is required. Care should be taken to make the incision longitudinal so that any subsequent radical surgery or postoperative radiation fields can include it.

A full blood count, liver function tests, chest radiograph, plain radiographs of the tumour bearing region and liver ultrasound are the initial investigations. CT and MRI (Fig. 28.1) scanning are important in defining the local extent and operability of the tumour. They are also useful in detecting any subsequent local recurrence. CT of the thorax is advisable if chest radiograph is normal and radical therapy is contemplated, since it may demonstrate small volume lung metastases. The staging system commonly adopted includes size, grade and metastases (Table 28.2).

Treatment

A multidisciplinary approach is required since surgery, radiotherapy and chemotherapy may all have a role to play, depending on the stage, site, grade and size of the tumour. The management of soft tissue sarcomas is controversial. Few would dispute the primary role of radical surgery. If the surgical resections are clear, the local recurrence rate is lower (5%). The extent of the resection will depend upon the site of the tumour. The more proximal the tumour in the limb, particularly in the groin, the more difficult a complete excision becomes. For the same reasons radical surgery of retroperitoneal sarcomas is rarely feasible. The primary tumour should be resected with one anatomical plane clear of the tumour at all stages. This is known as *compartmentectomy* (Fig. 28.2). The resection should

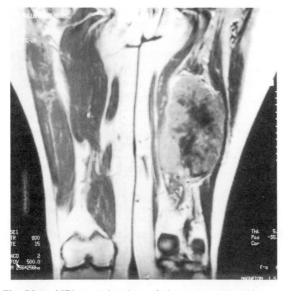

Fig. 28.1   MRI scan showing soft tissue sarcoma with central necrosis in the hamstring compartment of the thigh. (Courtesy of Dr L Turnbull, MRI Unit, Sheffield.)

Table 28.2   Staging system of soft tissue sarcomas

TNM	Clinical findings	Stage	
Tumour size		Ia	G1 T1 N0 M0
		Ib	G1 T2 N0 M0
T1	Tumour less than	IIa	G2 T1 N0 M0
	5 cm in diameter	IIb	G2 T2 N0 M0
T2	Tumour 5 cm or	IIIa	G3 T1 N0 M0
	more in diameter	IIIb	G3 T2 N0 M0
		IIIc	Any G, T1-2 N1 M0
T3	Tumour invading	IVa	Any G, T3, any N, M0
	bone, major vessels	IVb	Any G or T, M1
	or nerves		
Nodes			
N0	No histologically		
	verified metastasis		
	to regional nodes		
N1	Biopsy proven regional		
	lymph node metastases		
Metastases			
M0	No distant metastases		
M1	Distant metastases		

G, histological grade (1, 2 or 3).

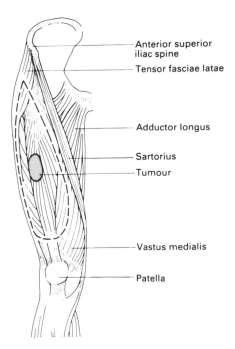

Anterior superior iliac spine

Tensor fasciae latae

Adductor longus

Sartorius

Tumour

Vastus medialis

Patella

Fig. 28.2 Compartmentectomy. The diagram illustrates the wide surgical excision of soft tissue situated, in this case, in the rectus femoris. (Reproduced with permission from Souhami & Tobias, Cancer and its Management, Blackwells, 1986.)

include all the skin and subcutaneous tissue near to the tumour, any previous excision or biopsy scars and areas containing blood clot from previous biopsies. The tumour itself should never be actively contacted during resection. Metallic clips at the margins of the excision are helpful in planning the limits of post-operative irradiation.

Adjuvant therapy

For well-differentiated tumours less than 5 cm in size which have been widely excised with clear surgical margins, no further therapy is necessary in most cases. The same applies following an amputation. However postoperative radiotherapy is indicated in the follow-ing circumstances to reduce the probability of local recurrence (see above):

— Limb-conserving or limited surgery (see below)
— Gross residual tumour or inadequate excision margins
— Grade 2 or 3 histology
— Tumours 5 cm or more in any dimension
— Virtually all tumours in the head and neck (because of impossibility of adequate excision).

Limb-conserving surgery

If limb-conserving surgery is undertaken (i.e. removal of the tumour mass with narrower excision margins), postoperative radiotherapy is given to deal with micro-scopic residual disease. In this way a more functional limb with a more satisfactory cosmetic result can be achieved. Conservative surgery is contraindicated where high dose radiotherapy is poorly tolerated (see below).

Primary radical radiotherapy

Radical radiotherapy alone is indicated for patients unfit for surgery but otherwise in reasonable general condition, those who refuse surgery or where the anatomical site precludes it (e.g. retroperitoneum). Preoperative adjuvant radiotherapy is recommended for very large sarcomas.

Contraindications to radical radiotherapy. The high doses of radiotherapy required for sarcoma are poorly tolerated by highly stressed areas of the lower limb, e.g. Achilles tendon, or in the ribs where patho-logical fractures may occur. Radical radiotherapy to the Achilles tendon is inadvisable, especially in young and active patients, since rupture may occur.

Target volume

Definition of the target volume requires information from the surgeon, pathologist and radiologist. The surgeon should be encouraged to place radio-opaque clips at the margins of the resection. The pathologist should comment on the adequacy of the resection. Very often it is necessary to ask the surgeon to carry out a further excision before postoperative radio-therapy is undertaken. The radiotherapist needs to discuss with the radiologist the position of the tumour, local extent and any residual disease as seen on CT and MRI.

The target volume will vary with the grade of the tumour. For well-differentiated (grade 1) tumours a 5 cm margin above and below the site of the original tumour is adequate. For moderately and poorly dif-ferentiated tumours (grades 2 and 3), a 10 cm margin should be allowed. The target volume is reduced later in the treatment (see below) to include the length of the scar with a margin of security at either end of 2 cm for boosting with electrons.

Where there is macroscopic residual disease, the volume cannot be reduced in the same way as when the excision margins are clear. In this situation, a 5 cm margin around the tumour is sustained throughout treatment.

Technique

This will vary with the site of the tumour. For the limbs and retroperitoneum, a parallel opposed pair of fields, often wedged, will provide a satisfactory dose distribution in most cases. In the shoulder region tangential fields may be needed to reduce the volume of lung irradiated. Tangential fields are also appropriate for superficial trunk lesions to spare the bowel. For tumours in the buttock, a direct posterior field and two wedged lateral fields will reduce the dose to the rectum. In the head and neck, the principles of planning and respect for the tolerance of critical structures such as the spinal cord are the same as for squamous carcinoma of the head and neck. Target volumes tend to be smaller than below the clavicles and so higher doses can often be delivered with acceptable morbidity. Computer planning is desirable to obtain a homogeneous distribution of dose within the target volume.

Stability of the limb is best assisted by a shell and appropriately positioned bolus bags. Bolus is applied to the scar to ensure it receives the maximum dose to minimise the risk of scar recurrence. Sagittal lasers are especially useful in lining up the limbs.

Care is taken to avoid irradiating the whole circumference of a limb to reduce the likelihood of lymphoedema as a late complication. This is achieved by adjusting the width of the field to leave a longitudinal strip of unirradiated tissue outside the target volume. In the proximal part of the limb, especially in the thigh, this strip occupies a large proportion of the limb.

When the retroperitoneum is irradiated, part or the whole of one kidney may need to be included in the target volume. Shielding of the other kidney by lead blocks on the anterior and posterior fields may be necessary, depending upon the site of the tumour.

Dose and energy

Since soft tissue sarcomas are only moderately radiosensitive, a higher dose than normal is needed.

Limbs

No gross residual disease

1. Large volume
   50 Gy in 25 daily fractions over 5 weeks at megavoltage (6–10 MV photons)
2. Boost volume
   16 Gy in 8 daily fractions over $1\frac{1}{2}$ weeks

(1) and (2) deliver a total dose of 66 Gy in 33 fractions over 6.5 weeks to the tumour bearing area.

Gross residual disease
66 Gy in 33 daily fractions over 6.5 weeks at megavoltage (6–10 MV photons) or up to 70 Gy in 35 fractions over 7 weeks, if volume permits in the boosted area

Implantation. Because of the low radiosensitivity of sarcomas, an implant may be used in appropriate circumstances to give a high dose to the boost volume, or to gross residual disease.

Retroperitoneum. Dosage is limited by small bowel tolerance.
45 Gy in 20 daily fractions over 4 weeks

Head and neck
60 Gy in 25 daily fractions over 5 weeks

Acute reactions. Skin reactions are often a problem. This is because very high doses are needed in the boost volume and are sometimes given to graft areas with surface bolus. Dry desquamation normally develops and is treated as for other skin reactions (p. 298). Moist desquamation is more likely to occur in the axilla, groin and perineum and is treated with gentian violet.

Late reactions. Atrophy of the skin and subcutaneous tissues and fibrosis within the muscles are common. Stiffness of a limb may be partly due to fibrosis of the intermuscular septa and partly due to fibrosis in the joint capsule.

Osteoporosis of bone is common since bone is frequently included in the target volume. Occasionally, particularly if the bone is invaded by tumour, radionecrosis may occur. In the ribs this may cause pathological fractures.

Radiation induced sarcoma is very rare. It has been estimated at 0.2% in patients who have been irradiated for breast cancer.

Palliative radiotherapy

Palliative radiotherapy is indicated for the relief of symptoms of local and metastatic disease.

Soft tissue disease

Technique
A single field or parallel opposed pair of fields or direct electron field are used.

Dose and energy
35–37.5 Gy in 10 daily fractions over 2 weeks (4–10 MV photons or electrons of appropriate energy)

Alternatively weekly doses of 3–5 Gy can be given to enable some growth restraint.

Bone metastases. For dose see page 512.

Chemotherapy

There is insufficient evidence to support giving routine postoperative adjuvant chemotherapy to high risk patients with high grade or bulky tumours. For metastatic disease, chemotherapy has limited efficacy. The most active drugs are adriamycin, ifosfamide and DTIC. Chemotherapy is rarely curative so it should be reserved for symptomatic metastases not relieved by radiotherapy. Toxicity should be minimised.

Results of treatment

In the best hands conservative surgery and radiotherapy can achieve over 90% local control and 5-year survival in stage I disease. For stage II disease local control is 85–90% and survival 90% (IIa) and 65% (IIb). For stage III local control is similar to stage II but survival is lower, 85% (IIIa) and 45% (IIIb).

If there is only microscopic residual disease following surgery, overall survival is 65%, falling to 30% when there is gross residual disease.

BONE TUMOURS

Benign and malignant tumours may arise in bone. The pathological classification is shown in Table 28.3. Bone tumours represent 0.4% of all cancers and all cancer deaths. Primary bone tumours are rare, only 1% of bone tumours, compared with 99% which are secondary deposits. The main malignant tumour which forms bone is osteosarcoma; that forming cartilage is chondrosarcoma. Malignant tumours arising from the bone marrow are myeloma (Ch. 26), Ewing's sarcoma and lymphoma (Ch. 26).

OSTEOSARCOMA (OSTEOGENIC SARCOMA)

This is the commonest and most malignant primary bone tumour. It arises in bone-forming cells (osteo-

Table 28.3 Classification of bone tumours

A. Tumours forming bone
  1. Benign,—e.g. osteoma
  2. Malignant—osteosarcoma
B. Tumours forming cartilage
  1. Benign,—e.g. enchondroma
  2. Malignant—chondrosarcoma
C. Giant cell tumour (generally benign)
D. Tumours of the bone marrow—myeloma, lymphoma and Ewing's sarcoma
E. Other tumours

---

blasts) and is commonest between the ages of 10 and 20 years. There is a second peak incidence in the elderly, as a complication of Paget's disease of bone. The male to female ratio is 1.6:1.

The cause of the usual adolescent's tumour is unknown but both internal and external sources of radiation can cause osteosarcoma. However there is also an increased incidence (400-fold) of osteosarcoma in patients with bilateral retinoblastomas, presumably due to the same genetic abnormality or mutation of the Rb tumour suppressor gene developing outside the irradiated areas.

Pathology

Osteosarcoma is commonest near the knee in the metaphysis of the distal femur or proximal tibia. In the elderly, its distribution matches Paget's disease.

Macroscopically the tumour is usually haemorrhagic. It expands the bone, destroying both the cortex and the medulla. The periosteum is frequently raised giving rise to the radiological features of Codman's triangle where the raised periosteum meets the cortex. Extension into the soft tissue follows. Blood-borne metastases to the lungs occur early. Bone metastases, though less frequent, also occur, although less frequently than lung metastases. Microscopically there are malignant osteoblasts laying down small pieces of irregular osteoid tissue. There are a variety of histological appearances. The two main varieties are osteoblastic and telangiectatic (containing irregular blood vessels). The third variety is parosteal sarcoma. It arises from the surface of the bone and does not involve the medullary cavity.

Clinical features

The commonest presenting feature is pain, usually with swelling and a limp. Sometimes pathological fracture may follow minor trauma. Cough and dyspnoea may indicate lung involvement.

Diagnosis and staging investigations

Plain radiographs and CT scan (Fig. 28.3) of the affected part may show the typical features of bone destruction and soft tissue extension. The cortex may be raised with a 'sunburst' appearance. Full blood count, liver function tests and chest radiograph (for lung metastases) are required.

A CT or MRI scan is necessary if surgery is contemplated to assess the involvement of the medullary cavity and the extent of soft tissue involvement. CT is

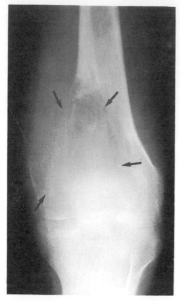

A

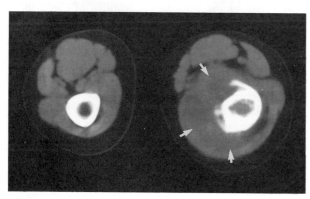

B

Fig. 28.3 **A** Plain radiograph and **B** CT scan of the femur showing bone destruction from an osteogenic sarcoma (arrows). Compare normal CT appearance on opposite side. (Courtesy of Dr R Nakielny, Sheffield.)

also helpful in assessing whether the capsule of a limb joint has been breached. An isotope bone scan may show increased uptake at the site of the tumour, in the adjacent bone (due to increased vascularity), in bone metastases and in bone-forming metastases in soft tissues. A biopsy should be carried out to confirm the diagnosis. It is important that the position of the biopsy is chosen so that the whole biopsy scar can be excised with the tumour to include potentially surgically contaminated tissue along the track of the biopsy. The initial biopsy for histological confirmation and in cases of high clinical and radiological suspicion, so-called

'clearance' biopsies to assess the distance of spread along the bone shaft, should be performed as the first procedure with a view to subsequent limb-sparing surgery. Ideally both biopsy and definitive surgery should be performed by the same surgical team. The limb prosthesis has to be planned several weeks ahead of limb-sparing surgery.

Treatment

The management of osteosarcoma requires a multi-disciplinary approach including orthopaedic surgeon, oncologist, pathologist and physiotherapist.

Surgery

There has been an increasing trend since the early 1980s to conserve limb function as far as possible and avoid the mutilation of an amputation. Limb preservation involves removing the tumour and replacing the bone defect with a custom-made artificial prosthesis (Fig. 28.4). Careful preoperative assessment is necessary and referral to a specialist centre (Birmingham and London in the UK) is desirable. To obtain a margin of normal tissue above the tumour may involve removing the whole femur. However it is now possible to carry out a total femoral replacement.

Contraindications to limb conservation are: (1) extensive soft tissue infiltration, (2) invasion of neurovascular bundles, and (3) involvement of the ankle joint. Similar principles apply to the upper limb.

Resection of lung metastases. Lung metastases are occasionally isolated and, in the absence of metastases elsewhere, surgical resection should be considered. Results are best in lung metastases of late onset. Surgery is contraindicated if there is pleural involvement.

Chemotherapy

Adjuvant chemotherapy is needed to deal with micrometastatic disease. The most useful drugs are Adriamycin, cisplatin, methotrexate and ifosfamide. Once the diagnosis has been established by the initial biopsy, preoperative chemotherapy is started to reduce and hopefully sterilise the tumour before radical surgery. Examination of the operative tumour may show extensive tumour necrosis. However it is often difficult for the pathologist to say whether the tumour is still viable. If chemotherapy seems to have achieved a response, then the same regime can be used postoperatively. If there is no response, an alternative regime is chosen.

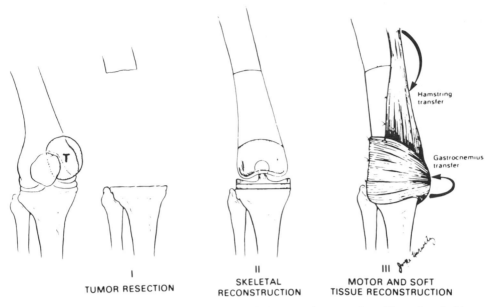

I
TUMOR RESECTION

II
SKELETAL
RECONSTRUCTION

III
MOTOR AND SOFT
TISSUE RECONSTRUCTION

Fig. 28.4   Schematic diagram of the three phases of a limb sparing procedure. (Reproduced with permission from Perez & Brady 1987.)

Radiotherapy

The indications for radiotherapy are: (1) palliation of pain from the primary tumour in the presence of metastatic disease or of bony metastases, and (2) radical treatment of inoperable sites (e.g. skull, vertebrae, ilium and sacrum). However proximity of critical structures, such as the spinal cord, often limits the dose that can be delivered.

Palliative radiotherapy of primary tumour

Technique
A parallel opposed pair of fields is suitable for limb primaries.

Dose and energy
35 Gy in 10 daily fractions over 2 weeks (4–6 MV photons or cobalt-60)

Radical radiotherapy

Technique
This will vary with the site of the primary. For tumours arising in a vertebra, a posterior oblique wedged pair (Fig. 26.10) with or without an unwedged direct posterior field provides a satisfactory dose distribution. For the ilium, parallel opposed fields suffice.

Dose and energy
Megavoltage is required. The choice of dose will be

determined by critical organ tolerance. In the spine above L2 it will be limited by spinal cord tolerance to **47.5 Gy in 25 daily fractions over 5 weeks**. In the ileum the dose delivered is limited by small bowel tolerance to a central tumour dose of **45 Gy in 20 daily fractions over 4 weeks**.

Results of treatment

The survival of osteosarcoma has improved with the development of more effective adjuvant chemotherapy. Average survival is 50% at 3 years. Osteoblastic and telangiectatic tumours have a similar prognosis. Parosteal sarcomas have a better prognosis and may be cured by surgery alone.

EWING'S SARCOMA

Ewing's sarcoma is the second commonest bone tumour. In the UK its incidence is 0.6 per million. The peak age is between 10 and 15 years. It is slightly commoner in males. It is very rare in Blacks.

Pathology

Ewing's sarcoma probably arises from connective tissue within the bone marrow. The commonest sites in order of frequency are the pelvis, femur, tibia, fibula, rib, scapula, vertebra and humerus. In contrast to osteogenic sarcoma, a higher proportion of these tumours occur in the flat bones of the trunk. About 40% occur in the axial skeleton. Microscopically there are sheets of uniform undifferentiated, small, deeply-staining round cells. The tumour needs to be distinguished from other small round cell tumours, including non-Hodgkin lymphoma, Hodgkin's disease, neuroblastoma and metastatic carcinoma. 90% will absorb a special stain for the presence of glycogen (periodic-acid Schiff (PAS)). This stain is not specific for Ewing's sarcoma since it may also be positive in neuroblastoma.

There is local spread along the marrow cavity causing bone destruction. However the epiphyseal plates are rarely breached. Blood-borne spread is early and common. About 50% will have lung metastases and 40% bone metastases and/or widespread bone marrow infiltration at presentation. Lymph node metastases are uncommon (less than 10%). Spread to the CNS may occur, usually late in the course of the disease.

Diagnosis and staging

Full blood count may show anaemia (leucoerythro-blastic, if there is bone marrow infiltration) and a mildly raised white cell count. ESR is often moderately elevated. Liver function tests may be abnormal (raised lactate dehydrogenase (LDH) or alkaline phosphatase).

A biopsy of the tumour is required. As in osteogenic

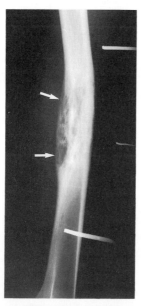

Fig. 28.5 Plain radiograph of the femur showing typical appearance of Ewing's sarcoma of bone. (Courtesy of Dr R Nakielny, Sheffield.)

sarcoma, care is taken to ensure the biopsy lies within the incision for any later proposed definitive surgical procedure. Plain radiographs of the primary are taken in two planes (usually anteroposterior and lateral). In long bones this may show the typical multilayered 'onion-skin' (Fig. 28.5) appearance of the periosteal reaction and often a large adjacent soft tissue mass. Pathological fracture occurs in 5% (less frequently than osteogenic sarcoma). CT scanning gives more detail of the local extent of the tumour and is useful in planning the site for a biopsy and sub-sequent surgery. MRI is superior to CT in assessment of the extent of infiltration within the medullary canal. A bone scan is necessary to screen for bone metastases.

A bone marrow and trephine are needed to exclude marrow infiltration.

Clinical features

Presentation is usually with a rapidly developing and painful swelling. Neurological symptoms may accom-pany this if there is nerve compression. Fever occurs in about 30% of patients.

Treatment

The choice of treatment will depend largely upon the site of the primary. Close liaison is required between orthopaedic surgeon and oncologist. Treatment should, as with osteogenic sarcomas, only be carried out by an experienced team.

Management differs from osteogenic sarcoma for three main reasons. First, Ewing's sarcoma is more chemosensitive. Secondly, Ewing's sarcoma occurs more frequently in the central than in the peripheral skeleton. Radical excision in the central skeleton is often not feasible because of limited access and the presence of adjacent vital structures (e.g. pelvic vessels). Thirdly, Ewing's sarcoma is more radiosensitive and can be controlled by radical radiotherapy when com-bined with adjuvant chemotherapy in about 75% of cases. However the likelihood of local tumour control is less if the primary tumour is large (9 cm or more). In these circumstances, unless the soft tissue component is very substantial, radical surgical removal of the whole bone (e.g. rib or fibula) is advised. If there is a bulky soft tissue component, initial reduction of its volume should be attempted with several cycles of chemotherapy before proceeding to surgery.

Where radical surgery to a limb would cause major functional impairment, a conservative approach, as in osteogenic sarcoma, can be adopted. A customised artificial prosthesis can be inserted at the end of the resected long bone. However amputation may be preferable for proximal tibial or distal femoral tumours in growing children because of reduced bone growth in the affected limb following local radiotherapy. The latter may give rise to limbs of unequal length and therefore a permanent handicap.

Radical radiotherapy

Target volume

It is not usually possible to deliver a radical dose uniformly to the whole bone unless it is very small because of toxicity to normal tissue. For this reason a 'shrinking field' approach is adopted with two consecutive phases based on the pretreatment volume. The initial volume is the tumour and a 5 cm margin of adjacent tissue. In long bones, an unirradiated strip of normal tissue containing lymphatics outside the tumour bearing area is left, if possible, to reduce the risk of lymphoedema as a late complication. In the second phase the volume is reduced to encompass the primary tumour with a 2 cm margin of normal tissue.

Technique

The choice of technique will vary with the site of the primary. For the limbs, a parallel opposed wedged pair of fields usually suffices. A 'shrinking field' technique is used for limb tumours. For pelvic primaries, it may be possible surgically to displace the bowel out of the radiation field, by inserting an absorbable mesh. For rib primaries, electrons of appropriate energy may be used to diminish the dose to the underlying lung.

Dose and energy

A high local dose (of the order of 50–60 Gy conventionally fractionated) to the bulk of the tumour must be delivered at megavoltage, using photons or electrons as appropriate. Patients should be included in nationally agreed protocols. The following regime is illustrative:

Phase 1: 40 Gy in 22 daily fractions over 30 days (4–6 MV photons)

Phase 2: 15 Gy in 8 daily fractions over 10 days (4–6 MV photons)

Acute and late reactions. These are the same as for soft tissue sarcoma (p. 504).

Palliative radiotherapy

Whole lung irradiation is useful in relieving cough and dyspnoea from lung metastases.

Technique

A parallel opposed pair of fields encompassing both lung fields is used.

Dose and energy

25 Gy in 20 daily fractions over 4 weeks (4–6 MV photons)

Chemotherapy

Adjuvant combination chemotherapy with agents such as vincristine, actinomycin D, Adriamycin, cyclophosphamide and more recently ifosfamide have proved effective. The search for the best combination is the subject of national and international studies.

Very intensive chemotherapy with autologous bone marrow transplantation for patients with poor prognostic factors is under investigation. Durable responses only seem to be obtained in patients in complete remission at the time of intensive treatment.

In the presence of metastases (e.g. in the lungs) cure can still be achieved in a small number of patients using the same agents as for adjuvant therapy.

Results of treatment

The outcome is better for patients with tumours of the peripheral rather than central skeleton. Up to 90% disease-free survival for peripheral tumours and 65% for central (axial) tumours has been achieved. Overall 5-year survival (and probably cure) is about 50%. Local recurrence occurs in about 10–15% of long bone primaries and 25–30% of pelvic tumours. The higher recurrence rate in the pelvis is probably due to the larger tumour size and the difficulty of irradiating the tumour homogeneously without damaging surrounding normal tissues.

CHONDROSARCOMA

Chondrosarcomas are malignant tumours of cartilage. They may arise in benign enchondromas or be malignant from the start. Adults aged 30–50 are affected. The commonest sites in order of frequency are the pelvis (50%), femur, humerus and scapula.

Macroscopically, the tumour is bulky, lobulated and semitranslucent. Microscopically, it is a sarcoma containing cartilage. Differentiation is variable. Poorly differentiated tumours (mesenchymal chondrosarcomas) behave more aggressively. In the well-differentiated form spread is slow locally. Blood-borne metastases occur late to the lungs.

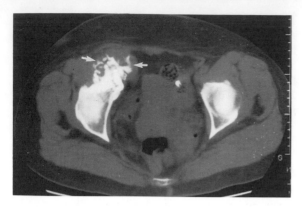

Fig. 28.6 CT scan of the pelvis showing a chondrosarcoma of the ileum (arrows). Note the flecks of calcification. (Courtesy of Dr R Nakielny, Sheffield.)

Clinical features

Presentation is usually with a slowly progressive painless swelling which eventually becomes painful.

Diagnosis and investigation

A biopsy is required. Plain radiography shows bone destruction and commonly abnormal flecks of calcification. CT scanning (Fig. 28.6) helps define the local extent.

Treatment

Radical surgery is the treatment of choice. Limb preservation may be possible. It is a very radioresistant tumour. Radiotherapy has only a palliative role for the relief of local symptoms, such as pain, and relatively high doses are required even for palliative effect.

Radiotherapy

Technique
A parallel opposed wedged pair of fields is suitable for the long bones. A three field technique for pelvic tumours using anterior and posterior wedged fields with an open lateral field may limit the dose to the bowel.

Dose and energy
60 Gy in 30 daily fractions over 6 weeks at megavoltage (4–6 MV photons)

Results of treatment

Five-year survival is about 50% over the age of 21 years but falls to 35% under that age. Younger patients tend to have tumours in the pelvis, where radical surgery is more difficult than in long bones. They also have more poorly differentiated tumours which metastasise more frequently.

OSTEOCLASTOMA (GIANT CELL TUMOUR OF BONE)

This is in most cases a benign tumour arising from osteoclasts. Occasionally it is malignant from the start or undergoes malignant transformation. It is commonest at the ends of long bones; 50% occur around the knee joint. Onset is usually between 20 and 35 years of age. Macroscopically osteoclastomas are eccentric expanding tumours which destroy bone. Microscopically there are giant cells of osteoclast type and a stroma of mononuclear cells. Spread is local and may eventually penetrate the joint. Blood-borne metastases are late and to the lungs (15%).

Clinical features

Presentation is with the gradual onset of pain and swelling, and sometimes pathological fracture.

Diagnosis and investigation

Plain radiographs typically show bone destruction by a multilocular cystic lesion expanding the cortex. Diagnosis is confirmed by open biopsy.

Treatment

Surgical excision or curettage is the treatment of choice for accessible sites. Radiotherapy offers an alternative for centrally placed tumours, e.g. in vertebrae, and for tumours in long bones where amputation may be undesirable in a young person. Chemotherapy has not been proven to be of value.

Radical radiotherapy

Target volume
If the primary tumour is at the end of the femur or in the upper tibia a margin of 4–5 cm normal bone proximally or distally, respectively, is needed. A smaller margin of 1–2 cm is given at the side of the tumour adjacent to the joint.

For tumours of a vertebral body, a margin of half a vertebral body above and below the affected vertebra is adequate.

Technique
For tumours in long bones, a parallel opposed pair of

fields is chosen. For vertebral tumours a posterior oblique wedged pair of fields is used to limit the dose to the spinal cord (Fig. 26.10).

Dose and energy

Relatively low doses (35 Gy in 15 daily fractions over 3 weeks) at megavoltage will control most tumours. If radiotherapy is the primary treatment, a higher dose is required (**50 Gy in 20–25 fractions over 4–5 weeks**). Care is taken to keep within spinal cord tolerance for vertebral tumours.

Results of treatment

Local recurrence following curettage is commoner, but following adequate excision prognosis is good, with 80% 5-year survival. Late sarcomatous change may occur, even at 15 years following radiotherapy. The role of radiotherapy in this malignant transformation is disputed.

SPINDLE CELL SARCOMAS

These include malignant fibrous histiocytoma (MFH), angiosarcoma and fibrosarcoma. They occur later (30–60 years of age) than osteosarcoma. Origin is both in the diaphysis and the metaphysis from the periosteum or the medullary cavity. Any bone may be affected. Microscopically there is variable collagen formation. Spread from the periosteum is to the soft tissues more than bone, and within the medullary cavity for endosteal tumours.

Clinical features

Pain and swelling are the main features.

Diagnosis and investigations

Plain radiography may show an area of bone similar in appearance to a bone infarct. A bone biopsy is necessary.

Treatment

Local excision is the treatment of choice with limb preservation if possible. Amputation may be necessary. Radiotherapy is only of palliative value. Adjuvant chemotherapy similar to that for osteogenic sarcoma is being evaluated.

Results of treatment

The prognosis is poor, with 5-year survival about 25%.

SECONDARY TUMOURS IN BONE

The great majority of bone tumours are not primary but are of metastatic origin. They represent 15–20% of the workload of a radiotherapy department. The most common primary sites are breast, lung, prostate, myeloma and kidney. The prognosis of bone metastases is generally poor, though the course of the disease may be relatively slow over a period of years, for example in some patients with breast cancer. Good symptomatic relief by a combination of analgesics and local radiotherapy can be achieved in most cases.

Clinical features and investigation

The usual presentation is with pain due to pressure on the periosteum or on nerve roots as they emerge from the spinal canal (Fig. 28.7). Early diagnosis is important before bone destruction has advanced so far as to cause pathological fracture or spinal cord compression.

Plain radiographs of the symptomatic area may show the deposits (osteolytic or osteosclerotic or both) or a pathological fracture. However a metastasis in a vertebral body has to have reached a size of about 2 cm before it will be visible on a radiograph.

A radioisotope bone scan (p. 185) is helpful in detecting bone metastases too small to be visible on plain radiographs and to detect deposits elsewhere in the skeleton. Multiple bone metastases are common, predominantly in the spine, ribs, pelvis and upper femurs. CT scanning of areas of the spine and sacrum where plain radiographs and bone scan are equivocal or normal may show bone destruction. If there is no known primary site, a CT guided biopsy may be necessary.

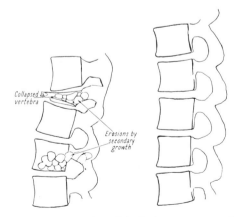

Fig. 28.7 Diagrammatic radiological appearances of normal vertebral column and secondary deposits from cancer (e.g. breast).

Treatment

The treatment of bone metastases includes analgesics, radiotherapy and occasionally surgery. Treatment is aimed at relieving pain as simply and quickly as possible. Analgesics are discussed in Chapter 33. The choice of treatment will depend on the site of the pain, its severity, complications such as spinal cord compression or pathological fracture, the underlying tumour and the general condition of the patient.

1. Site

Metastases in the spine are one of the commonest conditions that the radiotherapist irradiates. Careful clinical and radiological assessment is necessary to determine whether palliative radiotherapy is appropriate and, if so, which area is to be treated. Single fractions of 8 Gy to the affected vertebra and one normal vertebra above and below it are suitable for most thoracic and lumbar vertebrae (Fig. 28.8), with the exception of T12 and L1. The latter overlie the duodenum and fractionated doses (e.g. 20 Gy in 4 daily fractions) rather than single fractions are preferred, to reduce the incidence of radiation induced vomiting. Similarly, single fractions are not advised in the cervical spine due to the greater sensitivity of the spinal cord in this region. Orthovoltage generally has adequate penetration for the ribs and cervical spine. For most other sites megavoltage irradiation with cobalt-60 or a linear accelerator is needed. A simulator or portal film should be taken as a record of the area that has been treated. This is helpful if the patient re-presents at a later date with metastases within or adjacent to the previously irradiated area. In general, it is wise to allow 2 years to elapse before re-irradiating the spine and to fractionate the dose over a longer period of time (e.g. 20 Gy in 8 rather than 4 daily fractions).

Technique

Single fields are adequate for spinal (Fig. 28.8), sacral, rib and superficial skull deposits. For pelvic, long bone and base of skull deposits a parallel opposed pair of fields is used.

2. Pathological fracture

If there is a pathological fracture of a long bone, an

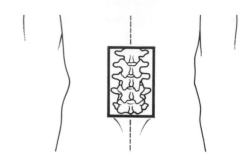

Fig. 28.8   Palliative single field (16 × 8 cm) to the lumbar spine (4–6 MV photons).

orthopaedic opinion should be sought on the feasibility of reducing and stabilising the fracture (Fig. 23.4). Pinning a fracture usually provides prompt pain relief and a return to mobility.

If there is evidence of spinal cord compression, surgical decompression of the cord may be necessary prior to fractionated radiotherapy (p. 491). Steroids should be given to patients with pain from nerve root infiltration and spinal cord compression.

Hemibody irradiation

If there are widespread painful bone metastases and the tumour is relatively radiosensitive (e.g. myeloma and prostate cancer), hemibody irradiation in a single fraction can be considered (see page 433 for technique and dosage).

Hormonal therapy

Hormonal therapy should be considered for patients whose tumours may be hormone responsive, such as breast and prostate tumours (see Chapters 23, 25 and 32).

Some patients are too unwell for even single fractions of treatment. Their pain should be controlled medically.

Results of treatment

About 75% of patients have worthwhile and often durable improvements in their pain following radiotherapy.

29. Cancer in children

Between the ages of 1 and 14 years malignancy is the main disease causing death. The annual incidence is 100 cases per million population in the UK. Most paediatric tumours (50%) occur under the age of 5 years.

Since the total number of cases is relatively small, it is best for treatment to be carried out in a few specialist centres. Experience has shown that the best results of treatment are achieved in this way. A multidisciplinary team of paediatric oncologist, radiotherapist and surgeon is required.

The commonest types of cancer are:

Leukaemia (mainly acute)	30%
CNS tumours	15%
Bone and soft tissue tumours	14%
Lymphomas	10%
Neuroblastoma	7%
Nephroblastoma (Wilms' tumour)	6%
Others	18%

Aetiology

In most cases the cause of malignancy in childhood is unknown. In a minority of tumours causative factors have been identified. For example intrauterine exposure of pregnant women to high doses of stilboestrol was associated with the development of adenocarcinoma of the vagina, a very rare tumour, in their children. The latent period following exposure to the drug varied from 4 to 22 years.

A number of patients with particular diseases are at higher risk of developing malignancy. There is, for example, an increased incidence of leukaemia in Down's syndrome. It is possible that chromosomal abnormalities account for nearly all cases of leukaemia. Wilms' tumour is 1000 times commoner than normal in children with a syndrome of congenital absence of the iris (aniridia), small head size, cataracts, mental retardation and urological abnormalities.

ACUTE LEUKAEMIA

This is the commonest cancer in childhood. It is of lymphocytic type (acute lymphoblastic leukaemia or ALL) in over 75% of cases. The annual incidence is 3.5 per 100 000 children. In the UK most cases occur between the ages of 2 and 7 years with a peak at 4 years. ALL is slightly commoner in boys (1.3:1).

The aetiology of leukaemia is unknown. There is, however, an increased incidence of ALL in children with chromosomal abnormalities (e.g. Down's syndrome and ataxia telangiectasia).

Clinical features

Most of the symptoms and signs of ALL are due to infiltration of the bone marrow, lymph nodes, liver and spleen by leukaemic cells. Common features are of anaemia (tiredness and pallor), skin haemorrhages and nose bleeds (due to low platelet count), fever and infection, ulceration of mucosal surfaces, and enlargement of lymph nodes, liver and spleen. There may be non-specific joint or bone pains. The CNS is involved at presentation in less than 5% of children.

Diagnosis and investigations

The diagnosis is made on bone marrow aspiration, in which leukaemic cells (lymphoblasts) can be identified. The peripheral blood count usually shows a low haemoglobin ($<10\,g/dl$), neutropenia ($<1.0 \times 10^9/l$) and low platelets ($<100 \times 10^9/l$). The total white count can be low, normal or elevated. Children with a total white cell count of over $100 \times 10^9/l$ at diagnosis have a poorer prognosis than children with lower white cell counts.

Treatment

Intensive cytotoxic therapy has considerably improved the prognosis of ALL. Treatment is divided into three phases: (1) induction of remission, (2) consolidation and (3) continuation therapy.

Induction of remission

In the first, induction phase of treatment the aim is to obtain a remission from the disease. This means (1) resolution of symptoms and signs (clinical remission) and (2) reducing the number of tumour cells in the bone marrow to <5% (haematological remission). None the less, even if a remission is obtained there are still a substantial number of leukaemic cells present in the body.

The most common induction regime used in the UK consists of:

Vincristine: 1.5 mg/m^2 i.v. weekly for 4 weeks
Prednisolone: 40 mg/m^2 orally per day for 4 weeks (and then tailed off)
Daunorubicin: 45 mg/m^2 i.v. daily on day 1 and 2 of induction
Asparaginase: 6000 units/m^2 (nine injections over 3 weeks)

Most patients in the UK are entered into national studies (United Kingdom acute lymphoblastic leukaemia (UKALL) trials).

Supportive therapy with platelet and red cell transfusions is often required. Intravenous antibiotics should be started at the first suggestion of any infection (usually a fever) because of the risk of serious infection. A number of different combinations of antibiotics are used. The most common include a third generation cephalosporin such as ceftazidime or a penicillin such as piperacillin in combination with an aminoglycoside (tobramycin or gentamicin). The use of prophylactic antibiotics is generally not encouraged in the management of acute lymphoblastic leukaemia because of concern over the production of resistant organisms (unlike the case with acute myeloblastic leukaemia where the majority of patients are given prophylactic antibiotics).

Tumour cell killing risks increasing serum uric acid levels due to the degradation of dead cells. Uric acid levels are monitored. Oral allopurinol (300 mg/m^2) is started before treatment to stimulate uric acid secretion and is continued usually for about 2 weeks. High blood uric acid levels may damage the kidneys (uric acid nephropathy).

About 95% of patients achieve a complete remission following 4 weeks of induction therapy.

Consolidation treatment

CNS directed treatment. The CNS is one of the sanctuary sites where tumour cells may lodge. They are unaffected by the drugs used in induction therapy since they are unable to cross the blood–brain barrier. Fifty per cent of patients will relapse in the meninges if no prophylactic treatment is given to the cranium. For this reason the whole cranium is irradiated and intrathecal methotrexate is given at intervals throughout induction and consolidation treatment and is based on CSF volume. Dosage will vary with age. Prophylactic cranial irradiation and intrathecal methotrexate reduce the risk of CNS relapse to less than 10%. Prophylactic cranial irradiation is not given to children under the age of 2 years.

Target volume

This includes the whole brain and the meninges. The lower posterior margin should cover the lower border of the second cervical vertebra (Fig. 29.1). The base of the skull can be seen on a lateral skull radiograph as a white line passing backwards from the base of the frontal sinus to the anterior clinoid process at the front of the pituitary fossa. This line is the lateral part of the anterior cranial fossa. Just below this line is a fainter line due to the cribriform plate of the ethmoid bone.

Technique

A shell is made with shaped lead blocks to allow adequate coverage of the cribriform plate and middle cranial fossa while blocking the eye and the face (Fig. 29.1). A rectangular field with its lower margin running along the line of the base of the skull and above the eye risks underdosage of the cribriform

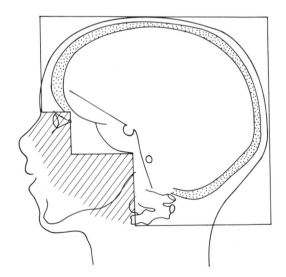

Fig. 29.1 Treatment volume for prophylactic cranial irradiation in acute lymphoblastic leukaemia.

plate where relapse may occur. A parallel pair of opposed lateral fields is used. For some children sedation or general anaesthesia may be required during irradiation.

Dose and energy
18 Gy central tumour dose in 10 daily fractions over 2 weeks (4–6 MV photons)

Acute effects. Most patients experience some degree of nausea and vomiting which may require antiemetics.

Occasionally a somnolence syndrome occurs, although this is now less common since the total dosage has been reduced from 24 Gy to 18 Gy. This is characterised by somnolence, headache, lethargy, fever, nausea, vomiting and diarrhoea 4–8 weeks after cranial irradiation. This syndrome is thought to be due to transient damage to the production of myelin, an important component of nerve cells. The incidence varies substantially from 10 to 80% but is low if total doses of <20 Gy in 10 daily fractions are given.

Late effects. Growth and development may be impaired due to irradiation of the hypothalamo-pituitary axis. Close surveillance of growth and development and referral to a paediatric endocrinologist for further investigation may be necessary. Problems with growth and development are rare with the doses used.

Continuation therapy

Maintenance therapy is required to prevent the disease from relapsing after the induction of a clinical and haematological remission. Two years of maintenance therapy is given.

The commonest regime for low risk (see below) patients is:

Oral 6-mercaptopurine 75 mg/m^2 daily.
Oral methotrexate 20 mg/m^2 weekly.
I.v. vincristine is given every 4 weeks with a 5-day course of oral steroids.

Complications of chemotherapy

The major complication during treatment is life-threatening sepsis. Intravenous antibiotics should be started at the first signs of infection or if the child is neutropenic. During and following chemotherapy the child is immunosuppressed and at risk of serious infections of chickenpox, measles and *Pneumocystis carinii*. Co-trimoxazole (Septrin) is given from the start of continuation therapy on alternate days as prophylaxis against *P. carinii* infection. Live viral vaccines should not be given. Chickenpox (varicella) or shingles (herpes zoster) should be treated by intravenous acyclovir.

Relapse

The CNS, testis and bone marrow are the commonest sites of relapse. The most frequent combination is the bone marrow and the CNS, particularly in ALL of T cell origin and those with a high initial white cell count (>100 × 10^9/l).

CNS relapse is difficult to treat since the prophylactic cranial irradiation and intrathecal methotrexate limit the amount of irradiation and intrathecal therapy that can be safely given without damaging the CNS. Intensive systemic chemotherapy (e.g. with methotrexate and cytosine arabinoside) is followed by craniospinal irradiation to a total dose of 30 Gy over 5 weeks. Isolated CNS relapse may be curable in about 30% of cases.

Bone marrow relapse within a year of the completion of maintenance therapy is rarely cured by additional chemotherapy. Bone marrow transplantation (p. 465) is considered for ALL in second or subsequent remissions. It may also be considered for 'bad risk' ALL in first remission, e.g. with white cell count >100 × 10^9/l.

Testicular relapse is a form of systemic relapse. It is characterised by a rapidly growing painless testicular swelling. It usually occurs about 3–4 months after the end of maintenance therapy if it is the only site of relapse. The diagnosis is confirmed by biopsy. If the biopsy is positive, the affected testis should be removed. If both testes are involved, only one testis should be removed. In both cases testicular irradiation and chemotherapy should be given. Irradiation is started after clinical resolution of the testicular mass on chemotherapy.

Testicular irradiation

Target volume
This includes the scrotum and both inguinal regions (Fig. 29.2).

Technique
An individualised lead cut-out is made. A single anterior electron field of appropriate energy is used.

Dose and energy
24 Gy in 12 daily fractions over 16 days (12–16 MeV)

Results of treatment

The 5-year survival rate for ALL improved from 30–40% in the early 1970s to 70–80% in the early 1990s.

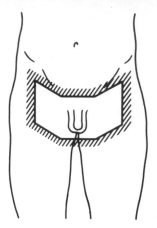

Fig. 29.2 Anterior electron portal for testicular irradiation in acute lymphoblastic leukaemia. (Reproduced with permission from Hope-Stone 1986.)

ACUTE NON-LYMPHOBLASTIC LEUKAEMIA

Acute non-lymphoblastic leukaemia (ANLL) is much less common that ALL in children but still represents 20% of childhood leukaemia. Acute myeloblastic leukaemia is the commonest type of ANLL. ANLL differs from ALL in being less responsive to chemotherapy, with lower remission rates and fewer long-term cures. More supportive therapy is needed against haemorrhage and infection.

Complete remissions can be induced in 85% of children with intensive chemotherapy. If an allogeneic donor is available, bone marrow transplantation is carried out in first remission. The benefit of autologous bone marrow transplantation has not been established. Maintenance therapy is not required for ANLL. If relapse occurs in the marrow, successful salvage therapy is rare.

Results of treatment

Overall 5-year survival is 40%.

NEUROBLASTOMA

Neuroblastoma is a malignant tumour arising from the sympathetic nervous tissue. It accounts for approximately 8% of childhood malignancy and is the commonest solid tumour in this age group; 50% occur under the age of 2 years and 75% under the age of 5. Occasionally it may be present at birth.

Pathology

Neuroblastoma arises from tissue of the neural crest

which forms the sympathetic nervous system. The sympathetic chain extends upwards from around the pelvic brim (5%) to the paravertebral region of the retroperitoneal tissues (70%), mediastinum (17%) and neck (8%). Neuroblastoma can develop at any of these sites. In the retroperitoneum the adrenal medulla accounts for 30% and abdominal side chain (10%) of tumours. The biological behaviour of this tumour is very variable. It may rarely undergo spontaneous regression with maturation into the adult non-malignant form (ganglioneuroma). Macroscopically the tumour appears as a soft, encapsulated vascular mass. Microscopically, in the least differentiated form, the tumour is composed of closely packed sympathetic nerve cells (sympathogonia) with many mitotic figures. In other parts of the tumour there may be formation of cells into rosettes. Ganglion cells may be identifiable in the better differentiated types. The tumour may stain positively for chromaffin, indicating cells of neural crest origin. Electron microscopy may show the presence of neurosecretory storage granules in the cytoplasm of the cell.

The tumour spreads locally (e.g. from the adrenal to the kidney and liver), to lymph nodes and to distant sites (especially bone and liver).

Clinical features

Neuroblastoma gives rise to a wide variety of symptoms and signs due to the many sites from which it may develop. In the abdomen, it may present with abdominal pain, anorexia and vomiting or with a painless mass in the abdomen or loin. In the pelvis, difficulty with bowel or urinary function may be associated with a mass palpable per rectum.

Thoracic tumours may present with dyspnoea, chest infection or dysphagia. In the neck, a mass may be palpable in association with signs of compression of the sympathetic chain, i.e. Horner's syndrome—drooping of the eyelid (ptosis), small pupil (miosis) and inward movement of the eye (enophthalmos).

In the paraspinal area, pain, tenderness, signs of spinal cord compression and bladder or urinary dysfunction are common.

The liver may be infiltrated (hepatomegaly, jaundice). Painful bone metastases, often with pathological fractures, are common. Retro-orbital deposits give rise to a protruding eye (exophthalmos). Skin metastases with a bluish colour are frequent. Lymph node metastases are mainly to cervical and supraclavicular nodes, particularly on the left side (Virchow's node from abdominal tumours). Lung metastases are uncommon (in contrast to Wilms' tumour).

Metabolic effects

The physiological activity of the sympathetic nervous system is mediated by complex organic substances called catecholamines. Metabolic breakdown products, e.g. homovanillic acid (HVA) and vanillylmandelic acid (VMA), are measurable in the urine. Raised blood levels give rise to the effects of stimulation of the sympathetic system (sweating, anxiety). Diarrhoea may rarely occur due to the production of a vasoactive peptide (VIP).

Diagnosis and staging investigations

The diagnosis is established by biopsy of the tumour mass, bone marrow examination and detection of excessive levels of urinary catecholamines, e.g. VMA.

Staging investigations include full blood count (anaemia, leucoerythroblastic if the bone marrow is infiltrated), blood urea and creatinine (raised if renal tract obstruction), electrolytes (low potassium from diarrhoea), liver function tests (for liver metastases), chest radiograph (lung metastases) or abdominal radiograph (mass, usually with calcification) and bone scan (multiple metastases).

CT scan and ultrasound are important in showing involvement of adjacent organs (e.g. liver and kidney), regional lymph nodes, extension from the abdomen into the chest or across the midline, and liver metastases.

A commonly used staging system is shown in Table 29.1.

Table 29.1 International staging system for neuroblastoma (Forbeck)

Stage	Clinical findings
I	Localised tumour confined to the organ of origin, complete gross resection, identifiable ipsilateral and contralateral nodes negative
IIa	Unilateral tumour with incomplete gross excision, identifiable ipsilateral and contralateral nodes negative
IIb	Unilateral tumour with complete or incomplete gross excision, positive ipsilateral nodes, negative contralateral nodes
III	Tumour infiltrating across midline with or without regional node involvement or unilateral tumour with contralateral regional nodes involved or midline tumour with bilateral regional node involvement
IV	Disseminated tumour to distant lymph nodes, bone, bone marrow, liver and/or other organs *except as defined in stage IVS*
IVS	Localised primary tumour (as defined for stage I or II) with dissemination limited to liver, skin or bone marrow

Table 29.2 OPEC chemotherapy regime for neuroblastoma

Vincristine (Oncovin) 1 mg/m² i.v.	Day 1
Cisplatin (platinum) 60 mg/m² i.v.	Day 2
VM-26 (Epipodophyll) 150 mg/m² i.v.	Day 3
Cyclophosphamide 600 mg/m² i.v.	Day 4

Repeated every 3 weeks for 6–10 courses

Treatment

A multidisciplinary approach is required since surgery, radiotherapy and chemotherapy may all have a role to play. Since 60–70% of all cases are metastatic at presentation, chemotherapy (Table 29.2) is indicated in all but the early stages (I and II). If the tumour has been completely excised in stages I and II and elevated catecholamine levels have returned to normal, there is usually no indication for postoperative radiotherapy or chemotherapy.

Stage III is treated by preoperative chemotherapy, excision and, if necessary, radiotherapy to residual disease.

Stage IV is treated primarily by chemotherapy. Local radiotherapy may be required to sites of bulk disease not resolving following chemotherapy, for palliation of painful metastases in skin, bone or liver, and for spinal cord compression (often after surgical decompression). Surgical excision of residual masses may also be helpful and avoids the potential damage to growing tissues from radiotherapy.

Stage I and II

For stages I and II local resection of the tumour, if possible, may be all that is required. Complete surgical resection is rarely possible because of the infiltration of local tissues. Radiotherapy may be given postoperatively to eradicate residual disease.

Target volume

This will include the primary tumour and adjacent spread, as identified by operative findings and radiological investigations (particularly CT), with a 1–2 cm margin of normal tissue.

Technique

In most circumstances a parallel opposed pair is adequate for radical irradiation.

Abdomen. In the abdomen care is taken to shield one kidney if all or part of the other is being irradiated. If the vertebral column has to be irradiated, it is important that the whole width of the vertebral body is included. Partial coverage will lead to unequal bone growth and deformity (scoliosis). The femoral heads and gonads should be shielded if possible.

Dose and energy

Neuroblastoma is a relatively radiosensitive tumour and modest doses may be adequate to obtain tumour shrinkage. This is particularly helpful in young children and infants where high doses are to be avoided to minimise impairment of growth and development.

Radical

Infants (below 2 years)
18–20 Gy in 15 daily fractions (4–6 MV photons)

Older children (2–10 years)
25–35 Gy in 15–20 daily fractions over 3–4 weeks followed, if within the tolerance of the tissues within the volume, by a boost to 40 Gy to bulk disease

Palliative

Bone metastases
15 Gy in 5 daily fractions over 1 week

Spinal cord compression
15 Gy in 10 daily fractions over 2 weeks

Liver metastases. Palliative radiotherapy may relieve the pain of distension of the liver capsule by metastases. **Central tumour dose of 4.5 Gy in 3 daily fractions over 6 days (treating alternate days)**

Skin metastases
Single fraction of 4 Gy at superficial or orthovoltage

Chemotherapy

A distinction needs to be made between the treatment of stages IV and IVS disease.

Stage IVS may resolve spontaneously or may respond to minimal treatment such as vincristine and cyclophosphamide or local radiotherapy to a dose of 4.5 Gy.

Stage IV requires multiagent chemotherapy. One of the most effective combinations, OPEC, is shown in Table 29.2. Resection of the primary tumour is often feasible after 6–10 courses. Following complete remission (i.e. no demonstrable tumour cells in the bone marrow) treatment with high dose melphalan and reinfusion of the patient's own bone marrow (autologous bone marrow transplantation) may be considered to prevent relapse. The harvested bone marrow can be treated with monoclonal antibodies attached to magnetic beads and passed through a magnet to remove any residual tumour cells before reinfusion.

Isotope therapy

Meta-iodobenzyl guanidine (MIBG) is a chemical similar in structure to noradrenaline. Its uptake by neuroblastoma cells is proportionate to the number of neurosecretory granules in the tumour. Disseminated neuroblastoma may absorb up to 40% of the administered dose. The use of MIBG for small volume residual disease following chemotherapy is being assessed.

Results of treatment

A number of prognostic factors which influence survival have been identified. They are the stage of the disease, age, site of the primary tumour and its degree of differentiation. Of these the stage is the most important.

The 2-year disease-free survival (and probable cure) is about 90% for stages I and II, 75% for stage IVS, 60% for stage II, 35% for stage III, and 25–30% for stage IV.

The prognosis for children under 1 year old is better than for older patients, whatever the stage.

Primary tumours in the cervical, thoracic and pelvic region have a better prognosis than abdominal tumours.

WILMS' TUMOUR

Wilms' tumour (nephroblastoma) is a malignant tumour of the kidney. It typically occurs in children between the ages of 1 and 5 years and arises from the renal parenchyma. Grossly the tumour is cystic, necrotic and haemorrhagic. There are three histological varieties with a poorer prognosis (anaplastic, rhabdoid sarcoma, and clear cell sarcoma) and two with a more favourable prognosis (multicystic nephroblastoma and nephroblastoma with fibroadenomatous structures).

Spread

Spread is local into the adjacent kidney, renal pelvis and ureter. Regional nodes are rarely affected. Blood-borne metastases occur typically to the lung.

Clinical features

The typical presentation is with a large swelling in the flank of a small pale infant. The mass is usually painless and fixed. Vigorous palpation should be avoided since

Table 29.3 Staging system for Wilms' tumour

Stage	Clinical findings
I	Tumour limited to the kidney and completely excised
II	Tumour extends beyond the kidney, but is completely excised
III	Residual tumour confined to the abdomen, e.g. peritoneal contamination or lymph node metastases
IV	Metastatic disease (e.g. lung, and occasionally liver or brain)
V	Bilateral renal tumours

this may rupture the tumour. Haematuria occurs in about 25% of cases. Occasionally presentation is with an acute abdomen requiring laparotomy. Hypertension occurs in up to 60% of cases but is rarely severe.

Diagnosis and staging investigations

The most commonly used staging system for Wilms' tumour is shown in Table 29.3.

Intravenous urography (IVU) may show the renal origin of the tumour. Typically it deforms the calyces and, if in the lower pole, may displace the ureter medially. IVU has been replaced in many centres by ultrasound and CT scanning. They are helpful in distinguishing between a cystic mass and a tumour and detecting small tumours in the other kidney. They may also show tumour thrombi in the inferior vena cava and liver metastases.

Full blood count (anaemia), urinalysis (protein, white cells and red cells) and chest radiograph (lung metastases) are required.

Treatment

Surgery, radiotherapy and chemotherapy are required alone or in combination and close liaison is required between specialists. The differentiation of the tumour is important in the choice of therapy. Well and moderately differentiated tumours are considered 'favourable' histology (85% of cases). Those with anaplastic or sarcomatous elements are 'unfavourable'.

Surgery

Surgical removal of the kidney is the initial treatment for stages I–III in most cases. Where the tumour is considered inoperable initial chemotherapy to render the tumour operable, if possible, may be required. At the time of surgery the abdomen is carefully examined to assess the extent of spread and to check that

the tumour is not bilateral. The regional nodes are biopsied. Residual tumour is marked with titanium clips to assist with planning of postoperative radiotherapy. If a postoperative CT scan is planned, metal clips are not recommended since they distort the CT images. A metal wire can be placed around the kidney and a peroperative radiograph taken to document the local disease. Peritoneal contamination from spillage from the tumour is noted.

Radiotherapy

The role of radiotherapy in Wilms' tumour is diminishing since late side-effects (impaired growth of bone and soft tissues) are inevitable if abdominal irradiation is given to cancericidal doses. Combination chemotherapy as an adjuvant after surgery is playing an increasing role since growth and development are not permanently inhibited. None the less, radiotherapy is a very effective treatment and reduced the mortality to about 50% when first introduced following surgery.

For stage I with 'favourable' histology no postoperative radiotherapy is required. In stage II, the role of radiotherapy is uncertain and is being evaluated in multicentre studies. It is probably unnecessary in stage II with favourable histology, particularly in children under the age of 2 years.

Postoperative radiotherapy is given to stage III with favourable histology. If the histology in stage III is unfavourable the decision to give postoperative radiotherapy will depend on the results of a 'second look' laparotomy after initial chemotherapy. If there is evidence of residual disease at laparotomy after initial chemotherapy, postoperative radiotherapy is given. If there is no residual disease, no postoperative radiotherapy is required.

In stage IV abdominal radiotherapy may be needed if a second laparotomy after biopsy and chemotherapy shows persistent abdominal disease.

Palliative radiotherapy to lung metastases may be helpful in shrinking lung metastases which are failing to respond to chemotherapy.

1. Primary tumour

Target volume

This should include the tumour bed, the regional nodes and the full width of the vertebrae (Fig. 29.3). The last of these is essential to avoid scoliosis from unequal bone growth. The lateral margin on the side of the tumour should extend to the lateral abdominal wall. If there is tumour spillage, the fields should encompass the area of spillage and not necessarily the whole abdomen. Only if there is wide peritoneal

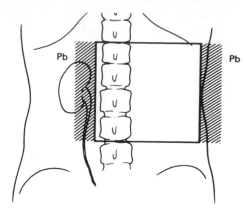

Fig. 29.3 Treatment volume for irradiating the renal bed in Wilms' tumour. (Reproduced with permission from Hope-Stone 1986.)

contamination does the whole of the abdomen need to be covered. Coverage of the whole abdomen extends from the dome of the diaphragm to the bottom of the obturator foramina of the pubic bones.

Care is taken to shield the kidney on the other side to limit its dosage to 12 Gy, whether locoregional or abdominal irradiation is given.

The liver should be shielded to reduce the dose to 20 Gy.

In girls the ovary on the opposite side to the tumour is shielded, as are the femoral heads and acetabula.

Technique

An anterior and posterior pair of fields is used.

Dose and energy

Total dose per week should not exceed 10 Gy. If the whole abdomen is irradiated this is reduced to 7.5 Gy (4–6 MV photons)

Stage III

Favourable histology
20 Gy in 20 daily fractions over 3 weeks

Unfavourable histology after positive 'second look' laparotomy
30 Gy in 20 daily fractions over 4 weeks

Stage IV to residual abdominal disease
20–30 Gy in 5–20 daily fractions over 1–4 weeks

2. Whole lung

Target volume
This includes the whole of the chest.

Technique
Anterior and posterior opposed fields are used. The humeral heads are shielded.

Dose and energy
12–15 Gy in 10 daily fractions over 2 weeks at megavoltage. A boost of 10 Gy is given in 3 daily fractions to small fields to encompass residual disease.

Acute reaction. Nausea and vomiting occur. White cell count and platelets fall but recover following radiation.

Late reactions. Vertebral growth is symmetrically impaired if the whole of the width of the vertebral body is included. Some degree of scoliosis may still occur due to fibrosis of the paravertebral soft tissues. Pneumonitis may follow 2–3 weeks after pulmonary irradiation. This complication may occur earlier if chemotherapy is delivered concurrently or radiotherapy is followed by chemotherapy with actinomycin D.

Chemotherapy

For patients with favourable histology—stage I: intravenous vincristine for 3 months; stage II: vincristine and actinomycin D for 6 months; stage III: vincristine, actinomycin D and doxorubicin for 1 year; stage IV: vincristine, actinomycin D and doxorubicin for 1 year.

For unfavourable histology more intensive chemotherapy is required. Etoposide or ifosfamide may be used.

Side-effects of chemotherapy. These are alopecia, vincristine neuropathy (Ch. 31), a syndrome of hepatic dysfunction and transient leucopenia, and thrombocytopenia (if concurrent hepatic irradiation and full dose actinomycin D).

Results of treatment

For patients with favourable histology the results are excellent: 2-year survival is 90% for stage I, 75% for stage II, 55% for stage III and 50% for stage IV. The prognosis for unfavourable histology has improved with the use of doxorubicin, with 2-year survival of 70%.

30. Non-malignant disorders

Cancer is not the only disease process in which radiation can be useful. It was inevitable that such a powerful form of energy should be widely explored in the early days before its dangers and limitations could be and were appreciated. Radiation was delivered to a very wide range of non-malignant conditions by enthusiasts in the pioneer days. Unfortunately a great deal of damage, some of it fatal, was done unwittingly before the serious consequences emerged. For example irradiation of the enlarged thymus gland in infancy used to be practised, and it caused gratifying shrinkage. Years later, however, carcinoma of the thyroid developed in some cases, undoubtedly induced by the effect of the rays on the immature thyroid cells. Similarly, some patients who received spinal irradiation to relieve spinal discomfort from ankylosing spondylitis, a chronic rheumatic disorder, later developed leukaemia and other tumours. The development of leukaemia in these patients discouraged many radiotherapists from treating this and other benign conditions with radiotherapy.

Where treatment appeared to be useful, e.g. in many non-malignant skin disorders, repeated dosage was commonly given for recurrent disease, since the cumulative effects of even low doses were for long not appreciated.

At present the indications for the use of radiotherapy for non-malignant conditions is much more limited. To a large extent this is due to the appreciation of radiation induced malignancy but it also reflects the availability of more effective non-radiotherapeutic treatments. None the less, there is considerable variation in the use of radiotherapy for benign disease between radiotherapy departments in the UK.

In general the use of ionising radiation for the treatment of benign disease should be discouraged and alternative therapies sought.

ENDOCRINE DISORDERS

Pituitary

Radiation is commonly used postoperatively following the surgical removal or debulking of pituitary tumours (see p. 484 for detailed description).

Ovary

The ovary, beside producing the ova or egg cells which unite with the sperm to form the next generation, secretes female sex hormones (e.g. oestrogen) which control secondary sexual characteristics and the various changes in the female organism. Towards the age of the menopause ovarian function may become irregular and cause intermittent excessive uterine bleeding (menorrhagia). If medical treatment fails, surgical hysterectomy is often advised. An alternative is to suppress ovarian hormonal secretion by radiation. This can be applied in two ways: internal and external.

Internal therapy

An intrauterine tube containing caesium, as used in uterine cancer, will irradiate and inhibit both the endometrium and the ovaries. A 50 mg tube applied for 40–48 hours will deliver about 5–10 Gy to the ovaries. General anaesthesia is needed, and this provides the essential opportunity for a thorough pelvic examination, uterine curettage and biopsy, to exclude malignancy as the cause of bleeding. This technique is very effective and still used, though it can lead to some degree of endometritis and uterine discharge. It is contraindicated in patients who are not fit enough for a general anaesthetic, usually due to poor cardio-respiratory function.

Induction of an *artificial menopause* in this way involves sterilisation of the patient. In almost all cases, this causes no problems and is in fact desirable. It is wise, however, to obtain the written informed consent of the patient who should be asked to sign a form stating that the effects of the treatment have been explained, understood and accepted.

In the past radiation was used to treat dysmenorrhoea and pelvic inflammatory disease. Such practice is to be condemned because of the risk of gene mutations affecting succeeding generations.

External therapy

External beam irradiation is the commonest means of inducing an artificial menopause. It is suitable for patients where general anaesthesia is contraindicated.

Target volume

The target volume is the true pelvis. A typical field size is 15 cm wide and 10 cm long.

Technique

A parallel opposed pair of anterior and posterior fields is used.

Dose and energy

There is some variation in the dose required to ablate ovarian function which is related to age and to individual factors. A larger dose is needed at and beyond the age of 35 years.

Under the age of 35: **12.5 Gy in 5 daily fractions (9–10 MV photons)**

Aged 35+: **4.5 Gy midplane dose in a single fraction (9–10 MV photons)**

Radioactive iodine and the thyroid gland

For the physical and technical aspects relating to this section reference should be made to Chapter 10.

The thyroid gland synthesises the hormones thyroxine (T4) and tri-iodothyronine (T3) which are essential for the maintenance of normal metabolism, utilising iodine from the diet. As with other endocrine function, the activity of the thyroid gland is controlled by the pituitary through the thyroid stimulating hormone (TSH) (p. 483). By substituting radioactive iodine, this unique affinity for the chemical provides a useful method of producing a high dose of radiation within a very small volume of tissue.

Thyrotoxicosis (hyperthyroidism)

This is a clinical state associated with raised levels of circulating T4 and/or T3. As a result there is an increase in the body's metabolism, manifested by agitation, palpitations, profuse sweating and weight loss. In some cases there is protrusion of the eyes (exophthalmos). The disease affects females more commonly and usually occurs in the 25–45 year age group. It is sometimes associated with a significant enlargement

of the thyroid gland (goitre). Occasionally when a large gland extends behind the sternum (retrosternal extension) there may be evidence of compression of the trachea.

The high affinity of the thyroid gland for iodine forms the basis of both diagnosis and treatment.

Myxoedema

Myxoedema (hypothyroidism) is a state of thyroid hormone deficiency, causing sluggish metabolism. Clinical features include tiredness, weight gain, hair loss, slow pulse and slow relaxing reflexes.

Investigation of thyroid function

The important in vivo tests of thyroid function are those associated with the uptake of radioactive iodine (iodine-131) or other isotopes (Technetium-99m). These may provide a measure of the physiological activity of the gland (tracer techniques) or of its size and position (imaging or scanning). Both of these tests require sophisticated apparatus and are in vivo. Blood levels of T4 and T3 and, if hypothyroidism is suspected, TSH are measured.

The tracer investigation. This can be carried out on an outpatient basis. The patient attends the isotope laboratory before breakfast and takes a very small dose of iodine-131 (0.55 MBq) through a straw. Four hours later the patient returns and lies on a couch, and a counter above the neck measures the radiation emitted from the gland. This gives a measure of the amount of iodine-131 which has been absorbed by the cells of the thyroid from the test drink, following its passage from the gut into the bloodstream. The count is repeated at 48 hours, when a blood sample is taken and the iodine-131 content of the blood proteins is measured.

Interpretation of the tracer test. The main relevant details are given in Chapter 10 and Figure 21.28B.

1. Gland. Normally the measured radioactivity rises gently to a plateau, reached soon after 24 hours, but the toxic gland removes iodine from the blood at such a rapid rate that the iodine-131 curve rises to a sharp peak in a few hours and then falls. Thus the measured uptake at 4 hours will identify most thyrotoxic cases.

2. Plasma. Normally the blood is cleared of iodine gradually and at 48 hours very little is left. However in the toxic cases there is a secondary rise due to secretion of newly formed hormone, incorporating some of the iodine-131. The 48-hour figures for protein bound iodine give almost conclusive evidence in most cases.

The thyroid scan. An image of the gland may be

obtained by giving the patient a small quantity of radioactive iodine or technetium (see above) and using a special detector called a rectilinear scanner. The latter will measure the activity within the gland at automated 1 cm intervals and produce a composite picture of the size and shape of the gland with areas of high and low activity clearly defined. The typical appearance of toxic multinodular goitre is shown in Figure 21.28B. Variation in shape and activity are easily detected and the test is invaluable in revealing retrosternal goitre, and particularly in the investigation of thyroid cancer (p. 357). The latter usually appears as a 'cold' area (Fig. 21.28A).

In vitro tests

1. Measurement of circulating T4 and T3 by chemical means (as distinct from the radioactive test).

2. Measurement of TSH. The level is low in thyrotoxicosis, as other mechanisms of thyroid stimulation are in operation in this disease, and increased in hypothyroidism.

3. T3 resin uptake. This reflects the amount of hormone binding to TBG (thyroid binding globulin). A resin is mixed with the patient's serum. There is competition between the resin and the unfilled binding sites on TBG. The amount of T3 retained in the resin after washing reflects the concentration of the unoccupied binding sites.

4. Free thyroxine index. This is calculated as: serum T4 × T3 resin uptake.

5. TRH test. When TRH (thyroid releasing hormone), one of the hypothalamic hormones, is given intravenously in the euthyroid person, it stimulates a rise in serum TSH levels. In hyperthyroidism there is little or no rise in TSH. Thus a positive response rules out primary hyperthyroidism.

In vitro tests are more important than tracer studies, so that the administration of radioactive material can very often be avoided altogether.

Treatment of thyrotoxicosis

A small proportion of patients with thyrotoxicosis will improve spontaneously, but active treatment is required in most patients. Essentially, treatment is concerned with the reduction of circulating thyroxine, either by partial destruction of the gland or by interrupting the synthesis of the hormone.

Destructive therapy may be achieved either by surgery (removal of most of the gland) or by using the specially radioactive iodine in carefully measured doses. Both methods have a place in the management of hyperthyroidism, but radioactive iodine therapy has the advantage of being relatively simple and devoid of serious side-effects and complications.

Medical control is achieved by antithyroid drugs such as carbimazole and propylthiouracil. Serious side-effects may occur (e.g. agranulocytosis with carbimazole). Drug therapy is usually used to render the patient euthyroid prior to surgery. It may be especially important where surgery or iodine-131 cannot be used because of other medical conditions, poor general condition or pregnancy.

Radioactive iodine therapy

The technique is simple. A dose calculated from the size of the gland and the uptake of radioactive iodine (in the tracer test) is given to the patient under the same conditions as for the diagnostic test. Unless the patient is ill, this can be arranged on an outpatient basis, although the patient should stay at the hospital for a few hours until the possibility of vomiting and other side-effects has subsided. The size of the therapeutic drink is of the order of 74–296 MBq which is usually sufficiently low to avoid the need for special precautions to prevent contamination and ensure the safety of staff. If the disease is not controlled by a single treatment, then more doses may be necessary, having allowed up to 12 months to elapse in order to assess the full effect of the first dose.

The drawback of this treatment is the progressive effects of the irradiation, which frequently leads to increasing atrophy of the gland with a slow decrease in the amount of circulating hormones, which can ultimately produce hypothyroidism.

This treatment is usually restricted to patients over the age of 40 because of the theoretical risk of inducing leukaemia or thyroid cancer. There is also the possibility of gene mutations in the reproductive cells of the ovary and testis.

RHEUMATIC DISORDERS
Ankylosing spondylitis

This is a disabling process, mostly in young men, with pain and stiffness, leading to 'poker back' rigidity. It usually begins in the sacroiliac joints, spreading later to the small joints between the vertebrae, and the costovertebral joints (where the ribs attach to the spine). The chronic inflammation leads eventually to ossification of ligaments, fusion of joint surfaces and bony ankylosis. Radiation usually gives dramatic pain relief and enables the patient to return to work.

Until 1955, deep X-ray therapy was widely and successfully used as the mainstay of treatment directed at either the sacroiliac joints alone or the whole spine. Total doses up to 30 Gy were applied. Then it was discovered that 10% of treated patients developed leukaemia, undoubtedly a late radiation effect. This led to the abandonment of the treatment by most radiotherapists, in favour of general measures, physiotherapy and drugs. There are still a few cases (e.g. a peripheral painful joint or boggy plantar fasciitis) where, if other methods fail, localised radiotherapy can be justified. The slight risks should be fully explained to the patient to whom the final choice is left. A full blood count should be taken before treatment to ensure no cellular abnormality is present.

Technique

A single field or parallel opposed pair is suitable for peripheral joints.

Dose and energy

2 Gy twice weekly to a total dose of 10 Gy (4–6 MV photons or cobalt-60)

Rheumatoid arthritis

Radiotherapy is rarely indicated. Occasionally instillation of yttrium-90 (185–277.5 MBq) is used to treat one or two large joints (e.g. the knee) if medical therapy including steroid injections has failed to control synovitis. It can be repeated once only. Because of the potential induction of second malignancy, patients under the age of 45 years should not be treated.

Villonodular synovitis

Yttrium-90 is also instilled into the knee joint to treat residual synovium in the posterior part of the knee joint, which is difficult to remove by synovectomy. The dose is the same as for rheumatoid arthritis.

DISORDERS OF THE EYE

Radiotherapy is rarely indicated in benign conditions of the eye. It is occasionally used in pterygium, corneal vascularisation and for thyroid eye disease. Care must be taken to avoid irradiating the lens and so avoid cataract formation. Similarly, the drainage of the aqueous must not be obstructed or glaucoma may occur.

Pterygium

Pterygium is a growth of fibrovascular tissue on the cornea. It is rare in the UK. It tends to grow slowly across the cornea and may impair visual acuity as it does so. Surgical excision is the treatment of choice for visual loss, local irritation and limitation of lateral gaze. Beta irradiation from a radioactive strontium-90 applicator is occasionally used immediately or a few days postoperatively to prevent the formation of episcleral vessels which may give rise to granulation tissue and recurrent pterygium. Beta irradiation is effective, although there are widely differing reported levels of benefit. Local recurrence rates with and without radiotherapy vary from 3–16% to 8–50% respectively.

Dose

7 Gy at the surface of the cornea once weekly for 3 treatments

Corneal vascularisation

The normal cornea is completely devoid of vessels. Ulcers or infection may lead to abnormal extension of tiny vessels from the surrounding conjunctiva to heal the lesion (Fig. 30.1). The new vessels are liable to persist, even if their purpose has been served, and with them any corneal scar is also liable to persist. If they can be obliterated, fading of the corneal opacity is encouraged. The aim of localised irradiation is to produce a reaction that seals the vessels. Small leashes of vessels are treated.

Dose

5 Gy weekly to a total of 4–5 treatments

KELOID SCARS

Keloid scars are sometimes irradiated following excision to reduce the incidence of recurrence. Therapy is usually given 7–10 days postoperatively once the

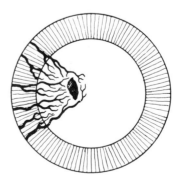

Fig. 30.1 Vascularisation in corneal ulcer.

wound is no longer at risk of dehiscence. Care should be taken not to irradiate keloid scars on the neck of children in case thyroid cancer is induced.

Target volume
The target volume is limited to the keloid scar without a margin of normal tissue.

Technique
Single direct field.

Dose and energy
10–12 Gy in 1–3 fractions (90–120 kV)

CEREBRAL ARTERIOVENOUS MALFORMATIONS AND ACOUSTIC NEUROMAS

Cerebral arteriovenous malformations (AVMs) are composed of a network of arterial and venous channels. The AVM itself does not contain normal brain tissue. AVMs account for 1–2% of all strokes. Fifty per cent present with intracranial haemorrhage. Other clinical features are headache, epilepsy, cranial nerve palsies, hydrocephalus and raised intracranial pressure. The risk of bleeding from an untreated AVM is 2–3% per year.

Acoustic tumours are benign tumours of the acoustic nerve. They are often bilateral. Progressive deafness and facial nerve palsy are common.

Cerebral arteriovenous malformations

Superficial AVMs can be removed surgically. Smaller AVMs, especially if deep seated, e.g. in the brainstem, are best treated by stereotactic focal irradiation. This can be delivered using a cobalt-60 gamma (Leksell) unit (Fig. 30.2), a linear accelerator or proton beam from a syncyclotron. This form of radiation treatment is known as 'radiosurgery', a term reflecting the original development of this technique by a neurosurgeon.

The only Leksell gamma unit in the UK is in Sheffield. The treatment head contains a hemispherical array of 201 cobalt sources. The beams from each source are collimated and focused to provide a small high dose volume. The fall-off in dose beyond the high dose volume is steep, allowing normal brain tissue surrounding an AVM largely to be spared. Different collimators are used (4, 8, 14 and 18 mm), sometimes in combination, depending upon the size and configuration of the AVM.

Treatment involves the fixing of a stereotactic frame to the head of the patient under local anaesthesia.

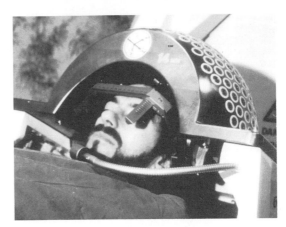

Fig. 30.2 Patient in treatment position in Leksell Unit. (Courtesy of Mr D Forster, Radiosurgery Unit, Sheffield.)

An angiogram (or occasionally a CT scan) is performed to identify the AVM. One or more collimators are selected to ensure the 50% isodose covers the fistulous component of the lesion (Fig. 30.3). With larger and irregularly shaped AVMs (>3 cm) some normal brain tissue is almost inevitably included in the treated volume. The dosimetry and coordinates of the centre of each treatment field are calculated by computer. The patient is treated prone or supine, depending on the optimal positioning of the collimator to cover the AVM. The coordinates in the vertical (z) and sagittal (y) planes are set on the stereotactic frame. The frame is secured within the treatment machine and the x axis set in the horizontal plane (x). Treatment is given in a single fraction. Treatment time is normally 15–30 minutes per field, depending on the activity of the

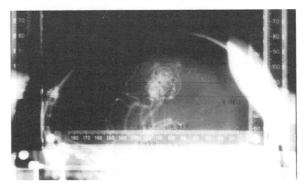

Fig. 30.3 Lateral view of planning angiogram showing temporoparietal arteriovenous malformation (AVM) and horizontal (y) and vertical (z) axes on the stereotactic frame. The AVM is encompassed by 50% isodose curves of 18 mm (anterior) and 8 mm (posterior) collimators. (Courtesy of Mr D Forster, Radiosurgery Unit, Sheffield.)

sources. A process of progressive thrombo-obliteration within the AVM is established.

Dose
20–25 Gy is given to the 50% isodose (peak dose 40–50 Gy) in a single fraction

Acoustic neuromas

The Leksell gamma unit can also be used to treat acoustic neuromas to avoid the need for surgery. A CT scan is performed with a stereotactic frame in place to identify the tumour.

Dose
16–18 Gy to tumour margin in a single fraction

Morbidity

Acute morbidity with gamma (Leksell) unit therapy is minimal. Major side-effects of treated AVMs (mainly focal neurological defects) occur in 3–4% of patients. Some of these deficits may be due to radionecrosis of normal brain included with the treatment volume. Eloquent areas of the brain seem particularly prone to radiation damage.

Trigeminal or facial nerve damage occurs in about 30% of patients irradiated for acoustic neuroma.

Experience with proton beam radiosurgery suggests higher morbidity (16%).

Results of treatment

About 50% of AVMs treated by the gamma unit are completely or almost completely obliterated 1 year after treatment and 84% by 2 years.

In selected acoustic neuromas (i.e. 3 cm or less) reduction in tumour size and preservation of hearing can be achieved in about 50% of patients.

Stereotactic multiple arc radiotherapy

Stereotactic multiple arc radiotherapy (SMART) can also be used to treat AVMs. A relocatable frame is secured on a base plate on the treatment couch to a dental impression of the patient's jaw. Early experience with SMART suggests that obliteration rates are comparable to gamma (Leksell) unit treatment.

Since the frame is relocatable, SMART can be fractionated. Fractionation is likely to improve the tolerance of normal brain to irradiation and tumour cell killing. Its applicability to small volume intracranial tumours is being evaluated.

31. Cancer chemotherapy

'Cancer chemotherapy' refers to the subject of cytotoxic (cell-poisoning) drugs. Hormone therapy is often considered under the same heading and is described in Chapter 32. The specialty of medical oncology has tended to be focused in teaching hospitals, often in departments involved in the clinical assessment of new chemotherapeutic agents. It has made important contributions to the treatment of the rarer malignancies such as Hodgkin's disease, the leukaemias, testicular teratoma and choriocarcinoma. Radiotherapists, medical oncologists and haematologists are trained in the use of chemotherapy. The responsibility for its supervision in any individual centre will depend on referral patterns and the experience and number of cancer specialists.

The major developments in medical oncology are relatively modern, dating from the 1940s. However in the 17th and 18th centuries, belladonna, antimony and arsenic were used to treat cancer. In the 19th century, in the 1860s, potassium arsenite was used without success to treat leukaemia.

The turning point came during the Second World War, from the investigation of poison gases. Even during the First World War, sulphur 'mustard' gas was noted to have a severe depressant effect on the bone marrow, and leucopenia was noted in those dying of mustard gas. In the 1940s the nitrogen mustards were found to cause gene mutations and chromosomal damage, leading to cell death at subsequent mitosis, in a manner similar to radiation. These agents were termed *radiomimetic* (i.e. imitating radiation). Profound effects on the bone marrow were observed. In 1942 a brief clinical remission was achieved in a patient treated with nitrogen mustard for lymphoma. The demonstration of some antitumour activity by nitrogen mustard prompted the development and testing of many thousands of agents. In 1948 an analogue of folate, aminopterin, was shown to cause remission in children with acute lymphocytic leukaemia. Despite the careful testing of many agents, only a very small proportion, about 30, have been sufficiently effective

to be adopted into clinical practice. Though small in total number, some agents (e.g. Adriamycin) have activity against a wide variety of malignancies.

Development and testing of anticancer agents

New cytotoxic agents are developed in four main ways. First, their efficacy may be detected from random screening for activity in cell lines of a group of chemical compounds. Secondly, they may be synthesised as modifications (analogues) of cytotoxic agents which are known to be effective. Thirdly, they may be created de novo to a specification which should confer particular anticancer properties. The second and third categories represent an increasing trend in the development of chemotherapeutic agents. Fourthly, there are chance discoveries of anticancer activity in drugs.

Once an agent has been shown, in its preclinical assessment, to have sufficient activity against animal tumours, with acceptable toxicity, it can be considered for clinical evaluation. In the UK approval of local ethics committees is required before clinical testing can begin. There are three phases of clinical assessment.

In *phase I* studies the main aim is to establish the maximum tolerated dose and the toxicity, but not the efficacy, of the agent under investigation. Such studies are performed with the informed consent of patients whose advanced disease has failed to respond to standard therapy.

If the agent shows acceptable toxicity in phase I studies, it may proceed to *phase II* studies designed to assess its antitumour activity. These are carried out on groups of patients with the same type of tumour. The selection of the tumour type will be guided by the response rates in different animal tumours and in phase I studies. The number of patients in each tumour category that need to be recruited in phase II studies will depend on the level of response of the best established agent. The new agent will need to show a higher response rate than established agents (or less toxicity for the same degree of response) to justify further testing.

In *phase III* studies the new agent is compared with an established treatment in a randomised trial. A group of patients with tumours against which the agent has shown activity in phase II studies is selected. The allocation of patients to the new or established treatment should be random. The response of the primary tumour, regional or metastatic spread is carefully documented.

PRINCIPLES OF CYTOTOXIC THERAPY

To understand the rationale of cytotoxic chemotherapy it is important to understand the features of tumour growth. These have been described in Chapter 15. Cytotoxic drugs act by interfering with the process of cell division (mitosis). Unfortunately these agents are not specific in acting against malignant cells and damage both normal and malignant proliferating cells. As with radiation a careful balance has to be kept between toxicity to the tumour and to the patient's normal tissues. What distinguishes normal and malignant cells is the failure of the malignant cell, unlike normal cells, to recover from cytotoxic damage.

Dose and frequency of administration

Initially single cytotoxic agents were given *continuously* in low dosage. Their administration was suspended when a response was obtained. When the tumour recurred, a second agent was administered in a similar manner. It was soon appreciated that this was relatively ineffective in controlling many tumours. In addition,

with continuous administration there was no opportunity for the normal tissues to recover. In many cases tumour regression and eradication were improved by administering the drug *intermittently* (e.g. 3–4-weekly) in much higher dose and allowing an interval for the normal and often dose limiting tissue to recover. Intermittent pulses or courses of treatment take advantage of the growth kinetics of malignant and normal tissues. In Figure 31.1 the effects of pulsed chemotherapy on a tumour and on the normal bone marrow can be seen. After each pulse, the normal and malignant cell populations decline due to killing of cells in mitosis. The lowest level of the blood count is known as the nadir. However, whereas the bone marrow recovers to its previous level, the malignant cell population does not. With each subsequent course this difference is accentuated. Larger doses per pulse than would be feasible with continuous treatment increase the fraction of tumour cells that can be killed per treatment.

The advantages of pulsed therapy may be summarised:

1. Maximum tumour cell killing occurs, while minimising toxicity.
2. Larger total dose maximises chance of cure.

It would be misleading to suggest that the 3–4-weekly schedules commonly used for the delivery of cytotoxic agents are necessarily optimal. However these frequencies have been derived from extensive assessments of different schedules. There is an increasing trend towards intensive weekly treatments.

If the interval between pulses is too short, toxicity may prevent the delivery of further pulses on schedule

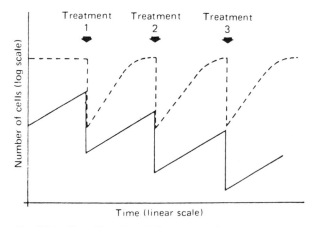

Fig. 31.1 The effect of multiple courses of cytotoxic therapy on normal and tumour cell populations. ---, normal cells; —, tumour cells. (Reproduced with permission from Priestman 1989.)

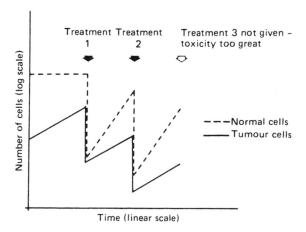

Fig. 31.2 The effect of multiple courses of chemotherapy with too short an interval for normal cell recovery. ---, normal cells; —, tumour cells. (Reproduced with permission from Priestman 1989.)

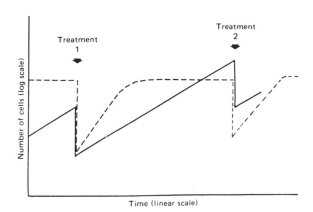

Fig. 31.3   The effect of multiple courses of chemotherapy with too long an interval, allowing increases in tumour cell population between courses. ---, normal cells; —, tumour cells. (Reproduced with permission from Priestman 1989.)

(Fig. 31.2). If the interval is too long, tumour may regrow between courses (Fig. 31.3).

The total dose that can be administered is limited by the tolerance of normal tissue. Toxicity is often cumulative and may be irreversible. For example the major dose limiting toxicity of the anthracyline, Adriamycin, is cardiotoxicity, which occurs if the total dosage exceeds 550 mg/m^2.

Higher than conventional doses of chemotherapy can be delivered if the primary organ toxicity is to the bone marrow and there is minimal toxicity to other organs. Bone marrow toxicity can be overcome by autologous bone marrow transplantation. Normal bone marrow is harvested from the patient before high dose chemotherapy. It is returned to the patient at the time of chemotherapy to support the bone marrow through the period of neutropenia and thrombocytopenia. High dose melphalan has been used, for example, to treat advanced cases of melanoma.

The route of administration is governed by the solubility, chemical stability and local irritant properties of the agent.

Oral. This is the simplest and most convenient route of administration. Examples are chlorambucil, cyclophosphamide and etoposide. Patients can take their tablets at home with intermittent outpatient visits to monitor treatment.

Unfortunately many cytotoxic drugs are unstable and inactivated in the stomach, rendering them ineffective.

Subcutaneous or *intramuscular* injection is avoided where possible since it can be painful, cause bruising in thrombocytopenic patients, requires hospital attendance and absorption may be unreliable. Bleomycin is often given by the intramuscular route.

Intravenous administration is the commonest route of administration of cytotoxic agents since it gives direct access to the systemic circulation. In addition continuous infusions can be given (e.g. 5-fluorouracil). Its risks are the introduction of infection and damage to the tissues around the site of administration if extravasation occurs. For this reason the antecubital fossa is best avoided. At this site extravasation is often difficult to detect. If it occurs, severe ulceration and contractures with major functional impairment may follow. Plastic surgery is often needed. Injections should be given into a vein on the back of the hand or on the radial side of the wrist.

Where very intensive chemotherapy is being given (e.g. acute leukaemia in children), peripheral venous sites may soon become thrombosed. The insertion of a catheter into the superior vena cava, usually under

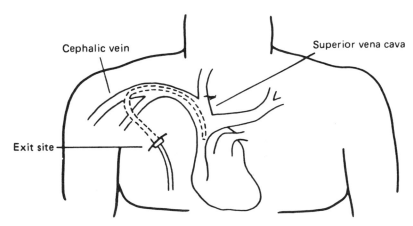

Fig. 31.4   Position of catheter for central venous infusion of cytotoxic drugs. (Reproduced with permission from Priestman 1989.)

general anaesthesia, and tunnelled subcutaneously allows comfortable and convenient access (Fig. 31.4).

Intrapleural chemotherapy is given to reduce the likelihood of recurrence of a pleural effusion. The effusion is tapped to dryness before the cytotoxic agent is instilled. It produces a chemical irritation of the pleura causing the two layers to become adherent to one another to prevent reaccumulation of the effusion. Bleomycin is most commonly used but is less effective than talc (Ch. 36).

Intraperitoneal chemotherapy has been given in diseases predominantly confined to the abdomen such as ovarian cancer. Higher concentrations within the peritoneal cavity can be achieved without causing severe systemic toxicity. It is only suitable for tiny microscopic foci of peritoneal disease. Its use is limited because of variability of drug absorption from the peritoneal surface and complications such as pain and bowel obstruction.

Intra-arterial administration is rarely used. It has the advantage of delivering the drug in high concentration to the tissues supplied by the artery. Its limitations are the complexity of administration and the difficulty in identifying correctly the arterial supply of the tumour. Its main use is in the infusion of chemotherapeutic agents into the hepatic artery of patients with liver metastases from colorectal cancer.

Intrathecal injection is used to deliver drugs in high dose into the CNS. Many cytotoxic drugs do not cross the blood–brain barrier and are therefore unable to kill tumour cells within the CNS. Methotrexate is the agent most commonly given by this route, e.g. in preventing CNS relapse in acute lymphoblastic leukaemia in conjunction with prophylactic cranial irradiation (Ch. 29).

Topical administration of cytotoxic agents is effective in a small number of tumours (e.g. nitrogen mustard in mycosis fungoides (Ch. 26) and 5-fluorouracil in Bowen's disease, a premalignant disease of the skin, and some superficial basal cell carcinomas).

Intravesical chemotherapy involves the instillation of cytotoxic therapy through a catheter into the bladder. In view of the limited depth of absorption, it is only appropriate for superficial tumours (Ch. 25). The drug (commonly thiotepa or mitomycin C) is left in the bladder for 1–2 hours before being drained. The main side-effect is a mild, short-lived chemical cystitis.

Factors influencing the efficacy of chemotherapy

A variety of host factors influence the response to chemotherapy, in addition to the intrinsic chemo-

sensitivity of the tumour and drug scheduling. These include the growth fraction of the tumour, the availability of the drug to the tumour and drug resistance.

Drug resistance

Resistance to chemotherapy may be intrinsic or acquired. Acquired resistance may have a variety of mechanisms. These include (1) changes in the cell membrane impeding drug transport (methotrexate), (2) repair of drug induced lesions (alkylating agents), (3) utilisation of alternative metabolic pathways (5-fluorouracil), (4) increased production of a target enzyme (e.g. dihydrofolate reductase binding to methotrexate), or (5) modification of the target enzyme, enabling it to recognise the difference between true and false metabolites. Irreversible binding between enzyme and cytotoxic drug (e.g. 6-mercaptopurine) is thus avoided.

Chemotherapy, as radiotherapy, is most effective in killing proliferating cells (p. 254). While the growth fraction is high in many chemosensitive tumours, such as the lymphomas and testicular teratomas, it is relatively low in many common tumours e.g. colorectal cancer.

In parts of the tumour the blood supply tends to be poor. As a result concentrations of drug reaching the tumour may be inadequate. In addition, as a result of the hypoxia induced by a poor blood supply, the growth fraction is reduced.

The reasons for drug resistance are not fully understood. It is common to find that a tumour responds to a particular drug or combination of drugs for a period of time and then ceases to do so. It is thought that within many tumour populations there are genetically determined drug resistant cells. When the chemosensitive cells have been killed, the resistant population may proliferate.

Adjuvant and neoadjuvant chemotherapy

Even when the primary tumour appears to be localised, clinically undetected metastases (micrometastases) may already have seeded to distant sites. The classical example is breast cancer where the lungs, liver and bone may be infiltrated by metastases. This is particularly so if the axillary nodes are involved at the time of primary surgery. Chemotherapy aimed at eradicating these micrometastases is called *adjuvant*. Other tumours in which the elimination of micrometastatic spread by adjuvant chemotherapy may be possible include osteogenic and Ewing's sarcoma of bone.

Adjuvant therapy is normally given shortly after surgical treatment of the primary. The rationale for early postoperative therapy is that (1) the growth fraction of metastases falls as they grow, (2) the probability of drug resistant cells emerging increases with time, and (3) areas of necrosis and hypoxic cells develop, due to impaired blood supply, and limit access to drugs.

Adjuvant combination cytotoxic chemotherapy (most commonly with cyclophosphamide, methotrexate and 5-fluorouracil (CMF)) confers a modest survival advantage in premenopausal women with breast cancer where the axillary nodes are involved. More impressive have been the improvements in survival in Wilms' tumour, Ewing's sarcoma and osteosarcoma in children.

Neoadjuvant therapy refers to delivering chemotherapy before surgery in order to reduce the tumour burden. By reducing the size of the primary tumour, the extent of surgery may be diminished. For example a large breast tumour that would require a mastectomy might, if reduced by chemotherapy, be amenable to local excision. An additional potential advantage is the killing of micrometastases at an earlier stage than conventional adjuvant therapy. However, if the tumour proves chemoresistant, toxicity will have been inflicted without any benefit. As yet neoadjuvant therapy is at an early phase of assessment and it is uncertain whether it will confer benefit in long-term survival.

CLASSIFICATION OF CYTOTOXIC DRUGS

The available agents may be divided into a few broad groups:

— Alkylating agents

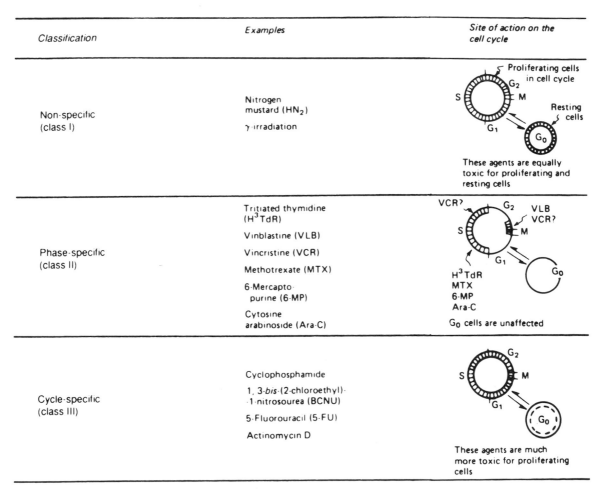

Fig. 31.5 Classification of anticancer agents according to action in cell cycle. (Modified from Calman, Smyth &Tattersall, Basic Principles of Cancer Chemotherapy, The Macmillan Press, 1980.)

— Antimetabolites
— Natural products
— Random synthetics
— Hormones (Ch. 32).

Some cytotoxic drugs act only on particular phases of the cell cycle (cell cycle specific), while others act throughout the cycle (cell cycle non-specific). These differences are summarised in Fig. 31.5.

The usual dosage, nadir white count and principal side-effects of commonly used cytotoxic agents are listed in Table 31.1.

Cytotoxic agents may interfere with precursors of nucleic acid synthesis, with DNA or RNA, or with specific proteins (Fig. 31.6).

Note. *Although guidelines on drug dosage have been included in the account of most commonly used agents, readers should consult the British National Formulary for guidance. Expert advice should be sought on all occasions, particularly for the more complex and toxic regimes.*

Alkylating agents

Mechanism of action

The main antitumour action of alkylating agents is the binding of an alkyl chemical group ($R\text{-}CH_2$) to DNA, so inhibiting its synthesis. They also bind to RNA and other cell proteins but these reactions are much less cytotoxic. The majority of alkylating agents have two available alkyl groups with which they can bind with DNA. Crosslinking may occur between a single strand of DNA or between two separate strands. Alkylating agents (e.g. nitrogen mustard) with this capacity to crosslink are called *bifunctional* and are more cytotoxic than alkylating agents with only one available alkyl group for binding to DNA.

Nitrogen mustard (mustine). Nitrogen mustard (mustine) was the first of the alkylating agents to be used. It was developed originally as a gas for chemical warfare. It was incidentally noted to be toxic to lymphoid tissue. It is chemically unstable and has to be given by rapid intravenous injection via a fast running drip.

Side-effects. Like mustard gas, it is a strong vesicant and is intensely irritant to the skin and other tissues. If it extravasates into the skin and subcutaneous tissues, it may cause painful thrombosis and phlebitis. In severe cases, this may lead to tissue necrosis requiring excision and skin grafting.

General effects are severe nausea and vomiting within the first 3 hours following injection but rarely lasting for more than 8 hours. Vomiting can usually be

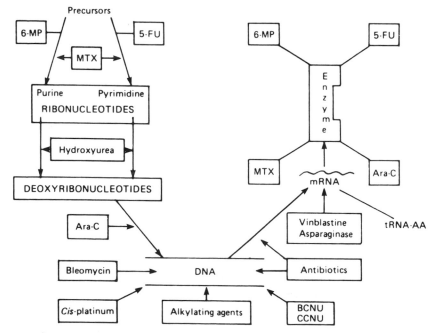

Fig. 31.6 Mechanism of action of anticancer drugs. (Reproduced with permission from Calman, Smyth & Tattersall, Basic Principles of Cancer Chemotherapy, The Macmillan Press, 1980.)

Table 31.1 Properties of cytotoxic agents

Agent	Dose	Nadir w.b.c—days	Toxicity type
Alkylating agents			
Nitrogen mustard	0.4 mg/kg i.v.	14–18	Bone marrow, nausea and vomiting, hair loss
Cyclophosphamide	300–600 mg/m² i.v.	5–10	Bone marrow, haemorrhagic cystitis, pneumonitis, cardiomyopathy, inappropriate ADH, alopecia, nausea and vomiting
Ifosfamide	1.5–2.5 g/m² i.v. for 3–5 days	5–6	Nausea and vomiting, encephalopathy, renal damage
Chlorambucil	10 mg daily p.o. alternate fortnights; 2–5 mg continually	10–21	Bone marrow
Melphalan	5 mg/m² for 5 days p.o.	28	Bone marrow, nausea and vomiting, mucositis, amenorrhoea
Busulphan	0.06 mg/kg per day p.o. (maximum 4 mg per day)	28	Bone marrow, lung fibrosis, skin pigmentation, adrenal failure, cataract
Thiotepa	0.5–10 mg daily	10–21	Bone marrow, nausea and vomiting, pain at injection sites
Antimetabolites			
Methotrexate	50 mg/m² i.v. 3–4-weekly; 12.5 mg intrathecal	10	Nausea and vomiting
			Bone marrow, alopecia, skin rashes, conjunctivitis, renal failure, liver damage, lung fibrosis, osteoporosis
6-Mercaptopurine	50–75 mg/m² p.o.	15	Bone marrow, liver damage
6-Thioguanine	2–2.5 mg/kg per day	7–14	Bone marrow, nausea and vomiting, liver damage
5-Fluorouracil	500–1000 mg/m² bolus or 24-hour infusion daily for 5 days 3-weekly	10	Bone marrow, nausea and vomiting, diarrhoea, oral mucositis, alopecia, skin rashes
Cytosine arabinoside	30–200 mg/m² i.v. or i.m. over 1–7 days	10	Bone marrow, nausea and vomiting, diarrhoea, oral ulceration, liver damage (reversible)
Natural products			
Vincristine	1–1.4 mg/m² i.v. (maximum 2 mg weekly in adults)	4–9	Neurotoxicity, inappropriate ADH
Vinblastine	6–8 mg/m² i.v. weekly or less frequently	10	Bone marrow, nausea, constipation, peripheral neuropathy, mucositis
Vindesine	3–4 mg/m² i.v. weekly	4–9	Bone marrow, neurotoxicity, alopecia
Antibiotics			
Adriamycin	40–70 mg/m² i.v. 3-weekly	10	Bone marrow, nausea and vomiting, alopecia, oral ulceration, cardiomyopathy
Mitomycin C	20–25 mg/m² i.v. 3–6-weekly	28	Bone marrow, nausea and vomiting, diarrhoea stomatitis, alopecia, renal damage, locally irritant
Bleomycin	1–15 mg/m² i.m.	—	Fever and chills, anaphylaxis, lung damage, skin pigmentation, alopecia
Mithramycin	0.3 mg daily i.v.	5–10	Thrombocytopenia, reduced clotting factors, nausea and vomiting, facial flushing, skin thickening. Note. These side-effects are not seen at doses used for malignant hypercalcaemia
Asparaginase	500–20 000 units/m² i.v.	—	Hypersensitivity reactions, pancreatitis, hypoglycaemia, liver damage, clotting defects
Cisplatin	20 mg/m² i.v. for 5 days or 100 mg/m² i.v. bolus 3–4-weekly	14	Nausea and vomiting, renal damage, deafness, peripheral neuropathy
Carboplatin	400 mg/m² i.v. 4-weekly	16	Bone marrow, nausea and vomiting
Procarbazine	50–200 mg/m² p.o. 4-weekly	25–36	Bone marrow, nausea and vomiting, CNS toxicity
Dacarbazine (DTIC)	100–200 mg/m² i.v. for 5 days	21	Bone marrow, nausea and vomiting, facial flushing, liver damage
Hydroxyurea	20–30 mg/kg continuously or 80 mg/kg every third day	7	Bone marrow depression, nausea and vomiting, diarrhoea, skin erythema

Table 31.1 (contd)

Agent	Dose	Nadir w.b.c—days	Toxicity type
CCNU	40–120 mg/m² p.o. 4–6-weekly	28	Bone marrow
Methyl CCNU	15–200 mg/m² p.o. 6–8-weekly	28	Nausea and vomiting
BCNU	40–120 mg/m² p.o. 4–8-weekly	28	Alopecia

reduced by prior antiemetic therapy. White blood count and platelets fall over 6–8 days with a nadir at 14–18 days. Hair loss and temporary amenorrhoea occur.

Main uses. Hodgkin's disease.

Cyclophosphamide (Endoxana). Cyclophospha-mide has the advantage that it is chemically stable and can be given orally in addition to intravenously. It is activated by the enzyme P450 in the liver. It is converted there to two active metabolites, acrolein and phosphoramide mustard. It is excretely solely in the urine. Dose adjustments are therefore necessary if kidney function is impaired.

Side-effects. Anorexia, nausea and vomiting are, unless high doses are used, much less severe than with mustine. Myelosuppression is the main dose limit-ing toxicity. The nadir is 5–10 days. Recovery occurs 10–14 days following administration. Platelets are less affected.

An acute haemorrhagic cystitis may occasionally occur at higher doses, or at lower doses if patients have renal impairment for any reason. Of these, dehydration is probably the commonest. The severity of cystitis varies from mild to severe. The cystitis is due to the irritant effects of urinary metabolites of the drug, particularly acrolein and 4-hydroxycyclophosphamide. Bladder fibrosis may follow.

Adequate hydration is essential before, during and after the administration of cyclophosphamide.

Rarely pneumonitis develops, similar to busulphan pulmonary toxicity. The onset is insidious. Typically this develops after prolonged therapy or continuous low dose treatment. Pathologically this is an alveolitis and may proceed to pulmonary fibrosis, respiratory failure and death. Steroids may help.

Cardiac damage may occur at high dose, ranging from asymptomatic minor abnormalities of the electro-cardiogram to severe cardiac failure.

Other side-effects are alopecia, inappropriate anti-diuretic hormone (ADH) secretion, oligo- or azoo-spermia and amenorrhoea. Both male and female infertility is usually permanent.

Mesna is used, reducing bladder toxicity at high dose (see under ifosfamide).

Drug interactions. Hepatic enzyme inducers (pheno-barbitone, phenytoin and chloral hydrate) increase the metabolism of cyclophosphamide and reduce its efficacy.

Cyclophosphamide potentiates the hypoglycaemic effects of sulphonylureas.

Main uses. Cyclophosphamide is useful against a wide range of malignancies including non-Hodgkin lymphomas, small cell lung cancer, ovarian cancer and soft tissue sarcomas.

Ifosfamide. Ifosfamide is structurally an analogue of cyclophosphamide. As with cyclophosphamide, it requires activation in the liver and is excreted in the urine. Unlike cyclophosphamide it cannot be given orally. It is always given intravenously with adequate hydration. Weight for weight, ifosfamide is less myelo-suppressive than cyclophosphamide.

Side-effects. Nausea and vomiting occur within a few hours of injection and last for about 3 days. It is dose related and can be very severe if high doses are used. Bone marrow suppression is moderate, affecting both white count and platelets. The nadir of the white count is at 5–10 days with recovery after 10–14 days. Alopecia is virtually universal. Central nervous toxicity may occasionally occur, particularly in patients who are inadequately hydrated, have impaired renal function or low serum albumin. The clinical features are of an encephalopathy with confusion, somnolence, lethargy and in severe cases coma and death. A sterile phlebitis may occur at the injection site. Necrosis may occur if there is extravasation.

Mesna in reducing bladder toxicity. In patients recei-ving ifosfamide therapy or, rarely, high dose (>1g/m²) cyclophosphamide, the risk of bladder toxicity can be minimised by giving oral or intravenous mesna. The sulphydryl group of this agent binds to metabolites (including acrolein) responsible for bladder toxicity. It converts them to compounds which do not damage the bladder.

Drug interactions. Hepatic enzyme inducing drugs have the same effects as on cyclophosphamide (see above).

Main uses. Soft tissue sarcomas, cervical cancer, testicular teratoma.

Chlorambucil. Chlorambucil has the advantages

of oral administration and little symptomatic toxicity. It is predominantly excreted in the urine. The dose may need to be reduced if there is renal impairment. It is normally given intermittently (e.g. 10 mg orally daily, alternate fortnights) or continually in a low dose (e.g. 2–5 mg orally per day).

Side-effects. The main dose limiting toxicity is to the bone marrow, causing leucopenia and thrombocytopenia. The nadir of the white count is normally at 14 days. Gastrointestinal toxicity, alopecia, pulmonary fibrosis and liver damage are uncommon. Hair is usually retained. Sterility, irreversible marrow damage and second malignancies occur.

Main uses. Hodgkin's disease, low-grade non-Hodgkin lymphoma, ovarian cancer.

Melphalan (L-phenylalanine mustard). Melphalan may be given orally or intravenously. Oral absorption may be erratic. Like chlorambucil it has few side-effects. It is the classical drug for high dose chemotherapy because of the absence of second organ toxicity (see under Principles of cytotoxic therapy).

Side-effects. The main dose limiting toxicity is bone marrow suppression, mainly affecting white count and platelets. The nadir is at 28 days. Nausea, vomiting and alopecia occur with higher doses.

Main uses. Multiple myeloma, ovarian cancer.

Side-effects. Nausea and vomiting, bone marrow depression, mucositis, amenorrhoea.

Thiotepa (triethylene thiophosphoramide). Thiotepa may be given by oral, intravenous or intracavitary routes. It has limited indications. It is mainly instilled into pleural effusions or ascites as a palliative procedure.

Side-effects. Bone marrow toxicity is dose limiting (leucopenia and thrombocytopenia). Nausea and vomiting and local pain at injections sites are the other most frequent side-effects.

Main uses. Intracavitary or high dose chemotherapy.

Busulphan. Busulphan is only given orally. It is selectively active against granulocytes. Its inactive metabolites are excreted in the urine.

Side-effects. Bone marrow depression. At low dose granulocytes are depressed with relative sparing of platelets. At higher dose platelets are also depressed. The nadir is at about 28 days and is prolonged. Recovery is slow, from 24 to 54 days.

Lung fibrosis may develop after prolonged treatment. Regular chest radiographs should be taken and pulmonary function regularly monitored. The drug should be stopped at the first signs of lung fibrosis and steroids commenced. Otherwise irreversible respiratory failure and death may occur.

Skin pigmentation occurs over pressure areas, axillae, skin creases and nipples, in a similar distribution to Addison's disease. Adrenal failure and cataract formation are rare.

Main uses. Chronic myeloid leukaemia, polycythaemia rubra vera.

Antimetabolites

Mechanism of action

Antimetabolites are structurally similar to normal metabolites involved in nucleic acid synthesis. They are divided into three groups: folate, purine and pyrimidine antagonists. They substitute for their normal purine and pyrimidine counterparts in metabolic pathways, resulting in abnormal nuclear material that fails to function normally, or bind to enzymes, so inhibiting protein synthesis.

1. Folate antagonists

Methotrexate is the classical example. A number of cofactors are necessary for the synthesis of purines and pyrimidines. The reduction of folic acid is essential for the production of these cofactors. A key reaction in this process is the reduction of dihydrofolic acid to tetrahydrofolic acid by means of an enzyme, *dihydrofolate reductase*. This is the main site of action of methotrexate. Methotrexate is structurally similar to folic acid and has a much greater affinity for dihydrofolate reductase than folic acid. Methotrexate therefore binds preferentially to dihydrofolate reductase and inactivates it. As a result tetrahydrofolates cannot be made and purine and pyrimidine synthesis is inhibited.

Methotrexate can be given orally, intravenously or at low dose intrathecally. About 50–60% of the drug in the serum is bound to protein. In conventional doses, it is excreted unchanged in the urine. It is widely distributed in body fluids. This is of importance because it may be retained in pleural effusions and ascites causing abnormally prolonged systemic toxicity. Such fluid collections should, if possible, be drained before methotrexate is administered.

High dose therapy. Methotrexate is one of the drugs for which there is evidence of increased effectiveness with higher doses in some sensitive tumours (e.g. small cell lung cancer and osteosarcoma).

Folinic acid 'rescue'. The metabolic block on the activity of dihydrofolate reductase can be bypassed by administering an intermediate metabolite, folinic acid (also known as citrovorum factor or leucovorin). Folinic acid is a tetrahydrofolate which provides an alternative source for continuing nucleic acid synthesis. It is also possible that folinic acid may act by displacing methotrexate from its binding to dihydrofolate reductase. In both these ways the cytotoxic action of methotrexate and its toxicity can be diminished. Folinic acid is only required when high doses (>100 mg) of methotrexate are used. It is delivered by the oral or intramuscular route 24–36 hours after the administration of methotrexate until the serum concentration of methotrexate is <10^{-7} mol/l. This is timed to allow the methotrexate to have its necessary cytotoxic action but to prevent further toxicity associated with persistently high blood levels of methotrexate. Starting folinic acid 40 hours or more after methotrexate has been given is ineffective. When high dose methotrexate is given, urine alkalinisation to pH 6.5–7.0, with oral or intravenous sodium bicarbonate or oral acetazolamide, and fluid hydration should be started beforehand.

Side-effects. The main side-effects of methotrexate are on the bone marrow and on the gastrointestinal tract. Anaemia, leucopenia and thrombocytopenia may develop rapidly. The nadir of the white count is at 10 days. Anorexia, nausea and vomiting are the first symptoms, followed 4–6 days later by oral and pharyngeal mucositis and diarrhoea. Skin rashes are common. Conjunctivitis may occur as a result of accumulation of the drug in tears. Renal failure may complicate high dose therapy. Liver damage (ranging from elevated liver enzymes to cirrhosis), lung injury (mainly fibrosis) and osteoporosis may complicate prolonged therapy. Alopecia is uncommon.

Drug interactions. (1) Drugs which are protein bound (e.g. salicylates, phenytoin, sulphonamides) may displace methotrexate from its binding with plasma protein, causing the serum levels of methotrexate and the risk of toxicity to rise. (2) Methotrexate potentiates the effects of anticoagulants such as warfarin.

Main uses. Non-Hodgkin lymphoma, acute lymphoblastic leukaemia, breast cancer, soft tissue and osteogenic sarcomas, head and neck cancer, choriocarcinoma.

2. Purine antagonists

6-Mercaptopurine. 6-Mercaptopurine is a purine antagonist. It has to be metabolised to an active form. It inhibits a number of enzymes involved in the synthesis of the purines, adenine and guanine. It is strongly bound to plasma proteins, metabolised in the liver and its metabolites are excreted in the urine.

It is normally given orally.

Side-effects. The main toxicity is on the bone marrow (leucopenia and thrombocytopenia) and the liver. The nadir for white count and platelets is at 15 days.

Raised serum bilirubin is the commonest feature of liver toxicity. This normally returns to normal on withdrawing the drug.

Interactions. Allopurinol inhibits the metabolism of mercaptopurine. If given concurrently the dose of mercaptopurine has to be reduced.

Main uses. Leukaemia, especially acute lymphoblastic.

6-Thioguanine. 6-Thioguanine is also a purine antagonist and is an analogue of guanine. It requires activation to an active form and may be given orally or intravenously.

Side-effects. The main dose limiting toxicity is to the bone marrow and is more marked when given intravenously than orally. Gastrointestinal intolerance is uncommon. Liver toxicity is less frequent than with mercaptopurine.

Drug interactions. If allopurinol is given with thioguanine the dose of thioguanine does not have to be reduced because its metabolism is not inhibited as it is with mercaptopurine.

Main uses. Acute and chronic myeloid leukaemia.

3. Pyrimidine antagonists

5-Fluorouracil. 5-Fluorouracil is a fluoropyrimidine (a combination of a uracil and fluorine) which inhibits DNA synthesis by inhibiting the main enzyme in pyrimidine synthesis and thus the formation of cytosine and thymine. In addition it is incorporated into RNA instead of uracil and inhibits RNA synthesis.

Absorption by the oral route is unpredictable and the drug is normally given intravenously. It can also be applied topically. Most of the drug is rapidly metabolised in the liver and excreted in the urine. Its action is potentiated if given in conjunction with folinic acid.

Side-effects. The main toxicity is to the gastrointestinal tract (diarrhoea, nausea and vomiting). Stomatitis occurring 5–8 days after treatment is usually an early sign of severe toxicity. Myelosuppression also occurs, with a nadir at 10 days. Less common side-effects are alopecia, skin rashes, and rarely an acute cerebellar syndrome.

Cytosine arabinoside. Cytosine arabinoside is an analogue of deoxycytidine. It is a competitive inhibitor of the enzyme DNA polymerase. Its principal action is as a false nucleotide competing for the enzymes which are responsible for converting cytidine to deoxycytidine and for incorporating deoxycytidine in to DNA. It is a cell cycle specific drug, only acting on proliferating cells.

It can be given by intravenous or subcutaneous routes. Most of the drug is excreted in the urine.

Side-effects. Bone marrow suppression, nausea, vomiting and diarrhoea, and oral ulceration are common. Reversible hepatotoxicity also occurs.

Main uses. Acute leukaemia (especially myeloid).

Natural products

These include mitotic inhibitors, antibiotics and enzymes.

1. Mitotic inhibitors

There are three valuable alkaloids from the periwinkle plant (*Vinca rosea*): vincristine, vinblastine and vindesine.

Mechanism of action

The vinca alkaloids inhibit the formation of the small tubules (microtubules) which make up the spindle on which the chromatids line up in metaphase. Cell division is therefore prevented.

Vincristine. Vincristine is given intravenously. It is excreted mainly via the bile and the faeces. Its toxicity may be enhanced in obstructive liver disease.

Side-effects. It is vesicant locally. Neurotoxicity is the main dose limiting toxicity. This is in the form of a sensorimotor peripheral neuropathy (paraesthesiae in fingers, muscle cramps, paralytic ileus, constipation). Vincristine should be stopped if there is any evidence of motor neuropathy. Less common is inappropriate antidiuretic hormone (ADH) production. Alopecia is rare.

Main uses. Lymphoma, leukaemia, breast cancer, sarcoma.

Vinblastine. Vinblastine is given intravenously. It is partly excreted in the bile and urine. The dose should be reduced in obstructive liver disease.

Side-effects. It is a sclerosant, causing a cellulitis if extravasation occurs. Bone marrow depression is the main dose limiting toxicity. The nadir for myelosuppression is 10 days. Neurotoxicity is less severe than with vincristine. Abdominal cramps, pain and constipation are common.

Main uses. Lymphoma, head and neck cancer, testicular teratoma.

Vindesine. The pharmacokinetics of vindesine are similar to the other vinca alkaloids.

Side-effects. Bone marrow suppression is the main dose limiting toxicity (leucopenia with sparing of platelets). Neurotoxicity is milder than with vincristine. Alopecia occurs.

Dose. 3 mg/m^2 i.v. weekly.

Main use. Malignant melanoma, lung cancer.

Epipodophyllotoxins. Epipodophyllotoxins are analogues of podophyllotoxin, an extract of the Mayapple. Podophyllotoxin is a spindle poison, binding to the microtubular proteins. It arrests cell division in the premitotic phase of the cell cycle (late G$_2$ and S). Etoposide (VP16) is the most widely used of this group.

It is a good example of a schedule dependent drug. It is more effective given over 5 days than on 1 day. It can be given orally or intravenously. It is mainly excreted in the urine.

Side-effects. The dose limiting toxicity is bone marrow suppression. The nadir is at about 16 days with recovery at 20–22 days. Nausea, vomiting and anorexia are relatively minor but more marked if etoposide is given orally. Alopecia is common. Mucositis and a mild peripheral neuropathy occur occasionally.

Note. Care should be taken not to give etoposide intravenously over less than 30 minutes, to avoid hypotension.

Main uses. Hodgkin's disease, non-Hodgkin lymphoma, leukaemias, small cell lung cancer, testicular teratoma, Ewing's sarcoma.

2. Antibiotics

Anthracyclines. Daunorubicin, doxorubicin (Adriamycin) and epirubicin are the principal anthracycline antibiotics. They are produced from different strains of fungi (streptomyces). The mechanisms of their cytotoxic action are not fully understood. They include insertion between opposing strands of DNA (intercalation), altering membrane permeability, alkylation, free radical formation and forming cytotoxic complexes with metals such as iron, copper and zinc. Their main effects are exerted during S phase of DNA synthesis.

Adriamycin is given intravenously. Its excretion is mainly via the liver. Reduction in dosage is essential in patients with liver dysfunction.

Side-effects. The toxicity is to the bone marrow, gastrointestinal tract and to the heart. The nadir of the white count is at 10 days. Epirubicin causes slightly less vomiting than the other two anthracyclines.

Daunorubicin and Adriamycin and, to a much lesser extent, epirubicin cause cumulative cardiotoxicity. The maximum recommended total dose of Adriamycin is 450–550 mg/m^2 and for daunorubicin 20 mg/kg. If cyclophosphamide, which is also cardiotoxic, is given at the same time as Adriamycin and daunorubicin, the total anthracycline dose is reduced to 450 mg/m^2. Acute cardiac toxicity is manifest by arrhythmias and abnormalities of electrical conduction. The chronic effect is a cardiomyopathy (pericarditis and congestive cardiac failure). Anthracyclines should be avoided if there is previous history of cardiac failure or ischaemic heart disease.

Interactions. Cyclophosphamide (see above).

Main uses. Lymphoma, breast cancer, sarcomas, lung cancer, Wilms' tumour, neuroblastoma. Acute myelogenous leukaemia (daunorubicin).

Non-anthracycline antibiotics

Actinomycin D. Actinomycin is only given intravenously. Its metabolism is minimal and its excretion slow in faeces and urine.

Side-effects. The dose limiting toxicity is myelosuppression. Oral ulceration, nausea, vomiting, diarrhoea, alopecia and skin rashes are common. It is very irritant if extravasation occurs.

Main uses. Wilms' tumour, rhabdomyosarcoma, osteogenic sarcoma, teratoma, Hodgkin's disease.

Mitomycin C. Mitomycin C is activated to an alkylating agent and forms cross-linkages with DNA. In addition it gives rise to free radicals. Both DNA and RNA are inhibited. It is mainly eliminated by metabolism in the liver. It is given intravenously or instilled into the bladder via a catheter.

Side-effects. The dose limiting toxicity is myelosuppression. The nadir is delayed, with nadir of white count and platelets at 3–8 weeks after administration. Anorexia, nausea and mild vomiting develop within 1–2 hours. Renal toxicity occurs, particularly if total dosage exceeds 100 mg. This is normally reversible if the drug is withdrawn. Interstitial pneumonitis is uncommon. Mitomycin C is highly irritant if it extravasates.

Main uses. Gastrointestinal, bladder and breast cancer.

Bleomycin. Bleomycin intercalates with DNA strands causing single and double strand breaks. It inhibits DNA synthesis, and, to a lesser degree, RNA synthesis. It is a cell cycle-specific agent (Fig. 31.5) with its main effects on G_2 and M phases. It is rapidly inactivated in the liver and kidney. Excretion is mainly in the urine. It is given intramuscularly, subcutaneously, intravenously, intrapleurally (for pleural effusions) and, rarely, intraperitoneally (for ascites).

Side-effects. The main toxicity is to the lung and is most likely to occur if the total dose exceeds 300 mg. Progressive fibrosis occurs. Presentation is with a nonproductive cough and dyspnoea. A chest radiograph initially shows pulmonary infiltrates which may proceed to fibrosis. Pulmonary function tests show a restrictive defect and reduced gas (carbon monoxide) transfer. Respiratory complications of general anaesthesia are increased.

Occasionally there may be an immediate life-threatening anaphylactic reaction. Fever and chills are common. Hypotension, renal failure and death may result from associated sweating and dehydration. These signs may not develop until several hours after administration.

Skin changes are common: pigmentation, erythema, and thickening of the nail bed. Alopecia is uncommon.

Myelosuppression is minimal.

Main uses. Head and neck and cervical cancer, teratoma, lymphoma, malignant pleural effusions.

Mithramycin. The mechanism of action is not fully understood. It is thought that its main cytotoxic action is due to binding to the exterior of the DNA molecule. It probably also intercalates directly into DNA. It is given as an intravenous infusion. In malignant hypercalcaemia it has a specific inhibitory action on osteoclast function. Because of its marked toxicity and the increasing use of bisphosphonates, its application is very limited.

Side-effects. It is a local irritant if extravasation occurs. Its main toxicity is due to thrombocytopenia and reduction of clotting factors resulting in bleeding. Bleeding may rapidly follow administration, even before the blood count drops. Anorexia, nausea, vomiting and diarrhoea are common. Facial blushing and subsequent thickening of skin folds occur in 30% of patients. Lung and renal damage may occasionally occur. Hypocalcaemia followed by transient rebound hypercalcaemia is rare.

Main uses. Malignant hypercalcaemia.

3. Enzymes

Asparaginase. Asparagine is an essential amino acid for protein and nucleic acid synthesis. Asparaginase is an enzyme produced from bacteria which degrades asparagine. Tumour cells, unlike their normal counterparts, have no or little asparagine synthetase, the enzyme necessary for making asparagine. When asparagine levels fall, both protein and nucleic acid synthesis are inhibited. Asparaginase remains largely confined to the vascular compartment, probably due to its large size. Urinary or biliary excretion is minimal.

A test dose is advised because of the risk of anaphylaxis. If the patient is found to be hypersensitive, an alternative preparation is available.

Side-effects. Nausea and vomiting are generally mild. Hypersensitivity reactions are common but life-threatening anaphylaxis is rare. Pancreatitis, hypoglycaemia, encephalopathy, abnormal liver function and clotting defects also occur.

Use. Acute lymphoblastic leukaemia.

Random synthetics

Cisplatin and carboplatin. Cisplatin and carboplatin inhibit DNA synthesis. Both act in a similar way to alkylating agents by forming cross-linkages between a pair of their chlorine atoms and the guanine molecules of opposing DNA strands (interstrand linkages), but differ in that they also bind to bases on the same

DNA strand (intrastrand linkages). Both drugs are predominantly excreted in the urine.

Side-effects. Cisplatin causes severe nausea and vomiting. This can be substantially reduced by giving high doses of intravenous metoclopramide. Cisplatin causes renal impairment. Pre- and post-treatment hydration is always used (with or without mannitol). Hypomagnesaemia is common and tetany sometimes occurs. Magnesium supplements arc oftcn rcquircd.

Hearing is also reduced due to damage to the auditory (8th cranial nerve), with characteristic high tone loss. Peripheral neuropathy also occurs.

Carboplatin has the advantage of much less emesis, ototoxicity, nephrotoxicity and neurotoxicity. The dose limiting toxicity is to the bone marrow, particularly to platelets. At present it is very expensive.

Main uses. Testicular teratoma and seminoma; ovarian and head and neck cancer.

Procarbazine. Procarbazine is a derivative of the hydrazine chemical group. Its precise mechanism of action is not known. Alkylation and free radical formation have been postulated. It seems to be cell cycle phase-specific, with its main cytotoxic effect on S phase (DNA synthesis). It is given orally and crosses the blood–brain barrier. The main route of excretion of its metabolites is in the urine.

Side-effects. Bone marrow suppression is the main dose limiting toxicity. The nadir of the platelet count is at 4 weeks followed by that of the white and red cell counts. The blood count has normally resolved by 6 weeks. Nausea, vomiting and diarrhoea start within a few days of administration. CNS toxicity has a wide variety of symptoms including dizziness, ataxia, headache, nightmares, hallucinations, somnolence and depression.

Interactions. (1) Tricyclic antidepressants and monoamine oxidase inhibitors, tyramine rich foods (e.g. cheese, wine and bananas) may precipitate hypertensive crisis. (2) CNS depressants (narcotic analgesics, phenothiazines and antihistamines, hypotensive agents (e.g. methyldopa) accentuate CNS depression. (3) Alcohol may increase gastrointestinal toxicity.

Main uses. Hodgkin's disease, brain tumours.

Dacarbazine (DTIC). The mechanism of action of dacarbazine is uncertain. It is metabolised to products which have alkylating properties and these probably account for its cytotoxic properties. It is given intravenously.

Side-effects. Myelosuppression is the principal dose limiting toxicity. The nadir is at 21 days. Acute nausea and vomiting occur commonly in the first 12 hours following administration. A flu-like illness may occasionally develop 7 days after administration and last 1–3 weeks. Facial flushing, paraesthesiae and liver toxicity also occur.

Interactions. Phenytoin and phenobarbitone may induce the metabolism of DTIC, reducing its efficacy.

Main uses. Malignant melanoma, sarcoma, lymphoma.

Hydroxyurea. Hydroxyurea is an analogue of urea. It inhibits the ribonucleotide reductase enzyme system that converts ribonucleotides to deoxyribonucleotides, inhibiting DNA synthesis (Fig. 31.6). It is given orally. It is mainly metabolised in the liver and excreted in the urine.

Side-effects. The main side-effect is bone marrow depression. Nausea, vomiting, diarrhoea or constipation, skin atrophy and dryness and erythema are common.

Interactions. Hydroxyurea potentiates the effects of irradiation. Radiation recall reactions may also occur (erythema and irritation in previously irradiated areas).

Main uses. Chronic granulocytic leukaemia.

Nitrosoureas (CCNU, BCNU, methyl-CCNU and streptozotocin). The nitrosoureas are a group of analogues whose main mechanism of action is thought to be alkylation. BCNU is the only member of the family with two alkylating groups and can crosslink DNA. In addition, the nitrosoureas inhibit a number of important enzymes in the synthesis and repair of DNA. They can be given orally or intravenously. Their high lipid solubility allows them to cross the blood–brain barrier into the CNS. They are extensively metabolised in the liver. Urinary excretion is slow.

Side-effects. (1) CCNU, BCNU, methyl-CCNU: nausea and vomiting frequently occur 4–6 hours after administration. Myelosuppression is dose limiting and delayed. The nadir of the white count is at 28 days. Alopecia and transient abnormalities of liver function are common. Kidney and lung damage are rare. (2) Streptozotocin: renal and gastrointestinal toxicity are dose limiting. Bone suppression is less marked compared with the other nitrosoureas.

Interactions. Hyperglycaemic action of streptozotocin increased by steroids.

Main uses. Brain tumours, lymphoma, carcinoid (streptozotocin).

SIDE-EFFECTS OF CYTOTOXIC CHEMOTHERAPY

The main normal tissues damaged by cytotoxic therapy are those with rapidly dividing cell populations: the bone marrow, the gastrointestinal epithelium, the hair and the germ cells of the testis. By contrast there is little effect on non-proliferating tissues such as skeletal muscle and nervous tissue. The short and medium term side-effects of commonly used cytotoxic drugs are shown in Table 31.2.

Bone marrow

The bone marrow contains stem cells from which develop red cells, white cells and platelets. Cytotoxic therapy exerts its inhibitory effects on cell division on the stem cell population. It has little effect on mature red cells, white cells or platelets.

The time of onset of anaemia, leucopenia and thrombocytopenia reflects the life spans of different mature cells. Leucopenia tends to occur first since the survival of white cells is about 5 days. Thrombocytopenia occurs next. Platelets survive 9–10 days. Anaemia occurs last since the red cell life span is considerably longer at 120 days.

The main risk of leucopenia is the increased susceptibility to infection. Septicaemia may be life threatening. Any infection should be promptly treated. Growth factors are now available for red cells and white cells to reduce toxicity (p. 571).

Table 31.2 Summary of short and medium term toxiciy of cytotoxic drugs

	Myelosuppression	Gastrointestinal toxicity	Neurotoxicity	Alopecia	Pneumonitis and/or lung fibrosis	Cardiotoxicity	Renal damage	Hepatotoxicity	Skin changes	Endocrine abnormalities	Haemorrhagic cystitis	Acute allergic reactions
Nitrogen mustard	3	2	1	1					1			
Cyclophosphamide	2	2		2	1	1		1	1	1	2	
Ifosfamide	2	2	2	2	1			1			3	
Melphalan	3	2		1	1				1			
Chlorambucil	2	1		1	1			1				
Thiotepa	2	1										
Hexamethylmelamine	2	2	2									
Busulphan	2				2				1	1		
Nitrosoureas	3	2		1	1			1	1			
Methotrexate	2	2	2	1	1		1	1	1			
5-Fluorouracil	2	2	1	1	1				1			
Cytosine arabinoside	2	2	1				1	1				1
6-Mercaptopurine	2	1						2				1
6-Thioguanine	2	1						1				
Vincristine	1	2	3	1					1			
Vinblastine	2	1	1	1					1			
Vindesine	2	1	2	1					1			
Doxorubicin	3	2		3		3			1			
Daunorubicin	3	2		2		3						
Epirubicin	2	1		2		2						
Actinomycin-D	2	2							1			
Mitomycin-C	2	2			1		1					
Bleomycin		1		2	3				1			1
Cisplatinum	2	3	2				3					1
Carboplatin	3	2	1				2	1				1
Mitozantrone	2	1		1		1		1				
Dacarbazine	1	2	1	1				1	1			1
Procarbazine	2	2	1					1				
Etoposide	3	2		2								1
Asparaginase	2	2	2	1	1		2	2		2		1
Amsacrine	3	2	1	1		1		1				
Hydroxyurea	2	1							1			

1. Occasional or minor side effect.
2. Common or moderately severe side effect.
3. Invariable or dose limiting side effect.
(Reproduced with permission from Priestman 1989.)

Gastrointestinal tract

The nausea and vomiting caused by many cytotoxic agents are multifactorial in origin. They are mainly due to stimulation of receptors in the gut (principally the small bowel). Other stimuli come from the cerebral cortex, the vestibular apparatus of the inner ear and an area of the brainstem (chemoreceptor trigger zone).

Drugs causing severe vomiting are:

— Cisplatin
— Nitrogen mustard
— Doxorubicin
— Actinomycin-D
— Dacarbazine.

Treatment. Nausea and vomiting can be reduced or abolished by a variety of agents (Table 31.3). Among the most effective are the anti-5-hydroxytryptamine (anti-5HT$_3$) antagonists such as ondansetron.

Oral mucositis is commonly caused by methotrexate, 5-fluorouracil and Adriamycin.

Treatment. The probability of mucositis from methotrexate can be reduced by folinic acid rescue (see under Methotrexate).

Diarrhoea may be caused by 5-fluorouracil and mitomycin C.

Hair

Hair loss (alopecia) is due to damage to hair follicles and is a reversible side-effect. Thinning of the hair is usually confined to the scalp. It usually begins about a month after the first dose of chemotherapy. The probability of alopecia varies from agent to agent and sometimes with dose (e.g. cyclophosphamide). Regrowth starts about 2 months after the end of treatment. New hair may differ in colour and texture.

Scalp cooling may limit the amount of hair loss with anthracylines at conventional dosage. At high dosage, its value is uncertain.

Complete loss of scalp hair is likely with:

— Adriamycin
— Etoposide
— Epirubicin
— Ifosfamide.

It is unlikely with:

— Cisplatin
— Chlorambucil
— Mitomycin C.

Alopecia occasionally occurs with:

— Methotrexate
— Mitozantrone.

Germ cells of the testis

The germinal epithelium becomes depleted following chemotherapy with many agents. It is most common in prepubertal boys. The sperm count falls. Sperm cells may disappear completely (azoospermia). Damage to the germinal epithelium is often cumulative. Combination chemotherapy is more likely to result in azoospermia with lower doses of drugs than is single agent therapy. Recovery of sperm production is difficult to predict. The higher the dose the lower and slower is the probability of recovery.

Table 31.3 Agents used in the treatment of nausea and vomiting

Agent	Dose
Corticosteroids (dexamethasone)	12–16 mg i.v.
Dopamine agonists	10–20 mg orally/i.v. (low dose)
Metoclopramide	10 mg/kg i.v. per 24 hours (high dose for Cisplatin)
Domperidone	10–20 mg 4–8-hourly oral/p.r.
Phenothiazines	5–10 mg oral/i.v./i.m./p.r. 8-hourly
Chlorpromazine	25 mg oral/i.v./i.m. 8-hourly
Cannabinoids	
Nabilone	1–2 mg oral 12-hourly
Butyrophenones	
Haloperidol	1–2 mg oral/i.v. 3–6-hourly
Benzodiazepines	
Lorazepam	2–4 mg oral 4-hourly
5HT$_3$ antagonists	
e.g. Ondansetron	8 mg i.v./oral, then 8 mg oral 12-hourly

In contrast to the ovary (see below) male endocrine function (i.e. testosterone production) is rarely affected.

Hodgkin's disease. Most men treated with MOPP or similar regimes (e.g. MVPP) for Hodgkin's disease are sterilised permanently. The ABVD regime (Ch. 26) has a much lower incidence of azoospermia (30%).

Testicular cancer. In patients undergoing combination chemotherapy with cisplatin, vinblastine and bleomycin, the probability of active spermatogenesis is about 80% 18 months after treatment. Spermatogenesis does not resume during the first 12 months of treatment.

Germ cell depletion is likely with:

— Chlorambucil (especially >400 mg)
— Cyclophosphamide (especially >6 g)
— Nitrogen mustard
— Procarbazine
— Busulphan.

It is unlikely with:

— Methotrexate
— Vincristine
— 6-Mercaptopurine
— 5-Fluorouracil
— Etoposide.

Prevention. Infertility may be overcome in some patients by sperm storage and cryopreservation before starting chemotherapy. Referral to an infertility clinic for counselling and sperm collection is necessary. Usually 2–3 specimens of semen are required over a 1–2 week period. Only if there are adequate numbers of motile sperm is banking worthwhile. Unfortunately many patients with germ cell tumours of the testis or Hodgkin's disease are infertile as a complication of their disease.

Female fertility

Female infertility is less likely than male infertility to be induced by chemotherapy. This is mainly because the number of ova is fixed before birth, in contrast to sperm which are continuously produced throughout adulthood. Chemotherapy may none the less be toxic to the ovaries, causing ovarian fibrosis, amenorrhoea, hot flushes and infertility. The probability of this occurring increases with age.

Single agent therapy

Ovarian function is more likely to be conserved in women under the age of 35–40, for a moderate dose of chemotherapy, than above this range. Periods are more likely to return within 6 months of chemotherapy under the age of 40 (e.g. in 50% of women after cyclophosphamide) than over 40.

Drugs most likely to cause infertility are:

— Cyclophosphamide
— Busulphan
— Melphalan
— Chlorambucil.

Drugs unlikely to cause ovarian failure are:

— Methotrexate
— 5-Fluorouracil
— 6-Mercaptopurine
— Etoposide.

Combination chemotherapy

Hodgkin's disease. Most information has been collected on patients undergoing MOPP (Ch. 26) for Hodgkin's disease. Ovarian failure occurs in 40–50% of women receiving this regime. Most women over the age of 30 will be sterilised. However under the age of 20 most will retain fertility. For example, 50% of women receiving alkylating agents (e.g. chlorambucil, cyclophosphamide) as part of combination chemotherapy are likely to be sterilised. Combination chemotherapy is more likely to induce sterility than single agent therapy.

Breast cancer. Women undergoing CMF chemotherapy for breast cancer are commonly sterilised.

Choriocarcinoma. Most women (over 85%) will retain their fertility after chemotherapy. This is because methotrexate, the main agent used, rarely causes ovarian failure.

Cardiac damage

Cardiac damage is uncommon, with the exception of Adriamycin and daunorubicin. The pathogenesis is ill defined. It may be due to the toxic effects of free radical formation, damage to cardiac membranes or intercalation of DNA base pairs. Previous cardiac disease and irradiation predispose to cardiotoxicity.

Lung damage

Pulmonary toxicity is uncommon but is associated with:

— Bleomycin
— Cyclophosphamide
— Busulphan
— Methotrexate.

The toxicity is usually cumulative and irreversible. Presentation is normally with non-productive cough and progressive dyspnoea. Chest radiography may show lung infiltrates progressing to fibrosis.

Neurological damage

The vinca alkaloids (particularly vincristine) are the commonest causes of neurotoxicity. This is in the form of a peripheral neuropathy (see under Vincristine).

Methotrexate may cause central nervous toxicity (dementia) if given by the intrathecal route, particularly if cranial irradiation is given concurrently (e.g. in the treatment of acute lymphoblastic leukaemia). 5-Fluorouracil may cause ataxia and ifosfamide encephalopathy.

Damage to the fetus

This is a very serious concern. Little information, however, is available about the effects of chemotherapy on pregnant women since chemotherapy is avoided if at all possible in these circumstances. In the few cases that have been reported, the evidence for a causal relationship is not firm. Most data on teratogenicity are derived from animal testing of anticancer agents. If chemotherapy has to be started during the pregnancy, the pregnancy may have to be terminated, depending on the medical condition and wishes of the patient and her partner.

Contraception. Care should be taken to ensure that patients are not or do not become pregnant during chemotherapy. Barrier contraceptive methods are advised.

Teratogenicity. The most serious risk of inducing a major, and often lethal, fetal abnormality (teratogenic effect) is during the first 8 weeks of pregnancy when the organ systems are developing. Examples of teratogenic effects are limb deformities and retinal defects. Patients are advised not to become pregnant during this period. At the end of this period the organs have formed. Fetal growth is then the major change. The risks of fetal damage diminish. The teratogenicity of methotrexate is best documented and it is contra-indicated during the first trimester.

Fetal growth retardation. Chemotherapy after the eighth week of pregnancy may cause fetal growth retardation. Anticancer agents can pass from the maternal circulation via the placenta to the fetus and cause the same side-effects as in the mother.

Premature delivery and low birth weight. These have been reported in some but not all pregnant women treated for leukaemia.

Genetic damage. Chromosomal damage by cytotoxic therapy is a theoretical risk but there is no clinical evidence to show that congenital abnormality in the offspring of patients who received chemotherapy is any greater than in the normal population. Studies of children born to women treated with chemotherapy for choriocarcinoma show no increased risk of congenital defects. Since the true risk is unknown, firm guidelines to couples on when they can safely attempt to have children after the end of chemotherapy cannot be given.

Advice to patients. Avoiding pregnancy for a year after the end of chemotherapy is a reasonable guideline.

Interaction with irradiation (radiation recall)

Patients who have been exposed to previous irradiation, when given certain cytotoxic agents (e.g. actinomycin D), may experience a repeated radiation reaction within the irradiated volume.

Psychological effects

Psychological difficulties may be related to malignant disease or a pre-existing psychological or psychiatric disorder. This applies to patients undergoing any form of conventional treatment for cancer. These are dealt with in Chapter 34.

The diagnosis of cancer, uncertainties about the future and the physical side-effects of chemotherapy frequently give rise to anxiety and depression. In extreme cases, suicide may be attempted. In women, change in body image (e.g. alopecia, weight gain or loss) can be very distressing. Marital and family dysharmony are common. A normal sex life may be interrupted because of loss of libido on the part of either patient or partner. Loss of self-esteem from prolonged periods off work with loss of earning capacity and fear of redundancy are also frequent.

Prevention and treatment. A clear explanation of the diagnosis and treatment and continuing counselling during and after treatment may allay many anxieties. Clinical staff need to be alert to the development of symptoms of an anxiety or depressive state. Referral to a clinical psychologist or psychiatrist is desirable for advice on management. Anxiolytic or antidepressant therapy may be helpful. Patients who are cured may still fail to rehabilitate psychologically to a normal working and home life. Constant reassurance is required, reinforced if necessary by investigations objectively confirming remission.

Day-care units or self-help groups of patients with and previously treated for cancer may help maintain morale and encourage rehabilitation. Sometimes patients with the same tumour (e.g. young men with testicular cancer) may provide mutual support during and after treatment, from the common experience of coping with chemotherapy.

Second malignancy

From the long-term follow-up of both adults and children treated with single agent and combination chemotherapy for malignant disease, there is clear evidence of a carcinogenic effect of chemotherapy.

Agents known to be carcinogenic in man

1. Alkylating agents—busulphan, chlorambucil, cyclophosphamide, melphalan, treosulfan, methyl-CCNU
2. Antimetabolites—azathioprine.

Some agents are carcinogenic in laboratory animals but not in man (e.g. bleomycin, Adriamycin, vinca alkaloids and cisplatin).

Mechanism of carcinogenesis. The exact mechanisms of carcinogenicity by anticancer agents are not known. The most likely is DNA damage. Alkylating agents bind to DNA and somehow interfere with its function, resulting in abnormal mitosis. This explanation is supported by the fact that agents which do not bind DNA (e.g. methotrexate) are not carcinogenic.

Effect of drug dosage. With some drugs the carcinogenic risk rises with total dose. For this reason chlorambucil is commonly discontinued after 6 months of treatment to reduce the likelihood of leukaemogenesis.

There is some evidence that prolonged low dose chemotherapy is more carcinogenic than higher doses given intermittently.

Type and incidence of second tumours

Acute non-lymphocytic leukaemia. The risk of developing leukaemia at 10 years following MOPP chemotherapy is 5–10%. It is maximal when chemotherapy is combined with radiotherapy. Prognosis is poor (<10% remission rates). Leukaemogenesis also occurs following melphalan and cyclophosphamide for ovarian cancer and multiple myeloma. Melphalan is more leukaemogenic than cyclophosphamide.

Non-Hodgkin lymphomas. These are commoner after treatment of Hodgkin's disease. The risk at 10 years following combination chemotherapy for Hodgkin's disease is 4%. If the patient has also received radiotherapy the risk is even higher (15%).

Solid tumours (e.g. sarcomas, bowel and lung cancer). These are also increased after MOPP chemotherapy for Hodgkin's disease. The cumulative risk of a solid tumour at 10 years is 7%.

Time of onset. The latent period for the development of acute leukaemia is 5.5 years and for solid tumours 9.5 years.

Prevention. Where two agents are equally effective against a particular tumour, the least carcinogenic should be chosen (e.g. cyclophosphamide rather than melphalan in ovarian cancer), but the chances of cure should not be compromised.

32. Hormones in oncology

The removal of certain of the body's own hormones or the addition of synthetic hormones can either stimulate, control or eradicate tumour growth.

HISTORICAL DEVELOPMENT

The relationship between hormones and cancer is an old one. An early milestone was the work of a Scottish surgeon, George Beatson, who removed the ovaries of two young women with breast cancer and found that the tumours subsequently regressed. It was thought at the time that the mechanism involved removal of some 'ovarian irritation' responsible for the breast lesions, but recurrence soon occurred. Although others repeated the procedure, the results were unpredictable and improvements only temporary. As a result the operation fell into disuse and its full significance was not appreciated until much later. It was 30 years later that the hormone oestrogen was isolated, whose source in the ovary Beatson had removed and which explained the temporary regression of the breast cancer.

Later, animal work again drew attention to hormonal factors, e.g. the incidence of spontaneous breast cancer was reduced by removing the ovaries (ovariectomy or oophorectomy). Other striking experiments produced breast tumours in mice by prolonged administration of ovarian hormones. Clinical interest revived in 1941 when Huggins in the USA reported favourable results of removing the testes (orchidectomy) in cancer of the prostate (p. 433). Much of the early work on endocrine therapy in cancer was empirical, involving the surgical or radiotherapeutic ablation of different endocrine glands. Such hormonal sensitivity is observed in a substantial number of patients with cancers of the breast, prostate and endometrium.

In the latter part of the 1960s the presence of *oestrogen receptors* was demonstrated in a number of breast tumour cells. It subsequently emerged that a response to endocrine therapy in some patients with breast cancer corresponded with the presence of these oestrogen receptors. Similarly, the absence of oestrogen receptors corresponded with a low probability of a response to endocrine therapy. Subsequently the presence of receptors for progesterone has been demonstrated on breast tumour cells. Some cells may have receptors for oestrogen or progesterone alone or a combination of both. The highest level of response (about 50–60%) is seen in patients whose breast tumours contain both receptors.

More recently it has been suggested that tumours control their own growth by producing their own (paracrine) growth factors. Some breast tumour cells have surface receptors for both oestrogen and for growth factors, e.g. epidermal growth factor (EGF). There is an inverse relation between EGF and oestrogen receptors. Cells with large numbers of EGF receptors generally have low numbers of oestrogen receptors and vice versa. In addition it has been shown that EGFs reduce the number of oestrogen receptors within the cell.

When an oestrogen receptor is stimulated, the result may be the synthesis and release of further growth factors which stimulate cell division and tumour growth. Alternatively, it may result in the synthesis of progesterone receptors which inhibit cell division and stimulate cell differentiation away from malignant development. It is not clear what determines the choice between these two responses. It may relate to relative hormonal levels. The production of growth factors is favoured by low oestrogen concentration and of progesterone receptors by higher oestrogen concentrations.

Tamoxifen stimulates breast cancer cells to produce transforming growth factor (TGFβ), an inhibitory growth factor which inhibits the production of stimulatory growth factors such as TGFα and platelet derived growth factor (PDGF). There are probably also oestrogen receptor independent actions on protein kinase C and NK (natural killer) cell activity.

HORMONES AS THERAPEUTIC AGENTS

There are a limited number of human cancers where hormone therapy is of value. These are in organs in which hormonal stimulation and control are known to be important, mainly prostate, breast, thyroid, and body of uterus. Quantitative and qualitative variation in clinical response is very wide. Remissions rarely last for more than a few years but symptomatic benefit may be substantial, and even dramatic, during this period.

While the administration of hormones avoids the morbidities particular to surgery, radiotherapy and cytotoxic chemotherapy, it is often accompanied by side-effects, which are sometimes unacceptable (e.g. masculinising effects of androgens in women with breast cancer) and can be dangerous (e.g. cardiovascular morbidity from stilboestrol for prostate cancer). A careful balance has to be struck between toxicity and benefit in tumour control.

Addition of hormones

Female hormones (oestrogens and progestogens)

1. Oestrogens

Synthetic rather than naturally occurring oestrogens are used since the naturally occurring are metabolised in the liver.

Action in females. Oestrogens are responsible for the enlargement of the breasts at puberty and during menstrual cycles, and for maturation and maintenance of secondary sexual characteristics and sexual organs.

Action in males. Oestrogens (1) inhibit the release of luteinising hormone (LH) from the anterior lobe of the pituitary gland, leading to a fall in testicular androgen production, and (2) possibly have a direct effect on the prostate gland.

Preparations

1. Diethylstilboestrol
   Indication: prostate cancer
   Dose: 1–5 mg orally daily
2. Ethinyloestradiol
   Indication: prostate cancer
   Dose: 0.1–0.5 mg t.d.s. daily
3. Phosphorylated methyloestradiol (Honvan)
   Indication: prostate cancer
   Dose: loading dose of 500–1000 mg daily for 5 days i.v., then 100–600 mg daily orally as maintenance

Side-effects

— Nausea and vomiting (50%)

— Fluid retention, sometimes leading to oedema, hypertension and cardiac failure
— Enlargement of the breasts
— Deepening pigmentation of the nipple and areola
— Uterine bleeding, from stimulation of the endometrium, even long after the menopause. This is also liable to occur if the oestrogen is stopped abruptly. Dosage should be tailed off gradually. The patient should be warned of possible bleeding to avoid alarm
— Thromboembolism
— Hypercalcaemia may be induced at the start of therapy.

In men:

— Loss of libido
— Shrinkage of the genitalia
— Enlargement of breast tissue (gynaecomastia).

2. Progestogens

The *corpus luteum* of the ovary secretes progesterone towards the end of each menstrual cycle. The main action of progesterone is the maturation of the endometrium ready for the implantation of the fertilised ovum. The mechanism of action of progesterones in breast and endometrial cancer is unclear. Probably the most important effect is its *antioestrogenic* action:

1. Increases the enzymatic conversion of oestradiol to the less potent oestrone, so reducing the level of available oestradiol to stimulate oestrogen receptors.
2. Reduces the number of oestrogen receptors.
3. Increases the number of progesterone receptors and cellular differentiation and inhibits cell division.
4. It seems to inhibit directly ovarian and adrenal production of sex hormones and has an important indirect action by inhibiting pituitary gonadotrophin production.
5. It may have a direct cytotoxic effect.

Side-effects

— Weight gain
— Sweating, muscle cramps, tremor (adrenergic effects)
— Fluid retention
— Increased blood clotting and risk of thrombosis (medroxyprogesterone acetate)
— Nausea, urticaria, carpal tunnel syndrome, thrombophlebitis, alopecia (megestrol acetate)
— Vaginal bleeding, amenorrhoea.

Preparations

1. Medroxyprogestone acetate
   Dose: 200 mg t.d.s. or 500 mg b.d. orally (breast cancer)
   Dose: 100 mg t.d.s. orally (endometrial cancer)
2. Megestrol acetate
   Dose: 160 mg once daily orally (breast cancer)

Male hormones or androgens

Testosterone and other androgens have masculinising and anabolic effects.

Side-effects

— Fluid retention
— Masculinising effects (increased body hair, deepening of the voice, increased libido)
— Increased well-being and appetite (anabolic effects).

Preparations

Nandrolone decanoate (decadurabolin)
Indication: advanced breast cancer
Dose: 50 mg i.m. 3-weekly

Antioestrogens

Tamoxifen is the most important synthetic anti-oestrogen preparation. It has two main actions:

1. Antioestrogenic: competitive binding to oestrogen receptors (ER).
2. Weak oestrogenic action, raising levels of sex hormone binding globulin which binds to freely circulating oestrogen and so reduces the amount of free oestrogen available to bind to oestrogen receptors. The binding of oestrogen to the oestrogen receptor reduces the synthesis of growth factors and stimulates the production of progesterone receptors. As a result cell division is arrested at the G_1 phase of the cell cycle (p. 254).

Lowering the free oestradiol levels stimulates the production of follicle stimulating hormone (FSH) from the pituitary. FSH then stimulates the ovarian production of oestrogen. In theory this latter effect of tamoxifen should contraindicate its use in premenopausal women with breast cancer because of the risk of oestrogen induced tumour growth. This theoretical risk has not been born out in practice.

Indications

1. Adjuvant therapy in early breast cancer in pre- and postmenopausal women.

2. Recurrent and advanced breast cancer.

Preparations
Tamoxifen
   Dose: 20 mg daily

Side-effects. These are infrequent. The following may occur:

— Nausea
— Hot flushes
— Dizziness
— Vaginal bleeding
— Fluid retention (very rare)
— Mild transient thrombocytopenia (very rare)
— Retinopathy (very rare)
— Acute hypercalcaemia in patients with bone metastases.

Antiandrogens

Preparations

1. Cyproterone acetate. This is a progestogenic anti-androgen. It has two actions. First, it reduces the production of testosterone in the testis by inhibiting the secretion of the pituitary gonadotrophins. Secondly, it competes with androgen receptors, from which it displaces testosterone.
   Indications: locally recurrent and metastatic prostate cancer
   Dose: 200–300 mg per day

Side-effects

— Tiredness
— Impotence
— Fluid retention
— Depression
— Gynaecomastia.

2. Flutamide. It is thought that flutamide competes for androgen receptors in the testis.
   Indications: locally recurrent and metastatic prostate cancer
   Dose: 250 mg orally t.d.s.

Side-effects

— Nausea
— Vomiting
— Depression
— Dizziness
— Hepatotoxicity.

Luteinising hormone releasing hormone (LHRH) analogues

LHRH is a protein which binds to receptors in the

anterior pituitary and stimulates the production of luteinising hormone (LH) and follicle stimulating hormone (FSH). The initial response is an increase in FSH and LH levels but within a few days there is a reduction in the number of pituitary LHRH receptors. The LH and FSH levels fall and correspondingly the levels of androgens and oestrogens produced peripherally fall.

Preparations

1. Goserelin acetate (Zoladex)
   Indication: recurrent and metastatic prostate cancer
   Dose: 3.6 mg subcutaneously every 28 days
2. Buserelin (Suprefact)
   Indication: recurrent and metastatic prostate cancer
   Dose: 100 µg by intranasal application six times a day

Side-effects

— Hot flushes
— Loss of libido
— Gynaecomastia
— Nausea.

An initial increase in testosterone may cause transient deterioration. Cyproterone acetate is sometimes given to prevent this during the first 2 weeks of treatment.

Adrenal hormones

The adrenal cortex produces three main groups of corticosteroid hormones: mineralocorticoids (regulating sodium balance), glucocorticoids (controlling carbohydrate and protein metabolism) and sex hormones (oestrogens, androgens and progesterone). The amount of glucocorticoid production is controlled by the levels of adrenocorticotrophic hormone (ACTH) from the anterior lobe of the pituitary gland. The naturally occurring glucocorticoids are cortisone and hydro-cortisone. Synthetic glucocorticoids are prednisone, prednisolone and dexamethasone. Of these, dexamethasone has the highest glucocorticoid potency, 25 times that of hydrocortisone. The relative glucocorticoid and mineralocorticoid potencies and common dosages are shown in Table 32.1.

Glucocorticoids have cytotoxic properties against specific tumours (e.g. lymphomas, breast cancers and leukaemias). Some of these tumours have been found to have *glucocorticoid receptors*. In acute leukaemia, better responses are seen in patients with higher levels of receptors than with lower levels. However the levels of glucocorticoid receptors do not seem to correlate with tumour response when cytotoxic agents are combined with steroids. Factors other than steroid receptor status may be important in mediating tumour response to steroids in breast cancer. It may be that steroids work by feedback inhibition on ACTH, so reducing circulating oestrogen levels. They reduce the production of androgens from which oestradiol is derived. In addition, steroids act as anti-inflammatory agents, reducing the oedema around secondary tumour deposits. At a cellular level steroids inhibit glucose transport and phosphorylation, inhibit protein synthesis and retard mitosis.

Glucocorticoids are of benefit for complications of malignant disease—cerebral oedema, chemotherapy induced vomiting, nerve root and spinal cord compression and some types of haemolytic anaemia. They are frequently used to treat hypercalcaemia, although the evidence for any hypercalcaemic action on non-hormone responsive tumours is scanty.

Side-effects are important and potentially life-threatening, especially after prolonged therapy, when adrenal suppression has developed. Sudden withdrawal of steroids for any reason or increased steroid requirements (e.g. due to infection or the stress of an operation) may result in acute adrenal insufficiency. For this reason all patients on steroids should carry a blue

Table 32.1 Relative potencies of natural and synthetic glucocorticoids

Drug	Relative potency		Typical dose (mg/day)
	Glucocorticoid	Mineralocorticoid	
Hydrocortisone	1	1	10–20*
Cortisone	0.8	1	10–20*
Prednisone	4	0.8	15–60†
Prednisolone	4	0.8	15–60†
Dexamethasone	25	0	2–16†

* Dose for replacement therapy where adrenal insufficiency is treatment induced, e.g. by aminoglutethimide.
† Dose for active treatment of malignancy.
(Modified from Priestman 1989.)

steroid card detailing their name, address and telephone number and that of their medical practitioner and their current steroid preparation and dosage. This card or a permanently worn bracelet or neck chain indicating that the patient is on steroids should alert medical staff in the event of the patient being too unwell to report that he or she is on steroids.

Side-effects

— Adrenal insufficiency
— Sodium and water retention (low serum potassium, fluid retention and cardiac failure)
— Cushingoid appearance (mooning of the face, 'buffalo' hump on upper back)
— Gastrointestinal upset (dyspepsia, peptic ulceration with or without perforation)
— Increased risk of infection
— Osteoporosis
— Hyperglycaemia
— Modification of tissue reactions (resulting in spread of infection, poor wound or ulcer healing)
— Skin changes (thinning of skin, bruising, acne)
— Psychosis
— Cataract formation
— Muscle weakness (especially thighs).

Inhibitors of steroid hormones

Aminoglutethimide is the most important inhibitor of steroid synthesis used in cancer therapy. It inhibits desmolase in the adrenal, which converts cholesterol to pregnenolone (Fig. 32.1). It is an inhibitor of the aromatase enzyme which converts androstenedione to oestradiol, principally in peripheral fat. It does not affect oestrogen production in the ovary and therefore is not of use in premenopausal women with breast cancer. It is given orally.

Side-effects

— Skin rashes occur in the majority of patients after 10 days of treatment. The patient should be warned about their probable occurrence and advised to start chlorpheniramine 4 mg t.d.s. to relieve the itching, but to continue aminoglutethimide. The rash subsides in most cases, even when the drug is continued.
— Dizziness ⎫
— Drowsiness ⎬ Features of central nervous toxicity
— Ataxia ⎭
— Agranulocytosis is rare but important.

Indications: locally recurrent or metastatic breast cancer in postmenopausal women
Dose: 125–500 mg orally b.d. and hydrocortisone 10–20 mg b.d.

At a dose of 125 mg b.d. the degree of adrenal suppression is insufficient to require hormone replacement with hydrocortisone. However steroids do reduce the incidence of side-effects from aminoglutethimide and their use is therefore recommended but not mandatory.

Removal of hormones

Ovaries. The chief source of the female hormone, oestrogen, may be removed surgically (oophorectomy/ ovariectomy). This is usually a minor procedure under

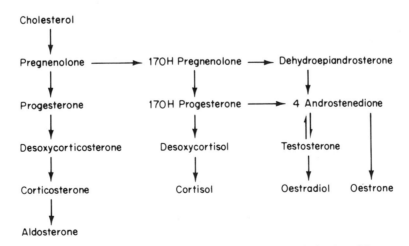

Fig. 32.1 Adrenal steroidogenesis. (Reproduced with permission from Sikora & Halnan 1990.)

general anaesthesia, necessitating only a few days in hospital. Alternatively the ovaries can be irradiated by a pelvic radiation field to stop them functioning (as for menorrhagia, see p. 521). Castrate hormonal levels are reached by 6 weeks.

Testes. The male hormone testosterone can be abolished by bilateral subscapular orchidectomy.

Adrenals. The glands may be removed by surgical adrenalectomy. This used to be done for advanced breast cancer but, because of the morbidity of the procedure, has been replaced by 'medical adrenalectomy' by aminoglutethimide (p. 549).

Pituitary. This is the master endocrine gland, as it controls all the others by its various secretions. Ablation may be achieved by surgical removal of a large part of the gland (transnasal hypophysectomy) or by radiation. Pituitary ablation for advanced breast cancer is now rarely practised with the development of antioestrogens (tamoxifen) and inhibitors of steroid synthesis (aminoglutethimide). However if the patient is not suitable for medical adrenalectomy and has demonstrated hormone responsiveness, pituitary ablation is worth considering. The best responses tend to be seen in patients with bone metastases.

Hypophysectomy/pituitary ablation by surgery/alcohol also has useful analgesic effects.

Transnasal hypophysectomy, if required, is a relatively straightforward procedure in skilled hands and has largely replaced pituitary ablation by interstitial implantation with yttrium-90 rods. The latter is carried out under radiographic control with a fluorescent screen. It is suitable for patients unfit for surgery. Long-term replacement therapy with thyroxine and hydrocortisone is required after surgical or radiotherapeutic pituitary ablation.

HORMONE THERAPY IN BREAST, PROSTATE, ENDOMETRIAL AND THYROID CANCER

The hormonal management of these tumours is discussed in Chapters 23, 25, 24 and 21 respectively.

33. Palliative and continuing care

In a regional oncology centre at least 50% of the work is concerned with palliative care for advanced disease. For such patients the main aim is the relief of physical and psychological distress. The period of *palliative and continuing care* incorporates the time from the diagnosis of incurable malignancy to death. The life expectancy of terminally ill patients may be a matter of a few days or weeks. Some patients with slow growing but incurable tumours such as breast cancer, soft tissue sarcomas and gliomas may survive months or even years.

Some patients may be in the terminal phase of their illness at the time of diagnosis. In others, curative therapy may have been attempted and failed or incurable local recurrence or metastases supervened.

The radiotherapist and oncologist should form part of a multidisciplinary team including general practitioners, specialists in palliative medicine, community nurses, anaesthetists, surgeons, medical social workers, dietitians, physiotherapists and clergy.

'NO PLACE LIKE HOME'

Most patients prefer to be cared for in their own homes where they are in familiar surroundings and close to family and friends. Every effort should be made to keep the patient at home and to support the family and friends in caring for the dying patient.

Professional help from the general practitioner, MacMillan or Marie Curie nurses or other support nurses, and voluntary workers can ensure a comfortable and dignified death at home for most patients. If this is not possible, admission to a hospital or hospice is required. Admission of terminally ill patients whose symptoms are not controlled at home should be accorded a high priority. Uncontrolled pain is distressing for both the patient and family.

A short period of hospital treatment may bring symptoms under control, or defuse a difficult situation at home. This may allow the patient to return home for the last days of life.

ORGANISATION OF PALLIATIVE CARE

The provision of palliative care and continuing care should be suited to the needs of each community. Of nearly 135 000 patients dying of malignant disease, 60% will die in an acute general hospital. Medical and nursing staff in general hospitals should receive training in symptom control. Specialist advice is available from visiting consultants in oncology or from anaesthetists in most general hospitals. Hospital palliative care support teams, modelled on home care teams, have been established to work both in the general hospital and in the community. A typical team would include a specialist in palliative medicine, a medical social worker, occupational therapist, secretary and chaplain.

Hospices

Since the early 1980s there has been a rapid expansion of the provision of purpose built hospices to care for the terminally ill. Hospices provide both inpatient and outpatient facilities, predominantly for adults. Most terminally ill children are managed by paediatric oncologists. At present there are two hospices in the UK specifically for children.

The hospice is often the base for a palliative home care team. Hospices are staffed by doctors and nurses experienced in palliative care. There are approximately 150 within the UK, funded by the NHS, voluntary bodies or a combination of both. They provide nearly 2200 beds. There are over 100 day hospices and home care teams. They care for about 30 000 patients per year, or a quarter of all patients who die from cancer and other terminal diseases. It is estimated that 40–50 hospice beds are required per million population. This figure has not yet been reached.

The provision of hospice care is not just a question of bricks and mortar. Some communities may feel that a home care service suits their needs better than a building. Geographical, financial and social factors are decisive. If patients and their relatives have to travel long distances to a regional oncology centre, a local hospice or home care service may be more appropriate.

Health authorities have taken over the running costs of many hospices. Health authorities and charitable bodies must ensure long-term funding of any hospice or home care service before it is inaugurated. A high nurse-to-patient ratio is needed to enable a high standard of patient care to be delivered. Twenty-five beds is regarded as an economic size. Close links are needed with various departments in a general hospital to provide specialist advice and facilities.

Hospices provide a more informal, less institutional and quieter environment than the noisy, busy surgical, medical or oncology ward. A high staff-to-patient ratio gives more time for the patients to talk to staff about their illness.

Palliative care medicine is now recognised as a separate specialty with specific training requirements. This should improve the provision of high standards nationally, and should encourage research into palliative care.

Admission of a patient for respite care may provide relatives with an opportunity for a much needed holiday and enable them to continue to care for a dying relative at home. Volunteer staff may visit to sit with the patient by day or night to give relatives an additional break.

Home care teams

About a third of patients will die at home. Teams of home care nurses trained in palliative care, commonly MacMillan nurses, provide additional support to the established services of the general practitioner and community nurses.

Day care centres

Many patients appreciate the support of others in a time of stress. Day centres may provide company and psychological and nursing support. In many such centres patients may attend whilst they are recovering from radiation reactions.

Family members may share care for some of the week with the day care centre. This may allow some patients to remain at home who would otherwise require hospitalisation.

SYMPTOM CONTROL

Pain, anorexia, nausea, vomiting, weight loss, dysphagia, dyspnoea and lack of energy are common symptoms in patients with advanced cancer. Patients with advanced cancer often have multiple symptoms.

Principles of management

As in any other branch of medicine the cause of symptoms should be established to provide a rational basis for treatment. While most symptoms will be caused by cancer, even a patient with advanced cancer may have a benign headache.

A careful history, clinical examination and limited investigations will establish the cause of most symptoms. Investigations should only be performed if their result is likely to influence management.

Symptoms are what the patient says they are. Whilst a patient may have multiple bony metastases in ribs and spine on bone scan, they may only be complaining of pain in one rib. One treats the symptoms, not the scan.

The priority is to establish which areas are really troubling the patient. Each symptom will need addressing in order of priority.

Pain is the most pressing symptom. Pain interferes with mobility and sleep and lowers morale in the whole family.

Some complications such as spinal cord compression require urgent assessment and treatment if neurological function is to be improved or retained (p. 491). Symptoms are often multiple. Each will need addressing in order of priority. Since the patient's life expectancy is short and symptoms are unpleasant and frightening, prompt assessment and treatment is required.

The patient should be constantly reviewed as symptoms may change daily in nature, site and severity. Experienced nursing staff, seeing the patients frequently and monitoring their physical and mental state, are the backbone of good palliative care.

Guidelines for treatment

Treatment should be aimed at specific goals, without upsetting the patient or attempting to prolong life inappropriately. The patient and family should be given a straightforward explanation of these aims, and of the reasons for a change in treatment.

Pain

Pain is a presenting feature in 30–45% of patients with cancer and occurs in 70% of those with advanced disease. In two-thirds of patients the pain is caused by the cancer itself.

Multiple sites of pain are common, with 80% of patients having more than one site. In one hospice the three commonest causes of pain were bone, nerve compression and soft tissue disease. The types of treatment for cancer pain are summarised in Fig. 33.1.

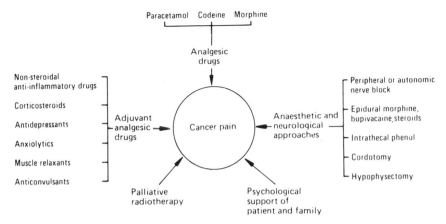

Fig. 33.1 The treatment of cancer pain. (Reproduced with permission from Baines, British Medical Journal, 1989.)

Assessment. Pain has both physical and psychological components. Anxiety or depression may accentuate the perception of pain and lower the pain threshold. Conversely, elevation of mood may raise the pain threshold. In addition to monitoring the physical attributes of pain, especially the site, character, frequency and intensity, the psychological state of the patient needs to be assessed and frequently reviewed.

Principles of analgesic treatment. The following guidelines should be followed:

1. Establish the cause of the pain.
2. Give a suitable analgesic on a regular and prophylactic basis.
3. Start with simple non-opioid analgesia and progress, if necessary, to opiates.
4. Use the oral route if possible.
5. Choose the minimum dose that controls the pain.
6. Increase the dose of opioid analgesia until the patient is pain free.
7. Deal with psychological factors which may be influencing the pain.
8. Consider the use of coanalgesics such as non-steroidal anti-inflammatory drugs (NSAIDs), steroids, and anti-depressants.
9. Consider non-drug treatments, such as radiotherapy, nerve blocks, splints and physiotherapy.
10. Regularly review the situation.

Escalation of analgesia

Mild and moderate pain

1. Paracetamol (1 g 4-hourly) and aspirin (300–1200 mg 4-hourly) are suitable for mild pain.
2. Aspirin or another NSAID such as flurbiprofen (50 mg t.d.s or q.d.s.) is useful for moderate pain.

3. NSAIDs often cause gastric upset which may be relieved by an oral antacid or an H_2-receptor blocker such as ranitidine (150 mg b.d.) or cimetidine (400 mg b.d.).

4. A low efficacy opioid such as codeine or dihydrocodeine (30–60 mg 4-hourly), sometimes usefully in combination with an NSAID, may be sufficient for moderate pain.

Severe pain

1. Strong opioids such as morphine or diamorphine are indicated for severe pain. Morphine or diamorphine are often usefully combined with NSAIDs in this situation.

2. Inexperienced practitioners may be reluctant to prescribe morphine for fear of psychological or physical dependence. If morphine is used appropriately, psychological dependence is not a problem. If the pain becomes less severe or subsides completely it is possible to wean the patient off morphine without precipitating the symptoms of physical dependence.

3. The dose of oral morphine sulphate may vary from as little as 5 up to over 100 mg 4-hourly. Long acting preparations of morphine sulphate, such as MST Continus tablets, enable dosage to be given twice daily only. Pain control is generally achieved more quickly if analgesic opioid requirements are established by titrating the dose of oral morphine sulphate every 4 hours.

4. Suggested increments are: 2.5, 5, 10, 15, 20, 30, 45, 60, 90, 120, 180, 240 and 320 mg. Doses beyond 320 mg 4-hourly are unlikely to achieve better pain control. Some forms of pain are intractable to usual doses of opioids. The role of psychological factors should be considered where escalating doses of morphine are not controlling the pain.

5. A larger dose of morphine at bedtime, one and a half to twice the daytime 4-hourly dose, may enable the patient to sleep through the night without being woken by pain, or by a nurse.

6. Once the daily total morphine requirement has been determined, the patient's dosage may be converted to a b.d. regime of a long-acting oral morphine preparation. For example a patient controlled on 20 mg 4-hourly has a daily morphine requirement of 120 mg, which could be given as 60 mg of MST b.d.

7. A regular laxative is necessary to prevent the inevitable constipation caused by morphine.

8. With the exception of children and the elderly, approximately 80% of patients are controlled on 20 mg of morphine 4-hourly. For patients with bone metastases, 60–90 mg 4-hourly are often needed, often combined with an NSAID.

9. Choice between morphine and diamorphine

a. The actions and side-effects of morphine and diamorphine (heroin) are similar. Diamorphine is metabolised to morphine and another active metabolite very quickly and before it reaches the central nervous system.

b. Although diamorphine is more potent than morphine, the efficacy of both drugs is the same. Diamorphine is preferred for injections (intravenous/subcutaneous/intramuscular) because it is more soluble than morphine.

c. For oral use, the conversion factor is 1.5, so that 10 mg of diamorphine is equivalent to 15 mg of morphine. For injection, 5 mg of injected diamorphine is equivalent to 15 mg of oral morphine, a conversion factor of 3.

10. Other routes of administration

a. If a patient is unable to swallow, then sublingual, subcutaneous, intramuscular and rectal routes are alternatives.

b. The sublingual route is suitable if the patient has adequate saliva. Buprenorphine, an opioid, 0.2–0.4 mg 8-hourly may be a useful equivalent to 60–240 mg of morphine daily. Both morphine and another potent opioid, phenazocine, may also be given by this route.

c. A continuous subcutaneous infusion of diamorphine via an indwelling butterfly needle, usually placed into the abdominal wall, is useful when oral medication is not possible due to nausea and vomiting, dysphagia, weakness or unconsciousness. Regular injections can largely be avoided. Diamorphine is delivered via a syringe driver, with most syringe drivers being calibrated in millimetres per 24 hours. With a standard 10 ml syringe a rate of 2 mm per hour is typical. The syringe can be topped up in hospital or, if qualified staff are available, at home. The infusion site usually has to be changed every 3 days.

d. Other drugs can be given via a syringe driver, in addition to diamorphine. These include antiemetics such as haloperidol, methotrimeprazine and cyclizine; and hyoscine for a 'death rattle'.

e. Intramuscular injections are sometimes necessary for the same indications as for the subcutaneous route. Diamorphine injections are given regularly every 4 hours if they are the sole form of opioid analgesia.

f. Morphine (10, 15, 30 and 60 mg suppositories) and oxycodone (30 mg and 60 mg) are strong analgesics that can be given by the rectal route. Oxycodone acts for longer (6–8 hours) than morphine (4 hours).

g. In patients who become very sedated on high doses of oral morphine required to control their pain, the insertion of an epidural catheter to deliver morphine may be considered. These are usually inserted by an anaesthetist.

The dose of morphine may be reduced from 240 mg 4-hourly to not more than 4 mg.

The central tranquillising effect of morphine is absent and an anxiolytic may be needed. There is a lack of constipation normally caused by oral morphine.

Complications include dislodgement or blockage of the catheter requiring reinsertion. However some catheters have remained in situ for up 250 days.

h. Nerve blocks

Nerve blocks are appropriate in a limited set of circumstances. The advice of an anaesthetist should be sought. When very high doses of narcotics are ineffective, or when the pain is very localised, nerve blocks may be helpful. The solution injected normally includes phenol and alcohol.

(i) Intercostal blocks are useful for rib metastases, chest wall infiltration and pathological fractures.

(ii) A brachial plexus block may relieve the pain of a Pancoast tumour or malignant infiltration of the plexus, commonly by breast cancer.

(iii) Coeliac axis block. Pain from pancreatic cancer can be relieved in up to 75% of cases. This procedure is associated with a risk of hypotension and hospitalisation is required for 24–48 hours after the procedure.

(iv) A pudendal block is helpful for perineal pain.

Nausea and vomiting

Nausea and vomiting trouble about 40% of patients who are terminally ill. The causes of these symptoms are legion and treatment should depend on the cause. They may be due to the cancer, its treatment or concurrent medical or surgical conditions. Common causes are summarised in Table 33.1.

Table 33.1 Causes of nausea and vomiting in malignant disease

Due to cancer	Due to treatment
Irritation of the upper gastrointestinal tract	Radiotherapy
Gastrointestinal obstruction	Chemotherapy
Constipation	Drugs, e.g.
Hepatomegaly	Opioids
Raised intracranial pressure	NSAIDs
Anxiety	Aspirin
Pain	Antibiotics
Hypercalcaemia	Carbamazepine
Hyponatraemia	Steroids
Uraemia	Oestrogen
	Iron
	Expectorant mucolytics

Other conditions
Peptic ulceration
Infection

(Reproduced with permission from Twycross & Lack 1990.)

Table 33.2 Causes of dysphagia* in malignant disease

1. Caused by cancer
   (a) Intraluminal
       Tumour in mouth, pharynx or oesophagus
   (b) Intramural
       Infiltration of the pharyngeal or oesophageal wall
   (c) Extraluminal
       External compression by mediastinal nodes or tumour
2. Neurological
   e.g. damage to brainstem or disruption of motor (5th, 7th, 9th–12th) or sensory (5th, 9th, 10th) pathways of cranial nerves
3. Caused by treatment
   (a) Radiation
       Loss of saliva; acute oral, pharyngeal or oesophageal reaction; radiation fibrosis in mouth/pharynx/ oesophagus (stricture)
   (b) Chemotherapy
       Oral mucositis
   (c) Surgery—radical resections, e.g. tongue flap repairs
4. Intercurrent conditions
   Benign oesophageal stricture; oral/pharyngeal/ oesophageal candidiasis

(Reproduced with permission from Twycross & Lack 1990.)

Drug induced vomiting is common. Haloperidol is the treatment of choice. In addition it has anxiolytic and antipsychotic properties. A dose of 1–1.5 mg is given stat and nocte. If the night dose is inadequate, it is increased to 3–5 mg. For radiation induced vomiting 5 mg is suggested. For chemotherapy or metabolic causes of vomiting 5–20 mg nocte or in divided doses is often necessary. Its side-effects are anticholinergic (e.g. dry mouth, constipation), extrapyramidal reactions and sedation. For further discussion of chemotherapy induced vomiting, see Chapter 31.

Metoclopramide (10 mg 4-hourly oral/intramuscular) is suitable if nausea and vomiting are due to physical or chemical irritation of the stomach. It increases gastric emptying, upper gastrointestinal peristalsis and contracts the lower oesophageal sphincter.

Prochlorperazine (5–10 mg 4–8-hourly), a phenothiazine, is preferred if the patient is anxious, since it is also sedative. Chlorpromazine (25 mg 6–8-hourly) is an alternative phenothiazine.

Dexamethasone (4 mg 6-hourly) is used to relieve nausea and vomiting due to raised intracranial pressure (Ch. 27). If this fails, cyclizine 50 mg b.d. is often helpful.

Dysphagia

Dysphagia encompasses any problem in moving liquids or solids from the mouth to the stomach. The process requires a normal mucosa, intact 5th, 7th and 9th–12th cranial nerves and coordinated function of smooth and skeletal muscle. The causes (Table 33.2) may be related to the tumour, treatment, neurological damage or intercurrent illness or a combination of these factors.

Treatment will depend on the cause. If the patient is able to swallow liquids but not solids, a liquidised diet is advised. If even fluids cannot be swallowed, an endo-oesophageal tube is needed. If the oesophageal aperture is 1 cm or more, a Clinifeed tube can usually be passed through the nose into the stomach using a guide wire. If this is not possible, insertion of a Celestin tube into the oesophagus under general anaesthesia should be considered. Intravenous fluids are often needed to correct the initial dehydration.

Oropharyngeal candidiasis is treated by oral antifungal agents (e.g. Nystatin, 100 000 u/ml, 1–5 ml 4-hourly). Treatment of the tumour by surgery, radiotherapy or chemotherapy or debulking by laser therapy may relieve obstruction.

Benign or radiation induced strictures can be dilated. Dilatation may have to be repeated if dysphagia recurs.

Anorexia

The origin of anorexia is often multifactorial. Causes include the underlying malignancy or its complications (e.g. bowel obstruction or pain), treatment by radiotherapy or chemotherapy, alteration in taste, oral ulceration, depression and anxiety.

The advice of a dietician familiar with the dietary problems of patients with cancer should be sought. Such advice can have a very positive effect on a patient's morale. Guidance is needed on the amount of liquid food (e.g. Buildup or Complan) required to supplement the normal diet in order to maintain body weight. Nasogastric feeding (see above) may be necessary if the patient is unable to swallow.

Treatment of the cause, alteration of diet and appetite stimulants may all help.

Loss of taste may be improved by adding seasoning to foods. Fish, poultry or eggs may provide protein when appetite for meat is lost. Flexibility and imagination in presentation and in the frequency, content and volume of meals are needed.

A trial over 7–10 days of oral steroids (prednisolone 15–30 mg mane) or dexamethasone 2–4 mg is worthwhile and sometimes improves the appetite.

Dyspnoea

Dyspnoea occurs in 50% of patients who are terminally ill. It is a frightening symptom. The anxiety that it generates (will I suffocate or stop breathing?) exacerbates the symptom. In many cases treatment of the underlying cause (e.g. tapping pleural effusion, relieving bronchial obstruction by radiotherapy (Ch. 22), correction of anaemia) is effective. Where anxiety is a factor an anxiolytic (diazepam 10 mg stat or 5–20 mg nocte) may help.

Morphine depresses both the respiratory rate and the sense of distress (2.5–5 mg orally 4-hourly). Where the patient is already on morphine for pain, the dose should be increased by 50% to relieve dyspnoea. Oxygen by mask or nasal spectacles reduces hypoxia. It is helpful in acute dyspnoea. Reassurance from staff, relaxation and breathing exercises can all assist.

For wheezing due to bronchial obstruction or lymphangitis carcinomatosa steroids are worth a trial (prednisolone 10 mg orally q.d.s.)

Anxiety and depression

It is said that anxiety and depression are experienced by at least a quarter of patients undergoing treatment for cancer. This is almost certainly an underestimate. The diagnosis is made more commonly by staff who have received psychiatric or psychological training. Since medical or psychological therapy may often help, close liaison with a clinical psychologist or psychiatrist should be established.

Patients often do not mention mental symptoms due to a sense of shame or because they think that the staff are only interested in physical symptoms. Alternatively, they may not realise that their symptoms are psychological rather than physical. Patients may reveal these symptoms to any member of staff, often to a dietician or physiotherapist, who is seen as an impartial confidant(e). Good communication between staff is needed to ensure that such information is passed on to medical and nursing staff.

Clinical features. The symptoms of anxiety may be divided into psychological and somatic. Psychological symptoms include weakness, dizziness, feelings of illness, insecurity and irritability. Somatic symptoms include palpitations, breathlessness, chest pain, headache, paraesthesia, fatigue, sweating, flushing, dry mouth and urinary frequency.

The main symptom of depression is low mood. This is commonly accompanied by loss of appetite and of sexual interest, inability to enjoy pleasurable events, insomnia, loss of energy and interest in work, slowing of movement and reduced facial expression, loss of self-esteem, anxiety, reduced ability to think and concentrate, suicidal thoughts, and bodily complaints including constipation, nausea and vomiting.

Distinguishing between the normal feelings of sadness and disappointment and clinical depression is often difficult. This again emphasises the need for access to expert psychological advice.

Fear induced by the diagnosis of cancer. The diagnosis of malignancy still induces widespread fear, irrespective of whether cure is possible. Most adult patients know someone who has died of malignancy. The experience understandably colours their own expectations of cancer treatment and of prognosis. Fears about unpleasant treatment, separation from family, change in body image, loss of job and income and career advancement are common. The loss of these aspects of normal life is like a bereavement reaction. This starts with a sense of disbelief and is followed by mental agonising, dejection and finally but not invariably an acceptance of the reality. Some patients cope by denying their illness.

Many of these fears can be overcome by a clear explanation of investigations, treatment and the prospects of cure or palliation. It is important to consider the whole patient and not simply their symptoms. An interest expressed in a patient's life (family, job or interests) may have a very positive effective on morale.

Prognosis. In regard to prognosis, it is often helpful to ask the patient how specific an answer he or she requires. Some patients find the knowledge of their probability of 5-year survival reassuring if it is high but depressing if it is low.

Financial worries. Concerns about the consequences of time off work for family and personal finances can often be alleviated. Guidance from a medical social worker can be given on eligibility for disability or attendance allowances or for help for relatives with travelling expenses to and from the hospital.

Efficient delivery of services. The management of cancer frequently involves a multiplicity of appointments for investigation and treatment. Delays incurred in waiting for investigations and uncertainties as to when tests or treatment will be carried out all contribute to the patient's anxiety. Prompt, courteous and informed answers from clinical and clerical staff all help to allay anxiety.

Communication with the general practitioner. The patient's general practitioner needs to be regularly briefed about his or her patient's progress, prognosis and plans for further management. The anxious patient may well have forgotten what the oncologist said in the initial consultation and often looks to the family doctor for explanation and reassurance. If the general practitioner is concerned about new symptoms in a patient, an early outpatient appointment should be arranged. If the patient is not well enough a domiciliary visit can be arranged. Such visits are reassuring to patient, family and general practitioner, even if no change in therapy is considered appropriate.

Medical treatment

Anxiety. Time spent discussing a patient's concerns about the diagnosis, investigation, treatment, prognosis or other issues can substantially reduce anxiety. Relief of physical symptoms such as pain, vomiting or constipation reassures the patient that clinical staff have the medical condition under control.

If the patient still remains anxious, anxiolytics, e.g. diazepam, a benzodiazepine, 2–20 mg orally nocte may be needed. If the patient also has pain of a severity to justify morphine, the anxiolytic effect of morphine may avoid the need for a benzodiazepine.

Depression. If depressive symptoms do not lift with explanation and reassurance, medical treatment is indicated. The most widely used are the tricyclic and related antidepressants. The choice of antidepressant will depend upon the clinical features of depression. The starting dose should be small and built up over 3–4 weeks to a maintenance dose. Clomipramine initially in a dose of 10 mg orally nocte and increased to 50–150 mg is useful in patients with associated obsessional features. It has some anticholinergic effects. Amitriptyline 25 mg orally nocte and increased to 50–75 mg has more sedative and anticholinergic effects.

Palliative surgery

Palliative surgery has a variety of useful roles. The decision to operate will take into account the severity of symptoms, the general condition of the patient, life expectancy and probability of benefit.

Operations include: (1) stabilising painful pathological limb fractures and restoring mobility; (2) toilet mastectomy for malodorous or bleeding advanced breast tumours; (3) decompression of spinal cord compression if pretreatment neurological deficit is not marked; (4) debulking of brain tumours or aspiration of cystic tumours to relieve raised intracranial pressure; and (5) colostomy for bowel obstruction or rectovaginal fistula.

34. Quality of life

In the last decade there has been a rapid expansion of interest in the nature and measurement of the quality of life of patients with cancer. Cancer touches a wide range of aspects of life: psychological, physical, spiritual and cultural. It is widely accepted that the diagnosis and treatment of cancer have a major disruptive effect on most patients' lives. The influence of psychological factors on patients with cancer is discussed in an earlier chapter (p. 556).

The concept of quality of life is not a new one. It is enshrined in the Hippocratic oath taken by doctors to do no harm to their patients. Clinical staff are well aware that surgery, radiotherapy and chemotherapy can have both transient and long-term unpleasant side-effects. There is increasing public awareness of quality of life as an issue in the choice of anticancer treatment.

Traditionally the outcomes of cancer treatment have been measured in terms of survival alone. However quality of life is increasingly being included in the assessment of outcome, although there is less agreement on its definition and measurement.

IMPORTANCE OF QUALITY OF LIFE AND ITS MEASUREMENT

The need for objectivity

Why is more objective, time-consuming and potentially costly assessment necessary? First, if quality of life is sufficiently important to influence treatment decisions and policies, it is worth the effort of measuring it as accurately as possible. Secondly, subjective impressions may result in capricious and misleading results. Thirdly, it helps to identify what aspects of health, illness and treatment do and do not concern patients. A knowledge of the important factors in a patient's quality of life may clarify the care and support that he or she needs.

Already quality of life assessments are included in the evaluation of the efficacy of a variety of trials of cancer therapy. Only 4% of cancer trials included a measurement of quality of life in 1975–76. Now most trials of new anticancer therapies will incorporate some form of quality of life assessment. This is likely to increase further if quality of life assessments are found to be practical, valid and reliable. To date there have been fewer quality of life assessments in radiotherapy and surgery than in chemotherapy. However they are very relevant to the assessment of all forms of cancer therapy.

Assessment of toxicity

With increasing survival following curative treatment for cancer, the importance of long-term sequelae are increasingly being appreciated. This is particularly pertinent to children where growth, intellectual function, mobility and endocrine function may all be affected.

Where the therapeutic intent is cure, patients will generally endure substantial side-effects (e.g. severe vomiting from cisplatin in the treatment of testicular teratoma). However, many treatments for advanced stages of common cancers (e.g. breast and colon) are still palliative. None the less, some therapies, particularly chemotherapy, inevitably cause toxicity if useful regression of disease is to be achieved. Toxicity is less of a problem with well-planned palliative radiotherapy.

The toxicity (morbidity) of treatment is inextricably linked to quality of life. One of the principles of good palliation (p. 281) is that minimal upset should be caused to the patient. Where two palliative treatments for cancer offer equal probabilities of disease regression, the one offering the patient the best quality of life is clearly preferable.

Choosing between alternative anticancer therapies

The initial focus of quality of life was in terminal care and advanced disease. However quality of life assessment has a much broader application to the comparison

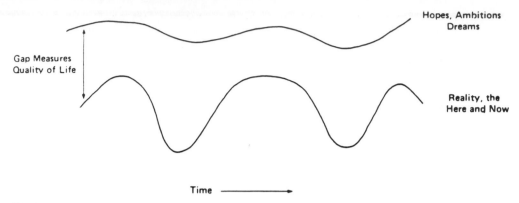

Fig. 34.1   Representation of the gap between reality and hopes, dreams and ambitions. (Reproduced with permission from Calman, Journal of Medical Ethics, 1984.)

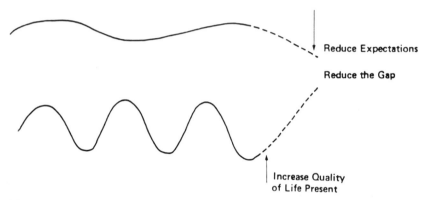

Fig. 34.2   The improvement in the quality of life represents either a reduction in expectations or a change in reality. (Reproduced with permission from Calman, Journal of Medical Ethics, 1984.)

of both curative and palliative treatments in cancer and to other diseases. For example, where cure rates of two treatments are similar (e.g. for stage I carcinoma of the cervix by surgery or radical radiotherapy), the quality of life of the patients on each treatment should strongly influence both patient and clinician in the choice of treatment.

A MODEL OF QUALITY OF LIFE

Calman has stated that: 'the quality of life can only be described and measured in individual terms, and depends on past experiences and future hopes and dreams and ambitions.' Life is of good quality when expectations are matched by their achievement. For poor quality of life the converse is true. Quality of life may vary over time, influenced by personal and therapeutic successes or failures. Calman's model provides a useful representation of quality of life (Fig. 34.1).

The upper line represents the hopes, ambitions and dreams of the individual. The lower line represents reality. Quality of life is measured by the gap between the two lines. Quality of life improves the closer each line is to the other and deteriorates the further apart they are. To narrow the gap, and so improve the quality of life, one has either to modify expectations or reality (Fig. 34.2). If reality exceeds expectation, the lines will cross (Fig. 34.3).

To illustrate this model: if a terminally ill patient

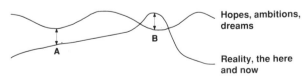

Fig. 34.3   Modification of Calman's model, showing expectation (top line) falling short of reality (lower line) at A and exceeding it at B.

anticipates, unrealistically, returning from hospital to live at home, quality of life will be poor if he or she remains in hospital. If the patient accepts that he or she is unable to go home but can realistically expect to be ambulant about the ward, quality of life may be higher. In terminal illness the patient needs limited but achievable goals for quality of life to be maintained at a reasonable level.

DEFINITION OF QUALITY OF LIFE

Ever since Aristotle wrote in his *Ethics* 'When it comes to saying in what happiness consists, opinions differ', there has never been a universally agreed definition of quality of life. Its definition will vary with the emphasis that each individual puts on each of its components.

Although definitions of quality of life vary, most would agree that it should include the following areas:

— Psychological functioning
— Physical and occupational functioning
— Social interaction
— Physical symptoms.

Psychological functioning

Stress and coping

It has long been thought that there is an association between an individual's life and illness or maladjustment. It is not possible to say what constitutes good coping behaviour in a given situation but there are indications of patterns of behaviour associated with poor coping (e.g. rumination, anger with oneself, alcohol abuse).

There is a growing body of evidence that factors such as the number and characteristics of major life events may influence the natural history of cancer.

Life events. A person's experiences can make an individual vulnerable to stress. This in turn may make the person more prone to feeling unable to cope. The physiological responses of anxiety may then influence, via the pituitary-adrenal axis, the patient's susceptibility to certain hormone tumours (e.g. breast cancer). Additional factors include not only the more major life events (e.g. bereavement and moving house) but the minor irritations of daily living (e.g. finding a parking place).

Social support. The degree of social support that the person perceives as being available can also affect the degree of stress and coping, and thus the quality of life.

Personality and cognitive processes. The psychological make-up of an individual (which is influenced by the person's own genetic make-up or experiences) has a considerable impact on the capacity to cope with major life events, such as cancer, and minor daily stresses. Individuals vary in the ways in which they cope with these stresses. Some may deploy problem-solving skills and weigh up the advantages and disadvantages before deciding on any particular course of action. Others find themselves paralysed by the seriousness of the diagnosis of cancer. Still others may cope by avoiding thinking about the diagnosis or denying its existence. The coping strategies used by individuals may vary over time, even though they may tend generally to have preferred styles of coping.

Patients' appraisal of the situation will depend on their thinking (cognitive) processes and their resources and options for coping. Their response to the diagnosis may be influenced by the probability of cure given by the clinician. If there is a reasonable prospect of cure, it may be possible to concentrate one's energy on achieving that outcome. If the tumour is incurable, 'fighting' the cancer may seem pointless.

Locus of control. Patients' perception of their quality of life also depends on whether they feel that they have any influence over their lives and treatment (*internal locus of control*) or feel that they are controlled by it or that what happens is entirely due to chance (*external locus of control*). Those who feel they can have some influence may take a more active role in complying with treatment regimes. They may, for example, do exercises to avoid postoperative complications of immobility (e.g. deep venous thrombosis or chest infection) which can reduce quality of life. Some may respond with fighting spirit, while others respond with little or none. Personality factors (feelings of mastery, self-esteem, strong commitments, religious beliefs and values) may also play a role.

Anxiety and depression. Anxiety and depression commonly affect patients with cancer and impair their capacity to cope. Worries about the effects of unemployment on the ability to meet personal and family financial commitments add to the anxiety generated by diagnosis, treatment and prognosis.

Physical and occupational functioning

Physical functioning

The local, regional and metastatic spread of cancer may result in considerable functional impairment and change in body image. Brain tumours may result in paralysis of one side of the body (hemiparesis) such that the patient is unable to walk and is confined to a wheelchair. Tumours of the frontal lobes may cause urinary incontinence due to interference with cortical control of continence. Bowel or bladder tumours may require a colostomy or urostomy, resulting in loss of normal control of bowel and bladder emptying, respectively.

Regional lymphatic spread to the axilla from breast cancer may result in a swollen, heavy and useless arm due to lymphoedema. Lymphoedema of the legs due to para-aortic node metastases or spinal cord compression (p. 490) may limit the patient's mobility.

Mutilating head and neck surgery may interfere with eating and swallowing. Mastectomy may be perceived as resulting in reduced femininity. Both pelvic radical radiotherapy and surgery may limit the normal sexual functioning of the vagina.

Occupational functioning

Cancer and its treatment may limit both the physical and mental capacity of a patient to carry out his or her previous job. Confusion or impaired memory due to brain disease may preclude the carrying out of the simplest tasks at work. Visual field defects or epilepsy may prevent the patient from driving. The patient may lose his or her job if dependent on a car to fulfil work commitments. Impaired sensation in the fingertips from the neurotoxicity of vinca alkaloids may prevent work requiring manual dexterity. Any impairment of the capacity to walk may limit access to places of work, particularly where stairs have to be climbed. Sometimes it is loss of energy from the effects of the disease or treatment, inability to concentrate, anxiety or depression, or lack of confidence which limit a return to work.

Social interaction

For most people interpersonal relationships are essential to their happiness. The support of family, friends and health care professionals can be of inestimable value to patients in enabling them to cope with cancer.

However their previous ability to socialise, whether as a spouse or parent or in peer groups, may be altered by their illness. This may result in loss of self-esteem. Marital dysharmony, breakdown and divorce are not uncommon results.

Patients may be reluctant to attend social gatherings because of embarrassment from disfiguring facial or breast surgery, weight gain or loss, or odour from a fungating tumour. Lack of physical energy and loss of earning capacity may also limit attendance and participation.

Members of the general public may believe that the cancer itself is contagious. As a result the company of the patient may be shunned. Refusing to eat or drink from cutlery or crockery used by the patient or to use bedclothes in which the patient has slept is not uncommon. Such behaviour reinforces isolation.

Physical symptoms

Symptoms such as nausea, vomiting, pain and immobility have a major impact on the quality of life. These may be features of the disease (e.g. pain from bone metastases) or of the treatment (nausea from chemotherapy or radiotherapy or difficulty swallowing from radical surgery for oral cancer). Chronic pain, for example, can dominate a patient's consciousness, making him or her a virtual prisoner. Nevertheless it should be stressed that good quality of life is more than just the absence of symptoms.

ASSESSMENT OF THE QUALITY OF LIFE
Problems in assessment

There are many difficulties in assessing quality of life. There are the usual problems of designing questionnaires. These include ordering and weighting the questions to avoid response bias and 'halo' effects. There are also difficulties particular to assessing quality of life. These include separating out factors due to the illness, its treatment or psychological factors (which are themselves influenced by the illness and its treatment) such as anxiety and depression. A further complication is that psychological factors such as stress and coping are difficult to define and therefore to assess. The design of assessment measures and the analysis and interpretation of results need to be carried out by staff with training in questionnaire design, research methodology and analysis and a good understanding of psychological assessment and of the physical effects of the illness and its treatment. Clinical psychologists have appropriate training in these areas and are well placed to collaborate with clinical oncologists in assessing quality of life.

There are interactions between all of the areas outlined above. For example a depressed psychological state may influence physical (retardation), social (isolation) and occupational functioning (unemployment). Both the disease and its treatment and the patient's response to them and the reactions of others may influence physical, psychological and social well-being.

Questionnaires and rating scales

The assessment of quality of life can be based on casual observations or on a more formal structured basis. At the simplest level the patient can be asked whether the quality of life is the same, better or worse than it was before treatment. However comparison between patients is impossible without some agreement on what elements of quality of life are being assessed and how they are defined and quantified. This has led to the development of more structured measures of assessment, which include questionnaires and rating scales.

Choice of test

The choice of assessment method for measuring the quality of life will depend on the aim, the aspects of quality of life considered most relevant and the time and personnel available to carry out the assessment. There are, for example, well-established scales of toxicity following chemotherapy. The most widely used is the WHO grading system. The performance status of the patient is commonly assessed using the Karnofsky or UICC scales (Table 34.1) before, during and after treatment.

Psychological assessment: linear analogue scales

Psychological assessment is an important part of assessing quality of life. One of the most frequently used methods of assessing this has been to use rating scales. Of these, the *linear analogue scale*, is perhaps the most popular. It can be used as a self-rating scale (i.e. it is the subject and not the observer who completes the scale). The subject is asked to make a mark

Table 34.1 Karnofsky and UICC performance status scales

Karnofsky	
100	Normal, no complaints
90	Normal activity, minimal signs or symptoms
80	Normal activity with effort, some symptoms
70	Caring for self, unable to work
60	Needs occasional assistance, but able to cater for most of needs
50	Needs considerable assistance and frequent medical care
40	Disabled, needs special care
30	Severely disabled, needs hospital care
20	Very ill, in hospital, needs supportive care
10	Moribund
0	Dead

UICC Grade	
0	Able to carry out normal activity
1	Able to live at home, with tolerable symptoms
2	Disabling symptoms but less than 50% of time in bed
3	Severely disabled, greater than 50% of time in bed but able to stand
4	Very ill, confined to bed
5	Dead

Table 34.2 Format of the Rotterdam Symptom Checklist

In this questionnaire you are asked about your symptoms. Would you please, for any of the symptoms mentioned, indicate to what extent you are bothered by it, by circling the answer most applicable to you. The questions are related to the past 3 days (the past week).

Have you, during the last 3 days (week) been bothered by:

Lack of appetite:	not at all	a little	quite a bit	very much
Irritability:	not at all	a little	quite a bit	very much
Tiredness:	not at all	a little	quite a bit	very much
Worrying:	not at all	a little	quite a bit	very much

(Modified from de Haes J C J M, Van Knippenberg F C E, Neijt J P 1990 British Journal of Cancer 62: 1034–1038

along a 10 cm line joining two extreme descriptions, for example:

'I feel sad most of the time' —— 'I feel happy most of the time'.

The mark represents how the patient is feeling at the time of or shortly before completing the scale. Linear analogue scales have been found to be a reliable and valid method of assessing mood and mood change in depressed patients. They allow small changes in rating to be recorded and are therefore applicable to situations where, as in cancer therapy, repeated assessments are required.

Questionnaires

A variety of questionnaires are available. Some focus on the physical and psychological symptoms. Others

Table 34.3 Symptoms (34) included in the Rotterdam Symptom Checklist

Lack of appetite	Feeling lonely
Irritability	Tension
Tiredness	Crying spells
Worrying	Abdominal aches
Sore muscles	Anxiety
Depressed mood	Constipation
Lack of energy	Diarrhoea
Low back pain	Heartburn/belching
Nervousness	Shivering
Nausea	Tingling hands or feet
Desperate feelings about the future	Difficulty concentrating
Difficulties sleeping	Sore mouth/pain when
Headaches	swallowing
Vomiting	Loss of hair
Dizziness	Burning (or sore) eyes
Decreased sexual interest	Deafness
Itching	Shortness of breath
	Dry mouth

(Modified from de Haes J C J M, Van Knippenberg F C E, Neijt J P 1990 British Journal of Cancer 62: 1034–1038 measure health more generally, encompassing physical, emotional and social factors. They are based on the concept that health is not simply the absence of illness.

If a comparison is being made between cancer and a different disease or a cost–benefit analysis is being attempted, the *Nottingham Health Profile* or *Sickness Impact Profile* are suggested.

If comparison is being made between cancer patients, a cancer specific test is needed. Of the cancer specific tests, the *Rotterdam Symptom Checklist (RSCL)* (Tables 34.2 and 34.3) is currently well regarded in terms of appropriateness, format, administration, scoring, structure, clinical usage, reliability and validity. It is intended to measure psychological and physical distress and takes about 8 minutes to complete.

If levels of anxiety and depression are to be included, the *Hospital Anxiety and Depression Scale (HADS)* is recommended. Both RSCL and HADS have the advantages of being relatively quick to complete and being acceptable to patients.

35. New developments in radiotherapy and oncology

CONFORMATION THERAPY (MULTILEAFED COLLIMATORS)

The collimation of the beam of the traditional linear accelerator allows a series of square or rectangular fields to be treated. These shapes do not necessarily correspond to the shape of the target volume, which is often spherical. However a new generation of linear accelerators is fitted with multileaf collimators (Fig. 3.24C). The position of each leaf can be independently controlled. This enables the treatment volume to encompass the configuration of the target volume more closely than is possible with square or rectangular fields produced by the jaws of conventional linear accelerators. The use of multileaf collimators should enable more normal tissue to be excluded from the treatment volume than was previously possible. The impact of conformation therapy on tumour control, survival and morbidity from radical radiotherapy is being evaluated.

ALTERED FRACTIONATION

Accelerated fractionation

Conventional daily fractions of radiotherapy over 3–6 weeks still fails to cure a substantial proportion of localised advanced cancers of the head and neck, brain and lung. This has stimulated laboratory and clinical studies into increasing the number of fractions given per day (*multiple daily fractions*) in an attempt to improve local tumour control.

Multiple daily fractions may be divided into *hyperfractionation or accelerated fractionation* and *superfractionation*.

Hyperfractionation refers to a fractionation schedule in which the number of fractions (*N*) is the same as in conventional fractionation. The overall treatment time is shorter since more than one (usually two or three) fractions are delivered each day. For example, in a hyperfractionated schedule 54 Gy might be given in three fractions per day of 1.5 Gy over 12 consecutive days, compared with a conventional regime of 60 Gy in 30 daily fractions of 2 Gy over 6 weeks. A slight reduction in dose (about 10%) has to be made in the hyperfractionated regime.

Superfractionation differs in that the overall treatment time is similar to conventional treatment but several smaller than normal fractions are given each day. In a superfractionated schedule 66 Gy might be given in 60 fractions (two per day) of 1.1 Gy over 6 weeks. The dose in a superfractionated regime is about 10% greater than in conventional fractionation.

In both hyperfractionated and superfractionated regimes, the interval between fractions is generally 3–4 hours.

Rationale for multiple daily fractions

The basis of multiple fractions is founded on five radiobiological factors of importance (Ch. 15):

Repair

Repair of sublethal damage is oxygen dependent. It is more likely to occur in well-oxygenated normal tissues than in hypoxic areas of tumours. An interval of 3–4 hours will facilitate the repair of sublethal damage in normal tisssue but not in hypoxic tumour cells.

Repopulation

In conventional radiation tumour repopulation may occur between daily fractions. It is thought that reducing the interval between fractions may limit tumour repopulation.

Redistribution

Radiosensitivity may differ by a factor of 2 or 3 depending on the phase of the cell cycle in which cells are irradiated. Maximal radiosensitivity occurs in G_2 and M phases. Increasing the number of fractions per day should increase the total number of cells lethally damaged in the more sensitive phases of this cycle.

Reoxygenation

The process of reoxgenation in some experimental animal tumours takes about 3 hours. This has been used as a guideline for the interval between multiple daily fractions. Prolonging the interval to 24 hours (as in conventional fractionation) may result in repopulation in some fast growing tumours.

Dose per fraction

There is some experimental evidence that the oxygen enhancement ratio (Ch. 15) decreases with smaller doses per fraction. Smaller doses per fraction may overcome the problem of radiation resistance due to hypoxic cells seen at conventional higher doses per fraction.

In addition it is thought that at low dose per fraction (of the order of 1 Gy) late normal tissue damage may be less than at higher doses per fraction. This may lead to a therapeutic gain, except in some tumours with very rapid doubling times.

Clinical results

Hyperfractionation

The most encouraging results of hyperfractionation have been in localised advanced head and neck cancer and non-small cell lung cancer (see below). No benefit has been shown in high grade gliomas. It is a more logical choice than superfractionation in tumours with a rapid doubling time.

Hyperfractionation tends to result in less skin reaction than conventional fractionation. Mucosal reactions tend to be more intense but subside more quickly.

Continuous hyperfractionated accelerated radiotherapy (CHART)

During a 3–6 week course of radical radiotherapy, tumour repopulation may be a cause of persistent disease. Traditionally in the UK radiotherapy has been delivered daily from Monday to Friday with a break on Saturday and Sunday. The weekend may provide a prolonged period for repopulation to occur.

The tolerance of normal tissue limits the size of single

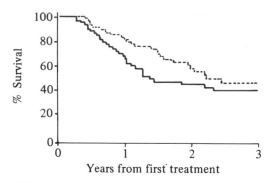

Fig. 35.1 Survival in T3 and T4 head and neck cancer treated by CHART (broken line) compared with conventional radiotherapy; $P = 0.048$. (Reproduced with permission from Saunders, Cancer Topics, 1990.)

daily fractions of external beam therapy. Shortening the overall treatment time but maintaining the total dose increases acute reactions. In general it does not increase late reactions. It has been found that giving several small fractions of radiation per day may give rise to a minor increase in acute reactions but a decrease in late reactions. To minimise the risk of repopulation it seems logical to shorten the overall treatment time, not to allow a gap in treatment over the weekend and to give several small fractions of radiation daily (Continuous Hyperfractionated Accelerated Radiotherapy [CHART]). A pilot study of CHART at Mount Vernon Hospital in the UK, of giving 54 Gy in three fractions per day for 12 consecutive days, demonstrated an improvement in local control and survival in patients with advanced (T3 and T4) head and neck cancer (Fig. 35.1) and in localised inoperable non-small cell cancer of the bronchus (Fig. 35.2). Results of a multicentre randomised trial comparing CHART and conventionally fractionated radiotherapy in head and neck cancer and inoperable non-small cell lung cancer are awaited. If benefit in tumour control and in reduced late morbidity is confirmed, considerable changes in local organisation and staffing of radiotherapy departments will be necessary.

Superfractionation

Superfractionation has improved the local control rates in Burkitt's lymphoma, a tumour with a very short doubling time, and in head and neck cancer. Conclusions must be tentative since these were non-randomised studies without a conventionally treated control group.

Superfractionation tends to cause a more marked skin reaction than does hyperfractionation for equivalent dose.

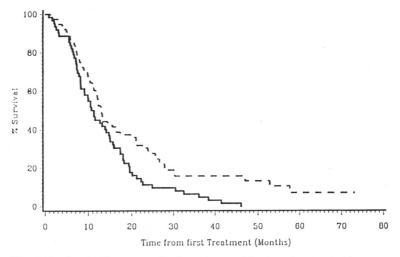

Fig. 35.2   Survival in non-small cell carcinoma of the bronchus treated by CHART (broken line, 76 cases) compared with conventional radiotherapy (62 cases); *P* = 0.0089. (Reproduced with permission from Saunders, Cancer Topics, 1990.)

PROTONS

There is increasing interest in the application of proton beams in the treatment of localised tumours. The physical characteristics of protons are described on page 206. They have three main advantages: (1) their absorption characteristics in tissue are more favourable than photons; (2) they have similar radiobiological characteristics to photons; and (3) the cost of delivering protons is less than that for heavier charged particles.

The most important physical advantage of protons is that there is no dose delivered deep to the target volume for each beam path. The dosage to normal structures outside the treatment volume is therefore minimised. By contrast, in conventional photon irradiation there is always an exit dose deep to the target volume, which may deliver substantial dose to normal tissues.

The proximity of critical structures limits the dose of photon irradiation to a variety of tumour sites. Examples are: (1) the spinal cord in cancers of the head and neck, lung and oesophagus; (2) the globe and optic nerve in tumours of the paranasal sinuses; (3) the small bowel in the irradiation of cancers of the cervix, endometrium, bladder and prostate; and (4) the kidney in retroperitoneal tumours. The application of planning techniques using protons might widen the range of tumours at these sites that could be treated radically, while reducing the morbidity to normal tissues (fibrosis, pathological fracture, renal, intestinal and spinal cord injury and radiation induced neoplasms).

As yet, clinical experience with protons has been limited to sites which are difficult to treat with photons because of the dose delivered to adjacent critical structures, e.g. ocular melanomas. Proton or qualitatively similar helium ion therapy has achieved control rates in excess of 95%, with the majority of patients retaining useful vision. Similar benefits have been shown in pituitary tumours. Chondrosarcomas of the base of the skull, which are difficult to treat because of the proximity of the brainstem, have been controlled in about 85% of cases. Proton beam therapy has also been used successfully to treat cerebral arteriovenous malformations (p. 526), although the obliteration rates are lower than with Leksell unit cobalt irradiation.

Clinical evaluation of protons is being carried out at centres such as Loma Linda in California (USA). The theoretical benefits of protons over photons in both morbidity and local control among the commoner cancers of the head and neck, lung, oesophagus, cervix and rectum has yet to be demonstrated.

HYPERTHERMIA

Hyperthermia refers to the application of heat to tumours. In practice this normally means the maintenance of a temperature within the tumour of about 43°C.

The rationale for its use, usually in conjunction with radiotherapy, is as follows. Hyperthermia has two mechanisms of action. First, it sensitises tumours to the effects of radiation and chemotherapy. Secondly, and probably the more important clinically, it has a direct cytotoxic effect. Many tumours have a poor blood supply. These anoxic conditions are associated with a low pH and render the tumour more prone to damage by hyperthermia. Since poorly vascularised tumours cool more slowly than well vascularised normal tissue, greater heating may be achieved in some tumours than in normal tissue for a given input of power.

An added advantage of hyperthermia is that it may damage tumour cells in the S phase of the cell cycle (p. 254), which are normally resistant to radiation alone. The total tumour cell kill may therefore be greater by combining heat and radiation than with either modality alone.

Thermotolerance

If hyperthermia is applied too frequently to tissues, resistance to its cytotoxic effects occurs. This is known as *thermotolerance*. For this reason hyperthermia treatments are normally separated by a gap of a week.

Treatment techniques

Heat can be delivered by ultrasound, microwave or radiofrequency waves. Each has its advantages and disadvantages but clinical results are similar whichever is used.

Hyperthermia may be applied locally, regionally or to the whole body. Most clinical hyperthermia is local or regional. Local hyperthermia is most commonly directed to (1) superficial advanced or locally recurrent breast tumours, (2) neck nodes in head and neck cancer, and (3) skin melanoma. Techniques for treating more deeply seated tumours (e.g. of the prostate and cervix) and for lung, oesophageal, brain and ocular tumours are under development.

For superficial lesions (e.g. 2 cm or less in thickness), the commonest indication for hyperthermia, the temperature is measured by thermocouples loaded into 1–2 plastic cannulas inserted within the tumour under local anaesthesia. The applicator is positioned over and in contact with the lesion. A temperature of 43°C should be maintained for about an hour. An alternative technique for superficial tumours is to use a scanning microwave applicator (Fig. 35.3). This tracks to and fro over but not in contact with the lesion. It has the facility for scanning over curved surfaces, a particular advantage for chest wall lesions. A typical temperature profile is shown in Figure 35.4.

Morbidity of superficial hyperthermia

Minor morbidity is in the form of temporary erythema and blistering which may occur over parts of the treated area in the week following treatment. Most heal quickly without treatment. Major local morbidity is rare.

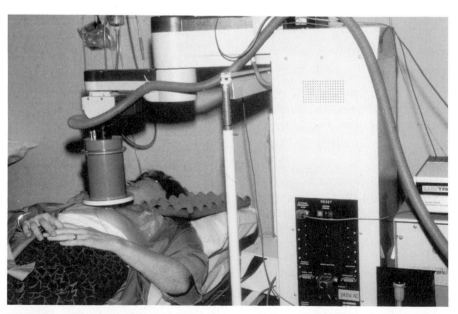

Fig. 35.3   A scanning microwave hyperthermia system for the treatment of recurrent breast tumours. The cylindrical applicator contains a microwave antenna scanned by a 6-axis robotic arm. (Courtesy of Dr J Conway, Sheffield.)

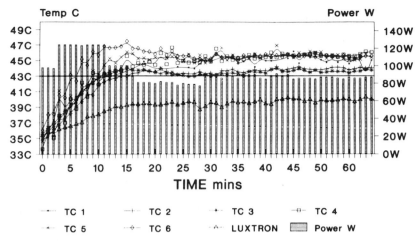

Fig. 35.4 Temperature achieved at six measurement sites during hyperthermia treatment of a breast tumour. (Courtesy of Dr J Conway, Sheffield.)

Results of treatment

Much of the early work on hyperthermia was carried out in non-randomised uncontrolled studies, often with small numbers of patients. However a review of studies in which heat was adequately delivered to locally recurrent breast cancer suggests a response rate of 60% from combining hyperthermia and radiotherapy, compared with 30% for radiotherapy alone.

If the randomised trials confirm the higher response rate of hyperthermia when combined with radiotherapy compared with radiotherapy alone, hyperthermia is likely to be more widely adopted in clinical practice.

SYSTEMIC RADIOTHERAPY

Radioisotopes have long been used in the treatment of well-differentiated thyroid cancer. Survival for 20 years or more is recorded with iodine-131 for lung metastases from thyroid cancer. However, until recently no other tumours had been identified in which systemic isotope therapy might control disease.

Interest has been rekindled by the development of new isotopes in the systemic treatment of a variety of metastatic malignancies, particularly of prostate cancer and the lymphomas. Radioisotope therapy might potentially replace total body irradiation (p. 465) in preparation for bone marrow transplantation.

Tumour physiology may either reduce or enhance radiolabelled antibody targeting of tumours. Increased interstitial pressure and reduced central vasculature reduce access to antibodies, whereas new vessel formation increases it.

The measurement of exactly what dose is delivered to the tumour is difficult.

The efficacy of Strontium-89 has been demonstrated in the relief of pain from bone metastases from prostate cancer (p. 434). It has potential as an adjuvant therapy in the treatment of poor prognosis disease.

The development of monoclonal antibodies (see later this chapter) has raised the possibility of targeting antibodies carrying radioisotopes to tumour cells. Iodine-131 is theoretically the ideal radioisotope for carrying a monoclonal antibody. It has an average beta energy of 0.183 MeV and a physical half-life of 8 days. These properties would be suitable for cytotoxic therapy. It emits gamma rays which are suited to tumour imaging and quantification. However, though easy to label, uncoupling from the monoclonal antibody is common and dose rates of only 0.05 Gy/hour have been achieved.

Yttrium-90 is a pure beta emitter of 0.037 MeV and has a physical half-life of 2.7 days. When conjugated to an antibody, it has been shown to achieve a fourfold greater dose rate than iodine-131.

Alpha emitters such as astatine-210 have the potential advantages of lack of the oxygen effect and a minimal distance of irradiation. In addition, there is no dose rate dependence for alpha particles.

In Hodgkin's disease ferritin is known to be synthesised by malignant T lymphocytes. Treatment with antiferritin antibody labelled with iodine-131 has achieved partial remissions in patients with relapsed Hodgkin's disease whose disease had failed to be controlled by chemotherapy. Remissions have been reported using iodine-131 antibodies to B cell lymphoma instead of total body irradiation.

Treatment of solid tumours, particularly colorectal

cancer metastatic to the liver, with iodine-131 labelled anti-CEA (carcinoembryonic antigen) antibody has been disappointing.

FOCAL BRAIN IRRADIATION

There is increasing interest in developing techniques for focal irradiation of small volumes of the brain. These include the Leksell gamma unit (p. 525), modified linear accelerators and interstitial implantation.

The term 'radiosurgery' was originally coined by neurosurgeons to describe single fraction focal brain irradiation by the Leksell cobalt gamma unit using a stereotactic frame. It is also commonly applied to focal brain irradiation by suitably modified linear accelerators. An alternative term, stereotactic multiple arc radiotherapy (SMART), is preferred by some radiotherapists to describe the use of linear accelerators in focal brain irradiation.

The aim is to enable high doses to be delivered to tumours or arteriovenous malformations (AVMs), avoiding the morbidity of wide field brain irradiation to radical doses. The efficacy of the Leksell unit in obliterating AVMs using a stereotactic frame and localisation by angiography (described on p. 525) is long established, but such machines are very expensive and, at present, only appropriate for single fraction irradiation. However for most malignant intracranial tumours fractionated radiotherapy is required to maximise tumour kill.

Many groups have adapted linear accelerators to irradiate tumours and AVMs localised by CT, MRI and angiography. Removable stereotactic head frames, fixed by a template to the patient's dentition for stability, have been developed. These allow acceptable reproducibility of daily set-up. Multiple non-converging arcs and dynamic rotation provide the best dose delivery, steepest fall-off outside the target volume, lowest skin dose (to avoid epilation) and low dose to the lens of the eye and to other radiosensitive organs (thyroid, breast and gonads). Preliminary experience of focal irradiation by modified linear accelerators of previously irradiated gliomas show acceptable tolerance. Clinical studies to assess its impact on local tumour control and survival of high grade gliomas are in progress.

An alternative is to implant the intracranial tumour with a radionuclide such as iodine-125 as a boost following external beam irradiation for well-defined high grade gliomas. The optimal combination of external beam and implant dose has yet to found to improve tumour control rate with acceptable morbidity.

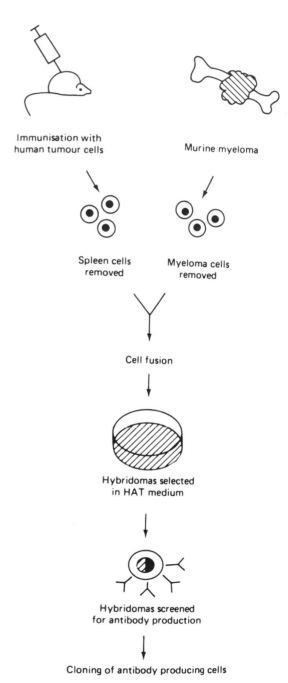

Immunisation with human tumour cells

Murine myeloma

Spleen cells removed

Myeloma cells removed

Cell fusion

Hybridomas selected in HAT medium

Hybridomas screened for antibody production

Cloning of antibody producing cells

Fig. 35.5 Production of monoclonal antibodies. HAT medium contains hypoxanthine, aminopterin and thymidine and only hybridoma cells contain the necessary enzymes to survive in this medium. (Reproduced with permission from Priestman 1989.)

HAEMATOPOIETIC GROWTH FACTORS

Less than the planned doses of chemotherapy, and, to a lesser extent, radiotherapy may be delivered because of treatment induced bone marrow depression. Myelosuppression is the main problem. A white blood count of less than $1 \times 10^9/l$ is associated with increased risk of septicaemia. This is a potentially fatal complication.

It is known that haemopoiesis, the process by which mature red cells, white cells and platelets develop from stem cells in the bone marrow, is controlled by a variety of growth factors. With the advent of gene cloning by recombinant technology, these growth factors can be produced in large quantities. Of these growth factors, *granulocyte colony stimulating factor* (G-CSF) and *granulocyte macrophage colony stimulating factor* (GM-CSF) are now available. G-CSF stimulates neutrophil production, with a lesser effect on monocytes. GM-CSF stimulates neutrophils, eosinophils and monocytes. Neither G-CSF nor GM-CSF affect platelet production. Their application is being evaluated in the following areas: (1) reduction of treatment induced neutropenia, (2) treatment of established neutropenic infection, (3) avoidance of dose reduction of chemotherapy, and (4) intensification of chemotherapy to obtain higher tumour response rates. It has already been shown that G-CSF and GM-CSF reduce the incidence of neutropenia and septicaemia in patients receiving chemotherapy for small cell lung cancer.

BIOLOGICAL RESPONSE MODIFIERS

Biological response modifiers such as interferon and interleukin-2 have been shown to have anticancer activity against melanoma and renal cell cancer. These tumours are resistant to conventional cytotoxic chemotherapy. Unfortunately these agents are toxic and expensive. Their impact on local control and survival is being evaluated in clinical trials. They are recommended for use only in specialised centres.

MONOCLONAL ANTIBODIES

In 1975 Milstein and Kohler showed that when antibody-producing B lymphocytes are fused with myeloma cells, the resulting hybrid cells (hybridomas) are capable of producing a limitless supply of the antibody (Fig. 35.5). If the B lymphocytes had previously been stimulated to produce a specific antibody, the hybridoma produced a clone of cells making the same antibody. This gene technology opened the way for raising and targeting antibodies against surface antigens of tumour cells. The antibody could carry an agent toxic to the tumour cell (cytotoxic agents, toxins (e.g. ricin) or radionuclides) to eradicate the tumour population. Theoretically this is a very attractive technique, both for the diagnosis and killing of cancer cells.

Panels of monoclonal antibodies have been used successfully by pathologists on histological specimens to classify non-Hodgkin lymphomas and to distinguish lymphomas from carcinomas in biopsies of undifferentiated tumours. Monoclonal antibodies to ovarian, breast and colon cancer cells have been labelled with a radioisotope (iodine-131), injected into patients and their localisation in tumour deposits identified by rectilinear scanning using a gamma camera. Imaging using radioisotopes is described in Chapter 9.

However there are many practical difficulties. The first is that tumour antigens specific to man have yet to be identified. Although many tumours have a greater concentration of particular surface antigens than normal cells, exposure to monoclonal antibodies raised against these antigens will damage normal cells as well as tumour cells. Where these antibodies are carrying very toxic agents, e.g. ricin, which are fatal in small quantities, absolute specificity to tumour cells must be obtained before they could be used in patients. One avenue being explored is raising monoclonal antibodies to tumour cell products (e.g. CEA) as opposed to the tumour cell itself. The advent of monoclonal antibodies in the routine treatment of cancer is, however, still some years away.

36. Medical complications of malignant disease

Cancer can cause a huge variety of medical and metabolic problems. These can be due to the physical presence of the tumour causing obstruction of, for example, the bile duct or a ureter, secretion of fluid into a body cavity such as the pleura (an effusion) or local invasion of adjacent structures. In addition, cancers frequently predispose the patient to infection and may cause constitutional disturbances which are not due to the local effect of the tumour but are collectively known as paraneoplastic syndromes. The problems of invasion into neighbouring structures are

discussed in Chapter 14. In this chapter we discuss the problems caused by effusions, infection and paraneoplastic syndromes (Table 36.1) in malignancy.

EFFUSIONS SECONDARY TO MALIGNANT DISEASE

Normally, the pleural, pericardial and peritoneal spaces contain only a few millilitres of fluid to lubricate the inner and outer surfaces. However, in cancer the normal capillary and lymphatic vessels can become damaged

Table 36.1 Endocrine and paraneoplastic manifestations of malignancy

System	Manifestation		
Endocrine	Hypercalcaemia		Parathyroid hormone related peptide
	Water retention		Inappropriate ADH secretion
	Cushing's syndrome	due to	ACTH
	Hypoglycaemia		Insulin-like proteins/somatomedins
	Gynaecomastia		Human chorionic gonadotrophin
	Thyrotoxicosis		Human chorionic gonadotrophin
Neurological	Peripheral neuropathy		
	Cerebellar ataxia		
	Dementia		
	Transverse myelitis		
	Myasthenia gravis		
	Eaton–Lambert syndrome		
Haematological/vascular	Anaemia		
	Polycythaemia		
	Red cell aplasia		
	Thrombophlebitis		
	Thromboembolism		
	Disseminated intravascular coagulation		
	Non-bacterial endocarditis		
Musculoskeletal	Polymyalgia rheumatica		
	Arthralgia		
	Clubbing		
	Hypertrophic pulmonary osteoarthropathy		
Dermatological	Pruritus		
	Various skin rashes		
Renal	Nephrotic syndrome		

and the hydrostatic pressures which regulate the transfer of fluid from one compartment of the body to another are disturbed. A build-up of fluid at any of these three sites can cause unpleasant symptoms which require treatment. Although effusions are usually a sign of advanced malignancy and treatment is only palliative, intervention is worthwhile and can provide useful benefit and improvement in quality of life.

Pleural effusions

The commonest malignancy to cause a pleural effusion is carcinoma of the bronchus. In addition, metastases from carcinoma of the breast, other adenocarcinomas and lymphoma may also quite frequently cause pleural effusions. Clinical detection is not possible until at least 500 ml has accumulated, and typically the effusion comprises 1000–4000 ml of fluid. This is usually straw coloured but may be blood-stained and will cause increasing shortness of breath, a dry cough and sometimes pain as it increases in size.

Drainage of the fluid is required for relief of symptoms. This can be performed through a needle inserted into the pleural space, which provides good emergency management, but, to prevent recurrence of the effusion, either effective treatment of the underlying cancer is required or the effusion must be drained to dryness. To achieve this a flexible drainage tube needs to be inserted into the pleural space and the fluid allowed to drain via a sealed drainage system which prevents air from replacing the fluid. Drainage should be relatively slow as sudden removal of large volumes of fluid causes distress to the patient and can precipitate pulmonary oedema. After 24–48 hours, when the effusion has drained to dryness, it is usual to inject a drug or chemical into the pleural space to effect a pleurodesis. This will inflame the pleural surfaces to encourage sticking together of the two layers and the development of fibrosis. Tetracycline and bleomycin are the most commonly used agents and will prevent recurrence of the effusion in 50–75% of patients. If recurrent effusions remain a problem after this approach, referral to a thoracic surgeon may be worthwhile to drain the fluid under general anaesthetic and insufflate talcum powder, a more effective method of achieving a pleurodesis.

Pericardial effusions

Pericardial effusions are much less common than pleural effusions. Again the same tumour types are usually responsible but probably less than 1% of cancer patients will develop a symptomatic collection of pericardial fluid. When this does occur the build-up of fluid restricts normal cardiac function and produces symptoms and signs of cardiac failure, first affecting the right ventricle, which as it worsens subsequently impairs left ventricular function, a condition known as cardiac tamponade.

Patients with tamponade are unable to lie flat, have chest discomfort, oedema and breathlessness. When cardiac tamponade develops, urgent drainage of the pericardial fluid can be life-saving and is indicated if the patient is otherwise in reasonable health. Pericardial drainage is technically more difficult than pleural drainage and is best performed by a cardiologist with ultrasound control to ensure safe placement of the drainage catheter. Treatment of the underlying malignancy will usually prevent recurrence but, if this is not possible, injection of sclerosants into the pericardial space can be helpful. For symptomatic recurrent pericardial effusions, the formation of a pericardial window by a thoracic surgeon may be indicated.

Peritoneal effusions (ascites)

In cancer, ascites is usually caused by widespread peritoneal seedling metastases which exude protein-rich fluid. Liver metastases may contribute to the problem through hypoalbuminaemia or portal hypertension. Ascites is the most common secondary to carcinomas of the ovary, gastrointestinal tract, breast and pancreas. Patients present with abdominal distension which becomes progressively uncomfortable, limits food intake and splints the diaphragm, making breathing difficult. Diagnosis is by clinical examination and is confirmed by ultrasound and aspiration cytology.

Treatment is by tube drainage (paracentesis) and should be performed relatively slowly, generally not exceeding a rate of 500 ml/hour. Drainage to dryness is not realistic and therefore sclerosants are less effective for ascites than for pleural effusions. Diuretics are commonly prescribed to prevent reaccumulation but are rarely effective in relieving established ascites. Intraperitoneal radioactive colloids or chemotherapy are sometimes of benefit and agents such as thiotepa, mitozantrone and carboplatin have been used with some success. For recurrent ascites surgical procedures should be considered if medical treatments have failed to control the underlying disease. A peritoneovenous shunt can be inserted which drains the fluid through a one-way valve into the venous system. Interestingly, despite drainage of large numbers of malignant cells into the circulation, metastatic disease in the lungs and other sites do not appear to be more common.

METABOLIC AND ENDOCRINE MANIFESTATIONS OF MALIGNANCY

Hypercalcaemia

Hypercalcaemia is a complication in around 5% of patients with advanced malignancy, and is particularly common in patients with carcinomas of the breast, lung and multiple myeloma. Three mechanisms are involved. Firstly, metastatic cancer cells in bone stimulate osteoclasts, the normal bone cell which breaks down bone, to destroy bone faster than the osteoblast, the normal bone cell which builds bone, can repair the damage. Secondly, the tumour may secrete proteins into the circulation which have similar effects on bone but also promote the kidney to reabsorb more calcium from the urine than is appropriate. Finally, dehydration or damage to the kidney, as commonly occurs in multiple myeloma, can be important.

Hypercalcaemia causes many symptoms including lethargy, nausea, thirst, constipation and drowsiness. Because the symptoms are non-specific and commonly encountered in many patients with advanced cancer, the diagnosis can be easily missed. Treatment, however, will rapidly improve the patient's condition and relieve the unpleasant symptoms. This can be reliably achieved without side-effects by rehydration of the patient and inhibition of bone breakdown by one of the class of drugs called bisphosphonates. A single short infusion of pamidronate or clodronate will restore the serum calcium to normal in 80–95% of patients.

Inappropriate secretion of antidiuretic hormone (ADH)

This syndrome results in retention of fluid by the kidney and is characterised by a low serum sodium. This causes weakness and confusion, occurring most commonly in patients with small cell lung cancer. Treatment is by fluid restriction, drugs such as de-meclocycline which inhibit the action of ADH, and chemotherapy for the underlying malignancy.

Other endocrine manifestations of malignancy

Many cancers produce hormones and peptides with biological activity. These include ACTH, which may result in the features of Cushing's syndrome, hypoglycaemia from production of insulin-like substances and gynaecomastia from tumour production of human chorionic gonadotrophin (HCG).

Hyperuricaemia and tumour lysis syndrome

An acute metabolic disturbance may result from the rapid destruction of a tumour following chemotherapy. This is particularly likely to occur in childhood leukaemia and rapidly growing lymphomas. As chemotherapy kills the cancer, the cells release products of nitrogen metabolism, especially urea and urate, plus large amounts of potassium and phosphate into the circulation. The high urate concentration may result in urate crystal formation in the kidneys and lead to acute renal failure. High potassium levels can cause cardiac dysrhythmias and increased phosphate may cause tetany. The syndrome can be prevented by prescribing allopurinol to prevent the production of large amounts of urate and intravenous fluids to encourage the kidneys to excrete the products of cell breakdown.

INFECTION

Infections are a major cause of death in cancer. Not only do they occur frequently but they are often more severe than in other patients, less responsive to therapy and sometimes are produced by organisms which in normal health would not cause any problem. The susceptibility of cancer patients to infection results from suppression of host defence mechanisms produced by the disease and its treatment. Infections are particularly frequent when the neutrophil count is suppressed by chemotherapy.

Advanced cancer and the treatments prescribed are associated with impaired neutrophil and lymphocyte function, depressed cell mediated and humoral immunity, and damage to skin and mucous membranes which allows organisms to enter the bloodstream more easily. *Escherischia coli*, pseudomonas, staphylococci and streptococci are the most frequent bacterial pathogens. Viruses such as herpes simplex and zoster (shingles), fungi, particularly candida, and protozoal infection of the lungs with pneumocystis are important non-bacterial causes of infection requiring specific treatment. Most of the infecting organisms come from within the patient, for example gut bacteria, and, providing sensible precautions are taken, infections transmitted from family or health care staff are of relatively minor importance.

If patients are infected while neutropenic, urgent admission to hospital and treatment with broad spectrum intravenous antibiotics are required as untreated septicaemia can be rapidly fatal. Occasionally, even in specialist cancer centres and despite efficient and aggressive treatment of infection, patients still die from overwhelming infection following chemotherapy.

PARANEOPLASTIC SYNDROMES

Neurological

Cancers, particularly of the bronchus, are associated with a number of neurological syndromes which are unrelated to direct compression or infiltration of neural tissue. The mechanisms which give rise to these problems are poorly understood. They are uncommon and usually are possible to diagnose only by excluding the presence of malignant disease in the central nervous system or around nerve roots. The syndromes include numbness and weakness due to sensory and motor peripheral neuropathies respectively, paralysis from spinal cord damage, unsteadiness from cerebellar degeneration, dementia from cerebral damage and a form of muscle weakness which resembles myaesthenia gravis. These neurological conditions may be the first manifestation of cancer. Sadly, treatment for the underlying cancer frequently fails to produce much neurological improvement.

Hypertrophic pulmonary osteoarthropathy

Lung cancer is the principal cause of this condition in which the bones of the forearms and shins become inflamed and painful. Plain radiographs show characteristic appearances and usually the patient has a deformity of the nails known as clubbing. Anti-inflammatory drugs relieve many of the symptoms and the condition may improve if the underlying tumour can be removed or destroyed.

Other paraneoplastic syndromes

A variety of general effects of cancer are sometimes described as paraneoplastic phenomena, and almost every organ in the body can be affected by one of these syndromes. Fever, cachexia and anaemia are relatively common and may be the presenting symptoms of malignancy. In addition, thrombophlebitis and clotting disorders, arthritis, skin rashes, itching, muscle inflammation and renal impairment are uncommon but well-recognised complications of malignant disease.

Glossary

L = Latin   G = Greek   Fr = French

The ending 'oma' signifies tumour or neoplasm
The ending 'itis' signifies inflammation
The ending 'osis' signifies state or condition

Ablate (verb), *ablation* (noun). L. ab = from, away; latus = part of the verb 'to bear, take, carry'. Take away, remove.

Acromegaly. G. acron = point, megalos = great. Disease characterised by overgrowth, especially of the face and extremities.

Adenocarcinoma. G. aden = gland; karkinos = crab. A cancer of glandular tissue.

Adjuvant. L. juvare = to help. Treatment aimed at eradicating micrometastases.

AIDS. Acquired immune deficiency syndrome caused by the human immunodeficiency virus (HIV).

Ala nasi. L. = wing. The curved outer wall of each nostril.

Allogeneic. Relating to tissue transplant between individuals of a single species.

Alopecia. G. alopekia = fox-mange, a bald spot. Loss of hair, baldness.

Alveolar (adjective), *alveolus* (noun). Diminutive of alveus = a hollow. Used for the tooth sockets in the jaw bones; also for the surface tissue of upper and lower jaws; terminal ducts of the small bronchi and the sac-like dilatations where gas exchange occurs; also the terminal secretory parts of glands; hence 'alveolar' carcinoma.

Amenorrhoea. G. men = month; rhoia = a flowing. Absence of normal menstruation, cessation of periods.

Amyloid. G. amylon = starch; eidos = resemblance. An acidophilic protein with great affinity for the stain Congo red, deposited typically as extracellular deposits in vascular or reticuloendothelial tissue.

Anaphylaxis. G. ana = back; phylaxis = protection. An increased susceptibility to injected foreign material,

protein or non-protein, brought about by a previous introduction of it.

Anaplasia (noun), *anaplastic* (adjective). G. ana = again; plassein = to form. Reversion of cells to a more primitive, embryonic-like type with increased reproductive activity, including malignancy.

Androgen (noun), *androgenic* (adjective). G. andros = male, man; gen = produce. Generic term for an agent, usually a hormone (e.g. testosterone and androstenedione), that stimulates the activity of accessory sex organs, encourages development of male sex characteristics (e.g. deepened voice, growth of beard) and promotes protein synthesis and growth.

Angiography. G. angeion = vessel; graphein = to write. Radiological investigation in which radio-opaque contrast medium is injected into the arterial system to identify abnormalities of the vessel wall, pathological new vessels, arteriovenous malformations or vascular tumours (e.g. glomus).

Angioma. G. angeion = vessel. Tumour, usually of blood vessels (haemangioma); also of lymphatic vessels (lymphangioma).

Ankylosing spondylitis. G. ankylosis = stiffening of a joint; ankyloein = to crook; spondylos = vertebra. Chronic inflammatory arthritis of the sacroiliac joints and spine. Stiffening or fusion occurs of the intervertebral joints; in advanced cases there is gross forward bending of the spine ('question mark' posture).

Anorexia. G. anorexis = longing. Lack of appetite.

Antrum. L. = cave. Usually to maxillary antrum.

Aplastic. G. a = not; plassein = to mould or form. Anaemia due to lack of formation of blood cells, especially red.

Arachnoid. G. arachne = spider. Arachnoid membrane is one of those of the brain and spinal cord, between the dura mater and the pia mater.

Areola. Diminutive of area (L), i.e. a small area. Used of the pigmented ring around the nipple.

Arrhenoblastoma. G. arren = male; blastos = germ, sprout. Tumour of gonadal cells of the ovary, liable to produce androgenic hormones and masculinisation (see Androgen).

Aryepiglottic. G. Epi = on; glottis = tongue. Aryepiglottic fold of mucous membrane stretching between the side of the epiglottis and the apex of the arytenoid cartilages (Fig. 21.12B).

Arytenoid. G. arytaina = a cup; eidos = form. Arytenoid cartilages lie on the lateral part of the upper border of the cricoid cartilage at the back of the larynx.

Ascites. G. askites—askos = belly. Effusion in the peritoneal cavity.

Astrocytoma. G. astron = star; kytos = a receptacle, cell. The microscopic appearance of the cell (one of the neuroglial cells) is star-shaped.

Ataxia telangiectasia. Familial syndrome of progressive cerebellar ataxia with oculocutaneous telangiectases.

Atrium (plural *atria*). L = cavity, entrance.

Autologous. G. autos = self; logos = discourse. Refers to the withdrawal of the patient's own bone marrow and its reinfusion after high dose chemotherapy.

Axial (adjective). L = axis. Relating to or in the central part of the body, in the head and trunk as distinguished from the extremities.

Basal cell naevus syndrome (Gorlin's syndrome). Autosomal dominant disorder, typified by multiple basal cell carcinomas, pitting of the palms and soles and other defects (e.g. cysts in the mandible).

BCG. Bacillus of Calmette (1863–1933) and Guerin (1816–1895), two French bacteriologists. A variety of tubercle bacillus, used as a vaccine for immunisation against pulmonary tuberculosis.

Bence Jones. London physician and chemical pathologist, 1814–1873; described a substance now known to be a protein of either kappa or lambda light chains, which appears when the urine is warmed and disappears when the urine is brought to boiling point.

Bilharziasis. A genus of worms—bilharzia (now called schistosomiasis). B. is the resultant disease after infestation.

Biopsy. G. bios = life; opsos = vision. Examination of tissue taken from a patient during life.

Blast. G = bud. Used of immature or primitive cells, e.g. precursors of adult blood cells.

Blood–brain barrier. A selective mechanism of controlling the passage of substances from the blood to the cerebrospinal fluid and brain.

Bowen's disease. Premalignant disease of the skin with reddish plaques; may progress to invasive carcinoma after many years.

Brachytherapy. G. brachys = short. Treatment by sealed radioactive sources inserted into body tissues (interstitial) or body cavities (intracavitary).

Bremsstrahlung. German bremse = brake; strahlung = radiation. 'Braking radiation' produced by the sudden slowing down of electrons by atomic collisions. They are exactly analogous to ordinary X-rays generated by the impact of electrons in the tube when they are suddenly halted by the target.

Bronchogenic. G. bronchos = windpipe; gen = beget, produce. Arising in a bronchus. (Compare Osteogenic, arising in bone.)

Buccal. L. bucca = cheek. Used mostly for the oral aspect.

Cachexia (noun), *cachectic* (adjective). G. kakos = bad; hexi = condition. Wasting in chronic disease.

Carcinoma. G. karkinos = crab. A malignant epithelial tumour.

Carina. L. = keel. Refers to the point of division of the two main bronchi.

Cataract. G. kataractes = waterfall, portcullis (sliding gate). The medical use, applied to the lens of the eye, is a figurative extension of this.

Cauda equina. L. cauda = tail; equus = horse. The lower spinal nerves (between 2nd lumbar and 2nd sacral vertebrae) lie loosely resembling a horse's tail.

Cheilitis. G. cheilos = lip. Inflammation of the lips.

Chiasm. G. chiasma = a cross-shaped mark. Optic chiasm is the decussation or intersection of the optic nerves just above the pituitary fossa.

Cholestatic. G. chole = bile; statike = bringing to a standstill. Refers to obstruction to the flow of bile, one of the forms of jaundice.

Choriocarcinoma. G. = membrane that encloses the fetus in the womb. It consists of several layers, of which the outermost is the *trophoblast*. (G. trophe = food; blasto = germ) with projections that become embedded in the uterine mucosa. The metabolic exchanges between mother and fetus take place through these. *Syncytiotrophoblast* is a multinucleated outer layer of the trophoblast. *Cytotrophoblast* is the deeper layer next to the mesoderm.

Chromophobe. G. chroma = colour; phobos = fear. Old term referring to sparsely granulated or degranulated cells in some forms of pituitary adenomas.

Cicatrising. L. cicatrix = scar, the fibrous tissue which replaces destroyed normal tissue.

Clinoid. G. klinein = lean. The upper angles of the pituitary fossa are formed in front and behind by the clinoid processes.

Clone (noun), *clonal, clonogenic* (adjectives). G. klon = shoot; gen = beget, produce. Refers to cells which are identical in structure and function, originating from a single cell.

Colloid (al). G. kolla = glue; eidos = form. A colloidal solution differs from an ordinary solution. The molecules are so large that they do not pass freely through the membranes of the body. They tend to remain confined to one of the body's cavities if injected (e.g. colloidal gold-198 into the peritoneum).

Colostomy. G. kolon = large intestine; stoma = mouth. (Making of) an artificial anus by an opening into the colon, brought on to the abdominal wall.

Colpohysterectomy. G. colpos = fold, hollow; hystera = uterus; tome = cutting. Removal of the uterus through the vagina.

Corpus callosum. L. corpus = body; callosus = hard. Midline neural connection between the frontal lobes of the brain allowing easy spread of gliomas in a 'butterfly' distribution.

Corpus luteum. L. corpus = body; luteum = egg yolk. Structure into which the ruptured ovarian follicle develops immediately following ovulation during the menstrual cycle, with associated production of progesterone.

Cortex. L = bark. Outer covering, e.g. of bone or adrenal gland.

Cribriform. L. cribrum = a sieve. As in cribriform plate, which separates the frontal lobe of the brain and the nose.

Cricoid. G = like a ring. Cartilage lying below the thyroid cartilage in front of the 6th cervical vertebra.

Cryopreservation. G. cryos = frost. Preservation of the body's cells or tissues by maintaining them at very low temperatures (e.g. sperm) for future use.

Cryosurgery. Surgery using decreased temperature, either locally or generally.

Cuirasse. French = leather, a defensive breastplate. *Cancer-en-cuirasse*—extensive malignant invasion of the skin of the chest wall.

Curettage. French 'curer' in the sense of 'to clear, cleanse'. A *curette* is a small instrument in the form of a loop, ring or scoop, with a sharpened edge and long handle, to scrape the interior of a cavity in order to remove tissue for histology or treatment.

Cyanosed. G. kyanos = blue. With livid skin due to deficient oxygenation of the blood. Also applied to local capillary stagnation in lips, nose, hands and feet due to cold without anoxia of the blood.

Cystoscopy. G. kystis = bladder; skopeein = to see. Inspection of the interior of the bladder by a miniature sort of telescope passed along the urethra.

Cystotomy. G. kystis = bladder; tome = cutting. Cutting into and opening of the bladder through the abdominal wall.

Cytology. G. kytos = receptacle, cell; logos = discourse, study. The science of the structure and function of cells.

Cytotrophoblast. See Choriocarcinoma.

Demyelination. G. de = down; myelos = marrow. Loss of myelin, the substance forming the medullary sheath of nerve fibres.

Desquamation. L. de = from; squama = scale. Shedding of the epidermis in scales or flakes.

Diabetes insipidus. G. dia = through; bainein = to go; L. in = not; sapidus = well tasted. Disorder of posterior lobe of the pituitary due to reduced production of antidiuretic hormone (ADH) leading to copious dilute urine.

Dilatation and curettage. See Curettage. Widening of the central canal of the cervix by metal dilators (sounds) and removal of tissue from the uterine cavity.

Diuretic. G. dia = through; ouron = urine. Diuresis is excretion of urine in excess of normal, induced by drugs. Such a drug is a diuretic.

Down's syndrome (or *mongolism*). Syndrome associated with mental retardation and mongoloid facial features in which there are three (trisomy) instead of the usual pair of chromosomes. The extra chromosome is considered to be number 21.

Dura (mater). L = hard (mother). The tough outer membrane enclosing the brain and spinal cord.

Dysgerminoma. From L. and G. for 'two' in the sense of 'twain, asunder'. Dys = bad, difficult, the opposite of 'eu' = well (eugenic, euthyroid). L. germen = bud, sprout. A rare tumour of the ovary, of gonadal germinal cells, corresponding to seminoma of the testis.

Dysmenorrhoea. G. dys (see above); men = month; rhoia = flow. Difficult or painful menstruation.

Dysphagia. G. dys = bad; phagein = to eat. Difficulty in swallowing.

Dysphonia. G. dys (see above); phone = voice. Hoarseness, difficulty or pain in speaking.

Dysplasia (noun), *dysplastic* (adjective). G. dys = ill; plassein = to mould. Refers to alteration in size, shape and orientation of epithelial cells, often in association with chronic irritation or inflammation (e.g. cervix, skin, oesophagus).

Dyspnoea. G. dys (see above); pnoea = breathing. Difficult breathing, shortness of breath.

Ectoderm (al). G. ecto = outside; derma = skin. The outer of the three primary layers of cells in the embryo. (The others are the mesoderm and the endoderm.)

Electron-affinic. G. elektron = amber. L. ad = to; finis = boundary. Attracting electrons, a property of radiosensitising compounds of hypoxic cells.

Electrophoresis. G. phoresis = carrying in. The movement of particles in an electric field toward one or other electric pole, anode or cathode.

Enchondroma. G. en = in; chondros = cartilage. Single or multiple masses of cartilage in any bone, most commonly in the fingers (Ollier's disease).

Endarteritis. G. endo = within; arteria = windpipe. Inflammation of the inner lining of an artery. May lead to obstruction of the vessel and ischaemia beyond it (*endarteritis obliterans*, L. ob = over; littera = letter).

Endocrine. G. endo = within; krinein = to separate. Applied to glands of internal secretion.

Endometrium. G. endo = within; metra = womb. The internal lining of the uterus.

Endoscopy. G. endo = within; skopein = to see. Inspection of the interior of a channel or hollow organ.

Endosteal. G. endo = within; osteon = bone.

Enophthalmos. G. en = in; ophthalmos = eye. Recession of the eyeball within the orbit.

Eosinophil (ic). G. eos = dawn; phileein = to love. Eosin is an (acid) rose-coloured dye. 'Acidophil' is an alternative name. Used of cells that take up acid (in contrast to basic stains). Eosinophils are white blood cells containing granules that stain with acid dyes. Eosinophilic is also an old term for certain pituitary tumours due to staining properties.

Ependymoma. G. ependyma = garment. The name was given by the great German pathologist Virchow to the lining membrane of the cerebral ventricles and central canal of the spinal cord.

Epidermis. G. epi = on; derma = skin. The outer (epithelial) layer of the skin.

Epididymis. G. epi = on; didymos = twin. A structure attached to the back of the testis, consisting mainly of coils of the excretory spermatic duct.

Epilation. L. e = out; pilus = hair. Removal of hair.

Epiphysis. G. epi = upon; physis = growth. An extremity of a long bone, originating in a centre of ossification separate from that of the shaft. The *epiphyseal plates* are areas of active growth.

Epithelium. G. epi = on; thele = nipple. Applied originally to the thin skin covering the nipples. Now used of the non-vascular layer covering all free surfaces, internal and external (skin, mucous and serous membranes) and all the structures, e.g. glands, contained therein.

Erythroblast(ic). G. erythros = red. See Blast. Primitive immature red blood cell.

Erythroplasia of Queyrat. See Erythroblastic. Premalignant condition, typically with red crusting patches on the prepuce or glans of the penis.

Eustachian tube. Joins the middle ear and the nasopharynx.

Euthyroid. G. ev = well; thyreoeides = shield-shaped. Normal thyroid function.

Exenteration. G. ex. = out; enteron = bowel. Removal of viscera.

Exophthalmos. G. ex = out; ophthalmos = eye. Protrusion of the eyeball. See Proptosis.

Extramedullary. L. extra = outside. See Medullary.

Fistula. L = pipe, tube. An abnormal passage leading from a cavity, e.g. abscess, or hollow organ to the surface, or from one cavity to another, e.g. rectum to vagina (rectovaginal).

Fluorescein. L. fluor = flow. A dyestuff fluorescing bright green, used in the diagnosis of corneal lesions; also used intravenously for determining the circulation time in man.

Follicular. L. follis = wind bag; the diminutive folliculus = little bag or sac. Microscopically the thyroid shows glandular tubes lined with cells. On cross-section they form little cavities, vesicles or follicles, with the secretory cells lining the walls and the secretion in the lumen. Follicular carcinoma may closely resemble normal thyroid tissue and be difficult to distinguish; or the follicles may be large and irregular.

Fornix (plural fornices). L. = arch, vault. For example at the sides of the uterine cervix.

Fossa. L = ditch. Pit or depression, e.g. pituitary fossa.

Frenulum. L. diminutive of frenum = bridle. The frenulum of the tongue is a fold of mucous membrane passing from the undersurface of the tongue in the midline to the floor of the mouth.

Fundus. L. = bottom. The base of an organ, i.e. the part remote from the external opening.

Ganglioneuroma. G. ganglion = tumour in a tendon sheath; still used in this sense. Another modern sense is enlargement or knot on nerve, from which nerve fibres radiate; also aggregation of nerve cells. G. neuron = nerve. A tumour of adult sympathetic nerve cells.

Gardner's syndrome. Genetic syndrome (polyposis of the colon, osteomas and sebaceous cysts), predisposing to thyroid cancer.

Genome. A complete set of chromosomes derived from one parent; the total gene complement of a set of chromosomes.

Glaucoma. G. glaukoma = cataract. Disease of the eye, characterised by increased tension within the eyeball and failing vision.

Glioma. G. glia = glue. Neuroglia ('nerve glue') is the specialised connective tissue or binding cells of the central nervous system.

Glomerulonephritis. L. glomus = clew of yarn (i.e. gathered into a ball). Inflammation of the glomeruli of the kidney.

Glossitis. G. glossa = tongue. Inflammation of the tongue.

Goitre. L. guttur = throat. A chronic enlargement of the thyroid gland.

Gonadotrophic. G. gone = seed; trophe = nourishment; hence gonad = germ or sexual glands. *Gonadotrophins* are hormones, e.g. pituitary follicle stimulating hormone (FSH) and luteinising hormone (LH), which stimulate the endocrine secretion of the gonads.

Granulation. L. granulum, diminutive of granum = grain. Granulation tissue is composed of capillaries and fibroblasts and inflammatory cells forming tiny fleshy projections on the surface of a wound in the process of healing.

Granulocyte. As above + kytos = cell. Mature polymorphonuclear leucocytes containing granules in the cytoplasm which take up acid (eosinophil or acidophil) basic (basophil) or neutral (neutrophil) stains.

Granulosa. The inner lining of the ovarian follicle, from which the ovum develops, is called 'membrana granulosa' (granular membrane), and the constituent cells 'granulosa cells'. They do not show granules microscopically and the origin of the name is obscure.

Grenz. German = boundary. Grenz rays lie on the border between ultraviolet and X-rays.

Gynaecomastia. G. gynaeco = woman; mastos = breast. Excessive development of male mammary tissue, sometimes with secretion of milk.

Haematocrit. G. haem = blood; krinein = sift, separate (compare Endocrine). Centrifuge for separating cells of the blood from plasma. Also used for haematocrit value, i.e. the percentage figure of the relative cell volume in the blood.

Haematoporphyrin. G. haem = blood; porphyra = purple (dye). Dye concentrated by neoplastic cells and administered before exposure of tumour to laser therapy.

Haemolytic. G. haem = blood; lysis = dissolution. Breaking up of red blood cells.

Haemopoietic. G. haem = blood; poiesis = making.

Haemoptysis. G. haem = blood; ptysis = spitting. Spitting of blood from lungs or air passages.

Hashimoto's thyroiditis. Autoimmune disease predisposing to hypothyroidism and thyroid carcinoma and lymphoma.

Hemianopia. G. hemi = half; an = without; opsis = sight. Loss of half of a visual field.

Histiocyte. G. histion = web, tissue; kytos = cell. One of the cells of the reticuloendothelial system. Also called macrophage.

Histology. G. histos = web, tissue; logos = study. Microscopic study of tissues and organs, and of cells arranged in tissues. Contrast Cytology—study of individual cells.

Hydatidiform. G. hydor = water; hydatis = watery vesicle, i.e. with the form or appearance of a hydatid. A cyst containing watery fluid, especially that formed by the larva of a tapeworm.

Hydatidiform mole. L. and G. mole = meal. Polycystic mass resulting from proliferation of the trophoblast (see choriocarcinoma) and cystic degeneration of its projections into the uterine wall.

Hydronephrosis. G. hydor = water; nephros = kidney. Dilation of the pelvis of the kidney due to obstruction to the flow of urine at some lower level.

Hydroureter. G. hydro = water. Distension of the ureter with urine due to obstruction, e.g. by a tumour.

Hyperbaric. G. hyper = over, in excess; baros = weight. At a pressure greater than one atmosphere.

Hyperkeratosis. G. hyper = over, in excess; keras = horn. Overgrowth of the horny outer layer of the epidermis.

Hyperplasia. G. hyper = over; plasma = form, mould. An increase in the size of the tissues due to increase in total cell numbers.

Hyperuricaemia. G. hyper = over; ouron = urine. Excessive production of uric acid in the blood, e.g. due to breakdown of neoplastic tissue in response to chemotherapy.

Hyperviscosity. G. hyper = over; L. viscum = mistletoe (whose fruits contain a sticky substance). Increased thickness of the blood, e.g. due to increased content of abnormal protein, as in myeloma.

Hypogonadism. Deficient internal secretions of the gonad, male or female.

Hypophysectomy. G. hypo = under; physis = growth; tome = cutting. *Hypophysis*—applied to the pituitary which appears to grow from the base of the brain.

Hypothalamus. G. hypo = below. A group of nuclei at the base of the brain, above and connected to the pituitary gland.

Ileus. G. ileos = colic. Mechanical or adynamic obstruction of the bowel.

Infarction. Necrotic changes resulting from obstruction of an end artery and the area so affected.

Infratentorial. L. infra = below; tentorium = tent. Refers to a sheet of dura mater stretched between the cerebrum and the cerebellum.

Intrathecal. L. intra = within; theke = sheath. Refers to the loose sheath covering the spinal cord and its surrounding cerebrospinal fluid.

Intravesical. see vesicant.

Ipsilateral. L. ipse = self, same; latus = side. On the same side.

Ischaemia. G. ischo = check, restrain; haem = blood. Local anaemia due especially to narrowing or obliteration of blood vessels.

Keloid (or *Cheloid*). G. chele = claw; eidos = form, appearance. Hyperplastic fibrous tissue, especially after burns or wounds, with claw-like processes radiating from its extremities.

Keratinised. G. keras = horn. Cornified (L. cornu = horn) or made horny (Compare Hyperkeratosis).

Keratoacanthoma. G. keras = horn; akantha = thorn. Non-malignant keratinising (see above) tumour of epidermis. One of the normal epidermal layers is composed of prickle cells with tiny microscopic processes looking like thorns—hence 'acanthoma', a tumour of these cells.

Keratosis. See Hyperkeratosis.

Kinetics. G. kineo = set in motion. Cell kinetics refers to the activity of cells, e.g. dividing, resting or decaying.

Koilonychia. G. koilos = hollow; onych = nail. Malformation of the nails, in which the surface is spoon-shaped instead of the normal convexity.

Laminectomy. L. lamina = thin piece or plate; tome = cutting. Removal of the posterior part of one or more vertebral arches, to expose the spinal canal and gain access to the spinal cord.

Laparotomy. G. lapara = flank; tome = cutting. Opening the abdominal cavity to inspect or perform an operation on its contents.

Leiomyosarcoma. G. leio = smooth; myo = muscle. Sarcoma of smooth muscle.

Lesion. L. laesio = hurt, injury. Any abnormal change in the texture or functioning of an organ, e.g. any inflammation, wound, infection, tumour or other more or less localised abnormality.

Leucoerythroblastic anaemia. Replacement of the bone marrow with malignant cells resulting in immature myeloid cells and nucleated erythroid cells in the circulating blood.

Leucopenia. G. leuco = white; penia = poverty, shortage. Diminution of the normal number of white blood cells; the opposite of leucocytosis.

Leucoplakia. G. leuco = white; plakos = flat.

Disturbance of maturation of epithelium causing heaped-up whitish patches; usually in the mouth, but also in the vulva.

Leukaemogenesis. G. leukos = white; haima = blood; gen = produce. Induction of leukaemia e.g. by ionising radiation or chemotherapy.

Leukopheresis. G. leukos = white; phoresis = carrying in. Removal of white cells from the blood.

Leukopoietic. G. Leukos = white; poieein = to make. The production of white cells in the bone marrow.

Lumen. L = light. A cavity or space enclosed by the walls of a tube, cell.

Lymphangitis carcinomatosa. L. lympha = water; karkinos = crab. Infiltration of the lymphatics with tumour in the lung.

Macula. L. macula = spot. Darker region of the fundus of the eye on the temporal side of the optic disc.

MCP. Mining and Chemical Products Ltd. An alloy of bismuth, zinc and cadmium used to shield tissues from megavoltage irradiation.

Medullary (adjective), *medulla* (noun). L. medulla = marrow. 'Medulla' is used of any soft marrow-like element. Refers to part of the brainstem and inner area of the adrenal gland.

Medulloblastoma. See Medullary. G. blastos = sprout, shoot, germ. Medulloblast is a primitive type of glial cell (see Glioma). In this case it refers to a particular part of the cerebellar region.

Megakaryocyte. G. mega = big; karyon = kernel; kytos = cell. An exceptionally large cell in the bone marrow, from which blood platelets are derived.

Meiosis. G. meiosis = reduction. Refers to the process of cell division which results in the formation of gametes, composed of two nuclear divisions in quick succession resulting in the formation of four gametocytes each containing half the number of chromosomes present in somatic cells.

Melanoma. G. melas = black. Tumour derived from cells capable of forming melanin (seen e.g. in freckles). Pigment may or may not actually be formed; if not, the tumour is 'amelanotic'. (G. a = without).

Meninges. G. meninx = membrane. Any of the three membranes that surround the brain and spinal cord.

Menorrhagia. G. men = month; rhegnynai = to burst. Abnormally profuse or prolonged menstruation.

Mesodermal. G. meso = middle. See Ectoderm.

Metachronous. G. meta = after; chronos = time. Used for example of separate primary tumour occurring in the same or opposite breast some time after an initial primary breast tumour.

Metaphysis. G. meta = after; physis = growth. The

extremity of the shaft of a long bone where it joins the epiphysis.

Metaplasia. G. metaplasis = a moulding afresh. Transformation; formation of a type of tissue by cells normally producing another type of tissue, e.g. transitional epithelium of the bladder may be changed to squamous.

Metastasis. See Metaplasia. G. metastasis = change of place. Especially production of secondary tumours remote from the primary.

Mitosis. G. mitos = fibre. An elaborate process of cell reproduction composed of a sequence of nuclear changes that result in the formation of two daughter cells.

Mucosa. L. mucus = nose mucus. Short for 'membrana mucosa'—mucous membrane, an epithelial surface lubricated by secreted mucus.

Myasthenia gravis. G. mys = muscle; sthenos = strength. Disease characterised by weakness of muscles and exacerbated by fatigue.

Mycosis fungoides. G. myke = mushrooom, fungus; eidos = shape, form. A malignant lymphoma of skin producing fungating tumour masses.

Myelitis. G. myelos = marrow. Inflammation of (1) the spinal cord once regarded as spinal marrow, or (2) bone marrow.

Myeloma. G. myelo = marrow. Usually refers to plasma cell myeloma (or plasmacytoma), a tumour of plasma cells of the bone marrow. Plasma cells are involved in antibody production. When the lesions are diffuse the disease is 'multiple myeloma' or 'myelomatosis'.

Myxoedema. G. myxa = mucus; oidema = swelling. In advanced thyroid hormone deficiency there is infiltration of gelatinous fluid into the tissues, giving the feeling of hard oedema. The name was given in the mistaken belief that the infiltrate was mucus.

Nadir. Fr. nadir = opposite to. The point of the heavens diametrically opposite to the zenith: the lowest point of anything, e.g. of blood count.

Naevus (*Nevus*; plural *naevi*). L. = mole, spot, blemish. A general term applying to any congenital lesion, often pigmented, especially on the skin. The chief types are (1) angioma and (2) melanoma.

Necrosis. G. nekros = death. Death of any part of the body.

Neoadjuvant. G. neos = new; L. juvare = to help. Refers to chemotherapy given before surgical treatment of a tumour.

Neoplasia, Neoplasm. G. neo = new; plasia = formation. New growth, tumour (in the oncological sense).

Nephrotic syndrome. G. nephros = kidney. Renal disease characterised by gross loss of protein in the urine causing oedema.

Oestrogen. G. oestros = gadfly, sting, frenzy; gen = beget, produce. *Oestrus* (animal heat or rut) is that part of the female sexual cycle during which mating is accepted. The hormone that brings on oestrus is 'oestrogenic'.

Oligodendroglioma. G. oligos = few or small; dendron = tree. Oligodendroglia refers to cells of the neuroglia which have relatively few and short branches.

Oncogene (noun), *oncogenic* (adjective). G. oncos = tumour; gen = produce. Small discrete sequences of DNA in which genetic changes may lead to the induction of cancer.

Oncology. G. oncos = mass, bulk, tumour. The science of tumours in all their aspects.

Oophorectomy. G. oion = egg, ovum; phoros = bearing, carrying; ectoma = excision. Removal of the organ that bears the eggs (oophoron = ovary).

Orchidectomy. G. orchis = testicle; ectomy = excision. The orchis family of plants is so named after the resemblance of the tubers to the shape of a testicle. Surgical removal of testicle(s).

Os. L = mouth. Plural = ora (hence oral). Note. Another word with same spelling = bone (plural = ossa, hence ossicle, osseous).

Osteo. G. osteon = bone.

Osteoclast. G. klasis = fracture. A large multi-nucleated cell in bone marrow, concerned in absorption and removal of bone tissue.

Osteogenic. G. gen = produce. Means either formed from bone or forming bone.

Osteoid. See Osteo. Bone-like.

Osteolytic. G. lytic = dissolving, destroying. Destructive of bone.

Osteomyelitis. G. myelo = marrow. Inflammation of bone marrow.

Paget, Sir James. 1814–1899. Famous London surgeon. Several conditions are named after him, including (1) Paget's disease of bone (p. 505), a skeletal disease leading to thickening and softening of bone and bending of weight bearing bones, and (2) Paget's disease of nipple (p. 385).

Pancoast's syndrome. Pain in arm etc., due to nerve involvement by a tumour at the apex of the lung.

Pancytopenia. G. pan = all; kytos = cell; penia = poverty, scarcity. Reduction in red, white cells and platelets below normal.

Papilla (plural *papillae*). L = nipple. Diminutive of papula = pustule or pimple, probably from an older root 'pap' = swell. Any small nipple-like projection.

Hence *papillary*, *papilloma* (plural = papillomas or papillomata), *papilliferous* (bearing papillae), *papillomatosis*.

Para. G. = by the side of. The primary meaning refers to position e.g. parathyroid (alongside the thyroid).

Paracentesis. G. parakentesis = pierce. The perforation of a cavity by a hollow instrument to remove fluid.

Paracrine. G. par = by side of; krinein = to separate. A type of hormone function in which hormone synthesised and released from endocrine cells binds to its receptor in nearby cells and affects their function.

Parametrium (plural = parametria). G. metra = uterus (see Endometrium). The connective tissue and other structures between the lateral border of the uterus and the pelvic wall.

Paraplegia. G. plege = blow or stroke. The name was originally applied to a stroke involving one side, now called hemiplegia (hemi = half) but was later used to refer to involvement of the lower limbs.

Parasellar. See Para. By the side of the sella turcica (pituitary fossa).

Peau d'orange. French = peel of orange. In locally advanced breast cancer lymphatic obstruction causes oedema of the skin while the sweat ducts are tethered so that their orifices become noticeable. The resultant pitted appearance is likened to orange peel.

Peptic. G. pepsis = digestion. Relating to the stomach or gastric digestion.

Perichondritis. G. peri = around; chondros = cartilage. Inflammation of cartilage.

Periosteum. G. peri = around; osteo = bone. The thick fibrous sheath adherent to and surrounding a bone.

Petrous. G. petra = rock. Applied to the hard part of the temporal bone protecting the inner ear. Temporal is from L. for 'temple', that part of each side of the head being metaphorically regarded as 'temple of the head'.

Phagocytosis. G. phagein = to eat; kytos = a vessel. Ingestion by white cells of foreign particles, bacteria and cell debris.

Phimosis. G = muzzling. Contraction of the orifice of the prepuce (foreskin) so that it cannot be drawn back over the glans penis.

Photophobia. G. photos = light; phobos = fear. Shrinking from light e.g. due to malignant meningitis.

Piezoelectric. G. piezein = to press. Refers to electricity generated by pressure on certain crystals, e.g. quartz.

Pinealoma. L. pinea = pine cone. The pineal body is a cone-shaped structure behind the third cerebral ventricle. Tumour of pineal gland.

Piriform. L. pirum = pear. Pear-shaped.

Pituitary. L. pituita = mucus or phlegm. Nasal secretion was thought by the ancients to come through the skull floor from the base of the brain.

Plasma. See Serous/Serum.

Plasma cell. See Myeloma.

Polycythaemia rubra vera. G. poly = much, many; kytos = cell; haem = blood. An increase of blood cells in number, especially red cells. L. rubra = red; vera = true, genuine, i.e. in distinction from secondary polycythaemia (p. 469).

Proctitis. G. proctos = anus. Medically, used to refer mainly to the rectum. Inflammation of rectal mucosa.

Progestogen. L. pro = in favour of; gesto = bear; G. gen = produce. Applied to hormones causing changes in the endometrium to prepare it for the reception of the fertilised ovum.

Proptosis. G. pro = forward; ptosis = falling. Forward displacement of a part, especially protrusion of the eyeball (= exophthalmos).

Pseudomucinous. G. pseudo = false. Pseudomucin is a gelatinous material ressembling mucin.

Pseudopodium (plural *pseudopodia*). G. pseudes = false; podion latinised from the G. podos = foot.

Psoriasis. G. psora = itch. A skin eruption with reddish-brown scaly patches. Itching is actually not at all characteristic.

Ptosis. G. ptosis = fall. Drooping of the upper eyelid.

Pyelography. G. pyelo = trough, basin; refers to the pelvis (collecting basin) of the kidney. G. graphein = to write. Radiography of the urinary tract.

Pyometra. G. pyon = pus; metra = uterus. Accumulation of pus in the uterine cavity.

Pyriform. See Piriform.

Pyrogen. G. pyr = fire; gen = produce. An agent causing a rise in temperature. Especially a substance of unknown nature, but probably (foreign) protein, liable to be present in solutions injected intravenously.

Raynaud's phenomenon refers to spasm of the digital arteries with whitening and numbness of the fingers occurring secondary to another disease.

Reticulum, Reticulosis. L. diminutive of rete = net. Net-like structure.

Retrosellar. L. retro = behind. See Sella. Behind the sella turcica.

Rhabdomyosarcoma. G. rhabdo = rod, strip. Malignant tumour of striated (striped) muscle. Compare Leiomyosarcoma.

Riedel's thyroiditis. Form of thyroiditis in which the thyroid gland has a typically 'woody' feel, leading to hypothyroidism.

Salpingitis. G. salpinx = trumpet. Used to denote a tube with flared end, in particular the fallopian tube along which the ovum passes to the uterus.

Scirrhous (adjective). G. skirrhos = hard. Overgrowth of tough fibrous tissue in a tumour gives it a hard feel.

Sclerotic. G. scleros = hard. Sclerosis refers to hardening of chronic inflammatory origin, e.g. in the walls of arteries. The sclera is the white of the eye, a fibrous coat forming the outer surface of the eyeball, except for the cornea in front.

Scoliosis. G. skoliosis = obliquity. Lateral curvature of the spine.

Sella. L. = seat, saddle. The saddle-shaped part of the upper surface of the sphenoid (G. = wedge-shaped) bone which houses the pituitary. Also called 'sella turcica' = Turkish saddle, after its shape.

Seminoma. L. semen = seed (from the verb 'to sow'). Tumour of male germ cells, precursors of spermatozoa.

Sequestrum. L. sequester = depositary. Piece of bone that separates, e.g. from part of the mandible which has undergone radionecrosis.

Serous, Serum. L = whey, watery fluid. Serum is the fluid part of the blood which separates from the clot after coagulation. Distinguish from *plasma*, the fluid after the removal of blood cells, which is still coagulable. Serous membranes line the closed cavities of the body, especially pleural and peritoneal, and are moistened by exuded fluid similar to the serum.

Situ. L. situs = site. *Carcinoma-in-situ* = cancer cells 'in position', still in their tissue of origin (e.g. epidermis) before breaking through the basement membrane.

Somatic. G. soma = body.

Spondylitis. See Ankylosing spondylitis.

Spongioblastoma. G. spongia = sponge; blastos = germ. The spongioblast is a primitive neuroglial cell, a precursor of the astrocyte. Multiple cavities in the cytoplasm in microscopic preparations give it a sponge-like appearance.

Sporocyst. G. spora = seed; G. kystis = bladder. The cyst developed in the process of producing spores.

Squamous. L. squama = scale. Refers to the scaly part of epidermal and other surfaces.

Steatorrhoea. G. stear = suet; rhoia = flow. Fatty stool due to malabsorption of fat, e.g. due to pancreatic disease.

Stenosis. G. stenos = narrow. Narrowing of any channel.

Stilboestrol. G. stilbein = to shine. Stilbene is the chemical name of a complex hydrocarbon (used e.g. in dyes).

Stomatitis. G. stoma = mouth. Inflammation of the mucous membranes of the mouth.

Stridor. L. stridere = to creak. Harsh whistling sound of obstructed breathing.

Stroma. G = bed, mattress. The supporting framework, generally connective tissue, of an organ or structure, as opposed to the specific cells of the organ or neoplasm.

Submental. L. sub = beneath; mentum = chin. Below the chin and floor of mouth.

Suprasellar. L.= above. See Sella. Above the sella turcica (pituitary fossa).

Supratentorial. L. supra = above. See Infratentorial.

Synchronous. G. syn = together; chronos = time. Occurring at the same time.

Syncytiotrophoblast. See choriocarcinoma.

Synovial. A term apparently coined by the ancient Greek physician, Paracelsus. Relating to the membrane that lines joints.

Telangiectasia. G. telos = end; angion = vessel; ectasis = extension, dilatation. Dilatation of small or terminal blood vessels, especially in the skin, like tiny varicose veins, producing a purplish, blotchy, spidery appearance.

Tenesmus. G. = straining, from the verb 'to stretch'. A continual inclination to empty the bowel (or bladder), with painful spasm, but little or no discharge.

Teratogenic. See Teratoma. G. gen = produce. Causing malformations in children.

Teratoma. G. teras = monster. A tumour composed of various tissues (e.g. bone, teeth) not normally existent at the site.

Theca. G. theke = case, sheath.

Thrombocytopenia. G. thrombos = clot; penia = poverty, scarcity. Diminution in number of blood platelets.

Thymus. G. = warty excrescence. Refers to the lymphoid organ in the superior mediastinum and lower neck, present in childhood. It is of great importance in immunological development.

Tracheostomy. G. trachea = rough, i.e the rough artery; the ancients believed that it was an artery, and the cartilaginous rings give it a rough feel. G. stoma = mouth. Formation of an opening into the trachea, to relieve obstruction of the airway.

Translocation. L. trans = across; locus = place. Transfer of genetic material, e.g. from one chromosome to another.

Transurethral. L. trans = across, through; urethra from same root as 'urine'. Refers to a procedure such as partial prostatectomy carried out by instruments passed along the urethral channel.

Trigone. G. tri = three; gonia = angle. Triangle,

especially the triangular area at the base of the bladder between the openings of the two ureters and the urethra.

Trismus. G. trismos = creaking. Lockjaw; a firm closing of the jaw due to tonic spasm of the muscle of mastication from disease of the trigeminal (motor) branch of 5th cranial nerve.

Trophoblast. See Choriocarcinoma.

Tuberose sclerosis. Rare disease in which sclerotic glial masses in the brain are associated with mental deficiency.

Ulcerative colitis. Form of inflammatory bowel disease, predisposing in longstanding cases to malignant transformation.

Uraemia. G. ouron = urine. Toxic excess of urea and other waste products in the blood, due to impaired excretion.

Urea. Same root as 'urine'. The chief end-product of nitrogen metabolism in mammals, excreted in the urine.

Uveal tract. L. uva = grape. Refers to iris, ciliary body and choroid of the eye.

Uvula. L diminutive of uva = grape. A conical projection from the middle of the soft palate.

Vallecula. L. diminutive of vallis = valley. Space separating the opening of the larynx from the back of the tongue.

Vasectomy. L. vas = vessel; G. tome = cutting. In this context the vas is the duct conveying the testicle towards the urethra. Surgical removal of a segment of the spermatic duct for the purpose of sterilisation.

Vesicant. L. vesica = blister bladder. Anything that causes blistering. Intravesical. L. intra = within.

Von Hippel–Lindau syndrome. Rare condition characterised by vascular tumours in the retina (haemangiomas) and in the central nervous system.

Von Recklinghausen's disease. Genetic condition inherited as autosomal dominant in which there are numerous nerve tumours (neurofibromas) of the cranial or peripheral nerves. May undergo sarcomatous change.

Wertheim's hysterectomy involves a radical removal of the uterus, cervix and upper third of the vagina with parametria and uterosacral tissues, and pelvic lymphadenectomy.

Xerostomia. G. xeros = dry; stoma = mouth. Dry mouth induced by irradiation of the salivary glands.

Bibliography

PART 1

General radiation physics

Ball J E, Moore A D 1986 Essential physics for radiographers. Blackwell, Oxford

Gifford D 1984 A handbook of physics for radiologists and radiographers. John Wiley, Chichester

Hay G A, Hughes D 1983 First year physics for radiographers. Baillière Tindall, London

Johns H E, Cunningham J R 1983 The physics of radiology. Thomas, Illinois

Meredith W J, Massey J B 1977 Fundamental physics of radiology. Wright, Bristol

Wilks R 1987 Principles of radiological physics. Churchill Livingstone, Edinburgh

Radiotherapy physics

Alderson A R (ed) 1986 Dosimetry and clinical uses of afterloading systems. Report 45. Institute of Physical Sciences in Medicine, York

American Association of Physicists in Medicine 1983 A protocol for the determination of absorbed dose from high energy photon and electron beams. Medical Physics 10:741–771

Bomford C K, Dawes P J D K, Lillicrap S C, Young J 1989 Treatment simulators. Supplement 23. British Institute of Radiology, London

British Journal of Radiology 1983 Central axis depth dose data for use in radiotherapy. Supplement 17. British Institute of Radiology, London

Cohen M, Mitchell J S 1984 Cobalt-60 teletherapy: a compendium of international practice. International Atomic Energy Agency, Vienna

Dobbs J, Barrett A, Ash D 1992 Practical radiotherapy planning, 2nd edn. Arnold, London

Fowler J F 1981 Nuclear particles in cancer treatment. Adam Hilger, Bristol

Godden T J 1988 Physical aspects of brachytherapy. Adam Hilger, Bristol

Greene D 1986 Linear accelerators for radiation therapy. Adam Hilger, Bristol

Greening J R 1985 Fundamentals of radiation dosimetry. Adam Hilger, Bristol

Institute of Physical Sciences in Medicine 1988 Commissioning and quality assurance of linear accelerators. Report 54. IPSM, York

International Commission on Radiation Units and Measurements 1978 Dose specification for reporting external beam therapy with photons and electrons. Report 29. ICRU, Bethesda

International Commission on Radiation Units and Measurements 1984 Radiation dosimetry: electron beams with energies between 1 and 50 MeV. Report 35. ICRU, Bethesda

International Commission on Radiation Units and Measurements 1985 Dose and volume specification for reporting intracavitary therapy in gynaecology. Report 38. ICRU, Bethesda

International Commission on Radiation Units and Measurements 1988 Use of computers in external beam radiotherapy procedures with high energy photons and electrons. Report 42. ICRU, Bethesda

International Commission on Radiation Units and Measurements 1989 Tissue substitutes in radiation dosimetry and measurement. Report 44. ICRU, Bethesda

Klevenhagen S C 1985 Physics of electron beam therapy. Adam Hilger, Bristol

Lillicrap S C, Owen B, Williams J R, Williams P C 1990 Code of practice for high energy photon therapy dosimetry based on the NPL absorbed dose calibration service. Physics in Medicine and Biology 35:1355–1360

Massey J B 1970 Manual of dosimetry in radiotherapy. IAEA Technical Report Series 110. IAEA, Vienna

Meredith W J 1967 Radium dosage: the Manchester system. E & S Livingstone, London

Mould R F 1985 Radiotherapy treatment planning. Adam Hilger, Bristol

Pierquin B, Wilson J-F, Chassagne D 1987 Modern brachytherapy. Masson, New York

Trott N G (ed) 1987 Radionuclides in brachytherapy: radium and after. Supplement 21. British Journal of Radiology, London

Tsien K C, Cunningham J R, Wright D J, Jones D E A, Pfalzner P M 1967 Atlas of radiation dose distributions. IAEA, Vienna

World Health Organization 1988 Quality assurance in radiotherapy. WHO, Geneva

Radioisotopes

ARSAC 1988 Notes for guidance on the administration of radioactive substances to persons for purposes of diagnosis, treatment or research. HMSO, London

Frier M, Hardy J G, Hesslewood S R, Lawrence R 1988 Hospital radiopharmacy principles and practice. Report No 57. IPSM, York

Horton P W 1982 Radionuclide techniques in clinical investigation. Adam Hilger, Bristol

International Commission on Radiation Units and Measurements 1979 Methods of assessment of absorbed dose in clinical use of radionuclides. Report 32. ICRU, Washington

International Commission on Radiological Protection 1987 Radiation Dose to Patients from Pharmaceuticals. Publication 53. Pergamon Press, Oxford

Medical Internal Radiation Dose Committee Pamphlets 5, 10 and 11. Society of Nuclear Medicine, Maryville

Medicine (Administration of Radioactive Substances) Regulations 1978 (SI 1978 No 1006). HMSO, London

Parker R P, Smith H S, Taylor D M 1984 Basic science of nuclear medicine, 2nd edn. Churchill Livingstone, Edinburgh

Radioactive Substances Act 1960 HMSO, London

Sharp P F, Gemell H G, Smith F W (eds) 1989 Practical nuclear medicine. IRL Press, Oxford

Williams E D (ed) 1985 An introduction to emission computed tomography. IPSM, York

Radiation protection

Health and Safety Commission 1985 Approved code of practice: the protection of persons against ionising radiation arising from any work activity. HMSO, London

Health and Safety Executive 1985 The ionising radiations regulations. (SI 1985 No 1333). HMSO, London

Health and Safety Executive 1988 The ionising radiation (protection of persons undergoing medical examination or treatment) regulations (SI 1988 No 778). HMSO, London

Institute of Physical Sciences in Medicine 1989 Radiation protection in nuclear medicine and pathology. Report 64. IPSM, London

International Atomic Energy Agency 1985 Regulations for the safe transport of radioactive material, No 6 Safety standards. IAEA, Vienna

International Atomic Energy Agency 1986 Regulations for the safe transport of radioactive material, No 6 Suppl safety standards. IAEA, Vienna

International Commission on Radiological Protection 1971 Protection of the patient in radionuclide investigations. Publication 17. Pergamon Press, Oxford

International Commission on Radiological Protection 1977 The handling, storage, use and disposal of unsealed radionuclides in hospitals and medical research establishments. Publication 25. Pergamon Press, Oxford

International Commission on Radiological Protection 1977 Recommendations of the International Commission on radiological protection. Publication 26. Pergamon Press, Oxford

International Commission on Radiological Protection 1982 Protection against ionising radiation from external sources used in medicine. Publication 33. Pergamon Press, Oxford

International Commission on Radiological Protection 1982 General principles of monitoring for radiation protection of workers. Publication 35. Pergamon Press, Oxford

International Commission on Radiological Protection 1985 Protection of the patient in radiation therapy. Publication 44. Pergamon Press, Oxford

International Commission on Radiological Protection 1987 Data for use in protection against external radiation. Publication 51. Pergamon Press, Oxford

International Commission on Radiological Protection 1987 Protection of the patient in nuclear medicine. Publication 52. Pergamon Press, Oxford

International Commission on Radiological Protection 1991 Recommendations of the international commission on radiological protection. Publication 60. Pergamon Press, Oxford

Kathren R L 1986 Radiation protection. Adam Hilger, Bristol

Mackenzie A L, Shaw J E, Stephenson S K, Turner P C R (eds) 1986 Radiation protection in radiotherapy. Report 46. IPSM, London

National Radiological Protection Board 1990 Patient dose reduction in diagnostic radiology. NRPB, Didcot

Shrimpton P C, Wall B F, Jones D G et al 1986 A national survey of doses to patients undergoing a selection of routine X-ray examinations in English Hospitals. NRPB-R2000. HMSO, London

Ultrasound

Fish P 1990 Physics and instrumentation of diagnostic medical ultrasound. John Wiley, Chichester

Hussey M 1985 Basic physics and technology of medical diagnostic ultrasound. Macmillan, London

McDicken W N 1991 Diagnostic ultrasonics: principles and use of instruments, 3rd edn. Churchill Livingstone, Edinburgh

PART 2

Cancer

DeVita V T, Hellman S, Rosenberg S 1989 Cancer: principles and practice of oncology, 3rd edn. J B Lippincott, Philadelphia

Doll R, Peto R 1982 The causes of cancer. Oxford University Press, Oxford

Heller T, Davey B, Bailey L 1989 Reducing the risk of cancer. Hodder and Stoughton, Sevenoaks

Perez C A, Brady L W 1987 Principles and practice of radiation oncology. J B Lippincott, Philadelphia

Priestman T J 1989 Cancer chemotherapy: an introduction. Springer-Verlag, London

Sikora K, Halnan K E (eds) 1990 Treatment of cancer, 2nd edn. Chapman and Hall, London

Twycross R G, Lack S 1990 Therapeutics in terminal care, 2nd edn. Churchill Livingstone, Edinburgh

Radiotherapy

Dobbs J, Barrett A, Ash D 1992 Practical radiotherapy planning, 2nd edn. Arnold, London

Hope-Stone H (ed) 1986 Radiotherapy in clinical practice. Butterworth, London

Johnson R J, Eddleston B, Hunter R D 1990 Radiology in the management of cancer. Churchill Livingstone, Edinburgh

Pierquin B, Wilson J-F, Chassagne D 1987 Modern brachytherapy. Masson, New York

Pointon R C S 1991 The radiotherapy of malignant disease, 2nd edn. Springer-Verlag, Berlin

Radiobiology

Nias A H W 1988 Clinical radiobiology, 2nd edn. Churchill Livingstone, Edinburgh

Steel G C, Adams G E, Peckham M J 1989 The biological basis of radiotherapy. Elsevier, Amsterdam

Thames H D, Hendry J H 1987 Fractionation in radiotherapy. Taylor and Francis, Bristol

Vaeth J M, Meyer J L (eds) 1989 Radiation tolerance of normal tissues. Karger, Basel

Pathology

Rubin E, Farber S L 1988 Pathology. J B Lippincott, Philadelphia

Scherer E, Streffer C, Trott K-R 1991 Radiopathology of organs and tissues. Springer-Verlag, Berlin

Underwood J C E 1992 General and systematic pathology. Churchill Livingstone, Edinburgh

Walter S B, Israel M S 1987 General pathology, 6th edn. Churchill Livingstone, Edinburgh

Index